THE SUDDEN INFANT DEATH SYNDROME

CARDIAC AND RESPIRATORY MECHANISMS AND INTERVENTIONS

ANNALS OF THE NEW YORK ACADEMY OF SCIENCES
Volume 533

THE SUDDEN INFANT DEATH SYNDROME
CARDIAC AND RESPIRATORY MECHANISMS AND INTERVENTIONS

Edited by Peter J. Schwartz, David P. Southall, and Marie Valdes-Dapena

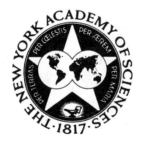

The New York Academy of Sciences
New York, New York
1988

Library of Congress Cataloging-in-Publication Data

The Sudden infant death syndrome.

(Annals of the New York Academy of Sciences, ISSN 0077-8923 ; v. 533)
Papers presented at a conference held on May 24–27, 1987; sponsored by the New York Academy of Sciences and others.
Includes bibliographies and index.
1. Sudden death in infants—Congresses. I. Schwartz, Peter J. II. Southall, David P. III. Valdes-Dapena, Marie A., 1921–   . IV. New York Academy of Sciences. V. Series. [DNLM: 1. Sudden Infant Death—congresses. W1 AN626YL v.533 / WS 430 S9427 1987]
Q11.N5 vol. 533 [RJ59] 500 s [618.92]   88-19549

ISBN 0-89766-462-0   66267
ISBN 0-89766-463-9 (pbk.)

BB
Printed in the United States of America
ISBN 0-89766-462-0 (cloth)
ISBN 0-89766-463-9 (paper)
ISSN 0077-8923

ANNALS OF THE NEW YORK ACADEMY OF SCIENCES

Volume 533
August 30, 1988

THE SUDDEN INFANT DEATH SYNDROME: CARDIAC AND RESPIRATORY MECHANISMS AND INTERVENTIONS[a]

Editors and Conference Organizers
PETER J. SCHWARTZ, DAVID P. SOUTHALL, and MARIE VALDES-DAPENA

CONTENTS

[a]This volume contains papers presented at a conference entitled The Sudden Infant Death
Syndrome: Cardio-Respiratory Mechanisms and Interventions, held on May 24–27, 1987, in Como,
Italy, and cosponsored by the New York Academy of Sciences; Centro di Fisiologia Clinica e
Ipertensione, Centro SIDS, Ospedale Maggiore, Università di Milano; the National Center for the
Prevention of Sudden Infant Death Syndrome; and the Division of Maternal and Child Health,
Department of Health and Human Services. The conference and this volume are, in part, a product
of the "Progetto Finalizzato Medicina Preventiva e Riabilitativa, Sottoprogetto Patologia Perinatale
e Sue Sequele" of the Consiglio Nazionale delle Ricerche, Rome, Italy.

Part V. Possible Role of Respiratory Mechanisms in SIDS

Major financial assistance was received from:

- CIBA-GEIGY
- DIVISION OF MATERNAL AND CHILD HEALTH, DEPARTMENT OF HEALTH AND HUMAN SERVICES (PHS GRANT NO. MCJ-009071-02-0)
- HEALTHDYNE
- KNOLL AG
- KONTRON INSTRUMENTS
- NATIONAL CENTER FOR THE PREVENTION OF SUDDEN INFANT DEATH SYNDROME
- NELLCOR INC.
- PABISCH

Additional financial assistance was received from:

- BURROUGHS WELLCOME CO.
- MARQUETTE INC.
- MEDTRONIC
- MERCK SHARP & DOHME
- WYETH LABORATORIES

Introductory Remarks

PETER J. SCHWARTZ,[a] DAVID P. SOUTHALL,[b] AND
MARIE VALDES-DAPENA[c]

[a]*Centro di Fisiologia Clinica e Ipertensione*
Istituto Clinica Medica II
Centro SIDS
Università di Milano
Milan, Italy
[b]*Cardiothoracic Institute*
Brompton Hospital
London SW3 6HP
United Kingdom
[c]*Department of Pathology*
School of Medicine
University of Miami
Miami, Florida 33101

In 1983 a conference of the New York Academy of Sciences was held in Europe for the first time.[1] The meeting was co-organized by one of us (P. J. S.) and was held in Florence. The success of that international conference prompted the Academy to plan an almost regular series of such assemblies to be held in Europe, in consideration of the significant portion of its membership who live on that continent. When the time seemed appropriate to the Conference Committee of the Academy for a conference on the Sudden Infant Death Syndrome (SIDS), the three of us were chosen to be the co-organizers. Simultaneously the National Research Council (C. N. R.) of Italy identified SIDS as a subject for "targeted research projects of national interest." On the basis of several considerations, including the beauty of the site, it was decided to hold that four-day meeting in Italy, and, specifically, on Lake Como.

In prior conferences and symposia on SIDS, significant progress was made in our understanding of the phenomenon, but the traditional format, involving presentations on almost all aspects of the subject, had unavoidably limited the possibility of extensive, in-depth discussion of specific issues. It was our goal, therefore, to focus most of the attention of this meeting on those two mechanisms that seemed most likely to contribute to the majority of SIDS deaths, i.e., the cardiac and the respiratory. The scientific program was then constructed around that nucleus. The first day included a set of state-of-the-art lectures on essential areas such as pathology, epidemiology, and the role of sleep, as well as important updates on problems related to the management of high-risk infants and the support of the affected families. The subsequent two days were devoted exclusively to the possible role of cardiorespiratory mechanisms; that arrangement made it possible for several speakers to present their often contrasting views on the same or similar aspects of SIDS. Furthermore, in addition to the traditional discussion period following each presentation, an unusually generous period of time was provided for general discussion at the end of each session. Thus, there was ample opportunity for in-depth analysis of the data and concepts presented, and the many expert SIDS investigators in the audience were able to interact constructively with the invited speakers. On the fourth day, a series of four closed workshops were held with the goal of defining, if possible, areas of consensus for both present knowledge and future research. This proved to be a complex task; the results are summarized in a special section of this volume.

SIDS is not only a puzzling scientific problem and one of the greatest challenges for contemporary medicine, it is also a tragic event with devastating psychosocial impact. Associations of parents of SIDS victims have been created to help cope with some of the many psychological difficulties the survivors experience. We thought that this truly international conference would represent a unique opportunity for those groups to meet, discuss their problems, exchange ideas, and feel less isolated. Accordingly, on the last day of the conference, while the closed workshops were taking place, those organizations met for a full day. We were extremely pleased that associations of parents from 13 countries participated in that unique event and that a record of the proceedings of their meeting could be included in this volume.

The participation of investigators, physicians, professionals, and laymen from so many different nations and continents represented, more than anything else, a sign that SIDS has become a major medical and social challenge without geographical boundaries. The fact that the speakers were staying at the gracious and secluded seventeenth century Villa d'Este afforded additional and extremely useful occasions for informal interaction and discussion. At the end of this stimulating meeting, we felt that our goal had been attained and that a more focused approach to SIDS was becoming a reality.

We would like to express our gratitude to the many people whose hard work, attention to detail, and anticipation of potential problems made this conference a success. A few deserve special mention. Mrs. Ellen Marks and her staff from the New York Academy of Sciences and Mrs. Giovanna Gattamelata and her staff from Studio G were invaluable in providing organizational assistance and in preventing or solving problems before and during the conference; Mr. Bill Boland and his staff, especially Ms. Janet Tannenbaum, provided expert editorial assistance in the preparation of this volume.

REFERENCE

1. GREENBERG, H. M., H. E. KULBERTUS, A. J. MOSS & P. J. SCHWARTZ, Eds. 1984. Clinical Aspects of Life-Threatening Arrhythmias. Ann. N. Y. Acad. Sci. Vol. 427. New York.

A Historical Perspective on SIDS Research

EILEEN G. HASSELMEYER[a] AND JEHU C. HUNTER

National Institute of Child Health and Human Development
National Institutes of Health
Bethesda, Maryland 20892

To put research concerned with the sudden infant death syndrome (SIDS) into perspective, it is essential to consider the nature of this problem. Unlike other, more tractable, medical conditions there are usually no obvious clues from the infants that something is awry before they are found dead. As with a mystery novel, the investigator is faced with a victim and must search for clues that will lead to a solution.

From the earliest efforts to solve the riddle of SIDS, investigators, who were few in number, sought to make sense of what they found during postmortem examinations. In the late 1700s through the late 1800s it was believed that an enlarged thymus pressed on the trachea cutting off the airway or the blood supply to the head.[1] As support for the thymic theory waned, the idea that SIDS infants had been "overlaid" or "stifled in bed," a theory which had never really been fully rejected, was again embraced by the medical profession and lay public. Even Templeman,[2] a Scottish medical examiner, whose description in 1892 of 258 cases of "suffocation" of infants bears a striking resemblance to postmortem and epidemiological descriptions of SIDS infants today, believed that these deaths by suffocation were due to ignorance, carelessness, drunkenness, and overcrowding among the lower classes.

Templeman's report that the greatest number of cases occurred between October and March and the highest incidence was among infants of poor socioeconomic circumstances who were between one and six months of age is consistent with epidemiological findings dating back several decades. An important difference is that it is quite clear that SIDS occurs in all socioeconomic groups, although, as with other medical problems, it is the poor who suffer the most.

The observations of infants at autopsy by Werne and Garrow[3-5] in the 1940s produced the first evidence that in many sudden and unexpected infant death cases, the cause of death appeared to be from natural causes, possibly involving an inflammatory response, and not suffocation. The observations of various investigators regarding seasonality, inflammation, frequent histories of a slight, upper respiratory infection prior to death, and essentially negative necropsy findings prompted the search in the 1960s for a viral etiology for SIDS.

With its establishment, the National Institute of Child Health and Human Development (NICHD) sought to stimulate interest in scientific studies by holding a research conference in 1963 at Seattle, Washington.[6] It was expected that the exchange of ideas during this conference would encourage research grant applications from the scientific community, but this did not occur. By 1969, NICHD was supporting only two projects that had SIDS as a primary focus.

A second NICHD-sponsored research conference[7] in Seattle, in 1969, expanded the

[a]Address correspondence to E. G. H., NICHD-NCNR, Bldg. 31B, Room 3B19, Bethesda, MD 20892.

TABLE 1. NICHD SIDS Research Emphasis Areas

1. Developmental neurophysiology, autonomic disturbances, and sleep state
2. Respiratory, laryngeal, cardiac functions, and responses to stimuli
3. Metabolic, endocrine, and genetic factors
4. Immunology and infection
5. Epidemiology
6. Anatomic pathology
7. Behavioral

areas of scientific explanation to encompass sleep, apnea, and the concept of "near miss" as pertinent areas for investigation. It was again expected that the conference would stimulate investigator-initiated applications for the study of SIDS; but the response was minimal. During fiscal years 1964–1971, thirteen research grant applications were submitted. Four were recommended for approval and funded; one of these was the 1969 conference.

An interesting aspect of the February 1969 conference, and a major factor in the evolution of the sudden infant death syndrome program in the United States, was the attendance at the conference, at their own expense, of parents of SIDS babies seeking answers for why their babies had died. They were disheartened by the lack of research activity on this most tragic medical problem. They organized; they wrote letters to the Congress; they called us; they visited us; they lobbied. Continuing parental pressure on the Congress in the early seventies resulted in NICHD taking a more directed approach toward support of SIDS research. Persistent parental lobbying also led to enactment of the Sudden Infant Death Syndrome Act of 1974 (P.L. 93–270). This act fixed by statute the responsibility of NICHD for the conduct of SIDS research; required the secretary of the Department of Health, Education and Welfare to carry out a program to develop public information and professional educational materials relating to SIDS; authorized the secretary to make grants and enter into contracts for projects to collect, analyze, and furnish information about the causes of SIDS and to provide information and counseling to families affected by SIDS; and required specific reports to the Congress or its committees concerning SIDS research, information and counseling projects, and internal budgetary requests.

Responsibility for expanding the National Institute of Child Health and Human Development's SIDS research effort was given to me (E. G. H.) in 1970 as the newly appointed Director of the Perinatal Biology and Infant Mortality Program. Mr. Hunter, then NICHD Assistant Director for Planning for Biological Sciences, was asked by the Institute Director to join with me in developing this directed SIDS research program.

Looking back now, 16 years later, the plan we developed seems rather simple and logical, but its implementation was a challenge. Some of the questions we asked were: What do we know about SIDS? What disciplines other than pathology and epidemiology could contribute to our understanding of the SIDS phenomena? How do we attract creative investigators from relevant disciplines to investigate the SIDS problem? What are the impediments to developing a directed research program?

Through a series of research planning workshops that began in 1971[8] an outline of emphasis areas emerged (TABLE 1). These areas of emphasis provided the framework upon which was built the NICHD SIDS research effort. This volume includes a number of reports pertaining to the NICHD Research Emphasis Areas One and Two. The remaining areas are discussed either directly or indirectly in various reports.

FIGURE 1 shows the number of SIDS research grants and contracts funded by NICHD from 1964 to 1986. The primary category represents the number of projects directly concerned with the study of SIDS; the related category represents those projects pertaining to the study of high-risk infancy; and the tertiary category includes projects that focus on the study of high-risk pregnancy.

As a result of the Institute's directed research efforts, the number of research projects directly related to the study of the sudden infant death syndrome (primary) peaked in 1977 with 41 funded projects. While the current number of NICHD projects primarily concerned with SIDS is not large, this does not indicate a lack of NIH interest. In addition to NICHD, other institutes are supporting research that is highly relevant to SIDS. An example is the recently published article by Giulian in the *New England Journal of Medicine* reporting evidence that the presence of a significant level of fetal hemoglobin in SIDS infants may be a useful postmortem marker.[9] This research was supported by the National Heart, Lung, and Blood Institute.

An important question for all of us is what has been accomplished since 1971? Some think not much because the etiology of SIDS has not been defined, and babies are still dying suddenly and unexpectedly. Others feel much has been accomplished even though we do not yet have a solution to the problem.

Of major importance is that in many countries, SIDS scientists and parents have brought to their nation's attention the problem of infants dying suddenly and unexpectedly. SIDS is now recognized as a major public health problem and a leading cause of post-neonatal deaths.

Of equal importance is the increased sensitivity of health care providers, public safety personnel, and the lay public to SIDS as a distinct medical entity. Recognition of this fact has resulted in a marked reduction in charges of infanticide brought against parents and baby sitters of SIDS infants. It has also led to a greater appreciation of the unique impact of these deaths on family members.

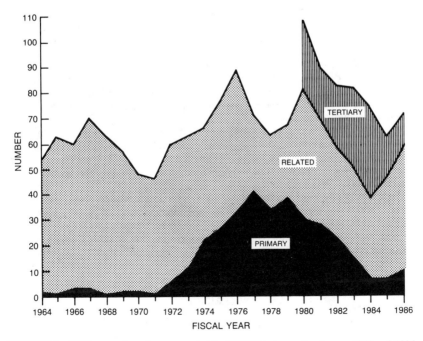

FIGURE 1. SIDS research projects supported by NICHD between fiscal years 1964 and 1986.

A significant accomplishment was inclusion in the ninth revision of the *International Classification of Diseases* of a separate code number (798.0) for sudden infant death that has made possible the acquisition of accurate statistics about SIDS incidence.

In 1971, when NICHD began its SIDS directed-research program, there was a paucity of scientists interested in the problem of SIDS. For the most part, scientists investigating the problem of infants dying suddenly and unexpectedly were predominantly pathologists and epidemiologists. There were some virologists but very few physiologists, obstetricians, and pediatricians. Over the years, many highly qualified scientists around the world, who had not previously been directly involved in research on the sudden infant death syndrome nor considered the relevance of their scientific work to SIDS, were attracted to the enigma of sudden unexplained infant death, became SIDS investigators, and contributed to advances in knowledge about the biology of fetal and early infant development.

As the pool of excellent scientists increased, so did the body of knowledge relevant to infancy and the sudden infant death syndrome. This new knowledge created a base of normative physiologic and developmental data for infants between birth and one year of age so that deviations from the norm that might be SIDS-related could be identified. As a result of research conducted in various countries, a significant amount of physiologic data pertaining to sleep physiology, arousal failure, infant apnea, vagal stimulation, respiratory obstruction, and cardiopulmonary function in normal and presumed "at-risk" infants has been developed. Some of that information will be presented in this volume. Other findings have already been published.

Through the recently completed Cooperative Epidemiologic Study of SIDS Risk Factors, the NICHD has developed a comprehensive base of information about SIDS infants, their mothers, and the environment. Data from this study have confirmed and extended the findings of earlier epidemiologic studies that were carried out with smaller sample sizes. The mothers of babies who subsequently died suddenly and unexpectedly experienced more health problems during the SIDS pregnancy. As newborn infants, these future SIDS victims exhibited an increased incidence of health problems during the early weeks of life.

We know now that, collectively, SIDS babies are not the healthy babies they were said to be in the early 1960s. As a group, these babies appear to have had subtle developmental deficits that contribute to their vulnerability and put them at risk of dying suddenly and without apparent cause. These hidden physiologic problems may be the result of a mix of environmental and genetic factors.

The improvement in our understanding of the SIDS phenomenon provides the basis for additional research efforts, which should help to more clearly identify in very early life those infants at increased risk for the sudden infant death syndrome. Identification of this subset of high-risk infants would permit health professionals to direct preventive efforts more effectively.

We are certainly much further ahead today in our knowledge about "apparently healthy" infants who die suddenly and unexpectedly than we were 16 years ago. Research pertaining to the syndrome is becoming more focused as scientists attempt to unravel the complexities of cardiorespiratory function, mechanisms, and control. Current research approaches appear reasonable in the light of information obtained from studies carried out in the recent past.

REFERENCES

1. SAVITT, T. L. 1979. The social and medical history of crib death. J. Florida Med. Assoc. **66:** 853–859.

2. TEMPLEMAN, C. 1892. Two hundred and fifty-eight cases of suffocation in infants. Edinburgh Med. J. **38:** 322–329.
3. WERNE, J. 1942. Postmortem evidence of acute infection in unexpected death in infancy. Am. J. Pathol. **18:** 759–761.
4. WERNE, J. & I. GARROW. 1947. Sudden deaths of infants allegedly due to mechanical suffocation. Am. J. Public Health **37:** 675–687.
5. WERNE, J. & I. GARROW. 1953. Sudden apparently unexplained death during infancy. I. Pathologic findings in infants found dead. Am. J. Pathol. **29:** 633–653.
6. WEDGWOOD, R. & E. P. BENDITT, EDS. 1965. Sudden Death in Infants. U.S. Department of Health Education and Welfare, Public Health Service Publication No. 1412.
7. BERGMAN, A. B., J. B. BECKWITH & C. G. RAY, EDS. 1969. Sudden Infant Death Syndrome. University of Washington Press. Seattle, WA.
8. WALPOLE, M. & E. G. HASSELMEYER. 1972. Research Planning Workshop on the Sudden Infant Death Syndrome. August 1971. Department of Health, Education and Welfare. Publication No. DHEW (NIH) 75–576. (First of a series of interdisciplinary research planning workshops.)
9. GIULIAN, G. G., E. F. GILBERT & R. L. MOSS. 1987. Elevated fetal hemoglobin levels in sudden infant death syndrome. New Engl. J. Med. **316** (18): 1122–1126.

Sudden Infant Death Syndrome in Epidemiologic Perspective: Etiologic Implications of Variation with Season of the Year

DONALD R. PETERSON,[a,b] EUGENE E. SABOTTA,[c]
AND DANIEL STRICKLAND[a]

[a]Department of Epidemiology
School of Public Health and Community Medicine
University of Washington
Seattle, Washington 98195

[c]Division of Health
State of Washington
Department of Social and Health Services
Olympia, Washington 98504

Deaths attributed to the sudden infant death syndrome (SIDS) typically occur more often during the autumn and winter than during the spring and summer in temperate zones of both the northern and southern hemispheres. Many respiratory diseases caused by infectious agents also occur more frequently during the colder and darker months of the year. Investigators in England and Australia report that the seasonal occurrence pattern of SIDS depends upon age-at-death; deaths during the first twelve weeks did not occur seasonally whereas deaths at older ages did.[1-3] Maternally endowed immunoglobulins diminish exponentially during early postnatal life; exposure to people, who might transmit infectious respiratory disease agents, usually increases as babies grow older. These considerations add credibility to the interpretation that SIDS deaths among older infants result from infections that occur more commonly during autumn and winter. On the other hand, data from Cook County, Illinois, did not reveal an association between season of death and age-at-death.[4,5] Evidence of infection from postmortem studies provides only partial support for the hypothesis.[6] Epidemic outbreaks of respiratory infections show little, if any, correlation with SIDS incidence.[7-9] Thus, the possible role of infectious respiratory disease agents in the etiology of SIDS remains at issue.

In this paper we examine the association of season of the year and SIDS occurrence on a larger scale, and in greater detail, than was done previously.

MATERIALS AND METHODS

We used information from birth and death certificates in linked computer files for the State of Washington over the calendar period 1975 through 1983 as our data base. We also used data from the National Institute for Child Health and Human Development (NICHD)

---

[b]Address correspondence to: D. R. P., 2637-108th Avenue N.E., Bellevue, WA 98004.

SIDS Cooperative Epidemiological Study (HOFFMAN et al., this volume), restricted to infants who died during the twelve-month period of January 1 to December 31, 1979, for comparison. We chose dates of the vernal and autumnal equinoxes to define season of the year. This definition separates time periods with longer, lighter days from those with shorter, darker days as well as other attributes of spring-summer (Mar 21–Sep 20) versus autumn-winter (Sep 21–Mar 20). We converted age-at-death to two-week increments to facilitate analysis. We used the chi square test to evaluate statistical significance.

RESULTS

During the period 1975–1983, postperinatal deaths (deaths from seven through 364 days of age) among residents of the State of Washington totalled 2,727. Of this number, 1,140 (41.8%) were ascribed to SIDS. SIDS occurrences during the autumn-winter

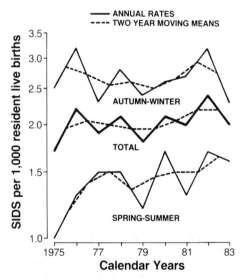

FIGURE 1. Comparison of total SIDS occurrences per 1,000 live births to residents of Washington State with season-specific SIDS death rates, 1975–1983.

amounted to 63.2% compared to 53.1% of 1,587 non-SIDS deaths ($\chi^2 = 32.64$, df = 1, $p < 0.001$). In the NICHD data, 58.7% of 569 SIDS babies died during the autumn-winter season.

FIGURE 1 shows the pattern of annual SIDS occurrence rates in Washington State over the nine-year period (labeled "Total" in the figure) compared to annual season-specific rates. We plotted two-year moving means of the annual rates to adjust for infants who died in the calendar year subsequent to their births. The trends of the "smoothed" rates run more-or-less parallel to one another and did not vary significantly over the interval. Plotting the rates on a logarithmic scale depicts equal, proportional changes as identical vertical displacements on the graph.

TABLE 1 addresses the association of age at death and season of the year in Washington State apropo of the infection hypothesis. We sorted subjects into four groups as shown in the table; two of the groups comprised infants whose births and deaths occurred within a six-month season (spring-summer or autumn-winter) and two whose births occurred in one season and deaths in the subsequent season. We did this on the premise that the full effect of season would accrue to those whose entire life spanned only one season. Axiomatically, when a birth and death occurs within a six-month season, the maximum age at death is 26 weeks; on average, such infants will be younger than babies for whom this stipulation does not apply. For this reason, we compared births and deaths within the spring-summer season with those within the autumn-winter separately from those born in one season and dying in a subsequent season. We found no statistically significant differences in the percentages over twelve weeks of age. TABLE 2 reveals similar distributions of the NICHD data, which do not differ significantly either.

FIGURE 2 shows the cumulative percentage distribution of SIDS in Washington State by age separately for those who died in the spring-summer season and in the autumn-winter. SIDS babies consistently died at an older age during the autumn-winter season than during the spring-summer season except at the upper ends of the age range (beyond 26 weeks). The median age for spring-summer deaths was 10.9 weeks compared to 12.5 for autumn-winter; the difference corresponds to 11 days. Analysis of the NICHD data in the same way revealed similar distribution patterns with medians of 10.5 weeks and 10.9 weeks, respectively; the difference translates to three days. As a further test of the

TABLE 1. Washington State SIDS: Season of Birth and Season of Death for Infants Over 12 Weeks of Age

Birth Season	Death Season (% of infants)	
	Spring Summer	Autumn Winter
Spring Summer	34.3	68.6
Autumn Winter	72.7	36.3

infection hypothesis, we analyzed additional variables that might relate to exposure and/or susceptibility to infection. TABLE 3 lists these variables and their relative frequency according to season of death, both for the Washington State and NICHD data sets. We examined each one in detail and found no statistically significant associations except for the seasonal differences shown for "ALL SIDS" in the table.

The NICHD data included information from which approximate gestational age could be calculated for each SIDS infant. Month of conception was estimated from gestational age and date of birth. FIGURE 3 reveals similar variations in month of conception and month of death. When analyzed with seasons defined by dates of equinoxes, 77.2% who died in autumn-winter were apparently conceived the previous autumn-winter; 74.9% of those who died in spring-summer were conceived in the corresponding season one year earlier.

DISCUSSION

The State of Washington was the venue for two international conferences on sudden deaths in infancy in the 1960s.[10,11] Certifications of cause of infant deaths indicate that by 1975, SIDS as a diagnostic entity, was in general use throughout the State; FIGURE 1

TABLE 2. NICHD Study of SIDS: Season of Birth and Season of Death for Infants Over 12 Weeks of Age

Birth Season	Death Season (% of infants)	
	Spring Summer	Autumn Winter
Spring Summer	28.0	66.9
Autumn Winter	53.8	31.4

reveals a relatively uniform rate pattern from 1975 through 1983. We cannot imagine how diagnostic or coding errors, to the extent that they may have occurred, would systematically bias the analyses described. The design of the NICHD study minimized the potential for errors of this sort.

Variation in season of death distinguishes SIDS from all other postperinatal deaths in the same birth cohort. Because of criticism of earlier studies,[12] we took season of birth into account in analyzing age-at-death in relation to season of death. The Washington State data included four infants born in spring-summer who lived through autumn-winter and died in the subsequent spring-summer, and 20 born in autumn-winter who died in the corresponding season subsequently. All of the analyses were performed both with and without these 24 subjects, with no evident difference in results. The data presented in this paper include these subjects, which introduces a slight bias in favor of older infants, but not enough to influence statistical significance. Our results do not support the hypothesis that death from infection among older SIDS infants produces seasonal variation in SIDS occurrence. We cannot explain why studies in the United States yield results different from those in the United Kingdom and Australia.

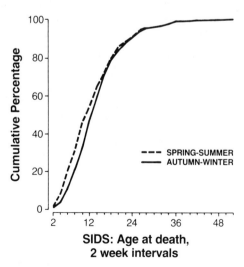

FIGURE 2. Comparison of season of death of SIDS subjects with cumulative percentage age distributions, Washington State, 1975–1983.

The lack of associations of salient SIDS risk factors listed in TABLE 3 runs counter to our original expectations. The size of the data base largely precludes non-detection of significant differences (Type 11 error).

The unique age distribution of SIDS victims spans the first six months of life and centers at about three months. Thus, season of death indexes the season of conception and early gestation in the previous year. Raring analyzed SIDS age distributions from seven different studies and concluded that the typical monomodal pattern was approximately log-normal. He concluded that this implied random variation in response to an antecedent factor.[13] These considerations suggest to us that some factor, peculiar to conception or early gestation, may play a significant etiologic role.

A recent report from Australia indicates that asymptomatic maternal thiamine deficiency may be such a factor[14]; seasonal variations in maternal intake of this nutrient could result in seasonal variation in SIDS. If this were the case, one would expect an association between season and adolescent, multiparous SIDS mothers. On a *de facto* basis, they comprise a socially, economically, and educationally disadvantaged subset of the childbearing population in which nutritional deficiency might be expected. Our results do not support this hypothesis either.

Seasonal variation of SIDS could, of course, be statistically significant but not etiologically significant as a result of more frequent conceptions during the autumn-winter season in the child-bearing population. However, the frequency of live births by month of occurrence in Washington State, when simply translated to month of conception nine months earlier, reveals only a slight increase in autumn-winter versus spring-summer (on the order of 1%). The corresponding variation for the NICHD SIDS subjects equaled 11.2%.

Alternatively, at conception, or shortly thereafter, some seasonally variable factor, perhaps hormonal, could initiate a process leading to failure of homeostasis in the infant a year later. The frequency distribution of SIDS babies by weight at birth, when compared to all live born infants, is significantly displaced toward the lower end of the birth-weight scale.[15] This observation supports the premise that some prenatal factor existed that precluded optimal intrauterine growth. Further evidence of impaired maturation is contained in a recent report that SIDS victims have elevated levels of fetal hemoglobin.[16] This hypothesis implies that SIDS results from some aberration, perhaps in DNA recombination, that produces a subtle developmental defect at the molecular level (enzymes, hormones, neurotransmitters). For example, during the first six months of infancy, maintenance of thermal equilibrium switches from mediation by norepinephrine

TABLE 3. Seasonal Distributions of Salient SIDS Risk Factors (% of Infants)

Factors	Washington State 1975–1983 $N = 1140$		NICHD Study 1979 $N = 569$	
	Spring Summer	Autumn Winter	Spring Summer	Autumn Winter
All SIDS	36.8	63.2	41.3	58.7
SIDS > 12 weeks	47.4	53.2	40.9	43.1
Mother < 20 years	29.0	29.4	29.8	32.0
Birth rank > 1	61.2	64.7	71.7	70.7
Mother = adolescent multipara	8.8	11.2	16.2	15.6
Birth weight < 2.5 Kg	20.2	15.8	26.8	22.8
Male sex	61.0	62.4	57.9	58.1
Black ethnicity	—	—	57.0	47.3

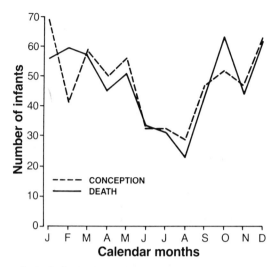

FIGURE 3. Comparison of month of death of SIDS subjects with their month of conception. NICHD study, 1979.

to epinephrine, with attendant metabolic perturbations. Thus, seasonality of SIDS could be a reflection of both the effect of the season of conception and of postnatal season on vital developmental responses to the environment. Such a concept provides a rationale for some reorientation of SIDS research.

ACKNOWLEDGMENTS

We thank Vicki Glasgo for manuscript preparation and Gerald Van Belle, Ph.D., for statistical consultation.

REFERENCES

1. FEDRICK, J. 1973. Sudden unexpected death in infants in the Oxford record linkage area. Brit. J. Prev. Soc. Med. **27:** 217–224.
2. BEAL, S. M. 1978. Seasonal variation in sudden infant death syndrome. Lancet **1:** 1257.
3. DEACON, E. L., M. J. J. O'REILLY & A. L. WILLIAMS. 1979. Some statistical and climatological aspects of the incidence of the sudden infant death syndrome. Aust. Paediatr. J. **15:** 248–254.
4. GOLDBERG, J. & R. J. STEIN. 1978. Seasonal variation in sudden infant death syndrome. Lancet **2:** 107.
5. GOLDBERG, J., R. HORNING, T. YAMASHITA & W. WEHRMACHER. 1986. Age at death and risk factors in sudden infant death syndrome. Aust. Paediatr. J. (Suppl. 1) **22:** 21–28.
6. WILLIAMS, A. L., E. C. UREN & L. BRETHERTON. 1984. Respiratory viruses and sudden infant death. Brit. Med. J. **288:** 1491–1493.
7. FOY, H. M. & C. G. RAY. 1973. Epidemiology of sudden infant death syndrome and lower respiratory tract disease in young children; a comparison. Am. J. Epidemiol. **98:** 69–71.
8. NELSON, K. E., M. A. GREENBERG, M. A. MUFSON & V. K. MOSES. 1975. The sudden infant death syndrome and epidemic viral disease. Am. J. Epidemiol. **101:** 423–430.

9. BONSER, R. S. A., B. H. KNIGHT & R. R. WEST. 1978. Sudden infant death syndrome in
    Cardiff; association with epidemic influenza and with temperature, 1955–1974. Int. J.
    Epidemiol. **7:** 335–340.
10. WEDGWOOD, R. J. & E. P. BENDITT. 1965. Sudden deaths in infants; proceedings of the
    conference on causes of sudden deaths in infants. DHEW PHS Publications. No. 1412.
    Washington, D.C. USGPO.
11. BERGMAN, A. B., J. B. BECKWITH & C. G. RAY. 1970. Sudden infant death syndrome;
    proceedings of the second international conference on causes of sudden death in infants.
    University of Washington Press. Seattle, WA.
12. FARBER, M. D. & V. CHANDRA. 1978. Seasonal variations in sudden infant death syndrome.
    Lancet **2:** 473.
13. RARING, R. H. 1974. SIDS; a note on the age distribution of the syndrome. *In* SIDS 1974;
    Proceedings of the Francis E. Camps international symposium on sudden and unexpected
    deaths in infancy. The Canadian Foundation for the Study of Infant Deaths. pp. 151–156.
    Toronto.
14. JEFFERY, H. E., B. V. McCLEARY, W. J. HENSLEY & D. J. C. READ. 1985. Thiamine
    deficiency—a neglected problem of infants and mothers—possible relationships to sudden
    infant death syndrome. Aust. N.Z. J. Obstet. Gynaecol. **25:** 198–202.
15. BERGMAN, A. B., J. B. BECKWITH & C. G. RAY. 1970. *In* Sudden infant death syndrome;
    proceedings of the second international conference on courses of sudden death in infants. pp.
    50–52. University of Washington Press. Seattle, WA.
16. GIULIAN, G. G., E. F. GILBERT & R. L. MOSS. 1987. Elevated fetal hemogloblin levels in
    sudden infant death syndrome. New Engl. J. Med. **316:** 1122–1126.

Risk Factors for SIDS

Results of the National Institute of Child Health and Human Development SIDS Cooperative Epidemiological Study

HOWARD J. HOFFMAN,[a,e] KARLA DAMUS,[b] LAURA
HILLMAN,[c] AND EHUD KRONGRAD[d]

[a]Biometry Branch
Prevention Research Program
National Institute of Child Health
and Human Development
National Institutes of Health
Bethesda, Maryland 20892
[b]Division of Community Health and Epidemiology
Department of Obstetrics and Gynecology
Albert Einstein College of Medicine
Bronx, New York 10461
[b]Division of Research and Epidemiology
Bureau of Maternity Services and Family Planning
New York City Department of Health
New York, New York 10007
[c]Department of Child Health
University of Missouri Hospital and Clinic
Columbia, Missouri 65212
[d]Division of Pediatric Cardiology
Department of Pediatrics
Columbia University School of Medicine
Babies Hospital
Columbia-Presbyterian Medical Center
New York, New York 10032

INTRODUCTION

The National Institute of Child Health and Human Development (NICHD) Cooperative Epidemiological Study of Sudden Infant Death Syndrome (SIDS) Risk Factors was initiated by the NICHD on the advice of leading pediatric researchers in this field and after careful consideration of the recommendations of a research planning workshop on future SIDS epidemiological studies.[1,2] The epidemiologists and biostatisticians who participated in the workshop recommended that any new large-scale, retrospective epidemiological study should: (1) focus on variables previously neglected in SIDS research,

[e]To whom correspondence should be addressed at: Biometry Branch, Prevention Research Program, NICHD, National Institutes of Health, Executive Plaza North, Room 630-S, 6130 Executive Boulevard, Bethesda, MD 20892.

13

(2) include follow-up interviews with mothers of SIDS cases and control infants, and (3) use more sophisticated methods of statistical design and analysis than previously employed. The participants also suggested that future retrospective, or case-control, studies include abstraction of routinely recorded maternal prenatal, delivery, and newborn medical records.

The resulting study, building upon these recommendations, was a multicenter, population-based, case-control study of over 800 SIDS cases and 1,600 control infants, using data collected at 6 study centers across the United States. It was believed that this broadly-based study could identify new risk factors for SIDS and could either confirm or reject several previously claimed risk factors. Earlier epidemiological studies had established several risk factors for SIDS, including higher incidence for infants between 1 and 4 months of age, males, blacks, parents of lower socio-economic status, young mothers with higher-order births, low birthweight and/or preterm infants, twins and other multiple births, cold weather months, and normal sleeping hours between midnight and 9:00 AM.[3-15] However, several other factors (for example, infantile apnea, maternal smoking during pregnancy, low maternal weight-gain during pregnancy, maternal anemia, preeclampsia or hypertension, short second stage of labor, short pregnancy interval and prior abortion or stillbirth, perinatal respiratory distress, lack of breastfeeding, prenatal and postnatal growth retardation, failure to obtain regular prenatal and postnatal medical care, and postneonatal illness) were less well documented in prior studies and remained to be investigated thoroughly.[8,9,12,16-19] Also, some factors emerged as important public health issues while the study was under way, such as the suggestion that SIDS could be linked to DTP immunization or could be the result of infant botulism.[20-23]

A critical consideration in developing the study design was the need to determine new risk factors which were specific to SIDS, over and above the risk factors which were generally associated with race and low birthweight. With this goal in mind, 2 living control infants were chosen for each SIDS case, and one of the control infants was explicitly matched for race and low birth weight. This paper presents an overview of maternal, neonatal, and postneonatal risk factors from the results of the NICHD SIDS Cooperative Epidemiological Study.

METHODS

Before the study began, problems in the classification of SIDS from death certificates led the National Center for Health Statistics to issue in 1975 new supplemental nosology guidelines for SIDS deaths to be used with the eighth revision of the *International Classification of Diseases;* this greatly improved the reporting of SIDS as a primary cause of death in the United States.[24-25] Also, as a result of the Sudden Infant Death Syndrome Act of 1974 (Public Law 93-270), Congress authorized the secretary of the Department of Health, Education and Welfare (DHEW) to establish information and counseling centers to collect and analyze data on SIDS and furnish information to families affected by SIDS.[2] As a result, when the NICHD SIDS Cooperative Epidemiological Study was begun in 1978, there was already in place at most of the study centers an existing SIDS Research, Counseling, and Information Program administered through the Office of Maternal and Child Health, DHEW, which greatly facilitated the identification of eligible SIDS cases for the study.

The NICHD SIDS Cooperative Epidemiological Study collected data at 6 geographically defined study centers with a total live-birth population of approximately 10% that of the entire United States. There were 3 relatively large study centers—Chicago, New York City, and California (8 counties)—which contributed 31%, 24%, and 21% of the 838 cases, respectively. Three smaller study centers—upstate New York (20 counties), St. Louis, and Seattle—contributed 10%, 8%, and 6% of the cases, respectively. The data analyzed in this report, however, come from the 757 singleton SIDS cases judged by a panel of 3 expert pathologists to have been either "definite" or "probable" SIDS cases after a thorough review of microscopic slides, gross autopsy reports, and death investigation reports.

Data were collected from eligible SIDS cases who died in the period from October 1978 through December 1979. A case was defined as "any infant who died suddenly and unexpectedly, and who upon postmortem examination was designated as an eligible sudden infant death case by a medical examiner or coroner, and who met all the eligibility criteria and none of the exclusion criteria." Eligibility criteria were that the death (1) occurred during the specified 15-month time period, (2) occurred within the geographic region of a study center, and (3) was designated as an eligible SIDS case by a medical examiner or coroner using the standardized necropsy protocol. Exclusion criteria were (1) no autopsy performed, (2) major deviations from standardized necropsy protocol occurred during the postmortem examination, (3) the death was of an infant younger than 14 days, or older than 24 months of age, or (4) the death of the infant occurred in a hospital after the infant was in the facility for more than 24 hr immediately prior to death.

Study procedures were agreed upon by a steering committee composed of the principal investigators at each study center and the NICHD program staff with responsibility for the scientific management of the study. A centralized data coordinating center managed the data processing, quality assurance, and interaction with project coordinators at each study center. A common necropsy protocol was developed for the study, based on the report by Jones and Weston,[26] which included a standard set of diagnoses for exclusion of infants whose deaths could be attributed to known causes. Also, a separate pathology coordinating laboratory ensured the uniform processing of pathology specimens and coordinated with the panel of 3 expert pathologists both the microscopic review of slides and the review of gross autopsy and death investigation reports.

For each of the SIDS cases, 2 living age-matched control infants were selected. Each of these control infants was randomly selected from a pool of eligible controls identified by birth certificates. The distributions of age of the infant at death for the SIDS cases or age of the infant at the time of the maternal interview for control infants were very similar: there was less than a 2-day difference in the mean age for the SIDS cases and either set of control infants. The first set of controls, control A infants, were matched only for age. The second set, control B infants, were matched in addition for low birthweight ($\leq$ 2,500 g) and race (black or non-black). For low birthweight SIDS cases, a control B infant was sought weighing within 250 g of the birthweight of the SIDS case. This close matching for low birthweight infants resulted in very similar rates of both very low birthweight ($<$ 1,500 g) and preterm births for SIDS cases and control B infants.

Statistical significance has been determined using chi-square tests on incidence data and fourfold tables. Also, exact one-sided tests for binomial proportions were performed for the matched comparisons in 2 × 2 tables. Both the standard odds ratio estimate for unmatched analysis and McNemar's estimate for matched-pairs analysis have been used to calculate relative risk for SIDS cases versus control A and control B infants.[27–28] Multivariate analysis results for unmatched and matched data appear elsewhere and are not presented in this report.[29] More detailed descriptions of the study design and procedures used in the pathologists' review of cases have also been published previously.[30–32]

RESULTS

Of the 838 eligible SIDS cases enrolled in the NICHD SIDS Cooperative Epidemiological Study, 800 were singleton births and 38 (4.5%) were multiple births. The numbers contributed by each of the 6 study centers are shown in TABLE 1. The SIDS incidence per 1,000 live-born infants is also shown for each study center. Overall, the SIDS incidence rate for the NICHD SIDS Cooperative Study was 1.75, which compares to an incidence of 1.51 for the entire United States, based on vital statistics in 1979. The excess SIDS incidence in the study was attributable to the higher incidence found for black births as compared to the national data (3.65 vs. 2.82); the incidence rates for non-black births were nearly identical (1.10 vs. 1.25). The incidence of SIDS varied from a high of 3.48 in Chicago, which was twice the average for the study, to a low of 0.86 in upstate New York, which was only half the incidence rate observed for the whole study.

The percentage of all postneonatal deaths attributable to SIDS in this study is also shown in TABLE 1. Overall, 37.9% of all postneonatal infant deaths were ascribed to SIDS. Although both the California and Seattle study centers reported a relatively high

TABLE 1. Number of SIDS Cases and Selected Vital Statistics Indices for Each Study Center

Study Center	SIDS Cases Eligible for Study (n)	Black Live Births[a] (%)	SIDS Deaths[a] (% total postneonatal deaths)	SIDS Rate[a] (no. per 1,000 live births)
Chicago	258	50.7	46.4	3.48
California	179	9.1	40.6	1.66
Seattle	47	7.0	48.5	2.00
New York City	203	36.1	33.4	1.52
Upstate New York	84	9.9	26.1	0.86
St. Louis	67	26.0	33.3	1.29
Totals	838	25.2	37.9	1.75

[a]Based on 1979 U.S. vital statistics for resident live births and postneonatal infant deaths within the geographic boundaries of each of the 6 study centers.

proportion of all postneonatal deaths to be due to SIDS (40.6% and 48.5%, respectively), the incidence rate for these 2 centers was not nearly as high as in Chicago, in part because of differences in the racial composition at the 3 sites. New York City and St. Louis both contributed a relatively high proportion of black SIDS cases to the study, but the SIDS incidence rate in these 2 urban areas was below the average for the study as a whole.

Of the 800 eligible singleton SIDS cases recruited into the study, 757 (94.6%) were determined to be "definitely" or "probably" SIDS cases after extensive review by a panel of 3 expert forensic or pediatric pathologists. The age distribution at death for the 757 SIDS cases and the age distribution of the corresponding sets of control infants at the time of the maternal interview are shown in TABLE 2. All SIDS cases dying between the ages of 2 weeks and 2 yr were eligible for the study. However, only 2% of SIDS cases were over 1 yr of age. The vast majority of SIDS cases, 88%, were less than 5.5 months of age (24 weeks). The age matching for control A and control B infants produced nearly identical age distributions for both sets of control infants, as demonstrated in TABLE 2.

The additional matching for birthweight and race in the control B infants removed the association with most newborn risk factors, as shown in TABLE 3. Although low birthweight and preterm delivery are highly significant risk factors in the comparisons of

TABLE 2. Distribution of Age at Death for Pathologically Defined Singleton SIDS Cases and Age at Time of Maternal Interview for Control Infants

Age at Death or Maternal Interview	SIDS Cases		Control A		Control B	
	n	%	n	%	n	%
2–5 weeks	118	15.6	98	12.9	94	12.4
6–11 weeks	311	41.1	312	41.2	307	40.6
12–23 weeks	239	31.6	252	33.3	259	34.2
24–51 weeks	73	9.6	78	10.3	80	10.6
52–103 weeks	16	2.1	17	2.2	17	2.2
Totals	757	100.0	757	100.0	757	100.0

SIDS cases with control A infants, neither is significantly increased in the comparisons with control B infants. Similarly, small-for-gestational age, based on standards defined for full-term infants only, was significantly increased in the comparison with control A infants but not with control B infants.[33–34] Also, low Apgar scores and black race are significantly increased only for the comparisons with control A infants. However, since male sex was not controlled by matching, this factor is significantly higher for SIDS cases compared to both sets of control infants.

Maternal Risk Factors

The strength of various maternal risk factors is indicated in TABLE 4. Those factors analyzed from the information obtained in the maternal interview are shown in the top half of the table, ranked by increasing odds ratio for SIDS cases compared to control A

TABLE 3. Relative Risk of Selected Newborn Factors for SIDS Cases Compared to Control Infants

Newborn Risk Factors	SIDS vs. Control A Odds Ratio	SIDS vs. Control B Odds Ratio	Frequency Among SIDS Infants (%)
Low birthweight ($\leq$ 2,500 g)	4.6[a]	1.0[b]	24.0
Very low birthweight ($\leq$ 1,500 g)	17.8[a]	1.0[b]	4.5
Preterm birth (< 37 weeks)	4.6[a]	1.1	18.2
Very preterm birth (< 33 weeks)	15.6[a]	1.3	5.8
Small-for-gestational age[c]	2.5[a]	1.2	26.6
Apgar score at 1 min < 7	2.0[a]	1.0	12.7
Apgar score at 5 min < 7	3.5[a]	0.9	4.1
Male sex	1.4[d]	1.5[d]	59.7
Black race	2.5[a]	1.0[b]	53.6

[a]Level of significance, $p < 0.001$.

[b]These odds ratios are equal to 1.0 due to study design, since control B infants were matched to SIDS cases for low birthweight and race.

[c]Small-for-gestational age was defined using the norms published by Miller and Merritt[33] for full-term infants (37–43 weeks gestational age).

[d]Level of significance, $p < 0.005$.

TABLE 4. Relative Risk of Selected Maternal Factors for SIDS Cases Compared to Control Infants

Maternal Risk Factors	SIDS vs. Control A Odds Ratio[a]	SIDS vs. Control B Odds Ratio[a]	Frequency Among Mothers of SIDS Cases (%)
Mother's interview			
Alcohol use during pregnancy	1.1	1.0	61.2
Parity $\geq$ 2	1.5[b]	1.8[b]	38.1
Mother's age < 20 yr	2.3[b]	1.6[b]	31.5
Late onset (third trimester) or no prenatal care	2.5[b]	2.5[b]	22.5
High crowding index in infant's home	2.7[b]	2.2[b]	43.1
Mother's education < 12 yr	2.7[b]	2.6[b]	56.7
Illicit drug use during pregnancy	2.9[b]	2.0[b]	25.6
Infant never breast-fed	3.1[b]	2.3[b]	73.7
Cigarette smoking during pregnancy	3.8[b]	3.4[b]	69.6
Mother not married	3.9[b]	2.5[b]	59.3
Mother's age < 20 yr at first pregnancy	4.4[b]	3.3[b]	75.4
Prenatal medical records			
Cesarean section delivery	1.0	1.2	16.8
Toxemia, preeclampsia, or hypertension	1.0	0.9	18.1
Vaginitis during pregnancy	1.1	1.0	24.6
Low prepregnancy weight (< 110 lb)	1.2	1.4[c]	15.8
Anemia during pregnancy	1.4[c]	1.4[c]	20.6
Trauma or injury during pregnancy	1.5	1.4	6.7
Weight gain < 20 lb at delivery	2.0[b]	1.7[b]	35.5
Urinary tract infection during pregnancy	2.4[b]	1.8[b]	15.8
Venereal disease during pregnancy	2.9[d]	1.8	4.6

[a]Odds ratios were calculated using the matching between SIDS cases and control A or control B infants, respectively.
[b]Level of significance, $p < 0.001$.
[c]Level of significance, $p < 0.05$.
[d]Level of significance, $p < 0.005$.

mothers. Among this group of factors, the most important are "cigarette smoking during pregnancy," "mother not married," and "mother's age less than 20 yr at first pregnancy," all of which have relative risk estimates of 3.8 or higher. In the comparisons between SIDS and control B (which were matched for race and low birthweight delivery), "mother not married" drops down to an odds ratio of 2.5, which is comparable to that of "mother's education less than 12 yr" and "late onset (third trimester) or no prenatal care." "Cigarette smoking during pregnancy" and "mother's age less than 20 yr at first pregnancy" remain as the 2 strongest risk factors, with relative risks of 3.4 and 3.3, respectively. It is notable that "alcohol use during pregnancy" was not associated with SIDS risk.

Maternal risk factors analyzed from information in the medical records are examined in the lower half of TABLE 4. No association was found with "cesarean section delivery," "toxemia, preeclampsia or hypertension," or "vaginitis during pregnancy." In fact, the medical risk factors were generally not as high as the social, behavioral, and demographic risk factors enumerated in the maternal interview. Associations of moderate strength (relative risks from 1.7 to 2.0 for SIDS compared to control B mothers) were found with "venereal disease during pregnancy," "urinary tract infection during pregnancy," and "weight-gain less than 20 lb at delivery" (i.e., relatively low weight-gain during pregnancy). Although the relative risks were only 1.4, "anemia during pregnancy" was statistically significant ($p < 0.05$) for SIDS cases in comparison to both control A and control B mothers and, similarly, "low prepregnancy weight (< 110 lb)" was statistically significant ($p < 0.05$) in comparison to control B mothers, because these 2 factors were relatively common in mothers of SIDS cases (20.6% and 15.8%, respectively). However, venereal disease, with a relative risk of 1.8, was noted in only 4.6% of the mothers of SIDS cases and did not quite reach statistical significance in the comparison with control B mothers ($p = 0.06$). Relatively low weight gain during pregnancy (less than 20 lb) was the most common of the 3 factors which were highly significant ($p < 0.001$), occurring in 35.5% of mothers of SIDS cases.

Neonatal Risk Factors

A number of conditions noted in the infant during the newborn nursery stay were examined for possible association with SIDS. TABLE 5 ranks these factors in order of increasing strength of their effect for SIDS compared to control A infants. All of the factors, except "jaundice" in the newborn, were statistically significant in the comparisons between SIDS cases and control A infants. "Newborn apnea" appeared to be the strongest risk factor, but this observation is potentially misleading because there were so few very low birthweight or premature control A infants. Moreover, the comparison of this factor between SIDS and control B infants, who were matched for low birthweight, shows that the effect disappears entirely. Hence, for examining risk, the most important comparison is between SIDS and control B infants, because this comparison differentiates

TABLE 5. Relative Risk of Neonatal Conditions for SIDS Cases Compared to Control Infants

Condition	SIDS vs. Control A Odds Ratio[a]	SIDS vs. Control B Odds Ratio[a]	Frequency Among SIDS Infants (%)
Jaundice	1.1	1.0	39.6
Bradycardia	1.4[b]	1.2	16.7
Tachycardia	1.6[c]	1.5[d]	24.2
Tremors	1.6[b]	0.9	7.0
Hypothermia	1.7[c]	1.3[b]	45.9
Tachypnea	1.9[c]	1.3[b]	25.6
Cyanosis	1.9[c]	1.5[d]	18.6
Poor feeding	1.9[c]	1.4[b]	13.3
Vomiting	2.0[c]	1.3	9.8
Pallor	2.3[c]	1.1	8.8
Irritability	2.6[c]	1.5[b]	14.4
Fever	2.6[c]	1.9[b]	6.3
Respiratory distress	2.8[c]	1.5[b]	16.7
Lethargy	3.1[c]	1.0	6.9
Abnormal cry	4.5[c]	1.5	6.4
Newborn apnea	7.2[c]	1.1	5.2

[a]Odds ratios were calculated using the matching between SIDS cases and control A or control B infants, respectively.
[b]Level of significance, $p < 0.05$.
[c]Level of significance, $p < 0.001$.
[d]Level of significance, $p < 0.01$.

TABLE 6. Incidence of Newborn Apnea in Each Gestational Age/Birthweight Category for SIDS Cases and Control Infants

	Birthweight (g)							
	800–1,499		1,500–2,499		≥ 2,500		Total, All Birthweights	
Gestational Age	n^a	% Apnea[b]	n^a	% Apnea[b]	n^a	% Apnea[b]	n^a	% Apnea[b]
Preterm infants (20–36 weeks)								
SIDS cases	28	50.0	78	23.1	26	0.0	132	24.2
Control A	2	0.0	18	16.7	13	0.0	33	9.1
Control B	31	58.1	70	20.0	19	0.0	120	26.7
Full-term infants (≥ 37 weeks)								
SIDS cases	1	0.0	61	0.0	520	1.0	582	0.9
Control A	0	0.0	26	0.0	686	0.3	712	0.3
Control B	1	0.0	71	2.8	548	0.0	620	0.3
All gestations								
SIDS cases	29	48.3	139	13.0	546	0.9	714	5.2
Control A	2	0.0	44	6.8	699	0.3	745	0.7
Control B	32	56.3	141	11.3	567	0.0	740	4.6

[a]Total number of infants within a gestational age/birthweight category (cell); e.g., the number of preterm SIDS cases weighing less than 1,500 g at birth was 28. Note that the numbers of SIDS cases and of control infants listed differ slightly between this table and Table 7 because some information was not recorded or reported for some infants.

[b]Percentage of the total infants in the indicated category who had apnea of 15 sec or longer duration noted on their newborn medical records; e.g., 50%, or 14, of the preterm SIDS cases weighing less than 1,500 g had apnea.

SIDS risk from risk associated with low birthweight (or race). In comparisons with control B infants, the most significant risk factors were "cyanosis" and "tachycardia," followed by "fever," "respiratory distress," and "irritability" (all with $p < 0.02$). Also, significant differences were noted for "hypothermia," "poor feeding," and "tachypnea" ($p < 0.05$). "Abnormal cry" did not attain statistical significance ($p = 0.07$), nor were any of the other risk factors statistically significant in comparisons with control B infants.

The number of infants with apnea during the newborn period is examined jointly by birthweight and gestational age categories in TABLE 6. Among preterm infants, i.e., those with gestational ages less than or equal to 36 weeks, apnea was fairly common, occurring in 24.2% of all preterm SIDS cases and 26.7% of all preterm control B infants. Among very small (birthweight less than 1,500 g) preterm infants, the percentage with apnea increased to 50.0% and 58.1% for SIDS and control B infants, respectively. There were too few very low birthweight control A infants (only 2 infants) to obtain a reliable rate for apnea of prematurity in these infants.

Among full-term infants, i.e., those with gestational ages of 37 weeks or greater, apnea in the newborn nursery was quite rare (TABLE 6). The apnea rate was less than 1% for either SIDS cases or control infants. For full-term infants weighing between 1,500 and 2,499 g, only 2 infants had newborn apnea, and both of these were control B infants. In conclusion, there were no differences between SIDS cases and control B infants (matched for low birthweight and race) in the rate of apnea observed in the newborn nursery.

Postneonatal Risk Factors

The occurrence of apnea observed by the mother after discharge from the nursery is examined in TABLE 7. Mothers were asked during the interview whether they had ever observed their infants to "turn blue or stop breathing." For each such episode, follow-up questions elicited further information. Overall, mothers of SIDS infants were more likely to have reported an apneic episode of this type, i.e., 7.7% of SIDS compared to 3.0% of control B infants ($p < 0.001$). This table also demonstrates that preterm infants were almost 3 times as likely to have an observed postneonatal apneic episode as full-term infants. Although more SIDS cases than controls were noted to have had postneonatal apneic episodes, these cases constitute only a small proportion of all SIDS cases. Also, the majority of all observed apneic episodes occurred while the infant was either awake or feeding, not during sleep.

TABLE 8 relates parental reports of infant illnesses and related conditions to the time interval prior to death for SIDS cases or the maternal interview for control infants. For example, 28.9% of SIDS cases had a cold in the 24 hr prior to death, but this percentage is not significantly greater than for either control A infants (25.9%) or control B infants (26.2%). If the percentage of infants with colds within the last 2 weeks, including the last 24 hr is examined, then 43.8% of SIDS cases, 35.7% of control A infants, and 38.8% of control B infants had colds within that time period, which is statistically significant for SIDS cases compared to control A infants ($p < 0.05$), but not compared to control B infants. Altogether, almost two-thirds of both the SIDS and the control infants had had a

TABLE 7. Incidence of Postneonatal Apnea ("Turned Blue or Stopped Breathing") in Each Gestational Age/Birthweight Category for SIDS Cases and Control Infants

| | Birthweight (g) | | | | | | | |
| | 800–1,499 | | 1,500–2,499 | | ≥ 2,500 | | Total, All Birthweights | |
Gestational Age	n^a	% Apnea[b]	n^a	% Apnea[b]	n^a	% Apnea[b]	n^a	% Apnea[b]
Preterm Infants (20–36 weeks)								
SIDS cases	25	20.0	75	16.0	25	16.0	125	16.8
Control A	2	0.0	20	5.0	13	15.4	35	8.6
Control B	32	12.5	72	6.9	19	0.0	123	7.3
Full-term infants (≥ 37 weeks)								
SIDS cases	1	0.0	64	4.7	521	6.0	586	5.8
Control A	0	0.0	26	0.0	695	3.3	721	3.2
Control B	1	0.0	72	5.6	560	1.8	633	2.2
All gestations								
SIDS cases	26	19.2	139	10.8	546	6.4	711	7.7
Control A	2	0.0	46	2.2	708	3.5	756	3.4[c]
Control B	33	12.1	144	6.3	579	1.7	756	3.0[c]

[a]Total number of infants within a gestational age/birthweight category (cell), e.g., the number of SIDS cases for whom information concerning the occurrence of postneonatal apnea was available and who were preterm and weighed less than 1,500 g at birth was 25.

[b]Percentage of the total infants in indicated category who had postneonatal apnea which was reported during the mother's interview; e.g., 20%, or 5, of the SIDS cases who were preterm and weighed less than 1,500 g at birth, and for whom information concerning the occurrence of postneonatal apnea was available, were reported to have had postneonatal apnea.

[c]Level of significance, $p < 0.001$.

TABLE 8. Selected Conditions by Time Interval before Death for SIDS Cases or Maternal Interview for Control Infants as Reported on Mother's Interview Form

Condition[a]	SIDS Cases (%)[b]		Control A (%)[b]		Control B (%)[b]	
Cold						
< 24 hr	28.9	} 43.8	25.9	} 35.7[c]	26.2	} 38.8[d]
< 2 weeks, > 24 hr	14.9		9.8		12.6	
> 2 weeks	22.9		23.1		24.9	
Never	33.2		41.2		36.4	
Cough						
< 24 hr	12.7	} 21.0	15.3	} 21.2[d]	16.7	} 26.6[e]
< 2 weeks, > 24 hr	8.3		5.9		9.9	
> 2 weeks	14.2		14.5		14.4	
Never	64.8		64.2		59.0	
Diarrhea						
< 24 hr	6.4	} 19.1	3.7	} 12.2[f]	3.7	} 12.0[f]
< 2 weeks, > 24 hr	12.7		8.5		8.3	
> 2 weeks	25.0		17.7		19.9	
Never	55.9		70.1		68.7	
Vomiting						
< 24 hr	7.9	} 14.6	3.2	} 7.7[f]	4.8	} 9.7[f]
< 2 weeks, > 24 hr	6.7		4.5		4.9	
> 2 weeks	14.3		9.5		9.5	
Never	71.7		82.8		80.8	
Colic						
< 24 hr	3.4		4.6		4.6	
< 2 weeks, > 24 hr	3.9		4.5		5.7	
> 2 weeks	10.8		13.6		13.8	
Never	81.9		77.2		75.8	
Bad fall						
< 24 hr	0.4		0.4		0.3	
< 2 weeks, > 24 hr	2.4		0.9		1.2	
> 2 weeks	7.6		4.0		2.5	
Never	89.4		94.7		96.0	
Seizure						
< 24 hr	0.6		0.0		0.0	
< 2 weeks, > 24 hr	0.1		0.0		0.0	
> 2 weeks	1.1		0.1		0.5	
Never	98.2		99.9		99.5	
Fever						
< 24 hr	5.8		2.9		2.8	
< 2 weeks, > 24 hr	7.5		8.9		9.3	
> 2 weeks	20.9		17.6		20.8	
Never	65.7		70.7		67.1	
Listless/droopy						
< 24 hr	7.8	} 10.5	1.1	} 3.8[f]	0.7	} 2.5[f]
< 2 weeks, > 24 hr	2.7		2.8		1.9	
> 2 weeks	4.6		3.7		4.0	
Never	84.9		92.5		93.5	

[a]Time period during which condition was observed, before infant's death (SIDS) or maternal interview (controls), is indicated. For each condition, only the most recent occurrence within the indicated time periods is included in this table.

[b]Percentage of total infants in indicated category in whom condition was observed.

[c]Level of significance, $p < 0.05$.

[d]N.S.

[e]Level of significance, $p < 0.01$.

[f]Level of significance, $p < 0.001$.

cold sometime since birth. Thus, these data do not show a strong association between colds in infants and SIDS. Also, control infants tended to have more "cough" than SIDS cases, which was significant for the comparison with control B infants. No statistically significant differences were found with "colic," "fever," "bad fall," or "seizure" for the last 2 weeks. However, "diarrhea" and "vomiting" were both highly significantly associated with SIDS deaths within the last 2 weeks, including the last 24 hr, prior to death ($p < 0.001$). "Listless or droopy" appearance was also increased for SIDS cases in the last 2 weeks and, especially, within the last 24 hr prior to death ($p < 0.001$).

TABLE 9 examines "diarrhea" and "vomiting" further to see whether they occurred in association with other symptoms of infectious disease, fever or colds. Infants were categorized as follows: those reported with diarrhea only, those reported with vomiting only, and those reported with a combination of both vomiting and diarrhea during the last 2 weeks (including the last 24 hr) prior to death (SIDS cases) or maternal interview (controls). In each category, about half of the infants also had a cold during this time period. The prevalence of fever increased in association with the occurrence of vomiting and, especially, in association with the occurrence of both vomiting and diarrhea. The pattern of association for diarrhea and/or vomiting with colds or fever was similar, however, for both SIDS and control infants. Thus, although the nature of the illness did not appear to be different from that of the controls, SIDS cases were more likely to have had a gastrointestinal illness (probably of viral origin, since colds were also quite common in these infants) during the last 2 weeks before death.

Other reported illnesses or conditions were examined in relation to "listless or droopy" appearance, which was also increased in SIDS infants compared to control infants in the last 2 weeks before death (SIDS cases) or maternal interview (controls). About two-thirds of the infants who were reported as listless or droopy in the last 2 weeks also had colds, as shown in TABLE 10. It is notable that this proportion did not differ between SIDS cases and control infants, even though many more SIDS infants were reported as listless or droopy. Similarly, other illnesses or conditions (cough, fever,

TABLE 9. Association of Diarrhea and/or Vomiting with Fevers or Colds during the Last Two Weeks before Death for SIDS Cases or Maternal Interview for Controls

Condition	SIDS Cases		Control A		Control B	
	n	%	*n*	%	*n*	%
Diarrhea	105	50.0	73	55.7	70	49.0
With fever[a]	17	16.2	12	16.4	11	15.7
With cold[a]	59	56.2	30	41.1	33	47.1
Vomiting	73	34.8	39	29.8	52	36.4
With fever[a]	15	20.6	13	33.3	14	26.9
With cold[a]	40	54.8	22	56.4	27	51.9
Both diarrhea and vomiting	32	15.2	19	14.5	21	14.7
With fever[a]	18	56.3	8	42.1	7	33.3
With cold[a]	20	62.5	9	47.4	12	57.1
Totals[b]	210	29.3[d]	131	17.3[c,d]	143	18.9[c,d]

[a]Percentages shown for fever or cold refer to the percent of infants with the specified condition (diarrhea, vomiting, or both) who also had either a fever or a cold during the last two weeks, as reported on the mother's interview.
[b]Total number of infants in each group (SIDS or control) with diarrhea and/or vomiting.
[c]Level of significance, $p < 0.001$.
[d]Percent of infants in each group (SIDS or control) with diarrhea and/or vomiting.

TABLE 10. Association Between Listless/Droopy and Selected Other Conditions during Last Two Weeks before Death for SIDS Cases or Maternal Interview for Controls

Associated Condition	SIDS Cases[a] $(\%)^d$	Control A[b] $(\%)^d$	Control B[c] $(\%)^d$
Cold	64.0	69.0	68.4
Cough	37.3	41.4	42.1
Fever	30.7	44.8	42.1
Diarrhea	40.0	31.0	21.1
Vomiting	37.3	27.6	31.6
Total[e]	10.5	3.8[f]	2.5[f]

[a]A total of 75 infants in this group were reported to have a listless/droopy appearance during last 2 weeks.

[b]A total of 29 infants in this group were reported to have a listless/droopy appearance during last 2 weeks.

[c]A total of 19 infants in this group were reported to have a listless/droopy appearance during last 2 weeks.

[d]Percent of total infants with listless/droopy appearance who also had indicated associated condition during last 2 weeks.

[e]Percent of total group (SIDS or control) reported to have listless/droopy appearance during last 2 weeks.

[f]Level of significance, $p < 0.001$.

diarrhea, and vomiting) all occurred with about the same frequency for SIDS cases and control infants. This pattern of internal consistency gives credence to the mother's reported observation of listless or droopy appearance. Although recall bias is certainly a concern, it would appear that SIDS mothers understood the terminology of "listless or droopy" and used these terms in a manner comparable to control mothers. Since 8% of SIDS cases were listless or droopy in the last 24 hr prior to death compared to less than 1% of control B infants in the corresponding time period (TABLE 8), the relative risk for this systemic condition is 12.7, which is the highest relative risk shown for any single factor and SIDS with respect to control B.

DISCUSSION

At the SIDS epidemiological research planning workshop convened in 1972, the participants expressed the view that identification of SIDS-specific risk factors through epidemiological studies alone would be quite unlikely, given the low incidence and the associated measurement difficulties.[1] The study by Peterson and colleagues[35] of SIDS and other major causes of infant deaths for King County, Washington, during the period 1969–1977, using vital records information, also supported this prediction that new SIDS-specific risk factors would be difficult to identify. For example, in that study only the age at death for SIDS cases distinguished them from all other causes of death. Thus, low maternal age with multiparity was associated with deaths due to respiratory distress syndrome as well as SIDS, and the seasonal pattern of deaths was similar for SIDS and deaths due to infection. These findings and similar results demonstrated by other researchers suggested that epidemiological studies may be expected to identify only factors which could act in a secondary fashion rather than as primary or causal agents.[10,36-37] Also, most epidemiologists agreed that low birthweight was an intermediate factor, affecting both SIDS and overall infant mortality, as well as resulting from many of the same maternal risk factors already associated with SIDS and other causes of infant mortality.

Against this background, the NICHD SIDS Cooperative Epidemiological Study was designed to determine the strength of associations between SIDS and potential risk factors of both a general nature and, to the extent practical, a SIDS-specific nature. Thus, the case-control design included both an age-matched living control infant, control A, randomly-selected from birth certificates, as well as an age-matched living control infant, control B, matched also for low birthweight and race. The control B infants were to be used to distinguish SIDS risk from factors which were more generally due to low birthweight or black race. As shown in this paper, several SIDS-specific risk factors (e.g., maternal smoking, newborn tachycardia, and diarrhea/vomiting) did emerge, at least to the extent that the association cannot be explained by low birthweight or black race *per se*. Another risk factor in this category, which has not been discussed in this paper, was the failure of SIDS cases to be immunized for diptheria-tetanus-pertussis (DTP), or with oral polio vaccine (OPV), as often as their age-matched control infants.[30] However, the strong associations which many other risk factors showed when SIDS cases were compared to control A infants either were weakened considerably, or disappeared altogether, when the factors were examined with respect to control B infants. Newborn apnea, as abstracted from the medical records of infants during their stay in the nursery, is a good example of the latter type of potential risk factor.

The failure to find an association between SIDS and colds in this well-controlled study was unexpected in view of the consensus that a mild respiratory infection is a common and important underlying factor in a large proportion of SIDS cases. Earlier studies have shown an association between colds and SIDS deaths for infants 12 weeks of age and older, especially for those deaths which occurred during winter months.[38-40] In the NICHD SIDS Cooperative Epidemiological Study, SIDS cases who were 12 weeks of age and older did tend to have more colds within the last 2 weeks compared to control A infants (relative risk [rr] = 1.8; $p < 0.05$) and, to a lesser degree, compared to control B infants (rr = 1.5; $p = 0.06$). However, there was no clear association between colds and age at death either with season (winter months) or male sex of SIDS cases, as has been suggested. Further information on seasonality and SIDS risk from the NICHD SIDS Cooperative Epidemiological Study has been presented by Peterson.[41]

An increased prevalence of diarrhea and/or vomiting in SIDS cases has been suggested in some prior studies.[36,42] Lack of breast-feeding has also been shown to be a risk factor for SIDS both in the NICHD SIDS Cooperative Epidemiological Study and in some previous studies.[9,19,43] Based on the recent findings of Eaton-Evans and Dugdale[44] that breast-feeding is protective against diarrhea and/or vomiting in the first 6 months of life, the relationship between breast-feeding and the mother's report of diarrhea and/or vomiting during the last 2 weeks before death or interview was further examined. For infants between the ages of 2 and 11 weeks, "never breast-fed" and "reported diarrhea and/or vomiting within the last 2 weeks" were strongly associated ($p < 0.02$) for SIDS cases (rr = 2.9), control A infants (rr = 2.5), and control B infants (rr = 4.2). For older infants, the relationship was not consistent, although SIDS cases between 12 and 23 weeks old showed an increased relative risk of 1.6 that was not significant.

The relationship of "never breast-fed" to "colds within the last 2 weeks" was also examined. Previous reports which controlled for socio-economic status and related factors[45-46] have suggested both that breastfeeding is protective, and that it is not protective, for upper respiratory and other common infections during the first few months of life. Infants between 2 and 11 months of age showed a consistent pattern of increased colds within the last 2 weeks if never breast-fed (SIDS, rr = 2.0; control A, rr = 2.2; control B, rr = 1.7); however, this was statistically significant only for control A infants. Thus, the NICHD SIDS Cooperative Epidemiological Study provides evidence that breast-feeding is protective against gastrointestinal infections, and has a tendency for protection against other infections, in both SIDS cases and living control infants. The fact that only 9.8% of SIDS cases were mostly or only breast-fed compared to 27.7% of control A infants and 22.3% of control B infants suggests that fewer SIDS infants received the benefit of the protective effect of breast-feeding.

The association found in this study between diarrhea and SIDS also suggests the possibility of an electrolyte imbalance as a contributing factor in some SIDS deaths, as has occassionally been suggested.[47] However, recent studies using postmortem vitreous humor have been unable to confirm the suggestion of a disturbance in electrolytes.[48] The NICHD SIDS Cooperative Epidemiological Study made no attempt to replicate these studies.

The information on apnea presented in this report was summarized previously at the NIH Consensus Development Conference on Infantile Apnea and Home Monitoring.[49] The NICHD SIDS Cooperative Epidemiological Study has provided clear evidence that newborn apnea (or apnea of prematurity) is not a risk factor for SIDS, because the rates of occurrence were nearly the same for SIDS cases and the age-, race-, and low birthweight-matched control B infants. Such information should prove valuable to physicians and parents of premature infants, who must decide how to manage these infants after discharge from the nursery.[50]

Based on the data presented here, the importance of postneonatal apnea as a risk factor for SIDS is still arguable. Although postneonatal apnea was statistically significant, it was noted in only a small proportion of SIDS cases. Also, since the data were obtained by parental interview without any objective means of verification, the increased risk may be due to recall bias. Steinschneider[51] demonstrated that infants with a history of postneo-natal apnea would be expected to have increased apneic episodes while sick with colds or nasopharyngitis and thus would be more likely to die at such times. In our study, SIDS cases with a history of postneonatal apnea did indeed have more colds in the last 2 weeks of life compared to SIDS infants without a history of postneonatal apnea (58.2% versus 42.7%, respectively; $p < 0.05$). Although infants with a history of postneonatal apnea were not more common among older (≥ 12 weeks of age) as compared to younger (2–11 weeks of age) SIDS cases, the association between a reported history of apnea and having a cold in the last 2 weeks was increased in the older SIDS cases (66.7% vs. 50.0%). The apneic event, "turned blue or stopped breathing," is quite heterogeneous because it can occur during sleep, waking, crying, while feeding, etc.; and many such episodes may have gone entirely unnoticed. Also, the correlation between the reporting of apnea by parents and the assessment of a life-threatening event using electrocardiographic mea-surements has been shown to be poor.[52] Thus, because the prevalence of apnea in SIDS cases is rather low and very few of the infants with reported apnea were brought to medical attention by their parents, the role of postneonatal apnea as a risk factor for SIDS has yet to be clearly established.

None of the risk factors documented in this paper are of sufficient strength to enable identification of SIDS infants prior to their death. Instead, a descriptive profile has emerged that associates several maternal, neonatal, and postneonatal factors with increased SIDS risk. Maternal factors such as inadequate prenatal care, smoking, low weight-gain, anemia, use of illicit drugs, venereal disease, and urinary tract infection all suggest that the *in utero* environment of SIDS infants prior to birth is less than optimal. Furthermore, the number of postneonatal regular medical care visits and the number of immunizations was less in SIDS cases as compared to control infants, suggesting that postneonatal care was also less than optimal.[30,43] The higher incidence of low birthweight and preterm deliveries, plus more subtle differences in the newborn signs and symptoms, such as, tachycardia, cyanosis, and fever, suggest that the SIDS newborns are different from control infants at birth, although only in subtle ways when compared to control infants matched for race and low birthweight. Prenatal and postnatal growth retardation have been addressed in previous studies, with the finding that differences do exist between SIDS cases and control infants.[17,34,53] The increased rate with which mothers of SIDS cases had urinary tract infections during pregnancy, as shown in this study, has also been found in previous studies.[18,54-55] However, further investigations of the neuropathology of SIDS cases will be required to establish whether neurological impairment in SIDS infants is closely associated with maternal urinary tract infection.[56-57] Finally, in this paper, illnesses in the last 2 weeks of life, especially gastrointestinal illness, and a droopy or listless appearance of the infant within the last 24 hr prior to death have been shown to be strongly associated with SIDS.

ACKNOWLEDGMENTS

A large number of individuals contributed to the success of this study. In particular, we wish to acknowledge the principal investigators and project coordinators from each of the study centers, plus other project staff and consultants: Julius Goldberg, Ph.D., and Ronald Hornung, M.S., Loyola University of Chicago; Jess Kraus, Ph.D., and Marilyn Misczynski, M.A., University of California at Davis; Donald Peterson, M.D., and Nina Chinn, R.N., University of Washington; Jean Pakter, M.D., Ehud Krongrad, M.D., and Patricia Hanson, R.N., Medical Health Research Association of New York; Dwight Janerich, D.D.S., Susan Standfast, M.D., and Diane Aliferis, M.A., New York State Health Department; Laura Hillman, M.D., Barbara Puder, R.R.A., and Sharon Hollander, M.A., Maternal and Child Health Council of St. Louis; **Data Coordinating Center:** Gerald van Belle, Ph.D. (Director), Marjorie Jones, M.A., Catherine Nanney, M.S., Mary Jane Almes, M.A., and Donald Kunz, B.S., University of Washington; **Pathology Coordinating Laboratory:** Boyd G. Stephens, M.D., and Donna J. Allison, Ph.D., San Francisco Office of the Chief Medical Examiner and Coroner; **Pathology Study Panel Members:** Marie A. Valdes-Dapena, M.D., University of Miami School of Medicine; Russell Fisher, M.D., Maryland Office of the Chief Medical Examiner and Johns Hopkins University Medical School; and James Weston, M.D., and Patricia McFeeley, M.D., New Mexico Office of the Chief Medical Examiner and University of New Mexico Medical Center; **Advisory Committee:** Henry L. Barnett, M.D. (Chairman), Albert Einstein College of Medicine and Children's Aid Society, New York City, NY; Ralph R. Franciosi, M.D., Children's Health Center Laboratory, Minneapolis, MN; William L. Harkness, Ph.D., Pennsylvania State University, University Park, PA; G. Eric Knox, M.D., Abbott Northwest Hospital, Minneapolis, MN; Richard R. Naeye, M.D., Milton S. Hershey Medical Center, Pennsylvania State University, Hersey, PA; James D. Neaton, M.S., University of Minnesota, Minneapolis, MN; and Zena Stein, M.B., New York State Psychiatric Institute, New York, NY; **Consultants:** Glen Bartlett, M.D., Ph.D., Milton S. Hershey Medical Center, Pennsylvania State University, Hershey, PA; Theodore Colton, Sc.D., Boston University School of Medicine, Boston, MA; David C. Hoaglin, Ph.D., Harvard University, Cambridge, MA; Lewis P. Lipsitt, Ph.D. Brown University, Providence, RI; William C. Orr, Ph.D., Presbyterian Hospital and University of Oklahoma Health Sciences Center, Oklahoma City, OK; Philip E. Sartwell, M.D., Harvard School of Public Health, Boston, MA; and Harold Morgenstern, Ph.D., Yale University, New Haven, CT; **NICHD Staff:** Eileen G. Hasselmeyer, Ph.D., R.N., Howard J. Hoffman, M.A., Charles R. Stark, M.D., D.P.H. (Project Officers); Jehu C. Hunter, B.S. (Study Coordinator); Harvey Shifrin, B.A. (Contracting Officer); Karla Damus, Ph.D. (Epidemiology Consultant); and Heinz W. Berendes, M.D. (Chairman, SIDS Study Review Panel).

In addition, we would like to thank all of the interviewers, public health nurses, medical records abstractors, and other staff at each of the participating centers. We are indebted as well to the many local coroners, medical examiners, and pathologists who contributed SIDS cases for this cooperative study. We also wish to thank Mr. Daniel Denman, NICHD, who contributed expert statistical and computational assistance in the preparation of the tables and Ms. Dorothy Day, NICHD, who typed the manuscript.

REFERENCES

1. STARK C.R. & P. FROGGATT. 1974. Epidemiological research. *In* Research Planning Workshops on the Sudden Infant Death Syndrome. DHEW Publication No. (NIH) 74-581. Vol. 5: 1–11. National Institutes of Health, PHS, Washington, D.C.
2. HASSELMEYER, E.G. 1988. A perspective on sudden infant death syndrome research development. *In* Sudden Infant Death Syndrome: Risk Factors and Basic Mechanisms. R.M. Harper & H.J. Hoffman, Eds.: 3–19. PMA Publishing Corporation. New York.
3. CAMERON, A.H. & P. ASHER. 1965. Cot deaths in Birmingham, 1958–61. Med. Sci. Law 5: 187–199.
4. PETERSON, D.R. 1966. Sudden unexpected deaths in infancy; an epidemiologic study. Am. J. Epidemiol. 84: 478–482.
5. STEELE, R. & J.T. LANGWORTH. 1966. The relationship of antenatal and postnatal factors to sudden unexpected death in infancy. Can. Med. Assoc. J. 94: 1165–1771.
6. STRIMER, R., L. ADELSON & R. OSEASOHN. 1969. Epidemiologic features of 1,134 sudden, unexpected infant deaths: A study in the Greater Cleveland Area from 1956–1965. J. Am. Med. Assoc. 209: 1493–1497.
7. HOUSTEK, D. 1970. Sudden infant death syndrome in Czechoslavakia: Epidemiologic aspects. *In* Sudden Infant Death Syndrome: Proceedings of the Second International Conference on Causes of Sudden Death in Infants. A.B. Bergman, J.B. Beckwith & C.G. Ray, Eds.: 55–63. University of Washington Press. Seattle.
8. KRAUS, A.S., R. STEELE, M.G. THOMPSON & P. DeGROSBOIS. 1971. Further epidemiologic observations on sudden, unexpected deaths in infancy in Ontario. Can. J. Public Health 62: 210–219.
9. FROGGATT, P., M.A. LYNAS & G. MacKENZIE. 1971. Epidemiology of sudden unexpected death in infants (cot death) in Northern Ireland. Br. J. Prev. Soc. Med. 25: 119–134.
10. KRAUS, J.F., C.E. FRANTI & N.O. BORHANI. 1972. Discriminatory risk factors in postneonatal sudden death unexplained death. Am. J. Epidemiol. 96: 328–333.
11. FEDRICK, J. 1974. Sudden unexpected death in infants in the Oxford Record Linkage Area: Details of pregnancy, delivery, and abnormality in the infant. Br. J. Prev. Soc. Med. 28: 164–171.
12. NAEYE, R.L., B. LADIS & J.S. DRAGE. 1976. Sudden infant death syndrome: A prospective study. Am. J. Dis. Child. 130: 1207–1210.
13. STANDFAST, S.J., S. JEREB & D.T. JANERICH. 1979. The epidemiology of sudden infant death in Upstate New York. J. Am. Med. Assoc. 241: 1121–1124.
14. PETERSON, D.R. 1980. Evolution of the epidemiology of sudden infant death syndrome. Epidemiol. Rev. 2: 97–112.
15. VALDES-DAPENA, M.A. 1980. Sudden infant death syndrome: A review of the medical literature 1974–1979. Pediatrics 66: 597–614.
16. STEINSCHNEIDER, A. 1972. Prolonged apnea and the sudden infant death syndrome: Clinical and laboratory observations. Pediatrics 50: 646–654.
17. PETERSON, D.R., E.A. BENSON, L.D. FISHER, N.M. CHINN & J.B. BECKWITH. 1974. Postnatal growth and the sudden infant death syndrome. Am. J. Epidemiol. 99: 389–394.
18. PROTESTOS, C.D., R.G. CARPENTER, P.M. McWEENEY & J.L. EMERY. 1973. Obstetric and perinatal histories of children who died unexpectedly (cot death). Arch. Dis. Child. 48: 835–841.
19. BIERING-SØRENSEN, E., T. JØRGENSEN & H. Jørgen. 1978. Sudden infant death in Copenhagen 1956–1971. I. Infant feeding. Acta Paediatr. Scand. 67:129–137.

20. HUTCHESON, R., JR. 1979. DTP vaccination and sudden infant deaths—Tennessee. Morbid. Mortal. Weekly Rep. **28:** 131–132.
21. BERNIER, R.H., J.A. FRANK, JR., T.J. DONDERO, JR. & P. TURNER. 1982. Diphtheria-tetanus toxoids-pertussis vaccination and sudden infant deaths in Tennessee. J. Pediatr. **101:**419–421.
22. ARNON, S.S., T.F. MIDURA, K. DAMUS, R.M. WOOD & J. CHIN. 1978. Intestinal infection and toxin production by clostridium botulinum as one cause of sudden infant death syndrome. Lancet **1:** 1273–1277.
23. PETERSON, D.R., M.W. EKLUND & N.M. CHINN. 1979. The sudden infant death syndrome and infant botulism. Rev. Infect. Dis. **1:** 630–634.
24. WEISS, N.S., D. GREEN & D.C. KRUEGER. 1973. Problems in the use of death certificates to identify sudden unexpected infant deaths. Health Serv. Rep. **88:** 555–558.
25. U.S., DEPARTMENT OF HEALTH, EDUCATION AND WELFARE. 1975. Sudden infant death syndrome. *In* Nosology Guidelines: Supplement to the Cause of Death Coding Manual. National Center for Health Statistics, Public Health Service. Rockville, MD.
26. JONES, A.M. & J.T. WESTON. 1976. The examination of the sudden infant death syndrome infant: Investigative and autopsy protocols. J. Forensic Sci. **21:** 833–841.
27. FLEISS, J.L. 1981. Statistical Methods for Rates and Proportions, 2nd ed. John Wiley & Sons. New York.
28. LILIENFELD, A.M. & D.E. LILIENFELD. 1980. Foundations of Epidemiology, 2nd ed. Oxford University Press. New York.
29. HOFFMAN, H.J., D.W. DENMAN, K. DAMUS & G. VAN BELLE. 1988. Comparison of matched versus unmatched analysis in a case-control study of SIDS risk factors. *In* American Statistical Association 1987 Proceedings of the Section on Social Statistics: 318–323.
30. HOFFMAN, H.J., J.C. HUNTER, K. DAMUS, J. PAKTER, D.R. PETERSON, G. VAN BELLE & E.G. HASSELMEYER. 1987. Diphtheria-tetanus-pertussis immunization and sudden infant death: Results of the National Institute of Child Health and Human Development cooperative epidemiological study of sudden infant death syndrome risk factors. Pediatrics **79:** 598–611.
31. HOFFMAN, H.J., J.C. HUNTER, N.J. ELLISH, D.T. JANERICH & J. GOLDBERG. 1988. Adverse reproductive factors and the sudden infant death syndrome. *In* Sudden Infant Death Syndrome: Risk Factors and Basic Mechanisms. R.M. Harper & H.J. Hoffman, Eds.: 153–175. PMA Publishing Corporation. New York.
32. VALDES-DAPENA, M. 1988. The morphology of the sudden infant death syndrome—An update, 1984. *In* Sudden Infant Death Syndrome: Risk Factors and Basic Mechanisms. R.M. Harper & H.J. Hoffman, Eds.: 143–150. PMA Publishing Corporation. New York.
33. MILLER, H.C. & T.A. MERRITT. 1979. Fetal Growth in Humans. Year Book Medical Publishers, Inc. Chicago.
34. VAN BELLE, G., H.J. Hoffman & D.R. PETERSON. 1988. Intrauterine growth retardation and the sudden infant death syndrome. *In* Sudden Infant Death Syndrome: Risk Factors and Basic Mechanisms. R.M. Harper & H.J. Hoffman, Eds.: 203–219. PMA Publishing Corporation. New York.
35. PETERSON, D.R., G. VAN BELLE & N.M. CHINN. 1979. Epidemiologic comparisons of the sudden infant death syndrome with other major components of infant mortality. Am. J. Epidemiol. **110:** 699–707.
36. FROGGATT, P., M.A. LYNAS & T.K. MARSHALL. 1971. Sudden unexpected death in infants (cot death) report of a collaborative study in Northern Ireland. Ulster Med. J. **40:** 116–135.
37. LEWAK, N., B.J. VAN DEN BERG & J.B. BECKWITH. 1979. Sudden infant death syndrome risk factors. Prospective data review. Clin. Pediatr. **18:** 404–411.
38. FEDRICK, J. 1973. Sudden unexpected death in infants in the Oxford Record Linkage Area. An analysis with respect to time and place. Br. J. Prev. Soc. Med. **27:** 217–224.
39. BEAL, S.M. 1978. Seasonal variation in sudden infant death syndrome. Lancet **1:** 1257.
40. NEWMAN, N.M. 1988. The epidemiology of the sudden infant death syndrome in Australia, with particular reference to Tasmania, 1975–1981. *In* Sudden Infant Death Syndrome: Risk Factors and Basic Mechanisms. R.M. Harper & H.J. Hoffman, Eds.: 53–71. PMA Publishing Corporation. New York.
41. PETERSON, D.R., E.E. SABATTA & D. STRICKLAND. 1988. Sudden infant death syndrome in epidemiologic perspective: Etiologic implications of variation with season of the year. Ann. N.Y. Acad. Sci. This volume.

42. STANTON, A.N., M.A.P.S. DOWNHAM, J.R. OAKLEY, J.L. EMERY & J. KNOWELDEN. 1978. Terminal symptoms in children dying suddenly and unexpectedly at home. Preliminary report of the DHSS multicentre study of postneonatal mortality. Br. Med. J. **2:** 1249–1251.
43. DAMUS, K., J. PAKTER, E. KRONGRAD, S.J. STANDFAST & H.J. HOFFMAN. 1988. Postnatal medical and epidemiological risk factors for the sudden infant death syndrome. *In* Sudden Infant Death Syndrome: Risk Factors and Basic Mechanisms. R.M. Harper & H.J. Hoffman, Eds.: 187–201. PMA Publishing Corporation. New York.
44. EATON-EVANS, J. & A.E. DUGDALE. 1987. Effects of feeding and social factors on diarrhea and vomiting in infants. Arch. Dis. Child. **62:** 445–448.
45. CUNNINGHAM, A.S. 1979. Morbidity in breast-fed and artificially fed infants, II. J. Pediatr. **95:** 685–689.
46. HOLMES, G.E., K.M. HASSANEIN & H.C. MILLER. 1983. Factors associated with infections among breastfed and babies fed proprietary milks. Pediatrics **72:** 300–306.
47. McGAFFEY, H.L. 1968. Acidosis may be clue to crib death. J. Am. Med. Assoc. **206:** 1440.
48. BLUMENFELD, T.A., C.H. MANTELL, R.L. CATHERMAN & W.A. BLANC. 1979. Postmortem vitreous humor chemistry in sudden infant death syndrome and in other causes of death in childhood. Am. J. Clin. Pathol. **71:** 219–223.
49. HOFFMAN, H.J., K. DAMUS, E. KRONGRAD & L. HILLMAN. 1987. Apnea, birth weight, and SIDS: Results of the NICHD cooperative epidemiological study of sudden infant death syndrome (SIDS) risk factors. *In* Infantile Apnea and Home Monitoring (Report of the National Institutes of Health Consensus Development Conference, September 29–October 1, 1986). NIH Publication No. 87–2905. Appendix B: 53–59. Department of Health and Human Services. Bethesda, MD.
50. SPITZER, A.R. & W.W. FOX. 1986. Infant apnea. Pediatr. Clin. North Am. **33:** 561–587.
51. STEINSCHNEIDER, A. 1977. Nasopharyngitis and the sudden infant death syndrome. Pediatrics **60:** 531–533.
52. KRONGRAD, E. & L. O'NEILL. 1986. Near miss sudden infant death episodes? A clinical and electrocardiographic correlation. Pediatrics **77:** 811–815.
53. NORVENIUS, S.G. 1987. Sudden infant death syndrome in Sweden in 1973–1977 and 1979. Acta Paediatr. Scand. Suppl. **333:** 1–138.
54. CARPENTER, R.G., A. GARDNER & P.M. McWEENY. 1977. Multistage scoring system for identifying infants at risk of unexpected deaths. Arch. Dis. Child. **52:** 606–612.
55. GOLDING, J., S. LIMERICK & A. MACFARLANE. 1985. Sudden Infant Death. Patterns, Puzzles and Problems. University of Washington Press. Seattle.
56. TAKASHIMA, S., D. ARMSTRONG, L.E. BECKER & J. HUBER. 1978. Cerebral white matter lesions in sudden infant death syndrome. Pediatrics **62:** 155–159.
57. LEVITAN, A. & F.H. GILLES. 1984. Acquired perinatal leukoencephalopathy. Ann. Neurol. **16:** 1–8.

A Pathologist's Perspective on Possible Mechanisms in SIDS

MARIE VALDES-DAPENA

Department of Pathology
School of Medicine
University of Miami
Miami, Florida 33101

INTRODUCTION

The first scientists in the United States to conduct systematic investigations of the sudden infant death syndrome (then known as crib death) were Drs. Werne and Garrow, pathologists at the Office of the Chief Medical Examiner in the Borough of Queens in New York City. Their first joint work on that subject was published exactly 40 years ago.[1,2] They stressed the presence of modest inflammation of the upper respiratory tract as having something to do with causation. Those of us who were young and inexperienced at the time were intrigued by their descriptions. What they were suggesting seemed incredible, i.e. the fact that seemingly healthy babies died on account of little more than minimal to moderate inflammation of the upper airway. To this day, I clearly recall reading the first of those articles in absolute disbelief that any such thing could happen. (I was working at the time in an academic institution and had never encountered a crib death.) Soon thereafter, however, I became an employee of the Office of the Medical Examiner of the City of Philadelphia; I saw what they had seen and I certainly had no better explanation to offer.

Like a certain popular American cigarette, scientists in general, and anatomic pathologists in particular, have come a long way in the intervening four decades. We all know much more about these babies than we used to. The details of ultimate mechanism of their deaths still elude us, but we have learned a great deal about who they are and where they come from. And much of that knowledge we owe to pathologists.

Probably the most important lesson we have learned in those forty years is the fact that there are even more subtle micropscopic changes in the tissues of these infants than Werne and Garrow had ever suspected. So subtle are they that the investigator is obliged to explore them by means of tedious microscopic measurements or morphometry and not in just a few cases but rather large numbers of both cases and controls in order to appreciate their very presence. It is that sort of endeavor, the stretching of ourselves, that has led to a new understanding of the morphology and possible mechanisms of the sudden infant death syndrome.

THE SO-CALLED TISSUE MARKERS OF CHRONIC HYPOXEMIA

It was Dr. Richard Naeye who first conceived of the notion of using microscopic morphometry to study these infant tissues. He entered into that project in the early 1970s to explore Dr. Alfred Steinschneider's hypothesis that idiopathic central apnea was responsible for many, or most, crib deaths. He reasoned that if these infants had been repetitively, episodically not breathing for prolonged periods of time, the resultant chronic oxygen deficiency ought to be perceptible microscopically in certain of their tissues. Thus, he examined seven critical potential anatomic sites for those alterations. In the end he had identified seven morphologic "markers" to support the apnea hypothesis: (1) abnormal thickening of smooth muscle in the walls of small pulmonary arteries; (2) hypertrophy of the free wall of the right ventricle; (3) abnormal relative retention of periadrenal brown fat; (4) increased hepatic erythropoiesis; (5) increased chromaffin tissue in the adrenal medulla; (6) gliosis in the brain stem in areas crucial to respiratory control; and (7) either hypo- or hyperplasia of glomic tissue in the carotid body.[3]

Dr. Naeye's final publication in that series appeared in 1976.[4] In the succeeding decade, numerous investigations have been undertaken in attempts to either confirm or refute his findings; the results have been variable. At the present time it would seem that three of them are holding up under scrutiny, namely the undue retention of periadrenal brown fat, the abnormal hepatic erythropoiesis, and, most importantly, the gliosis of the brain stem.[5] Still, the significance of these tissue changes is not at all clear. He assumed that they represented reflections of chronic hypoxia (markers 1 and 2) and hypoxemia (markers 3 through 7) secondary to repetitive episodes of central apnea, but, of course, that need not be so. If hypoxemia is involved in the mechanism, and it may well be, then it could as easily derive from anemia as from episodic apnea.

Of the three "markers" that have been confirmed, probably the most critical is the brain stem gliosis,[4] because the brain stem houses the control centers for a number of essential physiological functions, especially breathing, swallowing, and the beat of the heart. Naeye interpreted that lesion as probably causing central apnea and confined his exploration of the lesion to those centers crucial to respiratory control. Two major subsequent studies [6,7] did the same. The fact is, first of all, that the entire brain stem has not been assessed in this regard (there may be gliosis in other vital centers), and, secondly, the observed gliosis may be either the cause of some physiologic problem and/or the effect. Thus the observation gives rise to more questions than answers. However, all interested groups are gratified that work in this important area continues in the laboratory of Dr. Hannah Kinney of Boston Children's Hospital. She is using computer-generated, three-dimensional image analysis to reconstruct brain stems from both normal control infants and crib-death victims to establish, first of all, normal values for the various centers at various ages, and secondly, the extent of pathologic change in each. Her study, which is supported now by the National Institute of Child Health and Human Development, will continue for at least the next three years. We anticipate that, as a result of that work, we will ultimately know how much gliosis there really is and exactly where it is located, i.e. which brain stem centers are affected.

FETAL HEMOGLOBIN AND SIDS

In regard to the issue of hypoxemia and its possible relationship to the sudden infant death syndrome, a recent publication on the role of fetal hemoglobin in crib death deserves consideration.[8] Hemoglobin F (or fetal hemoglobin) is the predominant form in the erythrocytes of unborn babies; it carries more oxygen than does adult hemoglobin. The red cells of an infant born at term bear about 70% fetal hemoglobin. That relative value diminishes steadily thereafter so that at six months of age the normal infant has only a trace.

According to the recent study of Dr. Enid Gilbert's group in Madison, Wisconsin, 54 of 59 crib death victims had abnormal retention of hemoglobin F. (The five exceptions were all infants less than 46 weeks post-conceptual age, which is to say, less than six weeks post-natal age.) Interestingly, *none* of the 40 control infants (32 living and eight dead) had levels above the normal range. (Also worthy of note is the fact that virtually all of the control infants had levels above the mean.) The discrepancy between average levels for the two groups, cases versus controls, increased steadily with age; among those more than 50 weeks of post-conceptual age (37 cases and 19 controls) the difference was striking: 47.4 ± 3.6% versus 18.8 ± 3.1% ($p < 0.0005$).

Parenthetically, the manner in which these two curves move away from each other, progressively, during the first six months of post-natal life reminds one of two similar phenomena: one, the retention of periadrenal brown fat, which is ever more striking as the victim becomes older[9]; and two, the steadily increasing lag in growth parameters described by Naeye,[10] i.e. measurements for body weight, body length, and head circumference. His data showed all of those determinations to be in the 40th percentile (not the 50th or average) at birth, dropping steadily to the 20th percentile at 4 months (if the baby lived that long).

Dr. Gilbert and her co-workers believe that hemoglobin F will serve as a useful postmortem marker for crib death. (If that is so it will be the first time that pathologists have been able to make that diagnosis in a positive manner; heretofore, it has been a "diagnosis by exclusion," that is, simply an expression of the inability of the pathologist to identify an adequate explanation for the child's death.)

More importantly, they also suggest that abnormally high levels of hemoglobin F will single out the real "infant at risk" for crib death; that would make it the "wonder test" that everyone has been searching for, for at least the last decade. However, as in any such discovery, this work requires confirmation by other workers in other laboratories before it can be used in a practical way in either living patients or those who have died. The authors themselves note that, in an earlier investigation of this matter,[11] there appeared to be no difference between cases and controls in regard to relative levels of hemoglobin F. Dr. Gilbert suggests that the apparent discrepancy may be attributed to differences in the methods employed. In any case, this observation now requires confirmation by other workers. One hopes that the project will be addressed in the near future.

DYSPLASTIC, DYSMORPHIC, AND ANOMALOUS LESIONS

In recent years, the subject of dysplastic, dysmorphic, and anomalous lesions in crib death victims has attracted the attention of two independent groups of pediatric pathologists. Dr. Gordon Vawter and his colleagues at Boston Children's Hospital were the first to explore the matter.[12] They conducted a retrospective review of the autopsies involving 100 infants, six to 32 weeks of age, who had died unexpectedly at home. Fifty-seven of the deaths were unexplained; the other 43 were attributed to infection (21), trauma (10), and aspiration (12). Dysplastic lesions (nevi, hemangiomas, nodular renal blastema, and neuroblastoma) were present in 8 (14%) of the unexplained deaths and only 1 (2.3%) of the controls.

That same work was repeated shortly thereafter by a pair of Swiss investigators.[13] Using 130 of their own crib death autopsies and 133 controls cases (necropsies on infants who had died of recognized causes), Molz and Hartmann also found differences in the incidence of dysplastic lesions in the two groups, 10% among the SIDS victims and only 5% among controls.

Furthermore, this second and larger study showed striking contrasts between the two groups in regard to the comparative incidence of both dysmorphic lesions and anomalies. The dysmorphic lesions included hernias, club foot, and pectus excavatum. Nineteen percent of the crib death babies had dysmorphic lesions as contrasted with only nine percent of controls. The authors were interested in the incidence of minor anomalies such as Meckel's diverticulum, polydactyly, ectopic adrenal and pancreatic tissue, and minor cardiac defects such as atrial septal defects and small membranous ventricular septal defects. Thirty-four percent of the study group had such lesions as compared to only nineteen percent of the control group.

The above findings suggest that, as a group, infants who die of the sudden infant death syndrome probably have difficulties that precede not only their sudden deaths but their births as well. All of these lesions, i.e. dysmorphic, dysplastic, and anomalous, have their origins in intrauterine life. Their increased incidence in SIDS victims would seem to indicate that these infants have experienced some kind of subtle adverse intrauterine influence(s). It causes one to reflect on the possibility that similar subtle changes elsewhere in the body, such as, for example, the brain stem, might be associated with significant and perhaps hazardous functional alterations.

CYTOMEGALOVIRUS INFECTION AND SIDS

One other morphologic study of interest was presented this past year by Dr. Dale Huff of The Children's Hospital of Philadelphia.[14] Dr. Huff reviewed the microscopic sections from 401 consecutive autopsies (1980–1986) on infants two weeks to two years of age. Fifty-eight of them (14.5%) were crib deaths. He found cytomegalovirus (CMV) inclusions in 3% of the total group, 1.2% of those who had died of recognized causes and 12% of the SIDS victims. The difference is statistically significant ($p < 0.001$).

Furthermore, of the 11 infants in the total group who had evidence of CMV infection, 64% were crib death babies—even though their total number was only 17% of the number of infants in the non-SIDS group. The tissues containing the inclusions were those in which they are most often found in other cases, i.e. salivary gland, lung, kidney, liver, pancreas, epididymis, and adrenal. The author proffers no real explanation for this remarkable finding but suggests that some as yet "unrecognized factor may predispose infants to both CMV infection and sudden death."

THE NICHD MULTICENTER EPIDEMIOLOGIC STUDY

The National Institute of Child Health and Human Development designed and ultimately managed the largest scientific investigation of the epidemiology of the sudden infant death syndrome that ever has been or probably ever will be conducted. The original intent was to explore systematically the epidemiologic characteristics of 1,000 consecutive crib deaths, in each case immediately after autopsy. In every instance, the case was to be verified by a Special Pathology Panel who would review the pertinent historical information, the autopsy protocol, and 30–35 microscopic slides.

The cases were gathered during an 18-month period in six designated centers scattered about various parts of the country. All cases were routinely analyzed in their original offices but a specified set of formalin-fixed tissue samples were then sent to the Project's special histology laboratory in San Francisco where a complete set of microscopic slides was made for the panel. Those slide sets were shipped sequentially to the first, second, and then the third member of the panel. They were examined blindly and independently by each member and then sent back to the San Francisco laboratory. These examinations were done without any knowledge of the nature of the case. Although all cases actually submitted from the field were presumably examples of crib death, understandably, some of them turned out not to be. In addition, the biostatisticians in the planning group arranged for certain controls to be included, i.e. sets of slides from known cases of, for example, meningitis and pneumonia, for the purpose of checking on the performance of the panel members.

Reading those slides, approximately 30,000 of them, took the panel five years. At the end of that effort, they were treated to the real privilege of going through a second review, that time with all of the background information about the case, i.e. the history, reports of ancillary procedures, and the autopsy protocol together with his/her own diagnoses for the microscopic sections. (Because the slides had been read without any of that information, it was fascinating to go back over our interpretations.) The second review took approximately one year.

In 1984, the members of the panel were brought together by the Institute in a series of sessions to discuss and, if possible, resolve their differences. Ultimately not all differences were resolved. Cases were designated as being (1) unexplained, (2) probably unexplained, (3) unclear (when the panel either could not agree upon or could not be certain as to the definitive designation), or (4) explained. The "unclear" cases were set aside and not used for any of the final epidemiologic or morphologic determinations.

As might be expected, the number of cases in the final report is far short of 1,000. In some instances, pieces of the case, such as the autopsy protocol, were lost. In other instances the designation was "unclear," etc. In the end, the data for the epidemiologic study were based upon 757 certified crib deaths.

As morphologists, the panel has access presently to information about their own data on only the first 400 cases that entered the study as presumed typical examples of the sudden infant death syndrome. Because some of those cases were incomplete, it turns out that we can work now with a total of only 385. The following data are extracted from that set.

Two questions come to mind with regard to those data: (1) How often did the pathologist in the field, in the opinion of the panel, make a mistake with regard to case designation? and (2) Are there any microscopic features that seem to distinguish the SIDS from the non-SIDS cases?

Of the 385 cases for which we have statistics, the panel concurred in 300 or 78%.[15] In most of the remaining 22%, the panel could not agree upon or could not be certain as to a definitive designation for the type of death. In only six instances (1.6%) did the panel "turn the case around," so to speak, and sign it out differently. Those six final designations were: purulent meningitis, viral myocarditis, tuberous sclerosis, upper airway inflammation, starvation with dehydration and pneumonia, and dehydration with probable fluid and electrolyte imbalance. Three specific pathologic lesions were explored in search of distinctive microscopic characteristics of crib deaths, namely, pulmonary congestion, pulmonary edema, and thymic petechiae.

Pulmonary congestion, which has always been considered one of the characteristic features of the crib death autopsy, was noted in 99% of the SIDS victims but interestingly, in 100% of the six controls or "explained" deaths. Thus, there is no difference between the two groups and this feature turns out not to be a discriminator.

Similarly, pulmonary edema has long been recognized as a characteristic component of the sudden infant death necropsy. But the results of our work in this regard are the same as those with pulmonary congestion. Marked pulmonary edema was apparent microscopically in 75% of the crib deaths and 83% of controls. There is no significant difference between the two groups.

Thymic petechiae, on the other hand, are different. In data compiled from the combination of gross autopsy protocol and the interpretation of the microscopic slides, they were observed in 52% of the crib deaths and in none of the six explained deaths. Exciting as this difference seems, it must obviously be studied in the entire body of morpholgic material, i.e. all 757 cases. Those calculations are not yet available to us.

CONCLUSIONS

Despite everyone's expectations to the contrary, pathologists have made substantial contributions in the last ten years to the evolution of our understanding of this phenomenon. To summarize that which they have demonstrated one might make the following three statements: (1) There are differences between crib death infants and those who are not. (2) The differences probably have their origins in intrauterine life. (3) The differences may either participate in the ultimate mechanism of death or reflect other functional and/or structural differences which do so.

REFERENCES

1. WERNE, J. & I. GARROW. 1953. Sudden apparently unexplained death during infancy: I Pathologic findings in infants found dead. Am. J. Pathol. **29:** 633–675.
2. WERNE, J. & I. GARROW. 1953. Sudden apparently unexplained death during infancy: II Pathologic findings in infants observed to die suddenly. Am. J. Pathol. **29:** 817–827.
3. NAEYE, R.L. 1980. Sudden infant death. Sci. Am. **242:** 52–58.
4. NAEYE, R.L. 1976. Brain stem and adrenal abnormalities in the sudden infant death syndrome. Am. J. Clin. Pathol. **66:** 526–530.
5. VALDES-DAPENA, M.A. 1986. Sudden infant death syndrome. Morphology up-date for forensic pathologists—1985. Forens. Sci. Int. **30:** 177–186.
6. TAKASHIMA, S., D. ARMSTRONG, L. BECKER & C. BRYAN. 1978. Cerebral hypoperfusion in the sudden infant death syndrome? Brain stem gliosis and vasculature. Ann. Neurol. **4:** 257–262.
7. KINNEY, H.C., P.C. BURGER, I.E. HARRELL & R.P. HUDSON, JR. 1983. "Reactive gliosis" in the medulla oblongata of victims of the sudden infant death syndrome. Pediatrics **72:** 181–187.
8. GIULIAN, G.B., E. F. GILBERT & R.L. MOSS. 1987. Elevated fetal hemoglobin levels in sudden infant death syndrome. N. Engl. J. Med. **316**(18) 1122–1126.
9. VALDES-DAPENA, M., M.M. GILLANE & R. CATHERMAN. 1976. Brown fat retention in sudden infant death syndrome. Arch. Pathol. Lab. Med. **100:** 547–549.
10. NAEYE, R.L., B. LADIS & J.S. DRAGE. 1976. Sudden infant death syndrome: A prospective study. Am. J. Dis. Child. **130:** 1207–1220.
11. ZIELKE, R. & B.L. KRAUSE. 1982. Activity of 5 enzymes and fetal hemoglobin in RBC of infants dying from the sudden infant death syndrome. Fed. Proc. **41:** 1148 (abstract).
12. VAWTER, G.F. & H. KOSAKEWICH. 1983. Aspects of morphologic variation amongst SIDS victims. *In* Sudden Infant Death Syndrome. J.T. Tildon, L.M. Roeder & A. Steinschneider, Eds.: 133–144. Academic Press. New York.
13. MOLZ, G. & H. HARTMANN. 1984. Dysmorphism, dysplasia, and anomaly in sudden infant death (letter). N. Engl. J. Med. **311:** 259.
14. HUFF, D.S. 1986. Cytomegalovirus inclusions in 401 consecutive autopsies on infants aged 2 weeks to 2 years: A high incidence in patients with sudden infant death syndrome. Presented at the Interim Mtg. of the Soc. for Pediatr. Pathol. Dallas, TX. Oct. 17–19, 1986.
15. VALDES-DAPENA, M. 1988. The morphology of the sudden infant death syndrome: An update—1984. *In* Proc. 1984 International Symposium on the Sudden Infant Death Syndrome. Santa Monica, CA. Feb. 22–24, 1984. Pergamon Press. (In press)

Intrathoracic Petechial Hemorrhages: A Clue to the Mechanism of Death in Sudden Infant Death Syndrome?

J. BRUCE BECKWITH[a]

Department of Pathology
The Children's Hospital
Denver, Colorado 80218

Postmortem studies have revealed a repetitive spectrum of minor changes that lend substantial support to the view that SIDS is a clinico-pathological entity.[1-9] Among the most consistent of these findings are intrathoracic petechial hemorrhages (FIGURE 1). These distinctive lesions have been the subject of lively controversy among forensic pathologists for many years. They have been viewed by some as suggesting terminal respiratory obstruction,[1,4] but there has been considerable reluctance to accept this concept. In this paper, human and animal studies bearing on the question of petechiae as clues to the mechanism of death in SIDS will be reviewed.

INCIDENCE OF PETECHIAE IN SIDS

Perhaps the first writer to emphasize intrathoracic petechiae in sudden infant deaths was Fearn,[10] who in 1834 described two infants who had been found dead in bed without signs of antecedent illness, and in whom the only abnormality found during necropsy was the presence of numerous "spots of extravasated blood" over the surfaces of the thymus, lungs, and heart. While the first of these babies shared a bed with an adult, in the second case there seemed no possibility of external suffocation. Fearn ended his report with the plea that someone enlighten him as to the cause of these blood spots, as that might explain how these babes died so suddenly and inexplicably.

Many case reports in the 19th century mentioned that intrathoracic petechiae were prominent in infants found dead. Templeman's report,[2] for example, summarized the findings in 258 infant deaths in Dundee, Scotland, between 1882–1891, concluding that these were due to "overlaying," usually by a drunken parent sharing the bed with the infant. He supported his diagnosis of mechanical asphyxia by the regularity with which petechiae were found on the organs of the chest cavity.

Werne and Garrow,[3] in their pioneering step toward the establishment of SIDS as a medical entity, observed intrathoracic petechiae as one of the distinctive features of infants unexpectedly found dead after presumed sleep. They found them in 80% of such cases, while similar petechiae were rarely seen in infants dying of suffocation, carbon monoxide asphyxia, burns, or drowning.

---

[a]Address correspondence to: Department of Pathology, The Children's Hospital, 1056 East 19th Ave., Denver CO 80218.

Handforth's 1959 paper,[4] published long before SIDS was established as an entity, deserves special recognition. He reported a series of 12 babies under the age of six months, with a mean age of 9 weeks, who had been put to bed and found lifeless after intervals as short as 15 minutes. Intrathoracic petechiae were found in every case. Handforth was impressed with the petechiae as the most distinctive feature of the necropsy and proceeded to test the hypothesis that they denoted airway obstruction. He reproduced the petechiae in 20 rats by obstructing a tracheal cannula, monitoring the results with intraesophageal pressure readings. He concluded that airway obstruction was the likely mechanism of SIDS, proposing laryngospasm as a possible mechanism for this obstruc-

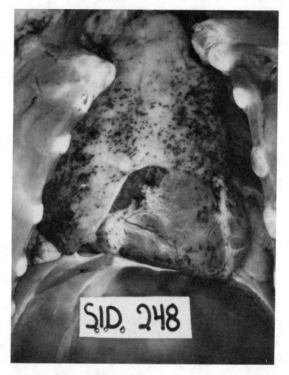

FIGURE 1. Intrathoracic petechiae in SIDS, showing numerous hemorrhages on surfaces of thymus and heart.

tion. Handforth's paper deserves recognition as one of the first to clearly delineate the features of SIDS, as well as being perhaps the first to report laboratory investigations into the mechanism of death in these cases, based upon his observations of intrathoracic petechiae.

While most authors have been content merely to mention that intrathoracic petechiae are unusually prominent in SIDS victims, a few have documented their frequency. TABLE I summarizes several such series.[3,4,11–15]

While the data in TABLE 1 refer only to the presence of petechiae, it is their *number and density* in many victims that is most impressive. In our study,[14] the petechial density

TABLE 1. Incidence of Petechiae in SIDS and Controls

Author reference	SIDS Cases	Petechiae	Non-SIDS Cases
Werne & Garrow[3]	31	25 (80%)	Absent or sparse in infant suffocation, CO asphyxia, drowning
Handforth[4]	12	12 (100%)	None
Jacobsen & Voight[11]	97	92 (95%)	Rare in infanticide, accidents
Geertinger[12]	80	63 (79%)	6 of 43 (14%)
Marshall[13]	162	114 (68%)	12 of 42 (29%)
Beckwith[14]	109	95 (87%)	16 of 38 (42%)
Krous[15]	100	85 (85%)	None
Total	591	486 (82%)	

was scored on the surfaces of the thymus, epicardium, and lungs. The thymus was the site of highest density. In 60 of 109 cases (55%), there were regions on the thymus with greater than 5 petechiae per square centimeter (TABLE 2).

DISTRIBUTION OF PETECHIAE IN SIDS

The distribution of petechiae may reveal important clues to their pathogenesis. When they are generalized, one looks for a systemic abnormality of vascular integrity or coagulation mechanisms. When they are localized, one looks for mechanisms to explain their localization. In the case of intrathoracic petechiae, then, it is incumbent upon us to account for the fact that petechiae are usually present on the surfaces of the thoracic cavity, yet occur rarely in other sites.

One of the most striking illustrations of the topographic distribution of these petechiae is their tendency to spare the dorsum of the cervical lobe of the thymus[14] (FIGURE 2). Of the three major organs in the chest, the heart and lungs are entirely intrathoracic, whereas the thymus usually extends a variable distance into the neck. The dorsal aspect of the cervical lobe is of particular interest, because a large venous trunk, the left brachioce-phalic vein, usually crosses the thymus on its dorsal aspect, at the thoracic inlet. This vessel is intimately related to the thymic capsule. In this position, it might serve to absorb negative pressure forces transmitted upward from the thorax. Such a "damping" factor could be expected to reduce the local effects of negative pressure at and above the level of the left brachiocephalic vein. This is in fact exactly what is seen in a majority of SIDS thymuses (TABLE 3).

Some petechiae are often seen on the ventral aspect of the cervical lobe, though usually they are less prominent than in the thoracic portion (FIGURE 1). Some transmission of negative pressure into this region would not be surprising in view of the familiar occurrence of suprasternal retractions in patients with obstructed inspiration. On the

TABLE 2. Petechial Density in SIDS versus Controls ($N = 109$)

Petechiae/cm^2	SIDS Cases	Controls
0	14 (13%)	22 (58%)
< 1	15 (14%)	2 (5%)
1–5	20 (18%)	11 (29%)
> 5	60 (55%)	3 (8%)

After Beckwith.[14]

ventral surface of the thymus, there is no anatomical barrier to pressure transmission such as exists on the dorsum.

The intrathoracic petechiae in SIDS are not restricted to the thymus, heart, and lungs. They may also occur on the parietal surfaces of the pleura and pericardium. For example, in 18% of 109 cases, we found them on the diaphragmatic pleura, but in none were they present on the abdominal surface of the diaphragm or elsewhere on the peritoneum.[14] Control cases, dying with meningococcemia or other septicemic conditions, regularly showed peritoneal petechiae.

Krous and Jordon[16] emphasized another interesting aspect of the distribution of petechiae in SIDS. They found that the epicardial and thymic, but not the pulmonary ones, tend to be most prominent on the surfaces of the involved organs. They suggested that this distribution was consistent with direct effects of negative pressure on the surfaces of heart and thymus, and indirect effects of negative pressure, via left ventricular afterloading, in the lungs.

We have observed another detail concerning the distribution of petechiae in SIDS, suggesting that pleural-pulmonary hemorrhages might differ pathogenetically from thymic-epicardial hemorrhages.[14] This is the fact that pleural petechiae in SIDS are often more prominent in areas of postmortem-dependent lividity, while those on the thymus and epicardium show no apparent effect of postmortem gravitational factors. The effect of postmortem position is especially notable for the larger, 1–5 mm "blotchy" hemorrhages, rather than the smaller, splinter-shaped hemorrhages seen on close inspection of the involved surfaces.

Cardiac arrest or failure cannot account for the distinctive distribution of petechiae in

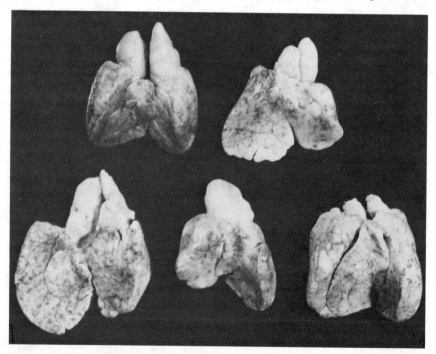

FIGURE 2. Dorsal view of thymus glands from five SIDS victims. Numerous petechiae on thoracic portion, with sparing of cervical portion.

TABLE 3. Relative Sparing of Cervical Lobe of Thymus in SIDS ($N = 109$)

Petechiae/cm^2	Cervical[a]	Thoracic
0	71 (65%)	14 (13%)
< 1	16 (15%)	15 (14%)
1–5	12 (11%)	20 (18%)
> 5	10 (9%)	60 (55%)

After Beckwith.[14]
[a]Cervical lobe = dorsal aspect of thymus, above lower border of left brachiocephalic vein.

SIDS, since the pattern does not fit any recognized segment of the vascular system. The suggestion that they are the result of increased intrathoracic negative pressure is consistent with this distribution. This thesis will be examined below.

INTRATHORACIC PETECHIAE IN NON-SIDS INFANT DEATHS

It is noteworthy that those series in which the incidence of petechiae in SIDS was compared to controls have consistently shown them in a much higher proportion of SIDS cases (TABLES 1 and 2). Our study[14] reported the highest incidence in controls (42% in thymus, 34% in pleura, and 40% in epicardium). However, our control population, composed both of "explained" and "possibly explained" cases, included a number of deaths from septicemia with *generalized* petechiae. The "possibly explained" group included a number of possible SIDS deaths that were excluded from the SIDS category because interpretation was debatable. In that study the numbers of petechiae were considerably lower in controls than in the SIDS group. TABLE 2, for example, compares the relative petechial density on the thymus in the two categories.

Intrathoracic petechiae are commonly seen in perinatal postmortem examinations. Not uncommonly, they are associated with cutaneous, visceral, and generalized petechiae. However, they may be conspicuously localized to the chest organs, notably in infants dying after abruptio placentae.[16] Perinatal deaths are usually complicated by complex, prolonged metabolic derangements including prolonged hypoxemia, acidosis, etc., which reduces their value in terms of unraveling agonal pathophysiology. For example, placental abruption is usually associated with hypofibrinogenemia and impaired oxygenation to the fetus. In this setting, the threshold for vascular rupture leading to petechiae may be lowered significantly, so that gasping *in utero,* for example, might generate forces sufficient to cause hemorrhage.

Of particular relevance to the thesis that respiratory obstruction might account for the petechiae of SIDS is the occurrence of petechiae in infants dying after documented airway obstruction.

Krous and Jordan[17] studied the distribution of petechiae in 50 cases dying of defined causes, including 33 under one year of age. Thirteen (26%) had petechiae limited to supradiaphragmatic structures. Nine of these were known to have upper airway obstruction. Thirty-seven (74%) had petechiae above and below the diaphragm. Only two were known to have had terminal upper airway obstruction, and each had a single adrenal petechia as the only infradiaphragmatic site. These authors concluded that petechiae limited to supradiaphragmatic surfaces were characteristic of upper airway obstruction.

The results from infants dying of accidental or intentional mechanical obstruction of the airway are conflicting. Many standard textbooks of forensic pathology describe intrathoracic and facial petechiae as being usual in deaths due to airway obstruction, but do not provide supporting data. Several authors have commented that the petechiae in suffocation are less commonly seen and much less numerous than in SIDS victims. Werne and Garrow[3] noted that intrathoracic petechiae were absent or sparse in infants dying of suffocation, carbon monoxide asphyxia, and drowning. Marshall[18] provided semiquantitative data from five cases of suffocation in plastic bags and six of aspirated foreign objects, and noted that petechiae were less numerous than in his cases of SIDS. We noted a possible explanation for this discrepancy during experiments with adult primates,[19] in which showers of petechiae were produced in one animal when the trachea was occluded *at the end of expiration,* whereas occlusion at partial or complete inspiration in two animals produced no petechiae.

HISTORICAL PERSPECTIVE:
PETECHIAE IN HUMAN FORENSIC PATHOLOGY

The 19th century French forensic pathologist, Ambroise Tardieu,[20,21] forcefully propounded the view that intrathoracic petechiae were characteristic of mechanical asphyxiation. He was careful to distinguish cases with generalized petechiae, which suggested systemic abnormalities such as toxemias and poisonings, from those with localized petechiae. When petechiae were limited in distribution to the thoracic cavity, and/or to the skin of the head and neck, Tardieu proposed they were diagnostic of mechanical asphyxiation. Since that time, these petechiae have often been referred to as "Tardieu's spots."

Paul Brouardel, who followed Tardieu as the doyen of French forensic scientists, published a monumental treatise on death by mechanical asphyxia in 1897,[22] which distilled the results of his extensive forensic experience and laboratory investigation into this subject. Some of his animal studies will be mentioned later. Brouardel took issue with some of Tardieu's conclusions concerning the significance of pleural and epicardial petechiae: (1) Intrathoracic petechiae occur in several types of violent deaths, including suffocation and hanging. However, in most cases of hanging, most strangulations, and many cases of unequivocal infant suffocation, they are absent. (2) They are produced experimentally in some species more readily than in others. For example, they are easily produced by suffocation of rabbits, but are more difficult to obtain in dogs. (3) In the suffocated human, they occur more often in the neonate than in older persons. (4) They can occur in certain clinical conditions, notably epileptic seizures, diphtheria, respiratory infections, and certain poisonings. (5) The presence of subpleural and subpericardial hemorrhages is an excellent sign of suffocation, but not a pathognomonic one. Tardieu was mistaken in concluding, on the basis of these alone, that a crime has been committed.

It is a tragic fact of history that many forensic scientists in subsequent decades ignored the last of these conclusions, with the result that countless convictions of homicide were based solely upon testimony that "Tardieu's spots" constituted unequivocal evidence of death by suffocation.

This unhappy situation was effectively terminated by an influential paper published in 1955,[23] reinforced by an equally influential editorial.[24] These authors denounced the view that thoracic petechiae are signs of suffocation. They suggested that petechiae may arise (or at least become more prominent) after death, and it was concluded that they have little or no pathophysiological significance. These papers have been widely quoted in modern forensic texts, and the opinions of the authors seem to have been generally endorsed. Certainly their view is preferable to the overzealous interpretation of petechiae as a sign of suffocation. But have we gone too far, in rejecting a thesis only because it was

TABLE 4. Important Variables to Consider in Experimental Petechial Studies

Animal species
Age of subjects
Type of asphyxia
nitrogen versus nitrogen/carbon dioxide
end-expiratory versus random airway occlusion
Petechial sites examined
lung only
chest only
all internal surfaces
Anesthetic used
Prior manipulations
Health of subjects

inappropriately applied in earlier times? The history of science contains many examples of theories that were initially overextended, followed by overrejection.

EXPERIMENTAL STUDIES OF INTRATHORACIC PETECHIAE

In view of the potential forensic importance of these petechiae, and their prominence in SIDS, it is surprising that so few investigators have examined this problem in the experimental laboratory. The few studies reported to date have yielded conflicting results. Some of the potential reasons for discrepant findings are listed in TABLE 4.

The pioneering work of Brouardel in the 19th century has been mentioned above.[22] He pointed out the importance of species and age differences in the ease with which these hemorrhages are produced. One of Brouardel's most interesting experiments involved the placement of a window in the chest wall of dogs, then asphyxiating them by the applying a mask of soft wax over the face. He observed that pleural petechiae did not form during the struggling phase, but that they suddenly developed at the precise moment of onset of the final (gasping) stage of asphyxia. He does not mention observations of the other intrathoracic surfaces in these experiments.

The first investigator to examine this topic experimentally in relation to SIDS was Handforth,[4] using 20 adult rats. He introduced a cannula regulated by a stopcock into the trachea, monitoring the effects of airway obstruction by an esophageal pressure recorder. He occluded the airway until respiratory efforts ceased, then reopened the stopcock. Some animals failed to recover, others apparently recovered spontaneously, and still others responded to resuscitative efforts. The survivors were sacrificed and they, like those that died initially, all showed intrathoracic petechiae. Handforth concluded that airway obstruction was the likely cause of the petechiae in SIDS.

Guntheroth et al.[25] sacrificed adult rats by six defined mechanisms, recording only the pleural surfaces. In the group of animals sacrificed by airway occlusion, there was no effort to obstruct the airway at end-expiration. Some animals in all six groups developed pleural petechiae, the incidence being lowest in the airway obstruction group and highest in the animals asphyxiated in 100% nitrogen. The same group was unable to replicate these results in a subsequent study,[26] using younger adult rats. In the latter study, they were able to produce petechiae in the nitrogen-asphyxiated animals after production of pneumonia by inoculation of Sendaivirus. The extent of pneumonia was not documented microscopically. Later, Guntheroth suggested that petechiae are the result of shearing forces between the lung and adjacent surfaces during gasping respiration.[27] The latter argument fails entirely to account for the distribution of petechiae in SIDS, since several of the surfaces of the thymus and heart that regularly show petechiae are completely shielded from the lung surface, yet the parietal pleura, in direct contact with the lungs, shows petechiae much more rarely than these organs.

Campbell and Read[28] produced numerous pulmonary petechiae in rabbits by repeated tracheal occlusion, and did not observe them when animals were sacrificed by apneic asphyxia induced by barbiturate. Electroshock to the heart, producing death by acute hypotension, and injection of nor-adrenaline produced pulmonary petechiae. Petechiae were not reported in extrapulmonary sites. These workers concluded that vigorous respiratory efforts were required for the genesis of pulmonary petechiae, but that circulatory factors may play a role.

Farber et al.[29] examined the effect of end-expiratory respiratory occlusion upon circulatory dynamics in rabbits. They found that pulmonary petechiae occurred readily when there was a large pressure difference between pulmonary wedge pressure and intratracheal pressure. They observed progressive increases in pulmonary wedge pressures with progression of asphyxia. They postulated that left ventricular afterloading as a result of intrathoracic negative pressure and/or decreased left heart compliance from the same mechanism could account for the pulmonary, but not the thymic or epicardial petechiae in SIDS. The same group[30] found that a single sustained end-expiratory tracheal occlusion in adult rats produced only rare petechiae, but that repeated occlusions produced numerous pulmonary petechiae. They found that injection of epinephrine followed by end-expiratory airway obstruction potentiated the formation of petechiae, and that this effect could be blocked by alpha-adrenergic and dopaminergic blocking agents. They postulated that hypoxia-induced endogenous catecholamine release might play a role in the pathogenesis of the pulmonary petechiae in SIDS.

Winn[31] examined the influence of age upon petechial formation and asphyxial responses in young rats. This study demonstrated a dramatic reduction in duration of gasping in rats asphyxiated in a mixture of nitrogen and carbon dioxide between birth and ten days of age. This study demonstrated that prolonged, deep gasping following hypoxic asphyxiation produced numerous petechiae on the lung surfaces and fewer on the other intrathoracic organs.

DISCUSSION

While final answers concerning the precise significance of intrathoracic petechiae are not justified by currently available information, a considerable amount has been learned concerning their pathogenesis. One important concept that should be considered in the design of experimental studies is that the pathogenesis of petechiae may differ in the low-pressure pulmonary circulation and in the systemic circulation of the thorax. Krous[15] has reviewed evidence that intrathoracic negative pressure may cause pulmonary petechiae by producing left ventricular dysfunction, resulting in back-pressure into the pulmonary veins. On the other hand, hemorrhages from structures in the systemic circulation may result more directly from the pressure gradient between the vessel lumen and the perivascular space. Many studies have documented systemic hypertension as a result of asphyxia.[27–29] The presence of increased intravascular pressure would seem likely to potentiate the effect of extravascular negative pressure, increasing the chances for rupture and hemorrhage from the systemic circulation in the chest.

The number and distribution of petechiae in SIDS support the view that intrathoracic negative pressures are involved in their genesis. But why are petechiae usually more prominent in SIDS than in most cases of accidental or homicidal infant suffocation? One possibility is that a greater magnitude of negative pressure is involved. We have suggested elsewhere[19] that if the fatal event occurs at end-expiration in SIDS, then greater negative pressures would be produced than if obstruction occurs at partial or complete inspiration. If it could be shown that SIDS deaths occur under circumstances where unusually high pressure gradients are produced between the intrathoracic vessels and their environs, this difference between petechiae in SIDS and in typical suffocation deaths could be explained.

An alternative explanation for this apparent paradox is that the vascular bed has been damaged by preceding abnormalities such as hypoxia, toxemia, hypertension, etc., so that a relatively modest degree of negative pressure could result in hemorrhages. Several experimental studies have suggested that repeated or prolonged respiratory efforts will produce petechiae where a single episode may not do so.[28,29]

While not all workers who have examined the pathogenesis of intrathoracic petechiae in experimental models would agree that occluded airways are required for their production, every study reported to date implicates respiratory efforts as being essential for their development; and most authors have emphasized that exaggerated respiration is necessary. Many have focused upon gasping in the final stages of asphyxial death as the probable mechanism in their models.

If nonspecific agonal gasping is the mechanism of petechiae in SIDS victims, it is difficult to account for the fact that the hemorrhages are usually more prominent than in deaths from other causes. Gasping is a common terminal phenomenon in dying patients, most of whom have antecedent hypoxia, acidosis, or other factors that would reduce capillary integrity. Therefore, if gasping causes the petechiae in SIDS, one would expect petechiae to be as numerous as those in many SIDS victims in a large proportion of postmortem examinations.

The pathophysiology of SIDS doubtless has features in common with other death mechanisms, but it seems clear from the number and prominence of petechiae that, as a group, SIDS victims seem to have experienced a final episode that either in nature or degree is relatively unique and is not experienced by the majority of dying humans.

SUMMARY AND CONCLUSIONS

(1) Intrathoracic petechiae are characteristic of most SIDS cases, and tend to be more numerous in these cases than in deaths from other causes, including mechanical asphyxia. (2) Their localization suggests that intrathoracic negative pressure plays a role in their genesis. (3) Several human and animal studies suggest that petechiae arising from the pulmonary circulation may differ from those originating from systemic vessels in the thorax. (4) Experimental studies suggest that vigorous respiratory efforts are responsible for their formation. This would seem to exclude respiratory paralysis as a mechanism for most SIDS deaths. (5) These petechiae are not consistent with cardiac arrest or failure as the primary agonal event in SIDS. (6) The fact that petechiae are more prominent in SIDS than in other deaths adds to the evidence that SIDS is not a "wastebasket" diagnosis, despite the imperfection of existing diagnostic criteria. (7) These petechiae do not prove that the final mechanism of most SIDS deaths is upper airway obstruction. However, they do provide substantial support for that thesis.

REFERENCES

1. BECKWITH, J. B. et al. 1970. Discussion of terminology and definition of Sudden Infant Death Syndrome. In Sudden Infant Death Syndrome. Proceedings of the Second International

Conference on Causes of Sudden Death in Infants. A.B. Bergman, J.B. Beckwith & C.G. Ray, Eds.: 14–22. University of Washington Press. Seattle.

2. TEMPLEMAN, C. 1892. Two hundred and fifty-eight cases of suffocation in infants. Edinburgh Med. J. **38**: 322–329.

3. WERNE, J. & I. GARROW. 1953. Sudden apparently unexplained death during infancy. I. Pathologic findings in infants found dead. Am. J. Pathol. **29**: 633–652.

4. HANDFORTH, C. P. 1959. Sudden unexpected death in infants. Canad. Med. Assoc. J. **80**: 872–873.

5. ADELSON, L. & E. R. KINNEY. 1956. Sudden and unexpected death in infancy and childhood. Pediatrics **17**: 663–697.

6. ADELSON, L. 1965. Specific studies of infant victims of sudden death. *In* Sudden Death in Infants. R.J. Wedgwood & E. P. Benditt, Eds.: 11–40. USPHS Publication 1412.

7. VALDES-DAPENA, M. 1982. The pathologist and the Sudden Infant Death Syndrome. Am. J. Pathol. **106**: 118–131.

8. BECKWITH, J. B. 1973. The Sudden Infant Death Syndrome. Curr. Prob. Pediatr. **3** (No. 8): 1–36.

9. STURNER, W. Q. 1977. Sudden unexpected infant death. *In* Forensic Medicine: Trauma and Environmental Hazards. C.G. Tedeschi, Ed.:1015–1032. Saunders. Philadelphia, PA.

10. FEARN, S.W. 1834. Sudden and unexplained death of children. Lancet **1**: 246.

11. JACOBSEN, T. & J. VOIGHT. Cited by Geertinger.[12]

12. GEERTINGER, P. 1968. Sudden Death in Infancy. Charles C. Thomas. Springfield, IL.

13. MARSHALL, T. K. 1970. The Northern Ireland Study: Pathology findings. *In* Sudden Infant Death Syndrome. Proceedings of the Second International Conference on Causes of Sudden Death in Infants. A.B. Bergman, J.B. Beckwith & C.G. Ray, Eds.: 108–117. University of Washington Press. Seattle, WA.

14. BECKWITH, J. B. 1970. Observations on the pathological anatomy of Sudden Infant Death Syndrome. *In* Sudden Infant Death Syndrome. Proceedings of the Second International Conference on Causes of Sudden Death in Infants. A.B. Bergman, J.B. Beckwith & C.G. Ray, Eds.: 83–107. University of Washington Press. Seattle, WA.

15. KROUS, H. F. 1984. The microscopic distribution of intrathoracic petechiae in Sudden Infant Death Syndrome. Arch. Pathol. Lab. Med. **108**: 77–79.

16. POTTER, E. L. & J. M. CRAIG. 1975. Pathology of the Fetus and the Infant. 3rd edit. p. 96. Year Book. Chicago.

17. KROUS, H. F. & J. JORDAN. 1984. A necropsy study of distribution of petechiae in non-Sudden Infant Death Syndrome. Arch. Pathol. Lab. Med. **108**: 75–76.

18. MARSHALL, T. K. 1970. Pathology Discussion. *In* Sudden Infant Death Syndrome. Proceedings of the Second International Conference on Causes of Sudden Death in Infants. A. B. Bergman, J. B. Beckwith & C. G. Ray, Eds.: 122–127. University of Washington Press. Seattle, WA.

19. BECKWITH, J. B. 1970. Pathology Discussion. *In* Sudden Infant Death Syndrome. Proceedings of the Second International Conference on Causes of Sudden Death in Infants. A. B. Bergman, J. B. Beckwith & C. G. Ray Eds.: 120–122. University of Washington Press. Seattle, WA.

20. TARDIEU, A. 1897. Étude Médico-Légale sur l'Infanticide. J.-B. Baillière. Paris.

21. TARDIEU, A. 1879. Étude Médico-Légale sur la Pendaison, la Strangulation, et la Suffocation. 2nd edit. J.-B. Baillière. Paris.

22. BROUARDEL, P. 1897. La Pendaison, la Strangulation, la Suffocation, la Submersion. J.-B. Baillière. Paris.

23. GORDON, I. & R. A. MANSFIELD. 1955. Subpleural, subpericardial, and subendocardial hemorrhages. A study of their incidence at necropsy and of the spontaneous development, after death, of subpericardial petechiae. J. Forens. Med. **2**: 31–50.

24. SHAPIRO, H. A. 1955. Tardieu spots in asphyxia. J. Forens. Med. **2**: 1–4.

25. GUNTHEROTH, W. G., D. BRAZEALE & G. A. McGOUGH. 1973. The significance of pulmonary petechiae in crib death. Pediatrics **52**: 601–603.

26. GUNTHEROTH, W. G., I. KAWABORI, D. G. BRAZEALE *et al.* 1980. The role of respiratory infection in intrathoracic petechiae. Am. J. Dis. Child. **134**: 364–366.

27. GUNTHEROTH, W. G. 1983. The pathophysiology of petechiae. *In* Sudden Infant Death

Syndrome. J. T. Tildon, L. M. Roeder & A. Steinschneider, Eds.: Academic Press. New York.

28. CAMPBELL, C. J. & D. J. C. READ. 1980. Circulatory and respiratory factors in the experimental production of lung petechiae and their possible significance in the Sudden Infant Death Syndrome. Pathology 12: 181–188.

29. FARBER, J. P., A. C. CATRON & H. F. KROUS. 1982. Pulmonary petechiae: Ventilatory-circulatory interactions. Pediatr. Res. 17: 230–233.

30. KROUS, H. F., A. C. CATRON & J. P. FARBER. 1984. Norepinephrine-induced pulmonary petechiae in the rat: An experimental model with potential implications for Sudden Infant Death Syndrome. Pediatr. Pathol. 2: 115–122.

31. WINN, K. 1986. Similarities between lethal asphyxia in postneonatal rats and the terminal episode in SIDS. Pediatr. Pathol. 5: 325–335.

The Role of Sleep and Arousal in SIDS

M.B. STERMAN

Sepulveda V.A. Medical Center
Sepulveda, California 91343
and University of California, Los Angeles
Los Angeles, California 90024

J. HODGMAN

Los Angeles County and
University of Southern California Medical Center
Los Angeles, California 90033

INTRODUCTION

Perhaps the most significant fact about sleep as it relates to SIDS is that it is physiologically very different from wakefulness. More specifically, the several *states* of sleep reflect a progressive sequence of physiological changes resulting in a continuous and recurrent flux in functional organization. These dynamic changes clearly serve important objectives in the biological economy; however, they also influence and exacerbate any existing deficiencies in that economy.

For example, in the case of epilepsy, the states of sleep produce a profound and diagnostically significant increase in abnormal EEG discharge.[1,2] In particular, the stages of non-REM sleep are frequently accompanied by an "activation" of EEG paroxysmal patterns. Actually, this is better described as a "release" of extant epileptic pathology, since it is thought to result from the well-documented neuronal disinhibition in telencephalic structures during non-REM sleep.[3]

In fact, it is useful to think of the neuronal disinhibition during sleep in general as a condition in which higher nervous structures are actively, if temporarily, relieved of responsibility for the oversight of more basic regulatory functions. This active process would seem to be essential for the restoration of forebrain functions. The temporary loss of a higher level support system, however, is another way in which the occurence of normal, biologically essential sleep can have deleterious consequences if all is not right at lower levels of organization. It is in this sense that developmental factors related to sleep could potentially influence events leading to SIDS.

This possibility became a focus of attention in the last decade when it was determined that most deaths attributed to SIDS occurred during periods of presumed sleep. During this same period the field of sleep research was providing evidence for a significant clinical syndrome in adults characterized by prolonged apnea associated with marked hypoxemia and increased pulmonary and systemic arterial pressure.[4] Cardiopulmonary function during wakefulness, however, appeared within normal limits. The so-called apnea hypothesis of SIDS[5] was launched in earnest when it was reported that some SIDS victims had exhibited high rates of short-duration apnea during sleep[6] and when histological evidence suggested that SIDS victims had experienced pathological hypoxia and hypoxemia prior to death.[7,8]

As shall be reviewed below, there is a body of evidence suggesting that infant groups identified as high risk for SIDS indeed do show physiological characteristics consistent with a mild, chronic hypoxia. However, some investigators have argued against this conclusion,[9] and the possibility of a causal relationship between prolonged apnea and SIDS has been put in serious doubt on the basis of more recent evidence.[5,10] Nevertheless, the potential for a dangerous interaction between an existing susceptibility and the dynamics of sleep-state maturation in early infancy remains viable as an etiologic factor in SIDS.

NORMAL DEVELOPMENTAL STAGES AND SLEEP MATURATION

In order to explore possible interactions appropriately, it is essential to review what has been learned about the maturation of normal sleep in the infant. The last several decades have produced an extensive literature in this area. As a result of a comprehensive study supported by the National Institute of Child Health and Development in our laboratory, we have had the opportunity to contribute significantly to that literature. Accordingly, the data reviewed here will draw heavily from our study, which was one of the most carefully conducted investigations of this kind ever attempted. This study of polygraphic variables in normal sleep-state development was designed to provide control data for comparison with a matched population of presumed high-risk infants recruited from families with a previous SIDS experience, so-called subsequent siblings.

Polygraphic data were evaluated from 20 normal, full-term infants at one week after delivery and at monthly intervals thereafter until six months of age. Recordings were non-invasive and included EEG, ECG, respiration, eye movements, and somatic activity. Data were collected continuously across the night from approximately 8:00 PM to 8:00 AM the next morning, and subjected to both visual and computer analysis.[11,12]

The states of sleep in the infant are conventionally referred to as active sleep (AS) and quiet sleep (QS), in recognition of their immaturity in comparison to the corresponding rapid-eye-movement (REM) and non-REM states seen in the adult. We had proposed earlier, on the basis of studies of intrauterine somatic activity, that state organization begins during fetal development with the emergence at approximately 20 weeks gestational age of a quiet-active cycle mediated by brain stem organization.[13] Subsequent findings supported this conclusion in demonstrating definitive periodicities in the heart rate and heart rate variability in late gestation, which were independent of maternal measures and corresponded closely to those observed directly in the same infants after birth.[14] It is this basic cycle that confers a 60-minute periodicity to virtually every physiological variable in the infant. This physiological periodicity is apparently a very early priority in nervous system development. The substrates for state organization are thus fundamental to development and appear to be endogenous to the maturing fetus. However, the early AS-QS cycle in the fetus is eventually incorporated into a sleep and waking cycle, which appears after birth with the maturation of forebrain neuronal organization.

The most overt change in physiological organization during infancy was found to be the emergence of this sleep-waking cycle, brought about by a lengthening and redistribution of both wakefulness and quiet sleep, as noted also by others.[15,16] The amount of active sleep decreased almost reciprocally to these changes. Sustained episodes of QS emerged and, together with remaining longer episodes of AS, began to constitute a period of sleep dominated by the QS state, constructed of stages resulting from the recurrent appearance of AS, and consolidated increasingly into the nighttime hours. At the same time, brief periods of wakefulness gradually disappeared from the night, with sustained epochs appearing at longer intervals and eventually dominating the daytime hours. Thus, a circadian sleep-waking cycle became superimposed over a preserved and stabilized ultradian rest-activity cycle. This post-natal reorganization was achieved primarily within the first 12 weeks of infancy.

A different perspective on post-natal maturation was provided by examining trends in developmental changes registered by individual physiological measures. These are summarized in FIGURES 1 and 2. Two distinct patterns were observed. During AS (FIG. 1), most measures showed a two-stage linear developmental sequence during the 24 weeks of study. These included a period of rapid change between 1 and 12 weeks and a period of slow change or stability thereafter. A similar pattern was seen in some measures during QS (FIG. 2); however, in this state a number of key variables showed a three-stage pattern of change. This consisted of a significant trend in one direction between 1 and 4 weeks of age that reversed abruptly between 4 and 12 weeks of age, and again stabilized thereafter. This same pattern was seen for heart rate during AS. We believe that this three-stage pattern discloses an important phase in forebrain maturation that is both critical to the consolidation of QS and relevant to our perspective on sleep and SIDS. Accordingly, we propose a scheme of post-natal development that contrasts with established concepts by recognizing, in particular, a period of "post-neonatal adaptation" between one and three months of age (FIG. 3).

It was suggested earlier[17] that physiological organization during the fetal stage of development is adapted to the unique requirements of that period. At birth, certain functions may be sustained in fetal status by maternal endowments (i.e., endocrine, immunological, etc.). The result is a unique physiology in the early neonatal period that in some ways is paradoxically more mature than at later ages. However, the loss of maternal endowment and the altered requirements of independent extrauterine existence promote a spurt in neuronal maturation[18] leading to a rapid physiological reorganization, the characteristic priorities of which result in the dynamic changes of the post-neonatal adaptation stage of development. The infant develops its own substrates for independent function during this period. By three months of age, truly a critical period in human development, this reorganization is essentially complete and a period of more gradual, if not more complex, development ensues.

The events that best summarize the dynamic changes in sleep and waking states during the post-neonatal adaptation phase of early development are: (1) a marked increase in the amount and duration of QS during the night; (2) a corresponding decrease in the frequency and interval between AS and waking episodes, with a consolidation of sustained waking into the daytime hours; (3) a sharp reduction in respiratory and heart rates during sleep; and (4) the emergence of cortical EEG spindle activity during QS.

This brief review of early developmental milestones in the maturation of sleep provides a useful theoretical perspective. In many ways the newborn resembles a decorticate preparation, in which everything above the brain stem has been removed. Sensory and motor activity is limited primarily to reflex function, affective response is stimulus specific and undirected, and state organization is limited to an accelerated cycling of active and quiet states, with the former dominating.[19,20] The first months of post-natal life are characterized by a rapid maturation of forebrain elements and the development of functional connectivity between cortex and lower structures.[18] Simultaneously, consolidated and reciprocal states of wakefulness and sleep emerge. The unique regulation of the newborn period is thus replaced by a more dichotomous, forebrain-mediated wakefulness and sleep.

It is important to recognize what this conceptualization implies. Prior to the early maturation of these states, there is no specific modulation of sensory, motor, and visceral functions in relation to states of wakefulness or sleep. It is only after the maturation of an active forebrain sleep-induction system has occurred that a functionally consolidated, circadian sleep-waking cycle becomes associated with the temporary loss of higher level support alluded to earlier. If the resulting suppression or altered regulation of visceral functions is to have any impact on physiological deficiencies, it is at this point that such an impact might occur. We believe that this accounts for the unique fact that most SIDS deaths occur between 2 and 3 months of age.

PREDISPOSING FACTORS IN SIDS

As stated earlier, there is considerable evidence that many SIDS victims are derived from a population of susceptible infants. Signs of existing pathology are modest and their confirmation limited by the low incidence of SIDS and a continuing controversy surrounding the definition of high risk in surviving infants. Nevertheless, findings from a variety of investigative sources have suggested subtle respiratory and cardiac abnormalities. Many are by now familiar with the histological studies of Naeye and associates[8] in SIDS victims, which provided morphologic evidence for chronic hypoxia. Additionally, there is the consistent finding of increased respiratory rates during sleep, first reported by our group in subsequent sibling infants,[21] and later observed by others in this risk group[22] as well as in near-miss and other risk groups.[23,24] Increased respiratory rates were actually confirmed in some infants who later became SIDS victims.[23,25] It should be pointed out that increased respiratory rates were documented in high risk and eventual SIDS victims as early as one week of age in some of these studies.[25,26] A link to chronic hypoxemia was provided also by the finding that kittens exposed to hypoxic conditioning showed an elevated respiratory rate and sometimes died of respiratory failure during QS.[27] Finally, the recent finding of elevated fetal hemoglobin levels at autopsy in SIDS[28] could also be construed as evidence for a compromise of oxygen supply to the developing fetus.

Findings implying cardiac abnormalities are less clear. Several studies have reported abnormally increased heart rates during sleep in both subsequent sibling[29] and near-miss[30] infants. This observation is consistent with an alternative theoretical model for the etiology of SIDS, the "QT" hypothesis.[5] Briefly, it is proposed that some SIDS deaths may result from ventricular fibrillation elicited by precipitating events acting upon a maturationally unbalanced sympathetic innervation of the heart. Markers for such a sympathetic imbalance include, among others, a prolongation of the QT interval of the ECG and a higher than normal heart rate. An extensive prospective study of the QT interval in a large group of infants, nine of whom became SIDS victims, indicated that a markedly prolonged QT interval could be an important risk factor for SIDS.[5]

While there are a number of additional abnormal findings in the literature concerning SIDS, one in particular is of interest to us. This was the discovery of elevated thyroid hormone levels in post-mortem studies of SIDS victims.[31] Convincing evidence from the studies of Tildon and Chacon[32] suggests that thyroid activity is chronically elevated in SIDS victims (FIG. 4). This observation could not only account for many of the abnormalities noted above, but may also provide an explanation for some intriguing findings that emerged from our study of subsequent siblings of SIDS.

SLEEP DEVELOPMENT PATTERNS IN SUBSEQUENT SIBLINGS

In this study a group of 20 carefully identified subsequent siblings of SIDS infants were monitored both pre- and post-natally in a manner identical to that described earlier for our low risk control group. Data from strictly age-matched control and sibling infant groups were compared in order to identify potential differences in respiratory, cardiac, and sleep-state polygraphic measures. As mentioned above, this study disclosed that our group of siblings had elevated respiratory and heart rates and decreased apnea rates when

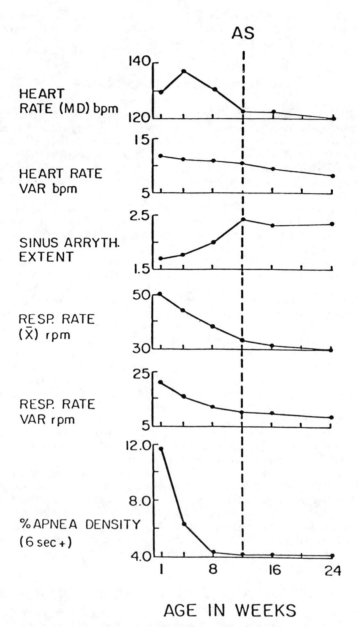

FIGURE 1. Developmental trends derived from data recorded during AS in 20 normal, full-term infants. Except for heart rate, these variables all show a two-stage post-natal sequence. It is proposed that this developmental pattern reflects an unaltered continuation of functional events initiated pre-natally.

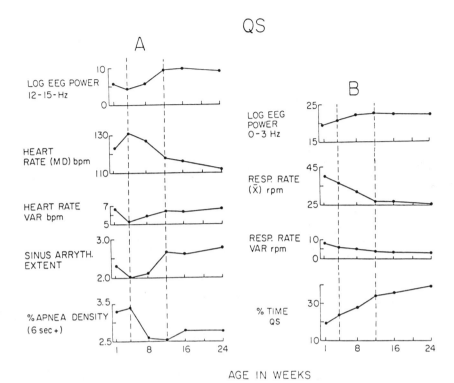

FIGURE 2. Developmental trends in polygraphic data from 20 normal, full-term infants recorded in all-night studies from 1 to 24 weeks of age. Data shown are group mean values sampled during QS episodes in the same portion of the night. Patterns from variables at A define a three-stage developmental sequence while those from variables at B indicate only two stages. It is proposed that the former reflect functional changes associated specifically with post-neuronal adaptation.

compared to controls.[21,26,29] Further, these differences were all significant within the first post-natal month.

Our findings in the realm of sleep-state development proved to be equally interesting. Comparison of the distribution of state patterns across the night indicated that the developmental lengthening of intervals between AS episodes and corresponding reduction of waking periods occurred significantly earlier in sibling infants.[33] In fact, siblings had a longer AS cycle by one week of age. Both cardio-respiratory and EEG measures showed manifestations of a circadian influence by the end of the first post-natal month in siblings, which was a month earlier than in controls.[34,35] Finally, the emergence of EEG sleep spindle activity, perhaps the most reliable index of non-REM sleep in adults, occurred earlier in siblings than in controls.[35] This discrepancy was significant by two months of age (FIG. 5). Collectively, these findings suggested that central nervous system maturational sequences were accelerated in this group of sibling of SIDS infants.

THE ACCELERATED MATURATION HYPOTHESIS

It has been known for some time that elevated levels of thyroid hormone during the perinatal period result in an accelerated cortical neuronal maturation with consequent

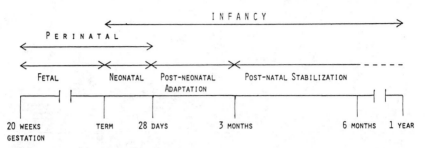

FIGURE 3. Proposed scheme for more dynamic characterization of stages in infant development. Traditional designation of perinatal and infancy periods is elaborated to recognize functional differences between fetal, neonatal, post-neonatal adaptation, and post-natal stabilization periods.

premature development of both EEG and behavioral response patterns.[36] Thus, the more recent discovery of elevated thyroid hormone levels in SIDS victims has provided a possible explanation for our findings. Increased metabolic activity could account for elevated respiratory and heart rates while the resulting facilitation of forebrain maturation would promote a more rapid state development. We refer to this as the "accelerated maturation hypothesis" of SIDS. Since none of our infants became SIDS victims,

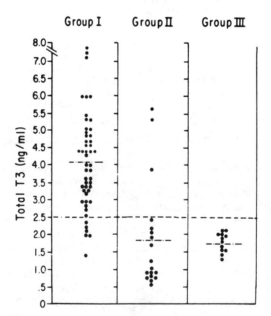

FIGURE 4. Triiodothyronine (T3) in SIDS and in non-SIDS control populations. The interrupted line depicts the upper limit of established euthyroid range. Each value represents the average of duplicate determinations for each individual infant. The mean for each group is represented by dot-dash lines. Group I = SIDS victims; Group II = autopsy controls; Group III = age-matched living controls. (From Tildon et al.[32] with permission from Academic Press.)

however, we can only speculate that this may be but one factor in the complex etiology of SIDS.

Although the hypothesis of accelerated maturation is appealing, several reports in the SIDS literature have arrived at the opposite conclusion. Haddad *et al.*[37] observed a significant reduction in quiet-sleep time at three months of age in "aborted SIDS" infants when compared to controls. They attributed this finding to a delayed maturation of sleep. However, these data were collected during midmorning sleep periods. As discussed earlier, the consolidation of sleep into the nighttime hours and an associated *reduction* of sleep during the day are classical signs of sleep-state maturation, as first elaborated by Kleitman[38] and confirmed by many others. Thus, these findings actually support the conclusion that sleep-state maturation is accelerated in high-risk infants.

CONTROL VS SIBLING EEG MATURATION (QS)
LEFT CENTRAL 12–15 Hz.

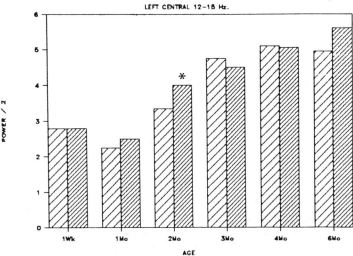

FIGURE 5. Power spectral density profiles for activity in the left central cortical 12–15 Hz band during the first quiet sleep episode of the night are shown here for control (wide crosshatch) and subsequent sibling (narrow crosshatch) infant groups ($N = 20$ per group) across the course of study. Note significant difference at 2 months of age (*), with siblings showing not only greater activity at this age but also a steeper rate of increment from values at 1 month. (From data in Sterman *et al.*[35])

Guilleminault and Coons[39] also suggested that state maturation was delayed in near-miss infants. This conclusion was based on data tabulated from the visual scoring of 24-hour polygraphic records. Despite the herculean effort represented by this study, dependence on subjective visual evaluation of highly variable infant polygraphic patterns is questionable. Using the kind of measures employed by these investigators, we found no state parameter differences between our sibling and control groups. In fact, a marked variability among infants was the most consistent finding in this evaluation. However, when computer-based quantitative analysis was applied to individual physiological measures, the objective differences outlined above were obtained. It should be pointed out that the risk groups and recording procedures used in this study were different from ours.

Nevertheless, we cannot consider these findings to be definitive by virtue of their lack of rigorous, objective analysis.

Another report concluding that maturation was delayed in high-risk infants is even more difficult to interpret. Gould[40] compared twins and other infants of presumed high risk for SIDS with "lower risk" controls in terms of sleep state and sleep EEG characteristics. He reports that overall amounts of QS and EEG activity in the sleep spindle frequency range were decreased in the high-risk subjects. These conclusions, while uninhibited, are also uninterpretable since the author provides no description of his subjects, no details concerning methodology, and no evidence of statistical analysis. Sleep-state measures were again based on subjective visual scoring of polygraphic data *obtained during daytime recordings!* The same problem as raised above for the Haddad *et al.* study, therefore, applies here. EEG findings were derived from percentage conversions of power spectral analysis data. To begin with, this is a highly complex technique that is subject to many procedural pitfalls and, accordingly, must be described in some detail for the reader to evaluate its validity. Further, percentage derivations of spectral densities can be very misleading since they reflect *relative* changes across the frequency spectrum rather than functional changes in a given frequency component. Finally, data obtained from daytime recordings, which again show the reverse of spectral findings during the night, are in fact supportive of an accelerated maturation!

ACCELERATED MATURATION AND AROUSAL

On the basis of these considerations, we prefer to conclude at present that the robust and quantitative findings in our sibling study, together with the link between SIDS and elevated thyroid hormone levels, constitute a reasonable basis for further consideration of an "accelerated maturation hypothesis" as at least one factor in the etiology of SIDS. Proceeding from this position, we propose that the early maturation of neural substrates for sleep and waking could result in a higher threshold for arousal at a critical period in autonomic regulatory maturation. As mentioned above, we observed an earlier reduction in nighttime spontaneous arousals in subsequent siblings than in controls. Others have reported increased arousal thresholds to hypercapnic breathing[42] as well as a profound reduction in hypoxic arousal[41,42] in near-miss infants during QS. Additionally, a number of studies, including our own, have documented a significant reduction in movements during QS in risk infants.[39,43]

One other finding from our infant studies is worthy of note here. A phasic-movement detection system was installed in the recording bed used in these studies and provided a continuous measure of phasic somatic activity across the night. When these data were compared in our control and sibling infants another interesting discrepancy was disclosed. The control infants showed a peculiar but very consistent increase in phasic activity during AS that began at 8 weeks, ended at 16 weeks, and peaked at 12 weeks of age (FIG. 6A). This increment was to some extent progressive through the night and was clearly greater in later AS epochs. A similar phenomenon was observed in the sibling group, but in this case emerged between 4 and 8 weeks of age (FIG. 6B).

This unusual finding has potentially important implications for an understanding of developmental dynamics relevant to SIDS. In adult sleep, phasic activity during the REM state increases progressively through the night.[44] This increase parallels a decrease in arousal threshold as sleep progresses.[45] It is also known that sedative-hypnotic drugs suppress phasic activity without affecting REM duration, while extended sleep results in an increase in this activity.[46] As a result of these and other considerations, Feinberg and associates have hypothesized that the magnitude of phasic activity during REM sleep labels the depth of sleep or, its reciprocal, the level of central arousal.[47]

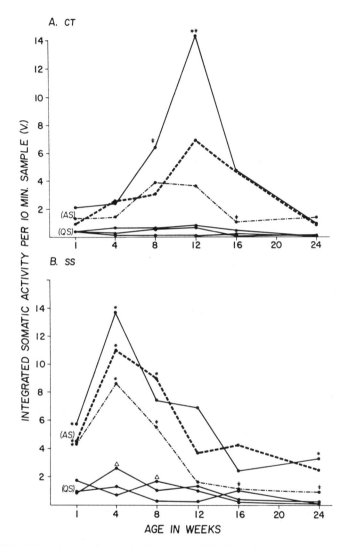

FIGURE 6. Minute-integrated mean phasic somatic activity during three 10-min samples across the night are shown here as sampled over the first 6 months of life in both quiet sleep (QS) and active sleep (AS) for two groups of 20 control (CT) and 20 subsequent siblings of SIDS (SS) infants. Ten-min samples were obtained during the first, middle, and last episode of each sleep state across the night. Statistical analysis indicated significant sample differences (‡) during AS only ($p<0.01$), where dot-dash curve = first sample, dash curve = middle sample, and solid line curve = last sample of the night. Significant group differences (*) were obtained at 1, 4, 8, 12, and 24 weeks of age, with motility elevated in the SS group. Somatic activity comparisons during QS reached 0.10 level of significance (△) at 4 and 8 weeks of age with increase noted during last episode of the night.

A) CONTROLS

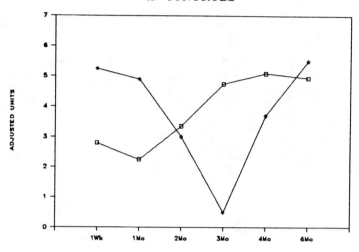

B) SUBSEQUENT SIBLINGS

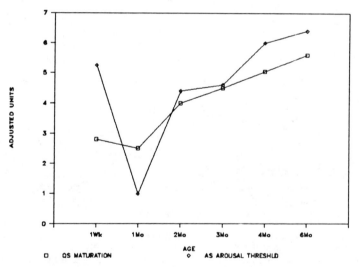

FIGURE 7. Comparison of post-natal developmental trends in two physiological measures obtained in our developmental study of sleep in subsequent sibling and matched control groups ($N = 20$ ea.). Data are configured to demonstrate potential consequences of maturational acceleration observed in sibling infants. Units on ordinate were adjusted for comparison. Quiet sleep maturation (□) is represented by the actual developmental function for EEG spectral density in the 12–15 Hz band. Arousal threshold (◇) is represented by the reciprocal of phasic somatic activity data recorded during active sleep, as discussed in text. Note drop in arousal threshold during emergence of functional quiet sleep state in controls, and developmental mismatch in siblings due to premature occurrence of this event.

If this very reasonable conclusion is correct, our data suggest that a specific decrease in central arousal threshold during sleep accompanies the functional transition represented by the post-neonatal adaptation period of infant development. We can speculate that maturational sequencing provides a transient facilitation of CNS arousal mechanisms to accommodate the progressive suppression of autonomic functions attendant upon the maturation of a forebrain-mediated sleep process. Once the brain stem mechanisms, which are more slow to mature, have caught up with this process, arousal thresholds return to previous levels. These proposed dynamics are diagrammed for control infants in FIGURE 7(A), based on actual data comparing adjusted scales of EEG sleep spindle development (QS maturation) with the hypothesized reciprocal of phasic somatic activity (arousal threshold).

A similar comparison of data from our group of sibling infants underscores the implications of a premature maturation of sleep and arousal mechanisms. The more rapid maturation of both processes leads to a developmental mismatch, with lowered arousal threshold occuring prior to the completion of the post-neonatal adaptation period. Consequently, a sleep-mediated suppression or deregulation of brain stem autonomic functions, which is still profound between two and three months of age, is not compensated by an increased potential for arousal. Under these circumstances the infant would be particularly vulnerable to any influence that either facilitated the depth or duration of QS or added further burdens to an already compromised autonomic regulation.

CONCLUSIONS

This discussion has reviewed evidence leading to the conceptualization of an accelerated maturation hypothesis concerning the etiology of SIDS. This theory, while one of many, has several appealing consequences. First, it provides for an integration of a number of epidemiologic and pathophysiologic findings in SIDS. Second, it accounts for the unique age distribution of SIDS. Finally, it would explain the frequently noted relationship between SIDS and such factors as upper respiratory infection and sleep deprivation or disruption. Perhaps the most appealing aspect of this hypothesis is that it should be relatively easy to examine experimentally.

REFERENCES

1. DALY, D. 1973. Circadian cycles and seizures. *In* Epilepsy: Its Phenomena in Man. M.A.B. Brazier, Ed.: 216–230. Academic Press. New York.
2. HAMEL, A.R. & M.B. STERMAN. 1982. Sleep and epileptic abnormalities during sleep. *In* Sleep and Epilepsy. M.B. Sterman, M.N. Shouse & P. Passouant, Eds.: 361–375. Academic Press. New York.
3. STERIADE, M. 1970. Asecending control of thalamic and cortical responsiveness. Int. Rev. Neurobiol. **12:** 87–144.
4. GUILLEMINAULT, C., A. TILKIAN & W.D. DEMENT. 1976. The sleep apnea syndrome. Annu. Rev. Med. **27:** 465–484.
5. SCHWARTZ, P.J. 1987. The quest for the mechanism of the sudden infant death syndrome: Doubts and progress. Circulation **75**(4): 667–682.
6. STEINSCHNEIDER, A. 1972. Prolonged apnea and the sudden infant death syndrome: Clinical laboratory observations. Pediatrics **50:** 646–654.
7. NAEYE, R.L. 1974. Hypoxemia and the sudden infant death syndrome. Science **186:** 837–838.
8. NAEYE, R.L., B. LADIS & J.S. DRAGE. 1976. Sudden infant death syndrome: A prospective study. Am. J. Dis. Child. **130:** 1207–1210.
9. BECKWITH, J.B. 1983. Chronic hypoxemia in the sudden infant death syndrome: A critical

review of the data base. *In* Sudden Infant Death Syndrome. J.T. Tildon, L.M. Roeder & A. Steinschneider, Eds.: 145–157. Academic Press. New York.

10. McGINTY, D.J. & M.B. STERMAN. 1980. Sleep physiology, hypoxemia, and the sudden death syndrome. Sleep 3(3/4): 361–373.

11. HOFFMAN, E., B. HAVENS, S. GEIDEL, T. HOPPENBROUWERS & J.E. HODGMAN. 1977. Long term, continuous monitoring of multiple physiological parameters in newborn and young infants. Acta Paediat. Scand. (Suppl. 26): 5–23.

12. HARPER, R.M., R.J. SCLABASSI & T. ESTRIN. 1974. Time series analysis and sleep research. IEEE Trans. Auto. Cont. 19(6): 932–943.

13. STERMAN, M.B. & T. HOPPENBROUWERS. 1971. The development of sleep-waking and rest-activity patterns from fetus to adult in man. *In* Brain Development and Behavior. M.B. Sterman, D.J. McGinty & A.M. Adinolfi, Eds.: 203–225. Academic Press. New York.

14. HOPPENBROUWERS, T., J.C. UGARTECHEA, D. COMBS, J.E. HODGMAN, R.M. HARPER & M.B. STERMAN. 1978. Studies of maternal-fetal interaction during the last trimester of pregnancy: Ontogenesis of the basic rest-activity cycle. Exp. Neurol. 61: 136–153.

15. ROFFWARG, H.P., J.N. MUZIO & W.C. DEMENT. 1966. Ontogentic development of the human sleep-dream cycle. Science 152: 604–619.

16. EMDE, R.N. & S. WALKER. 1976. Longitudinal study of infant sleep: Results of fourteen subjects studied at monthly intervals. Psychophysiology 13: 456–461.

17. HUMPHREY, T. 1964. Some correlations between the appearance of human fetal reflexes and the development of the nervous system. Prog. Brain Res. 9: 93–135.

18. SCHEIBEL, M.E. & A.B. SCHEIBEL. 1971. Selected structural-functional correlations in postnatal brain. *In* Brain Development and Behavior. M.B. Sterman, D.J. McGinty & A.M. Adinolfi, Eds.: 1–20. Academic Press. New York.

19. STERMAN, M.B., D.J. McGINTY & Y. IWAMURA. 1974. Modulation of trigeminal reflexers during the REM state in brain transected cats. Arch. Ital. Biol. 112: 278–297.

20. JOUVET, M. 1967. Neurophysiology of the states of sleep. Physiol. Rev. 47(2): 117–177.

21. HOPPENBROUWERS, T., J.E. HODGMAN, R.M. HARPER, D.J. McGINTY & M.B. STERMAN. 1976. Incidence of apnea in infants at high and low risk for sudden infant death syndrome (SIDS). Pediatr. Res. 10: 425–433.

22. CARSE, E.A., D.J. HENDERSON-SMART, P. JOHNSON, P. WHITE & A.R. WILKINSON. 1980. Transcutaneous oxygen tension measurements during the sleep of the newborn baby and infants. Arch. Dis. Child Neurol. 19: 134–138.

23. THOMAN, E.B., V.N. MIANO & M.P. FREESE. 1977. The role of respiratory instability in the sudden infant death syndrome. Dev. Med. Child Neurol. 19: 729–738.

24. FRANKS, C.I., J.B.G. WATSON, B.H. BROWN & E.F. FOSTER. 1980. Respiratory patterns and risk of sudden unexpected death in infancy. Arch. Dis. Child. 55: 595–599.

25. GORDON, D., D.H. KELLY, A. SOLANGE, A. UBEL, R. KENET, R.J. COHEN & D.C. SHANNON. 1982. Abnormalities in HR and respiratory power spectrum in SIDS. Ped. Res. 16: 350A.

26. HOPPERBROUWERS, T., J.E. HODGMAN, D.J. McGINTY, R.M. HARPER & M.B. STERMAN. 1980. Sudden infant death syndrome: Sleep apnea and respiration in subsequent siblings. Pediatrics 66: 205–214.

27. BAKER, T.L. & D.J. McGINTY. 1977. Reversal of cardiopulmonary failure during active sleep in hypoxic kittens: Implications for sudden infant death. Science 198: 419–421.

28. GULIAN, G.G., B.A. ENID, F. GILBERT & R.L. MOSS. 1987. Elevated fetal hemoglobin levels in sudden infant death syndrome. N. Engl. J. Med. 316: 1122–1126.

29. HARPER, R.M., B. LEAKE, T. HOPPERBROUWERS, M.B. STERMAN, D.J. McGINTY & J. HODGMAN. 1978. Polygraphic studies of normal infants and infants at risk for the sudden infant death syndrome: Heart rate and variability as a function of state. Pediat. Res. 12: 778–785.

30. LEISTNER, H.L., G.G. HADDAD, R.A. EPSTEIN, T.L. LAI, M.A.F. EPSTEIN & R. B. MELLINS. 1980. Heart rate and heart rate variability during sleep in aborted sudden infant death syndrome. J Pediat. 97: 51–55.

31. SCHWARTZ, E., L.S. HILLMAN & F. CHASALOW. 1982. Elevation of triiodothyronine (T3) in sudden infant death syndrome (SIDS): A marker of normal thyroid function at death. Ped. Res. 16: 307A.

32. TILDON, J.T. & M.A. CHACON. 1983. Changes in hypothalmic-endocrine function as possible factor(s) in SIDS. *In* Sudden Infant Death Syndrome. J.T. Tildon, L.M. Roeder & A. Steinschneider, Eds.: 211–219. Academic Press. New York.

33. HARPER, R.M., B. LEAKE, H. HOFFMAN, D.O. WALTER, T. HOPPENBROUWERS, J.E. HODGMAN & M.B. STERMAN. 1981. Periodicity of sleep states is altered in infants at risk for the sudden infant death syndrome. Science **213:** 1030–1032.

34. HOPPENBROUWERS, T., D.K. JENSEN, J.E. HODGMAN, R.M. HARPER & M.B. STERMAN. 1980. The emergence of a circadian in respiratory rates: Comparison between control infants and subsequent siblings of SIDS. Pediat. Res. **14:** 345–351.

35. STERMAN, M.B., D.J. MCGINTY, R.M. HARPER, T. HOPPENBROUWERS & J.E. HODGMAN. 1982. Developmental comparison of sleep EEG power spectral patterns in infants at low and high risk for sudden death. Electroenceph. Clin. Neurophysiol. **53:** 166–181.

36. SCHAPIRO, S. 1971. Hormonal and environmental influences on rat brain development and behavior. *In* Brain Development and Behavior. M.B. Sterman, D.J. McGinty & A.M. Adinolfi, Eds.: 307–334. Academic Press. New York.

37. HADDAD, G.G., E.M. WALSH, H.L. LEISTNER, W.K. GRODIN & R.B. MELLINS. 1981. Abnormal maturation of sleep states in infants with aborted sudden infant death syndrome. Pediat. Res. **15:** 1055–1057.

38. KLEITMAN, N. 1963. Sleep and Wakefulness. 2nd edit. pp. 131–147. University of Chicago Press. Chicago, IL.

39. GUILLEMINAULT, C. & S. COONS. 1983. Sleep states and maturation of sleep: A comparative study between full-term normal controls and near-miss SIDS infants. *In* Sudden Infant Death Syndrome. J.T. Tildon, L.M. Roeder & A. Steinschneider, Eds.: 410–411. Academic Press. New York.

40. GOULD, J.B. 1983. SIDS a sleep hypothesis. *In* Sudden Infant Death Syndrome. J.T. Tildon, L.M. Roeder & A. Steinschneider, Eds.: 443–452. Academic Press. New York.

41. MCCULLOCH, K., R.T. BROUILLETTE, A.J. GUZZETTA & C.E. HUNT. 1982. Arousal responses in near-miss sudden infant death syndrome and in normal infants. J Pediat. **101**(6): 911–917.

42. RODRIGUEZ, A.M., D. WARBURTON & T.G. KEENS. 1987. Elevated catacholamine levels and abnormal hypoxia in apnea of infancy. Pediatrics **79**(2): 269–274.

43. HOPPENBROUWERS, T., D. JENSEN, J.E. HODGMAN, R.M. HARPER & M.B. STERMAN. 1982. Body movements during quiet sleep (QS) in subsequent siblings of SIDS. Clin. Res. **30:** 257–264.

44. FEINBERG, I. 1974. Changes in sleep cycle patterns with age. J. Psychiat. Res. **10:** 283–306.

45. RECHTSCHAFFEN, A., P. HAURI & M. ZEITLIN. 1966. Auditory awakening thresholds in REM and NREM sleep stages. Percept. Motor Skills **22:** 927–942.

46. FEINBERG, I & A. KOEGLER. 1982. Hypnotics and the elderly: Clinical and basic science issues. *In* Treatment of Psychopathology in the Aging. C. Eisdorfer & W.E. Fann, Eds.: 75–96. New York.

47. FEINBERG, I. T.C. FLOYD & J.D. MARCH. 1987. Effects of sleep loss on delta EEG and REM density: New observations and hypotheses. Electroenceph. clin. Neurophysiol. (In press.)

The Relationship between Sleep and
Sudden Infant Death

JEFFREY B. GOULD, AUSTIN F. S. LEE,[a] AND
SUZETTE MORELOCK[b]

School of Public Health
Maternal and Child Health Program
University of California
Berkeley, California 94720

INTRODUCTION

Interest in the possible role of sleep in the pathogenesis of the sudden infant death syndrome (SIDS) stems from the close temporal relationship between the SIDS event and sleep. Bergman and associates report that 74% of 160 SIDS victims were found upon awakening in the morning and 14% at the end of an afternoon nap.[1] While time of discovery does not necessarily imply that SIDS occurs during sleep, most infants who are observed to die during the awake period have autopsy findings consistent with a non-SIDS etiology. One of the first physiologic studies to stress the importance of sleep to the pathogenesis of SIDS was Steinschneider's demonstration of excessive amounts of brief apnea in some near-miss infants who eventually died of SIDS.[2] This disturbed respiratory pattern, compatible with Naeye's reports of post-mortem tissue changes suggestive of chronic hypoxia,[3-5] was the basis of the sleep apnea hypothesis. Two models supported the concept of SIDS resulting from respiratory failure during sleep: apnea of prematurity, which results in large part from a failure of respiratory drive during sleep,[6] and Ondine's curse, a failure to increase ventilation in response to CO_2 during quiet sleep.[7] Subsequent studies have not demonstrated clear-cut failures of respiration during sleep in infants at high risk for SIDS.[8] Two prospective studies attempting to identify future SIDS cases on the basis of respiratory pattern during sleep have failed. Even in near-miss infants it has not been possible to identify those infants who will die from a future attack on the basis of respiratory pattern (i.e. apnea, periodic breathing, etc.) recorded during sleep.[9-12]

While it seems most unlikely that SIDS results from a serious defect in respiration that becomes unmasked by sleep, there is a great deal of evidence that suggests that in infants at risk for SIDS, mechanisms essential for the maintenance of homeostasis during sleep may be compromised.

Sleep is a complex neurophysiologic process consisting of the alteration of two behavioral states, quiet sleep and active (REM) sleep. In active sleep there are body movements, eye movements, and rapid and irregular heart and respiratory rates. There is also absence of antigravity tone and a low-voltage fast EEG. In the newborn, after 40 minutes of REM sleep there is a transition to quiet sleep characterized by the absence of body and eye movements and by slower and more regular cardiac and respiratory rates. During quiet sleep there is tonic antigravity muscle tone and a high voltage, slow EEG. This pattern then repeats itself. Early infancy is a period of rapid functional maturation

---

[a]Present address: Department of Mathematics, Boston University, Boston, MA.
[b]Present address: Boston University School of Public Health, Boston, MA.

and integration.[13-17] The neonate has a preponderance of REM sleep. Over the first three months the percentage of "phasic" REM decreases and the percentage of "tonic" quiet sleep increases. The increase in the percentage of quiet sleep is accompanied by a dramatic increase in the complexity of the EEG. By two to three months of age, sleep spindles emerge.[18] This activity in the range of 12 to 16 Hz makes it possible to classify infant sleep into adult sleep stages and signifies the development of thalamo-cortical interconnections between higher centers and the brain stem. The development of the integration of suprapontine and brain stem structures is considered critical for arousal and cardio-respiratory homeostasis.[19] The increased percentage of quiet sleep at two to three months of age is a consequence of this neurophysiologic maturation and indicates a functional increase in the ability of the CNS to sustain inhibition. During the awake state, the ability to sustain inhibition allows the maintenance of attention and is essential to the development of learning. With respect to sleep, the ability to sustain inhibition allows the coalescence of the multiple brief naps characteristic of the neonate into the more prolonged "adult" sleeping pattern that emerges in the two to three month-old infant. Although 24-hour sleep time has decreased by only one hour, by two to three months of age the longest sleep period lengthens to eight hours, the majority of sleep occurs during the night, and is spent primarily in the quiet state.

The ability to maintain state is made possible by the maturation of both CNS inhibitory capacity and by maturation of the ability to maintain homeostasis and effect arousal in the face of homeostatic failure. We believe that it is the interplay between the homeostatic demands of prolonged sleep and the ability of the maturing infant to meet these demands that is critical in the development of SIDS.[38] This hypothesis offers a physiologic explanation for the unique age distribution of the SIDS, which reaches a peak at two to three months.[20] After six to eight months, the homeostatic mechanisms critical to the pathogenesis of SIDS have matured sufficiently to withstand the stress of prolonged sleep even in the face of mild perturbations (i.e. a "cold") and the incidence of SIDS dramatically decreases.

RESEARCH STRATEGIES

Research into the possible role of sleep in the etiology of SIDS is greatly constrained by our complete lack of knowledge regarding its pathophysiology. Basic SIDS-oriented sleep research has addressed the issues of maturation, homeostasis, and neurophysiologic integration.[19,21,22] Infant studies' have compared sleep-state organization, maturation, state-specific cardio-respiratory patterns, and homeostatic respiratory mechanisms in infants epidemiologically at higher and lower risk for SIDS. The two most commonly studied groups are siblings of SIDS victims[16,17,23,24] and near-miss infants.[25-30] However, two recent reports raise the question of the suitability of sibs as a high risk study group. When one controls for maternal age and birth order Peterson's case control study of all SIDS in Washington state between 1969 and 1984 did not find a significantly increased SIDS risk in the siblings. Peterson and associates' estimates confirmed those derived from Norwegian data.[31,32] The authors conclude that the risk of SIDS in the sibs groups has been greatly overestimated due to over reporting and under enumeration.

Our studies at Boston University/Boston City Hospital (Supported by NIH Contract NO1-HD-3-2789) compared higher SIDS risk twins and lower SIDS risk singleton controls. A large number of studies have reported twins to be at high risk for SIDS and there are many reports of both twins dying on the same day.[33] Although the increased likelihood of a co-twin dying exists only for one month, the rate of SIDS in the co-twin has been estimated at 42/1,000.[34] The likelihood of both twins dying is similar in

TABLE 1. Infants Studied

	Twins	Controls
Number	58	24
% black	64.1%	79.9%
% male	41%	44.8%
Mean gestation age (wk)	36.6 ± 2.2	36.4 ± 2.1
Mean birth weight (g)	2,291 ± 542	2,427 ± 561
Number of polygraphic studies	236	97

monozygous and dizygous twin sets. This finding is in line with other studies that suggest SIDS is not a genetic disease in the strict Mendelian sense.[31,32,35] Indeed, the increased risk of SIDS in both members of a twin set regardless of zygosity suggests that they were exposed to a common environmental circumstance prenatally and postnatally.

In the analysis of our data, twins were also stratified with respect to the risk factors of race, sex, and gestational age. Race is a powerful risk factor for SIDS (5.1/1000 in blacks versus 1.2/1000 in whites[36]). The male disadvantage is more controversial and may only occur in whites.[1,37] Birth weight, on the other hand, is a powerful risk factor for SIDS that fits an exponential model.[36]

In the next section we will present our study of sleep-state maturation in twins and singletons followed by a discussion of the possible relationship of specific sleep states to the pathophysiology of SIDS.

METHODS

The study group consists of 29 twin sets born to low income families at the Boston City Hospital and 24 singleton controls (TABLE 1). All infants were free of congenital abnormalities and serious illness. None of the study infants had sleep apnea during infancy or subsequently died of SIDS. Polygraphic studies were obtained in an attempt to define the effects of genetic and environmental factors on sleep physiology. We obtained 333 studies at 36–38, 40–41, 43–45, 47–49, and 51–53 weeks after conception. Twin sets were evaluated within 24 hours during a morning and an afternoon nap.

Recordings were obtained following the technical guidelines set forth by Anders et al.[39] Infants were studied under standard environmental conditions. Electrodes were applied prior to feeding, the infant fed, placed in a prone position, and a two- to four-hour interfeeding sleep polygraph performed on a Grass Model 78-B polygraph with Model 7P511G amplifiers. The following recordings were made: Two channels of EEG (10–20 system: left frontal-left temporal, left central-left occipital), one channel of eye movements, one channel of submental EMG, one channel of EKG, one channel of respiration (nasal thermocouple), one channel of movement (via an air mattress-strain gauge system), and a 20-second time mark. Chart speed was 15 mm/sec, giving one polygraphic page per 20 seconds of real time. Behavioral observations were written directly on the polygraphic record. Electrode resistance was always under 10,000 ohms prior to recording.

Scoring and Sleep-State Determination

The basic scoring epoch was 20 seconds. Each of five parameters (EEG, EOG, EMG, respiration, and motility) was visually evaluated for each 20-second epoch. Using standard infant criteria,[39] parameters consistent with REM sleep were scored ''1'' and parameters consistent with quiet sleep were scored ''0'' (TABLE 2).

Sleep state was determined using a modification of the Rip-Van technique.[40] The total score for each 20-second epoch could range from ''0'' (all five criterial consistent with quiet sleep) to '' +5'' (all five criteria consistent with REM sleep). Sleep was considered quiet when the epoch scores were 0 for three consecutive epochs, REM when the epoch scores were 5 for three consecutive epochs, and indeterminate when the epoch scores were 1 to 4 and lasted at least three epochs. During epochs with apnea, respiration was not used as a state criteria and the above rules were modified accordingly. Only records with a total sleep time greater than 60 minutes were included for analysis.

RESULTS

TABLE 3 gives the descriptive statistics for the high SIDS risk and low SIDS risk group comparisons.

Sleep-State Ontogeny in Singletons: 37 to 52 Weeks Post-conception

Over the period of 37 to 52 weeks post-conception, the percentage of REM sleep decreases and the percentage of quiet sleep increases (FIG. 1). This increase in percentage of quiet and decrease in percentage of REM is similar to the results of other investigators.[14,41,42]

Singletons also demonstrate a significant linear decrease in the percentage of indeterminate sleep ($p < .001$) over the periods 37 to 52 weeks.

Twin Versus Singleton Sleep-State Comparisons

Both twins and singletons show a significant decrease in REM over the period 37 to 52 weeks (FIG. 1). Over the entire period, twins have higher levels of REM than

TABLE 2. Sleep-State Criteria

Criteria	Score
REM Sleep	
Rapid eye movements	+ 1
Irregular respiration	+ 1
Absent or phasic submental EMG	+ 1
Body, face, or extremity movements	+ 1
Low-voltage fast/mixed EEG	+ 1
REM sleep score	+ 5
Quiet Sleep	
No rapid eye movements	0
Regular respiration	0
Tonic submental EMG	0
No movements except occasional startle	0
High-voltage slow/trace alternate/mixed EEG	0
Quiet sleep score	0

TABLE 3A. Comparison of Percentage of Sleep State in Singletons Versus Twins and White Twins Versus Black Twins

| | | Study Week | | | | |
		37	40	44	48	52
REM	N	14	24	23	17	19
Singleton[a]	mean	30.8	25.1[c]	19.2	15.6	15.5
	S.D.	9.5	9.5	9.7	8.4	8.6
	N	39	55	63	32	47
Twin	mean	31.7	31.3	22.3	18.0	16.3
	S.D.	11.6	12.4	8.7	7.3	8.0
Quiet	N	14	24	23	17	19
Singleton	mean	9.4	19.6	26.5	37.3	46.5[d]
	S.D.	8.9	9.6	13.2	10.5	14.4
	N	39	55	63	32	47
Twin	mean	11.6	21.1	26.1	32.1	37.3
	S.D.	6.4	8.8	10.6	9.7	12.6
Ind	N	14	24	23	17	19
Singleton	mean	52.8	47.8[b]	45.7	40.9	35.5
	S.D.	16.0	15.2	16.8	13.4	13.3
	N	39	55	63	32	47
Twin	mean	50.0	40.3	43.8	43.0	42.3
	S.D.	11.4	13.8	14.1	11.2	13.0
REM	N	13	23	22	13	17
Non-black twins	mean	27.0[b]	30.9	24.0	18.3	13.2
	S.D.	15.0	13.5	9.3	8.7	5.6
	N	26	32	41	19	30
Black twins	mean	34.0	31.6	21.4	17.8	15.2
	S.D.	8.9	11.9	8.3	6.4	9.0
Quiet	N	13	23	22	13	17
Non-black twins[a]	mean	10.5	22.7	25.9	35.9	42.0[c]
	S.D.	5.6	8.8	10.4	5.5	7.7
	N	26	32	41	19	30
Black twins	mean	12.1	19.9	26.1	29.5	34.5
	S.D.	6.8	8.7	10.8	11.1	14.1
Ind	N	13	23	22	13	17
Non-black twins	mean	56.0[b]	39.2	41.5	37.6[b]	36.5[b]
	S.D.	10.7	14.1	12.8	10.7	8.3
	N	26	32	41	19	30
Black twins	mean	47.0	41.1	45.1	46.8	45.7
	S.D.	10.7	13.8	14.7	10.2	14.0

[a]Overall difference between groups $p < .05$, Ind = indeterminate.
[b,c,d]Study date difference between groups $p < .05, .01, .001$ (two tailed), respectively.

singletons ($p < .03$). The difference is most marked at 40 weeks and by 52 weeks there is a convergence in twin and singleton REM values.

For the quiet system there is no difference between twins and singletons between 37 and 44 weeks. Twins then experience a delay in their rate of maturation relative to the singletons and by 52 weeks have a significantly lower percentage of quiet sleep ($p < .001$). There was no difference in overall indeterminate sleep between the singleton and twins. In both groups the percentage of indeterminate sleep decreased from 37 to 52 weeks.

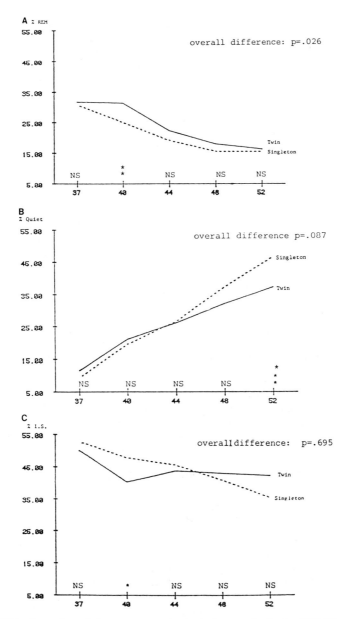

FIGURE 1. Comparison of sleep-state maturation in singletons and twins for REM (A), quiet (B), and indeterminate sleep (C). **Abscissa:** age post-conception (weeks); **Ordinate:** % of sleep time in indicated sleep-state.

Racial Differences in the Twin Sample

The twins were divided into black and non-black groups. The only REM difference was seen at 37 weeks, where blacks had higher levels of REM sleep (FIG. 2).

Quiet sleep was equal in blacks and non-blacks until 44 weeks. The rate of increase in non-blacks then became greater than in the blacks resulting in a significant increase overall ($p < .03$) and at 52 weeks ($p < .01$). Blacks also had higher levels of indeterminate sleep at 48 and 52 weeks (FIG. 2).

Several similarities emerge when one compares lower SIDS risk singletons and non-blacks to higher SIDS risk twins and blacks. Differences in the REM sleep occur at the early study dates and have been resolved by 52 weeks, while differences in the quiet sleep are more extensive and emerge at the later study periods.

Male–Female Comparisons

Although males had increased levels of indeterminate sleep at 37 weeks, the most significant difference was in quiet sleep. FIGURE 3 shows that across all study periods males have significantly less quiet sleep than females ($p < .025$). However, this difference appears to close by 52 weeks.

Term–Premature Comparisons

Our premature and term twins studied at the same post-conceptional ages had similar results in terms of most sleep measures (TABLE 3B). The only significant difference was the increased percentage of REM in term infants at 40 weeks, which corrected by 44 weeks. The marked similarity between premature and term infants studied at the same post-conceptional age is in keeping with other reports, and suggests that sleep-state ontogeny is secondary to basic neuroanatomical development (myelinization and dendritic aborization), which takes place on a post-conceptional timetable.

To summarize, in the above analysis comparisons in sleep-state organization and maturation were made between infants at higher risk (twins, black twins, male twins, premature twins) and at lower risk for SIDS (singletons, white twins, female twins, term twins). Higher levels of REM were seen in the twins at the early study dates. Black twins also have increased REM at 37 weeks. Even more striking was the decreased rate of quiet sleep maturation seen in twins versus singletons and black twins versus non-black twins.

Quiet Sleep at 52 Weeks

The finding of decreased percentage of quiet sleep in sub-populations at risk for SIDS prompted a more detailed analysis. The concept of "percent quiet" was initially introduced as a way of comparing quiet sleep activity in infants with differing total sleep time. Behind this concept is the notion that percent quiet is independent of total sleep time. Because sleep is a cyclic phenomenon consisting of the rhythmic alternation of the quiet and REM state, the number of sleep cycles observed during a sleep period becomes an important variable. For example, because infants enter sleep via the quiet state and the quiet state may last from 15–25 minutes, infants who sleep less than 60 minutes will appear to have a higher percentage of quiet-sleep activity. For this reason infants with total sleep times less than 60 minutes were not included in our analysis. Even when measuring sleep-state percentages over only a few sleep cycles, the results may not reflect

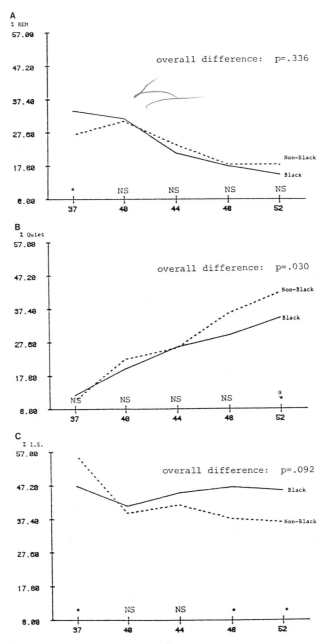

FIGURE 2. Comparison of sleep-state maturation in non-black twins and black twins for REM (A), quiet (B), and indeterminate sleep (C). **Abscissa:** age post-conception (weeks); **Ordinate:** % of sleep time in indicated sleep state.

TABLE 3B. Comparison of Percentage of Sleep State in Female Versus Male Twins and Term Versus Preterm Twins

| | | Study Week | | | | |
		37	40	44	48	52
REM	N	21	37	41	22	27
Female twins	mean	33.2	29.5	21.6	18.1	17.3
	S.D.	12.4	10.2	8.1	5.9	8.5
	N	18	18	22	10	20
Male twins	mean	29.9	35.0	23.7	17.6	14.9
	S.D.	10.7	15.8	9.6	10.2	7.2
Quiet	N	21	37	41	22	27
Female twins[a]	mean	13.3	21.8	28.3[c]	33.5	36.7
	S.D.	6.0	8.1	9.4	9.8	13.5
	N	18	18	22	10	20
Male twins	mean	9.6	19.6	21.8	29.1	38.0
	S.D.	6.4	10.2	11.4	9.1	11.6
Ind	N	21	37	41	22	27
Female twins	mean	46.1[b]	40.4	42.3	40.8	42.4
	S.D.	11.5	12.1	13.7	10.5	14.9
	N	18	18	22	20	10
Male twins	mean	54.5	40.3	46.6	42.2	40.1
	S.D.	9.8	17.2	14.6	10.2	11.5
REM	N	6	16	22	7	17
Term twins	mean	32.2	36.4[b]	23.0	18.4	15.3
	S.D.	14.2	14.9	8.9	11.8	7.3
	N	33	39	41	25	30
Premature twins	mean	31.6	29.2	22.0	17.9	16.9
	S.D.	11.3	10.8	8.6	5.8	8.4
Quiet	N	6	16	22	7	17
Term twins	mean	10.8	19.8	23.5	37.5	36.9
	S.D.	8.3	8.2	11.4	5.0	9.0
	N	33	39	41	25	30
Premature twins	mean	11.7	21.6	27.4	30.6	37.5
	S.D.	6.1	9.1	10.0	10.2	14.4
Ind	N	6	16	22	7	17
Term twins	mean	53.8	38.6	45.8	38.2	43.8
	S.D.	9.6	14.4	14.0	10.1	11.0
	N	33	39	41	25	30
Premature twins	mean	49.5	41.1	42.8	44.4	41.5
	S.D.	11.8	13.7	14.1	11.3	14.1

[a]Overall difference between groups $p < .05$.
[b,c]Study date difference between groups $p < .05$, $< .01$ (two tail), respectively. Ind = indeterminate sleep.

differences in the potential for quiet-sleep activity, but rather where in the sleep cycle the infant awakes. While this is not a problem in infants with multiple sleep cycles, it could bias the results obtained from relatively short interfeed naps. To overcome this problem we developed an alternative technique for estimating quiet-sleep activity based on regression analysis.

We found that quiet-sleep time in minutes is positively correlated with the length of

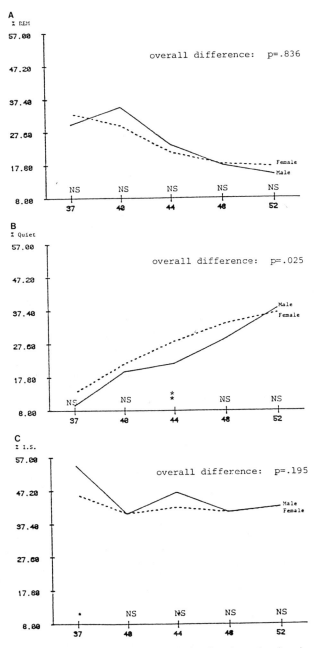

FIGURE 3. Comparison of sleep-state maturation in female twins and male twins for REM (A), quiet (B), and indeterminate sleep (C). **Abscissa:** age post-conception (weeks); **Ordinate:** % of sleep time in indicated sleep state.

TABLE 4. Stratification of Risk Groups for Sudden Infant Death on the Basis of Minutes of Quiet Sleep Excess at 52 Weeks of Age

Non-black singletons	$+9.2$ minutes
Black singletons	$+5.3$ minutes
Non-black twins	$+2.2$ minutes
Black twins	-5.8 minutes

total sleep ($\hat{Q} = a + b$TST, where TST equals total sleep time) at all study dates. Using the formula $\hat{Q} = 10.898 + .305$ total sleep time (R = .67, $p < .001$) it was possible to compute the expected minutes of quiet sleep at 52 weeks, based on that infant's total sleep time. The residual value, that is, the difference between the expected and the actual minutes of quiet sleep, allows one to quantitate the degree to which the infant has an excess ($+$) or deficit ($-$) of quiet sleep with respect to the entire population of infants, as their measurements formed the basis for the reference regression line. This technique was extended to our sub-populations at higher and at lower risk for SIDS, and the sub-population characterized in terms of its overall excess or deficit in the expected levels of quiet sleep.

To test our hypothesis that quiet sleep activity is decreased in high SIDS risk infants at 52 weeks, we have compared the amount of quiet sleep that is in error from that predicted by the total sleep time using the formula $e_Q = Q - \hat{Q}$, where Q is the total amount of sleep in minutes, $\hat{Q}$ is the amount of quiet sleep predictable from total sleep time, and e_Q is the amount of quiet sleep in minutes in excess of, or short of, the level of $\hat{Q}$ that is predictable from the total sleep time. Using Sheffe's test of multiple comparisons, a significant difference was found between twins and singletons. However, this difference can be partitioned out and represents a difference between Black twins and singletons (and also black twins and non-black twins) (TABLE 4). It is of further interest that the relative amount of error follows the expected relative risk. Black twins are at highest risk and white singletons at lowest. These results suggest that percent quiet sleep is a valid physiological correlate for SIDS risk at 52 weeks.

DISCUSSION

The Role of Sleep in the Pathogenesis of SIDS

Quiet Sleep

A major finding in our study was a decrease in the maturation of quiet sleep in sub-groups who are epidemiologically at increased risk for SIDS. Similar findings have also been reported in near-miss infants.[26,27] In addition to delayed maturation as measured by percentage of quiet sleep we have also described a maturational delay in the development of EEG sleep spindle activity during quiet sleep.[38]

The quiet system has been shown to be vulnerable to a variety of prenatal insults.[42–46] The majority of these studies were limited to the neonatal period (approximately 40 weeks) and demonstrated an "early" deficit in percentage of quiet sleep. Quiet sleep vulnerability has been felt to represent the vulnerability inherent in neurologic mechanisms that are in a state of development. "With various kinds of pre- and perinatal pathology the neonatal brain loses this recently acquired ability to coordinate all these parameters and/or to maintain the still very labile state of Quiet sleep . . . ."[45]

An important question is what is the source of pathology that results in quiet-sleep deficits in these infants. Chronic intrauterine and postnatal hypoxia is a reasonable candidate and could also be responsible for the pre- and postnatal growth retardation;[47] systemic[3-5] and CNS[5,48] findings seen at autopsy in many SIDS victims. While decreased maturation of the quiet-sleep system is indicative of its compromise, its role in the pathogenesis of SIDS most likely involves cardio-respiratory control mechanisms and/or arousal. In quiet sleep, respiration is dependent upon chemical control and chemical reflexes have the greatest effect.[49] A large number of studies have evaluated the integrity of these reflexes during quiet sleep in sibs of SIDS and near-miss infants. While there is a great deal of controversy in the overall interpretation of results due to methodological and subject differences, a recent review suggests that as a group these infants exhibit differences in respiratory control.[8] Compromise of respiratory control during quiet sleep has also been reported. In an analysis of pneumograms obtained in 17 of 11,100 infants who subsequently died of SIDS Kelly and associates observed that during quiet time the SIDS as a group had a significantly higher cardiac rate and a significantly increased level of periodic breathing.[12] Ten of the infants had been evaluated for a history of apnea and seven were sibs of SIDS without a previous history of apnea.

Arousal from quiet sleep in response to hypoxia and hypercapneic stress has been evaluated by several investigators in near-miss infants.[24,29,30] While it is difficult to compare these studies because of differences in methodology (stimulus levels, presentation schedules, use of chloral hydrate, amount of "non-respiratory" stimulation) they all demonstrate various abnormalities during quiet sleep. For example, Van der Hal and associates evaluating 56 near-miss infants found that while all control infants aroused to hypercapnea, the control infants aroused at a lower inspired pCO_2. Even more important was the observation that all control infants but only 38% of the near-miss infants aroused to hypoxia.[29] These findings indicate that during quiet sleep some infants at risk for SIDS exhibit abnormalities in the recognition or response to hypoxia.

Indeterminate Sleep

The percentage of indeterminate sleep is classically considered a measure of CNS disorganization, as during this "state" the observed physiologic parameters contain a mixture of "tonic forms" characteristic of quiet sleep and "phasic forms" characteristic of REM sleep. An increase in indeterminate sleep is seen in severely brain-damaged infants, in infants born to drug-addicted mothers (a group at high risk for SIDS[a]),[46] and as a result of sleep deprivation. When we further subdivide indeterminate sleep, it consists of transitions between states, tonic periods during REM, and phasic periods during quiet. Twin and singleton apnea levels have been reported as being transitional during the transitions, slightly lower in "tonic" REM, and slightly higher in "phasic" quiet. Similar "orderly" findings were seen for respiratory and cardiac rate and variability. These observations[38] do not support the concept of indeterminate sleep as a vulnerable period for cardio-respiratory homeostasis. In our twin study there were no striking differences in indeterminate sleep across our higher and lower risk subgroups.

---

[a]Ward and associates have described an increase in total sleep time, apnea, and periodic breathing, heart, and respiratory rates during sleep on overnight pneumograms of infants of substance-abusing mothers. Analysis by sleep state was not reported (58).

REM

REM or active sleep is characterized by phasic activity that superficially resembles the awake state. However, there is marked inhibition of both sensory input and spinal motor output during REM. This inhibition prevents dreaming adults from acting out dreams. Other consequences of this REM-specific inhibition, e.g., depression of the intercostal muscles, chest wall instability, and defective response to nasal obstruction[49,50] have important implications for premature infants with respiratory problems. During REM sleep, respiratory control appears to be dependent upon intrinsic drive mechanisms that are poorly understood. Both brief and prolonged apneas are seen most frequently during REM sleep.[57]

A major source of respiratory drive in many species is environmental temperature. While mammals are considered homeotherms, the ability to increase metabolic rate during hypothalamic cooling and the ability to increase respiratory rate during heating[51] are markedly diminished during REM sleep. During REM the precise thermoregulatory control seen in the awake and quiet sleep states is lost. Darnall and Ariagno have demonstrated that the premature infant may have intact thermoregulation during REM.[52] Therefore, with respect to SIDS it would be important to investigate if the developmental loss of REM thermoregulation takes place during the peak time period for SIDS.

Stanton, on the basis of febrile seizures,[59] and Harper on the basis of altered respiratory drive[18] suggest that the loss of thermoregulation during REM could be important in the pathogenesis of SIDS. In a recent report comparing twin SIDS victims to their surviving co-twins, a history of repeated profuse sweating during sleep was obtained in 9 of 42 victims. None of the surviving co-twins and none of the 84 control infants gave a history of night sweating ($p < .004$).[54] If valid, this finding is compatible with an abnormality involving temperature regulation or autonomic instability.

REM sleep has often been considered a vulnerable period for cardiac arrythmia on the basis of the repeated bursts of vagal and sympathetic activity[55] typical of the REM state. However, during quiet sleep there is a higher vulnerability of ventricular fibrillation and a lengthening of the qt interval. From a cardiac stand point both sleep states could have a potential role in SIDS a situation that is not resolved by clinical studies. For example, in the evaluation of near-miss infants Leistner et al.[56] described a decrease in the median RR interval, a decrease in the variability of the RR interval, and a decrease in the beat to beat variability (compared to controls) in both the quiet and REM sleep states.

In our study we found that twins and to a lesser extent black twins had higher amounts of REM sleep than singletons and white twins in the early study periods. This demonstrates that both REM sleep and quiet sleep have theoretic vulnerabilities and show laboratory disturbances in infants at higher risk for SIDS.

SUMMARY

Infants epidemiologically at high risk for SIDS demonstrate a variety of abnormalities in sleep-state organization, maturation, and sleep-state modulation of cardio-respiratory control mechanisms. These involve both the REM and quiet-sleep states and are seen in twins who have had no evidence of clinical cardio-respiratory compromise during infancy as well as in near-miss infants who have suffered serious cardio-respiratory failure. Although these infants have higher levels of REM sleep around 40 weeks, of special concern is the decrease in the maturation of the quiet system, which becomes evident after 44 weeks, and the reported quiet-sleep abnormalities in reflex control of respiration and arousal. The source of these abnormalities is environmental rather than genetic and most likely occurs prenatally. During the critical period for SIDS, infant sleep begins to coalesce from a series of naps to more prolonged night time sleep periods that last up to 8 hours. We believe that the ability to maintain physiologic homeostasis during prolonged sleep is a challenge facing infants who are epidemiologically at risk for sudden infant death. The challenge facing sleep research is the more complete understanding of the relationship between prolonged inhibition, homeostasis, arousal, and development.

REFERENCES

1. BERGMAN, A.B., C.G. RAY, M.A. POMEROY *et al.* 1972. Studies of the sudden infant death syndrome in King County, Washington: III. Epidemiology. Pediatrics **49:** 860–870.
2. STEINSCHNEIDER, A. 1972. Prolonged apnea and the sudden infant death syndrome: Clinical and laboratory observations. Pediatrics **50:** 646–654.
3. NAEYE, R.L. 1973. Pulmonary arterial abnormalities in the sudden-infant-death syndrome. N. Engl. J. Med. **289:** 1167–1170.
4. NAEYE, R.L. 1976. Brain-stem and adrenal abnormalities in the sudden-infant-death syndrome. Am. J. Clin. Pathol. **66:** 526–530.
5. NAEYE, R.L. 1980. Sudden infant death. Sci. Am. **242:** 56–62.
6. BROOKS, J.G. 1982. Apnea of infancy and sudden infant death syndrome. Am. J. Dis. Child. **136:** 1012–1123.
7. SHANNON, D.C., D.W. MARSLAND, J.B. GOULD *et al.* 1976. Central hypoventilation during quiet sleep in two infants. Pediatrics **57:** 342–346.
8. BRADY, J.P. & J.B. GOULD. 1984. Sudden infant death syndrome: The physician's dilemma. *In* Advances in Pediatrics. L.A. Barness Ed.: 635–672. Yearbook Medical Publishers.
9. WEINSTEIN, S.L., A. STEINSCHNEIDER, & E. DIAMOND. 1983. SIDS and prolonged apnea during sleep: Are they only a matter of state? *In* Sudden Infant Death Syndrome. J. Tyson-Tildon *et al.*, Eds.: 413–421. Academic Press. New York.
10. SOUTHHALL, D.P., J.M. RICHARD, E.A. SHINEBOURNE *et al.* 1983. Prospective population based studies into heart rate and breathing patterns in newborn infants: Prediction of infants at risk of SIDS. *In* Sudden Infant Death Syndrome. J. Tyson-Tildon *et al.*, Eds.: 621–652. Academic Press. New York.
11. DAVIDSON, S.L., T.G. KEENS, L.S. CHAN *et al.* 1986. Sudden infant death syndrome in infants evaluated by apnea programs in California. Pediatrics **77**(4): 451–458.
12. KELLY, D.H., H. GOLUB, D. CARLEY, & D.C. SHANNON. 1986. Pneumograms in infants who subsequently died of sudden infant death syndrome. J. Pediatr. **109**(2): 249–254.
13. LENARD, H.G. 1970. Sleep studies in infancy. Acta Paediatr. Scand. **59:** 572–581.
14. ANDERS, T.F. & E. HOFFMAN. 1973. The sleep polygram: A potentially usefully tool for clinical assessment in human infants. Am. J. Ment. Defic. **77:** 506–514.
15. PARMELEE, A.H. JR. 1974. Ontogeny of sleep patterns and associated periodicities in infants. Mod. Probl. Paediatr. **13:** 298–311.
16. HOPPENBROUWERS, T. & J.E. HODGMAN. 1983. Sudden infant death sydrome (SIDS). Public Health Rev. **11:** 363–390.
17. HOPPENBROUWERS, T. & J.E. HODGMAN. 1982. Sudden infant death syndrome (SIDS): An integration of ontogenetic, pathologic physiologic and epidemiologic factors. Neuropadiatrie **13:** 36–51.
18. WU, H.S., J.B. GOULD, A.F.S. LEE *et al.* 1980. Factors affecting sleep spindle activity during infancy. Dev. Med. Child. Neurol. **22:** 344–351.
19. HARPER, R.M. 1986. State-related physiological changes and risk for the sudden infant death syndrome. Aust. Paediatr. J. (Suppl.): 155–158.
20. PETERSON, D.R., G. VAN BELLE & N.M. CHINN. 1979. Epidemiologic comparisons of the sudden infant death syndrome with other major components of infant mortality. Am. J. Epidemiol. **110:** 699–707.
21. MCGINTY, D.J. 1983. The reticular formation, breathing disorders during sleep, and SIDS. *In* Sudden Infant Death Syndrome. J. Tyson-Tildon *et al.* Eds.: 375–400. Academic Press. New York.
22. RIGATTO, H. 1984. Control of ventilation in the newborn. Annu. Rev. Physiol. **46:** 661–674.

23. FLORES-GUEVARA, R., L. CURZI-DASCALOVA et al.: 1982. Respiratory pauses in normal infants and in siblings of victims of the sudden infant death syndrome. Kyoto Symposia (EEG) suppl. No. 36: 631–640.
24. BRADY, J.P. & E.M. McCANN. 1985. Control of ventilation in subsequent siblings of victims of sudden infant death syndrome. J. Pediatrics 106(2): 212–217.
25. STEINSCHNEIDER, A. & S. WEINSTEIN. 1983. Sleep respiratory instability in term neonates under hyperthermic conditions: Age, sex, type of feeding, and rapid eye movements. Pediatr. Res. 17: 35–41.
26. HADDAD, G.G., E.M. WALSH, H.L. LEISTNER et al. 1981. Abnormal maturation of sleep states in infants with aborted sudden infant death syndrome. Pediatr. Res. 15: 1055–1057.
27. GUILLEMINAULT, C. & S. COONS. 1983. Sleep: Sleep states and maturation of sleep: A comparative study between full term normal controls and near miss SIDS infants. In Sudden Infant Death Syndrome. J. Tyson-Tildon et al., Eds.: 401–411. Academic Press. New York.
28. HADDAD, G.G. & R.B. MELLINS. 1983. Cardiorespiratory aspects of SIDS: An overview. In Sudden Infant Death Syndrome. J. Tyson-Tildon, et al., Eds.: 357–374. Academic Press. New York.
29. VAN DER HAL, A.L., A.M. RODRIGUEZ et al. 1985. Hypoxic and hypercapneic arousal responses and prediction of subsequent apnea in apnea of infancy. Pediatrics 75(5): 848–854.
30. McCULLOCH, K., R.T. BROUILLETTE et al. 1982. Arousal responses in near-miss sudden infant death syndrome and in normal infants. J. Pediatrics 101(6): 911–917.
31. PETERSON, D.R., E.E. SABOTTA & J.R. DALING. 1986. Infant mortality among subsequent siblings of infants who died of sudden infant death syndrome. J. Pediatrics 108(6): 911–914.
32. IRGENS, L.M., R. SKJAERVEN & D.R. PETERSON. 1984. Prospective assessment of recurrence risk in sudden infant death syndrome siblings. J. Pediatrics 104: 349–351.
33. SMIALEK, J.E. 1986. Simultaneous sudden infant death in twins. Pediatrics 77(6): 816–821.
34. SPIERS, P.S. 1974. Estimated rates on concordance for the sudden infant death syndrome in twins. Am. J. Epidemiol. 100: 1–6.
35. PETERSON, D. R., N.M. CHINN & L.D. FISHER. 1980. The sudden infant death syndrome: Repetitions in families. J. Pediatrics 97: 265–267.
36. BLACK, L., R.J. DAVID et al. 1986. Effects of birth weight and ethnicity on incidence of sudden infant death syndrome. J. Pediatrics 108(2): 209–214.
37. KAPLAN, D.W., A.E. BAUMAN & H.F. KROUS. 1984. Epidemiology of sudden infant death syndrome in American Indians. Pediatrics 74(6): 1041–1046.
38. GOULD, J.B. 1983. SIDS: A sleep hypothesis. In Sudden Infant Death Syndrome. J. Tyson-Tildon et al., Eds.: 443–452. Academic Press. New York.
39. ANDERS, T., R. EMDE & A. PARMELEE. 1971. A manual of standardized terminology, techniques and criteria for scoring of states of sleep and wakefulness in newborn infants. UCLA Brain Information Service/B.R.I. Publications Office. Los Angeles, CA.
40. ANDERS, T.F. & M. ZANGEN. 1972. Rip-van: Sleep state scoring in human infants. Psychophysiology 9: 653–654.
41. DREYFUS-BRISAC, C. 1970. Ontogenesis of sleep in human prematures after 32 weeks of conceptional age. Dev. Psychobiol. 3: 91–121.
42. PARMELEE, A.H. JR. & E. STERN. 1972. Development of states in infants. In Sleep and the Maturing Nervous System. C.D. Clemente & D.P. Purpura, Eds.: 199–228. Academic Press. New York.
43. SANDER, L., P. SNYDER, H. ROSETT et al. 1977. Effects of alcohol intake during pregnancy on newborn state regulation: A progress report. Alcoholism 1(3): 233–241.
44. SCHULTE, F., U. LASSON et al. 1969. Brain and behavioral maturation in newborn infants of diabetic mothers. Neuropadiatrie 1(1): 36–55.
45. SCHULTE, F., G. HINZE & G. SCHREMPF. 1971. Maternal toxemia, fetal malnutrition and bioelectric brain activity of the newborn. Neuropadiatrie 2(4): 439–460.
46. SCHULMAN, C. 1969. Alterations of the sleep cycle in heroin-addicted and "suspect" newborns. Neuropadiatrie 1: 89–100.
47. PETERSON, D.R., E.A. BENSON, L.D. FISHER et al. 1974. Postnatal growth and the sudden infant death syndrome. Am. J. Epidemiol. 99: 389–394.
48. QUATTROCHI, J.J., N. BABA et al. 1980. Sudden infant death syndrome (SIDS): A preliminary study of reticular dendritic spines in infants with SIDS. Brain Res. 181: 245–249.

49. PHILLIPSON, E. 1978. Respiratory adaptations in sleep. Annu. Rev. Physiol. **40:** 133–156.
50. HENDERSON-SMART, D. & D. READ. 1976. Depression of respiratory muscles and defective responses to nasal obstruction during active sleep in the newborn. Aust. Paediatr. J. **12**(4).
51. PARMEGGIANI, P., C. FRANZINI & P. LENZI. 1976. Respiratory frequency as a function of preoptic temperature during sleep. Brain Res. **111:** 253–260.
52. DARNALL, R.A. JR. & R.L. ARIAGNO. 1982. The effect of sleep state on active thermoregulation in the premature infant. Pediatr. Res. **16:** 512–514.
53. McCULLOCH, K., R.T. BROUILLETTE, A.J. GUZZETTA *et al.* 1982. Arousal responses in near-miss sudden infant death syndrome and in normal infants. J. Pediatrics **101:** 911–917.
54. KAHN, A., D. BLUM, M.F. MULLER *et al.* 1986. Sudden infant death syndrome in a twin: A comparison of sibling histories. Pediatrics **78**(1): 146–150.
55. SCHWARTZ, P.J. 1983. Autonomic nervous system, ventricular fibrillation, and SIDS. *In* Sudden Infant Death Syndrome. J. Tyson-Tildon *et al.*, Eds.: 319–339. Academic Press. New York.
56. LEISTNER, H.L., G.G. HADDAD, R.A. EPSTEIN *et al.* 1980. Heart rate and heart rate variability during sleep in aborted sudden infant death syndrome. J. Pediatrics **97:** 51–55.
57. GOULD, J.B., A.F.S. LEE, O. JAMES *et al.* 1977. The sleep state characteristics of apnea during infancy. Pediatrics **59:** 182–194.
58. DAVIDSON-WARD, S.L., S. SCHUETZ, V. KRISHNA *et al.* 1986. Abnormal sleeping ventilatory pattern in infants of substance-abusing mothers. Am. J. Dis. Child. **140:** 1015–1020.
59. STANTON A.N. 1984. Overheating and cot death. Lancet **24:** 1199–201.

Problems in Management of Infants with an Apparent Life-Threatening Event[a]

A. KAHN, E. REBUFFAT, M. SOTTIAUX AND D. BLUM

Pediatric Sleep Unit
University Children Hospital
1020 Brussels, Belgium

The following notes discuss some aspects of the management of infants with an apparent life-threatening event. These are based on articles and some reviews published in the recent literature[1-3] as well as on local experience. These notes are therefore liable to be both interpretative and not exhaustive. It is hoped that they can nevertheless contribute to the information of those interested in the management of infants thought to have survived a possible life-threatening event.

INFANTS WITH AN APPARENT LIFE-THREATENING EVENT

Infants with an apparent life-threatening event (ALTE) are infants presented to medical attention because an acute and unexpected change in behavior alarmed the caregivers. The initial episodes appear to occur during quiet or active sleep, wakefulness, or feeding. They are most commonly described as some combination of apnea (central or obstructive), color change (usually cyanotic or pallid, occasionally erythematous), marked change in muscle tone (usually limpness, rarely rigidity), or choking or gagging. In most cases the observers reported that the episode was potentially life threatening, some times that the child had actually died. The term "apparent life-threatening event" (ALTE) was coined to describe the chief complaint and to replace the previously used "near-miss for SIDS" infants, debated as too precisely indicating an association with the sudden infant death syndrome (SIDS).[1,2]

It is not proven that infants with an apparent life-threatening event are really aborted SIDS cases, although some history-based studies have failed to outline significant differences between SIDS and ALTE victims.[4,5] Up to 9.5% of future SIDS infants had been found cyanotic or pale during sleep at least once and were stimulated by their parents, some weeks before death.[6] Infants were reported who eventually died from SIDS after having survived an ALTE.[7] In a retrospective study, we compared the histories of 65 infants with an ALTE with 95 SIDS victims.[4] The infants with an ALTE appeared to have benefited from more favorable circumstances and were discovered and rescued earlier than the infants who died. For instance, contrary to SIDS accidents, 82% of the ALTE occurred between 08.00 and 20.00 hr, when the caregivers were awake. However, it is difficult to conclude about the relationship between ALTE and SIDS. The validity of the parents' "life-threatening event" has often been questioned.[8] Furthermore, the proven heterogeneity of the ALTE group renders comparison between ALTE and SIDS difficult.[9]

[a]Supported by the Fondation Nationale de la Recherche Scientifique (Grant 3.4543.83).

Factors responsible for difficulties in comparing results among studies include varied types of presenting spells, varied terminology, inconsistent efforts to identify causes of the episodes, dependence on untrained observers, and lack of follow-up programs.

In our collaborative study conducted between January 1980 and 1987, 2,779 infants were referred for an apparent life-threatening event. They were sent by their pediatricians, other clinics, or were brought directly by their parents. The mean age of the patients was 13.3±7.3 weeks and 1,918 (69%) were boys. Detailed descriptions of the event and the child's and family's history were obtained. Further information was obtained from the family's pediatrician. A complete clinical investigation was then conducted to identify a possible cause for the event, including an all-night polysomnography. TABLE 1 illustrates the main clinical diagnostic groups. In up to 61% of the ALTE cases, a specific medical or surgical cause could be identified. Symptoms reported by the parents greatly

TABLE 1. Clinical Diagnoses of Infants Admitted for an ALTE between January 1980 and 1987 (N = 2,779)

Apparent Life-Threatening Episodes (ALTE)	N	Percentage
Known Origin	1695	(61)
Digestive	773	(46)
Gastroesophageal reflux, pyloric stenosis, aspiration, infection, congenital malformation, functional abnormality		
Neurological	509	(30)
Epilepsy, brain tumor, subdural hematoma, infection, vasovagal response, congenital malformation		
Respiratory	289	(10.4)
Infection, airway abnormality, congenital or acquired, congenital alveolar hypoventilation		
Metabolic and endocrine	41	(2.4)
Hypocalcemia, hypoglycemia, hypothyroidism, carnitine deficiency, Leigh syndrome, Reye syndrome, fructosemia, other food intolerance		
Cardiovascular	34	(2)
Cardiomyopathy, arrhythmia, infection, abnormality of major vessels, other congenital malformation		
Miscellaneous	49	
Smothering, drug effect, sepsis, accident, nutritional error		
No Known Origin		
apparently minor incident	695	(25%)
apparently severe incident	389	(14%)

contributed to establish most diagnoses.[10] As seen in TABLE 1, ALTE can be a symptom of many disorders including gastroesophageal reflux, infection, seizures, airway abnormalities, hypoglycemia or other metabolic problems, and impaired regulation of breathing during sleeping and feeding. Seizure-related apneas were only rarely observed (6 cases). Repeated EEG were necessary to disclose hypsarythmia in 4 infants, and in one 6-month-old boy with Aicardi syndrome. Smothering was encountered for 4 infants only. A 6-month-old infant had suffered from repeated episodes of hypoglycemia due to insulin injections by his mother who had severe emotional problems. Polygraphy showed central sleep apneas longer than 20 seconds in 3 infants with pulmonary cytomegalovirus or influenza infection. Obstructive apneas were seen in infants with hypothyroidism, Pierre Robin syndrome, cystic or vascular compression of the airway. All sleep studies normalized after appropriate treatments. Although apnea of prematurity makes up to 18%

of SIDS infants, it was excluded from the definition of ALTE, as it can have other prognostic implications.[2]

The "idiopathic ALTE" group is formed by 39% of the infants investigated. For these infants, we had no sufficient evidence to assign them to a specific diagnostic group despite an appropriate workup. In all but 50 of these cases (5%) the polygraphic studies gave normal results. Although some observations supported the occurrence of prolonged central apneas,[11] increased periodic breathing,[12] and obstructive apneas[13] in infants referred for an ALTE, ours and other studies failed to confirm that these respiratory characteristics were frequently found in infants from the ALTE group.[14-16] During sleep, oxygen tension, which was measured transcutaneously, was similar in these infants and in control infants.[16]

TREATMENT OF INFANTS WITH AN ALTE

When a specific cause for an ALTE is identified, an appropriate medical or surgical treatment was initiated. If no cardiorespiratory abnormality was found during polysomnography, no further surveillance was undertaken, although association with a medical entity does not establish causality for the ALTE.[1,2] For the infants with an "idiopathic ALTE" the outcome is not predictable. A study reported that those infants who responded only to resuscitation and have a subsequent similar episode, who are siblings of victims of SIDS, or who develop a seizure disorder during monitoring, have a risk of dying that is greater than 25%.[17] We divided the group of 1,084 infants with an idiopathic ALTE into two clinical subgroups depending on the apparent severity of the incident. For 695 infants, the initial incident was apparently benign, as no resuscitation was needed, apart from gentle stimulation. These infants were sent home without treatment. A second subgroup of 389 infants (14% of all ALTE) was considered as having had a life-threatening event because intensive resuscitation, vigorous and prolonged stimulation, mouth-to-mouth respiration, and/or cardiac massage were required. In 237 infants (61%) periodic breathing above 5% of sleep time, central apneas longer than 15 seconds, or obstructive apneas longer than 3 seconds were found. These severe forms of idiopathic ALTE were monitored at home, independently of polygraphic findings. These subgroups definition, however clinically useful, suffer possible limitations. Because of anxiety and lack of professional experience, the reports of caregivers can be subjective and difficult to appraise. Even experienced observers can overestimate the severity of the incident, as the child's unresponsiveness may be due to a deep sleep state, or underestimate it because of early intervention. Still, a precise history is of paramount importance as invasiveness of the medical evaluation and treatment depend on the index of clinical suspicion.

DRUG TREATMENT OF INFANTS WITH AN IDIOPATHIC ALTE

Newborn infants with apneas of infancy may benefit from the administration of respiratory stimulants like xanthines (theophylline or caffeine) or doxapram,[18] especially if the child is born premature and is still young. Such treatments were shown to normalize cardiorespirograms in infants,[19] but have not yet been shown to prevent the recurrence of ALTE or to improve survival from SIDS. These drugs are not free of side effects as xanthines were shown to favor gastroesophageal reflux[20] and caffeine has been associated with the development of seizures, possibly by lowering the seizure threshold in seizure-prone infants.[21] Long-term side effects of methylxanthines in infants are unknown. We treat infants with apnea of prematurity with xanthines, controlling their plasma levels of the drug.

HOME MONITORING PROGRAMS

Detractors of home monitoring argue that SIDS may not be preventable despite home monitoring,[22] that monitoring devices are expensive, that home monitoring could induce significant psychological trauma, and that injuries related to misuse of components of home monitors have occurred.[23] Deaths have also been reported on monitors.[17,24-26] Some occurred because of malfunction of the equipment, inappropriate type of monitor equipment, inappropriate alarm system, failure to hear the alarm, inadequate response, or non-utilization of the monitoring devices. Occasional reports indicate that some children could not be resuscitated despite adequate parental responses.

It has been suggested that home monitoring can effectively protect some infants considered at higher risk for SIDS.[22,27] Deaths were reported in infants considered at risk for sleep apnea and whose parents refused to monitor.[22,24,27] We still have no data to validate the protective effects of home monitoring, as the effectiveness of home monitoring programs has not yet been based on scientifically selected groups of patients. Alternatively, the effectiveness of home monitoring programs on the general incidence of SIDS in a given community should not be anticipated, as the proportion of SIDS victims with a history of apnea is less than 9%.

There are at present no definite criteria universally accepted to determine which child should be monitored. Infants are usually considered at risk because of the presence of clinical symptoms or on epidemiologic grounds. The routine monitoring of normal infants is generally not considered medically indicated.[1,2] The history of an idiopathic ALTE, especially when requiring vigorous stimulation or resuscitation, the identification of cardiorespiratory abnormalities (such as prolonged apneas or idiopathic obstructive sleep apneas) and the family history of two or more SIDS victims are frequently used criteria for instituting home monitoring. Likewise, certain diseases or conditions, such as central hypoventilation, can also favor the decision for home monitoring.[2]

If used, monitoring devices should include both respiratory and cardiac surveillance.[1,27-29] It should detect prolonged central apneas, as well as bradycardia due to obstructive apneas, cardiac arrhythmia, or autonomic dysfunction. The effectiveness of bradycardia alarms alone should be evaluated as prolonged apnea and hypoxia could develop before a significant bradycardia. If monitoring devices generally appear to be safe with the exception of a few isolated incidents, they are still far from perfect. Even the best cardiorespiratory devices commercially available are liable to false positive and false negative alarms. False positive alarms can result from low amplitude respiration or movement artifacts. During night polysomnographic recordings in our laboratory cardiorespiratory monitors gave 2.1 ± 1.1 false positive alarms per 100 hours of recording. False negative alarms may be due to cardiogenic artifacts, although such false negative alarms were only occasionally seen in our experience. These technical limitations together with the poor ability of care takers to objectively determine the true nature of an alarm make the evaluation of the effectiveness of home monitoring and parental interventions difficult.[8,9] Monitoring technology is still being developed and refined, including ability to produce a permanent record,[29] or measure oxygen saturation.[2]

TABLE 2 summarizes our collaborative study of infants with idiopathic ALTE monitored at home between January 1983 and 1987. It concerns 200 infants for whom monitoring was completed. When the cardiorespiratory monitors were prescribed, a complete supportive program was offered to the family, including continuous medical, psychological, and technical support. Parents and other caregivers were trained in observation, operation of the monitor, and infant cardiopulmonary resuscitation techniques. The monitors were controlled during night polygraphies. The cardiac alarms were set at 70 cpm, and the apnea alarms at 20 seconds. Repeated alarms were reported for 90% of the 200 "idiopathic ALTE" infants monitored. Most isolated apneas occurred at the beginning of monitoring (85% within the first six months). The number of apnea alarms declined progressively thereafter. By the 12th month of monitoring, alarms still occurred for only 12 children. After the 18th month, all alarms had stopped. Most cases of bradycardia alarms (61% of these), either isolated or associated with apneas, occurred between the 5th and the 8th month of monitoring. Bradycardias disappeared by the end of the first year of life. Most alarms happened at night, mainly during the second part of the night. These observations also apply to young infants still sleeping several hours during the day. Alarms were often separated by several days or weeks free intervals. A marked tendency to clustering of the alarms was noted over the days, with an increased number of alarms following infection, unusual stress, such as disrupted life or vaccinations, or fatigue. The administration of sedative drugs, like phenothiazines syrups appeared to favor the occurrence of the alarms. Cigarette smoke in the child's environment, controlled by measurements of the infants' urine cotinine concentrations, could not be related with a greater number of alarms. Most infants were stimulated at least once by their parents. Most interventions took place at the beginning of monitoring, and in some cases might

TABLE 2. Infants Monitored at Home for an Idiopathic ALTE (1980–1987)

	Number	Percentage
Number of infants monitored	200	
Age (wk)	13 ± 7.3	
Number of infants with alarms	180	90
Total number of alarms	9447	
apnea > 20 sec	6547	69.3
bradycardia < 70 cpm	1351	14.3
apnea and bradycardia	1549	16.4
Time of alarms		
19.01–24.00 hr	2862	30.3
24.01–0.700 hr	4082	43.2
07.01–19.00 hr	2503	26.5
Number of infants stimulated	177	88.3
Number of infants intensely stimulated	20	10.0
Duration of monitoring (wk)	35.8 ± 12.0	
Age at discontinuance (wk)	48.8 ± 16.4	

have been favored by parent anxiety. In 81% of the alarms, no intervention was required, as the infants were found with normal cardiorespiratory rhythms. Only 10% of the infants were "intensely" stimulated (e.g., vigorous, prolonged, and repetitive shaking, or mouth-to-mouth breathing). These resuscitations usually took place between the 4th and 7th month of monitoring. Although the reports by the parents indicated a serious event in these 20 cases, every infant resumed a normal appearance after resuscitation and none required hospitalization. The reported rate of "resuscitations" was much less than the 50% rate reported in other studies.[24]

In a retrospective analysis of 150 night polysomnograms recorded after the ALTE event, we saw no correlation between the presence of long central apneas or excessive periodic breathing and the frequency or apparent severity of the alarms. In 31 infants with obstructive sleep apneas, we observed more frequent alarms, bradycardias, stimulations, and "resuscitations" than in 119 infants with no obstructive apnea during polygraphic study ($p<.01$). Obstructive apneas, due to upper airway obstructions could be more dangerous than central apneas of similar duration because they induce more severe cardiac arrhythmias,[11] bradycardias and fall in oxygen tension.[11,16] These obstructions can be favored by abnormal control mechanisms during sleep.[11] They can be enhanced by the use of sedative drugs, like phenothiazines,[30] by chemoreceptive reflexes, upper respiratory infections,[31] as well as by airway occlusion due to a hypermobile mandible,[32] or by anatomic abnormalities of the airways.[33] No relation was seen between the infants' body position during sleep and the occurrence of sleep apnea or differences in transcutaneous oxygen or carbon dioxide tensions.[34] It has been shown that severe gastroesophageal reflux could induce severe symptoms such as coughing, choking, or apneas.[35] Like others,[36] we could find no causal relation between esophageal reflux and prolonged central or obstructive apneas by studying the night polysomnographies and lower esophageal pH in 10 idiopathic ALTE and 10 control infants. Statistical correlation could only be made with the occurrence of body movements and subsequent fall in pH values.

Compared to control infants, infants with an ALTE showed a decreased number of awakenings and less body motility.[37] The depressed arousal responses could result from previous sleep deprivation or fragmentation.[38] As a higher arousal threshold could oppose a homeostatic reaction to hypoxia, and hence increase the risk of SIDS, several studies were directed to the evaluation of arousal responses from sleep. Auditory stimulation during sleep has however failed to reveal a higher awakening threshold in similar infants.[39] Like others,[40] we were unable to significantly differentiate the ALTE infants from control infants through hypercarbic and hypoxic arousals challenges, although as shown by other groups, these tests can be abnormal in some ALTE infants.[41]

The two criteria chosen for discontinuing home monitoring were the same as those usually reported in the literature: the absence of a life-threatening event for 3 months despite a biological stress, such as nasopharyngitis or sleep disruption, and, possibly, normalization of a previously abnormal sleep study. Monitoring was interrupted by the end of the first year of age for 178 infants, and before the 22th month of life for the remaining infants. All 200 children with an idiopathic ALTE survived the first year of life. Contrary to other reports, no death occurred during monitoring.[24,26,42] All infants treated for a specific medical or surgical cause, apparently responsible for an ALTE, survived the first year of life. Likewise, no death was seen in the infants with an apparently minor ALTE incident and sent home without treatment or particular surveillance.

If home monitoring has been reported a source of support and reassurance for parents,[42-44] it can also be a source of stress. In our experience, the major psychological impact of home monitoring takes place during the beginning of surveillance and just after its discontinuance. In a prospective study, we compared 20 families with a child monitored to control families matched for age, parity, and social classes.[45] Most monitoring parents (17/20) complained of stress and sense of isolation. Mothers (19/20) developed psychosomatic complaints, such as insomnia or headaches. Older siblings (5/14) were reported to receive less attention from the parents. As reported by others, the mothers' problems persisted several months after monitoring was stopped.[44]

The marketing of "over-the-counter" monitors should therefore be strongly discouraged, as sufficient medical, technical and psychological supportive measures are not offered to the families. Furthermore, inappropriate types of monitors could be chosen.[1,2,29] To determine the frequency of infants monitored without medical advise and supervision we questioned all families presenting an infant to our University sleep clinic between September 1, 1986 and June 1, 1987. They were referred by their pediatrician because of sleep difficulties or to allay the parents' anxiety about sleep apneas. Sleep monitors had been purchased by the parents of 30/622 (4.8%) normal infants with no personal or family history of apnea, of 2/87 (2.2%) infants whose cousin died of SIDS, of 63/210 (30%) siblings of SIDS victims, and of 32/315 (10%) of infants with an ALTE. This prevalence of "over-the-counter" monitoring could of course be partly explained by the high anxiety of this selected group of parents asking for medical advice. A larger study should be undertaken to investigate the incidence of self-monitoring in the general population. Should the results indicate an increasing habit of monitoring without medical advice, the information could cast serious doubt about the validity of recent or future epidemiological studies on SIDS occurrence in various risk groups.

Because of possible family stress and for all the caveats relating to home monitoring discussed above, we resist pressure from parents and referring centers for entering all ALTE infants into our home monitoring program. Only those with a severe idiopathic ALTE, or those rare infants with life-threatening apneas related to other non-treatable conditions benefit from such program.

EXPERIENCE WITH ALTE INFANTS AFTER DISCONTINUANCE OF MONITORING

The evolution of the ALTE infants depends on the severity of the initial life-threatening event. For instance, if status epilepticus follows a hypoxic ischemic episode, prognosis can be poor. In milder cases, appreciation of the child's condition depends on the moment of examination after the event. Transitory abnormalities, such as weakened muscle tone, were observed in the weeks following an event.[46] In some infants, sequelae were seen in the form of fine or gross motor difficulties, hyperactivity, or slowness. It is still unknown whether the abnormalities are a primary cause of the incident or whether it appears secondary to the insult. Retrospective reports of diminished muscle tone or fatigue during feeding led to the suggestion that some SIDS victims were suffering from an underlying brain dysfunction.[47,48] Still, after studying the histories of 42 twins pairs with one SIDS infant we question the specificity of these symptoms.[6]

In a prospective study, we saw no significant difference in the neurodevelopmental performance of 27 previous ALTE infants studied five years after the inital incident and control children matched for age, sex, and social environment.[45] The previous ALTE infants had normal neurological examination, IQ, and language evaluations. They only showed greater frequencies of breath-holding spells (8/27), snoring (6/27), and minimal behavioral difficulties. Conflicting reports in the evaluation of outcome of these infants can be due in part to the small number of children studied and to the possible heterogeneity of the "ALTE" group.

OBSERVATIONS DURING MONITORING RELATED TO A POSSIBLE AUTONOMIC DYSFUNCTION IN ALTE INFANTS

Autonomic dysfunction has been postulated in SIDS, possibly leading to abnormalities of the autonomic regulation of respiratory and/or cardiovascular function. Both excessive sympathetic and vagal abnormalities have been suggested.[49] Some infants with an ALTE were shown to have abnormal heart rate changes during sleep apneas characterized by an excessive heart rate slowing,[11,15] or a decreased heart rate variability.[14] Some infants with an ALTE were also shown to have an increased heart rate,[7,50] a decreased heart rate variability,[50] and a small QT_c index.[51] The isolated bradycardias seen during home monitoring could also illustrate the presence of an autonomic dysfunction in some ALTE infants. In 35 infants with an ALTE, we prospectively performed a 10-second oculocardiac stimulation during quiet wakefulness.[52] The challenge revealed significantly prolonged asystoles in 10 of these infants (up to 12 seconds), compared to those measured in 69 normal controls (RR intervals under 2 seconds). This observation was interpreted as indicating an exaggerated cardioinhibition in a significant number of ALTE infants.

Unexplained episodes of profuse night sweat were repeatedly seen during sleep in 21% of future SIDS victims.[6] We therefore prospectively measured transcutaneous water evaporation rates in 39 ALTE infants, 85 siblings of SIDS victims, and 134 normal control infants.[53] Transepidermal water evaporation rate was measured from the forehead with the use of an Evaporimeter during one night polygraphic sleep recording. During NREM sleep 31% of the ALTE infants had significantly higher evaportation rates than the other infants (20.1 ± 1.9 vs. 11.3 ± 0.7 g/m^2/hr). These characteristics were not related to differences in environmental or rectal temperatures. They were attributed to a possible autonomic dysfunction in some ALTE infants.

GENERAL CONCLUSIONS

Our clinical experience agrees with most of the recent literature that infants with an ALTE form an heterogeneous entity. We could find a specific medical or surgical cause for the event in 61% of the cases. Only 14% of the infants with an apparently severe event entered a home monitoring program. The other infants were treated, whenever appropriate. All infants survived the first year of life. Home monitoring was shown to require continuous assistance to the parents and to create a significant stress to the families. We therefore limit home monitoring to infants for whom no better medical support can be offered. If it is still not known whether some idiopathic ALTE represents real aborted SIDS, the characteristics of the infants with an ALTE, before or at the moment of the event, as well as during home monitoring, cannot be differentiated from those reported for SIDS infants. Observations of infants with an idiopathic ALTE indicate that some infants present symptoms of a possible autonomic dysfunction. The follow-up of the infants five years after the ALTE event reveals no neurodevelopmental abnormality in most of the infants. A systematic exclusional study of the infants with an ALTE, together with appropriate treatment programs could thus provide the possibility of a good survival for most infants. These conclusions appear important as no other form of SIDS prevention is yet available.[1–3,54]

ACKNOWLEDGMENTS

We thank Professor H.L. Vis for constant encouragement. We recognize the scientific contribution, through our collaborative study, of Drs. M. F. Müller, M. Alexander, R. Denis (Brussels), A. Halut-Godin (Namur), and A. Bochner (Antwerpen).

REFERENCES

1. KAHN, A. 1986. Brussels International Workshop on Sudden Infant Death Syndrome, Brussels, Oct. 15–18, 1985. Draft report. Free University of Brussels.
2. Consensus statement. 1987. National Institutes of Health consensus development conference on infantile apnea and home monitoring. Sept. 29 to Oct. 1, 1986. Pediatrics **79:** 292–299.
3. HASSELMEYER, E.G. & J.C. HUNTER. 1985. Sudden infant death syndrome. Child Health **4:** 120–141.
4. KAHN, A., D. BLUM, P. HENNART, C. SELLENS, D. SAMSON-DOLLFUS, J. TAYOT, R. GILLY,

J. DUTRUGE, R. FLORES & B. STERNBERG. 1984. A critical comparison of the history of sudden-death infants and infants hospitalised for near-miss for SIDS. Eur. J. Pediatr. **143:** 103–107.

5. WENNERGREN, G., J. MILERAD, H. LAGERCRANTZ, P. KARLBERG, N.W. SVENNINGSEN, G. SEDIN, D. ANDERSSON, J. GRÖGAARD & J. BJURE. 1987. The epidemiology of attacks of lifelessness and SIDS in Sweden. Acta Paediatr. Scand. (In press).

6. KAHN, A., D. BLUM, M.F. MULLER, L. MONTAUK, A. BOCHNER, N. MONOD, P. PLOUIN, D. SAMSON-DOLLFUS & E.H. DELAGREE. 1986. Sudden Infant Death syndrome in a twin: a comparison of sibling histories. Pediatrics **78:** 146–150.

7. KELLY, D.H., H. GOLUB, D. CARLEY & D.C. SHANNON. 1986. Pneumgrams in infants who subsequently died of sudden infant death syndrome. J. Pediatr **109:** 249–254.

8. KRONGRAD, E. & L. O'NEILL. 1986. Near miss sudden infant death syndrome episodes? A clinical and electrocardiographic correlation. Pediatrics **77:** 811–815.

9. VALDES-DAPENA, M. 1980. Sudden infant death syndrome: a review of the medical literature 1974–1979. Pediatrics **66:** 597–614.

10. KAHN, A., L. MONTAUK & D. BLUM. 1987. Diagnostic categories in infants referred for an acute event suggesting near-miss SIDS. Eur. J. Pediatr. **146:** 458–460.

11. GUILLEMINAULT, C., R. PERAITA, M. SOUQUET & W.C. DEMENT. 1975. Apneas during sleep in infants: possible relationship with sudden infant death syndrome. Science **190:** 677–679.

12. KELLY, D.H. & D.C. SHANNON. 1979. Periodic breathing in infants with near-miss sudden infant death syndrome. Pediatrics **63:** 355–359.

13. GUILLEMINAULT, C., R. ARIAGNO, R. KOROBKIN, L. NAGEL, R. BALDWIN, S. COONS & M. OWEN. 1979. Mixed and obstructive sleep apnea and near miss for sudden infant death syndrome. II. Comparison of near miss and normal control infants by age. Pediatrics **64:** 862–891.

14. HOPPENBROUWERS, T., J.E. HODGMAN, K. ARAKAWA, D.J. MCGINTY, J. MASON, R.M. HARPER & M.B. STERMAN. 1978. Sleep apnea as part of a sequence of events: a comparison of three months old infants at low and increased risk for sudden infant death syndrome (SIDS). Neuropädiatrie **9:** 320–337.

15. GUILLEMINAULT, C., R. ARIAGNO, S. COONS, R. WINKLE, R. KOROBKIN, R. BALDWIN & M. SOUQUET. 1985. Near-Miss sudden infant death syndrome in eight infants with sleep apnea-related cardiac arrhythmias. Pediatrics **76:** 236–242.

16. KAHN, A., D. BLUM, P. WATERSCHOOT, E. ENGELMAN & P. SMETS. 1982. Effects of obstructive sleep apneas on transcutaneous oxygen pressure in control infants, siblings of sudden infant death syndrome victims, and near miss infants: comparison with the effects of central sleep apneas. Pediatrics **70:** 852–857.

17. OREN, J., D. KELLY & D.C. SHANNON. 1986. Identification of a high-risk group for sudden infant death syndrome among infants who were resuscitated for sleep apnea. Pediatrics **77:** 495–499.

18. BARRINGTON, K.J., N.N. FINER, K.L. PETERS & J. BARTON. 1986. Physiologic effects of doxapram in idiopathic apnea of prematurity. J. Pediatr. **108:** 125–129.

19. KELLY, D.H. & D.C. SHANNON. 1981. Treatment of apnea and excessive periodic breathing in the full-term infant. Pediatrics **68:** 183–186.

20. VANDENPLAS, Y., D. DE WOLFF & L. SACRE. 1986. Influence of xanthines on gastroesophageal reflux in infants at risk for sudden infant death syndrome. Pediatrics **77:** 807–810.

21. DAVIS, J.M., K. METRAKOS & J.V. ARANDA. 1986. Apnoea and seizures. Arch. Dis. Child. **61:** 791–806.

22. DAVIDSON WARD, S.L., T.G. KEENS, L.S. CHAN, B.E. CHIPPS, S.H. CARSON, D.D. DEMING, V. KRISHNA, H.M. MACDONALD, G.I. MARTIN, K.S. MEREDITH, T.A. MERRITT, B.G. NICKERSON, R.A. STODDARD & A.L. VAN DER HAL. 1986. Sudden infant death syndrome in infants evaluated by apnea programs in California. Pediatrics **77:** 451–455.

23. KATCHER, M.L., M.M. SHAPIRO & C. GUIST. 1986. Severe injury and death associated with home infant cardiorespiratory monitors. Pediatrics **78:** 775–779.

24. KELLY, D.H., D.C. SHANNON & K. O'CONNELL. 1978. Care of infants with near-miss sudden infant death syndrome. Pediatrics **61:** 511–514.

25. LEWAK, N. 1975. Sudden Infant Death syndrome in a hospitalized infant on an apnea monitor. Pediatrics **56:** 296–298.

26. MONOD, N., P. PLOUIN, B. STERNBERG, P. PEIRANO, N. PAJOT, R. FLORES, S. LINNETT, B. KASTLER, C. SCAVONE & S. GUIDASCI. 1986. Are polygraphic and cariopneumographic respiratory patterns useful tools for predicting the risk for sudden infant dath syndrome? Biol. Neonate **50:** 147–153.

27. KAHN, A., D. BLUM & L. MONTAUK. 1986. Polysomnographic studies and home monitoring of siblings of SIDS victims and of infants with no family history of sudden infant death. Eur. J. Pediatr. **145:** 351–356.

28. NELSON, N.M. 1978. But who shall monitor the monitor? Pediatrics **61:** 663–665.

29. Task force on prolonged infantile apnea. American Academy of Pediatrics. 1985. Prolonged infantile apnea: 1985. Pediatrics **76:** 129–131.

30. KAHN, A., D. HASAERTS & D. BLUM. 1985. Phenothiazine-induced sleep apneas in normal infants. Pediatrics **75:** 844–847.

31. ABREU E SILVA, F.A., U.M. MACFADYEN, A. WILLIAMS & H. SIMPSON. 1986. Sleep apnoea during upper respiratory infection and metabolic alkalosis in infancy. Arch. Dis. Child. **61:** 1056–1062.

32. TONKIN, S. 1975. Sudden infant death syndrome: hypothesis of causation. Pediatrics **55:** 650–660.

33. KAHN, A., D. BLUM, A. HOFFMAN, M. HAMOIR, D. MOULIN, M. SPEHL & L. MONTAUK. 1985. Obstructive sleep apnea induced by a parapharyngeal cystic hygroma in an infant. Sleep **8:** 363–366.

34. KAHN, A., A. SANGELEER & D. BLUM. 1985. Effects of sleep position upon transcutaneous gas tension in infants. Arch. Fr. Pediatr. **42:** 419–421.

35. HERBST, J.J., L.S. BOOK & P.F. BRAY. 1978. Gastroesophageal reflux in the 'near miss' sudden infant death syndrome. J. Pediatr. **92:** 73–75.

36. WALSH, J.K., FARRELL M.K. & W.J. KEENAN. 1981. Gastroesophageal reflux in infants. Relation ot apnea. J. Pediatr. **99:** 197–199.

37. HARPER, R.M., B. LEAKE, H. HOFFMAN, D.O. WALTER, T. HOPPENBROUWERS, J. HODGMAN & M.B. STERMAN. 1981. Periodicity of sleep states is altered in infants at risk for the sudden infant death syndrome. Science **213:** 1030.

38. GUILLEMINAULT, C., R. ARIAGNO, R. KOROBKIN, S. COONS, M. OWEN-BOEDDIKER & R. BALDWIN. 1981. Sleep parameters and respiratory variables in 'near miss' sudden infant death syndrome infants. Pediatrics **68:** 354–360.

39. KAHN, A., E. PICARD & D. BLUM. 1986. Auditory arousal thresholds of normal and near-miss SIDS infants. Dev. Med. Ch. Neurol. **28:** 299–302.

40. ARIAGNO, R., L. NAGEL & C. GUILLEMINAULT. 1980. Waking and ventilatory responses during sleep in infants near-miss for sudden infant death syndrome. Sleep **3:** 351–354.

41. HUNT, C.E. 1981. Abnormal hypercarbic and hypoxic sleep arousal responses in near-miss SIDS infants. Pediatr. Res. **15:** 1462–1464.

42. KELLY, D.H. & D.C. SHANNON. 1982. Sudden infant death syndrome and near sudden infant death syndrome: a review of the literature, 1964 to 1982. Pediatr. Cl. North Am. **29:** 1241–1261.

43. CAIN, L.P., D.H. KELLY & D.C. SHANNON. 1980. Parent's perceptions of the psychological and social impact of home monitoring. Pediatrics **66:** 37–39.

44. MCELROY, E., A. STEINSCHNEIDER & S. WEINSTEIN. 1986. Emotional and health impact of home monitoring on mothers: a controlled prospective study. Pediatrics **78:** 780–786.

45. KAHN, A., F. VERSTRAETEN & D. BLUM. 1984. Preliminary report on neurodevelopmental screening in children previously at risk for Sudden Infant Death syndrome. J. Pediatr. **105:** 666–668.

46. KOROBKIN, R. & C. GUILLEMINAULT. 1979. Neurologic abnormalities in near miss for sudden infant death syndrome infants. Pediatrics **64:** 369–374.

47. NAEYE, R.L., B. LADIS & J.S. DRAGE. 1976. Sudden infant death syndrome: a prospective study. Am. J. Dis. Child. **130:** 1207–1210.

48. STEINSCHNEIDER, A., S.L. WEINSTEIN & E. DIAMOND. 1982. The sudden infant death syndrome and apnea/obstruction during neonatal sleep and feeding. Pediatrics **70:** 858–863.

49. SCHWARTZ, P.J. 1976. Cardiac sympathetic innervation and the sudden infant death syndrome: a possible pathological link. Am. J. Med. **60:** 167–169.

50. LEISTNER, H.L., G.G. HADDAD, R.A. EPSTEIN, L.T. LAI, M.A.F. EPSTEIN & R.B. MELLINS.

1980. Heart rate and heart rate variability during sleep in aborted sudden infant death syndrome. J. Pediatr. **97:** 51–55.

51.   HADDAD, G.G., M.A.F. EPSTEIN, R.A. EPSTEIN, N.M. MAZZA, R.B. MELLINS & E. KRONGRAD. 1979. The QT interval in aborted SIDS infants. Pediatr. Res. **13:** 136–138.

52.   KAHN, A., J. RIAZI & D. BLUM. 1983. Oculocardiac reflex in near miss for Sudden Infant Death syndrome infants. Pediatrics **71:** 49–52.

53.   KAHN, A., C. VAN DE MERCKT, M. DRAMAIX, P. MAGREZ, D. BLUM, E. REBUFFAT & L. MONTAUK. 1987. Transepidermal sleep water loss in at risk for sudden infant death and control infants. Pediatrics. (In press.)

54.   SOUTHALL, D.P., J.M. RICHARDS, V. STEBBENS, A.J. WILSON, V. TAYLOR & J.R. ALEXANDER. 1986. Cardiorespiratory function in 16 full-term infants with sudden infant death syndrome. Pediatrics **78:** 787–796.

Drug-Addicted Mothers, Their Infants, and SIDS

TOVE S. ROSEN[a] AND HELEN L. JOHNSON[b]

[a]Department of Pediatrics
College of Physicians and Surgeons
New York, New York 10032
[b]Department of Early Childhood
Queens College
Flushing, New York

In the past decade we have seen an increasing number of newborns born to substance-abusing mothers. The pattern and incidence of drug abuse has changed in the recent years.[1-3] Previously, we saw babies born to mothers taking heroin, alcohol, methadone-maintenance, and "pills." At present the most used drugs are cocaine, marijuana with or without alcohol, and occasional heroin and PCP. All these drugs cross the placenta and enter the fetus. With this change in the drug abuse pattern, we are seeing an increase in the incidence of obstetrical complications such as abruptio placentae, premature labor, fetal distress, venereal disease,[4-7] and a higher admission rate of premature and asphyxiated infants in our neonatal intensive care units. There has been a surge of reports in both the medical and lay literature on the effects of cocaine on pregnancy and on the neonate. These reports have described neonates with decreased birth weight and length and head circumferences; central nervous system abnormalities and cerebral infarcts, a syndrome of increased tone, abnormal movements, irritability and increased deep tendon reflexes, abnormal EEGs and evoked visual potentials; and genitourinary abnormalities.[5-12] It should be remembered, however, that cocaine was one of several drugs abused by many of these mothers.

These same infants have a 5-10 times increased risk of dying of sudden infant death syndrome in comparison to the general population.[13,14] SIDS was the cause of death for 25% of infants who died in the first year of life and had been born to addicted women in New York City compared to 10% of the general population.[3]

We will report on data collected from three groups of mothers and their infants. The mothers were multidrug abusers, on methadone maintenance, or on no drugs of abuse. The primary drugs used were cocaine and marijuana with/without mild to moderate alcohol intake. Data on the perinatal period and the first 12 months of life will be presented.

SUBJECTS AND METHODS

In 1982, we began a study of 111 pregnant women from our prenatal clinic, with a history of multidrug abuse, methadone maintenance, and no substance abuse during the second and early third trimester of pregnancy. Written consent was obtained. The women who were substance abusers and on methadone maintenance were followed in the high risk prenatal clinic. Urines were collected at least five times during pregnancy from all subjects and tested for drugs of abuse. We screened for the following drugs: heroin, methadone, barbiturates, cocaine, benzodiazepines, PCP, and marijuana. Drug question-

89

TABLE 1. Maternal Characteristics

	Group I Methadone ($N = 25$)	Group II Multidrug ($N = 42$)	Group III Control ($N = 44$)
Age (M ± SE)	29.2 ± .8[a]	24.7 ± .8	25.5 ± .8
Gravida (M ± SE)	4.8 ± .5[a]	3.7 ± .3	3.5 ± .3
Para (M ± SE)	2.0 ± .4[a]	1.3 ± .2	1.4 ± .2
Positive Ob.Hx[b]	40%	36%	23%
PROM[c] > 16 hr	20%	14%	11%
Race:			
White	20%	5%	7%
Black	60%	57%	43%
Hispanic	20%	32%	50%
Smoking > 1 pack/day	90%[a]	83%[a]	14%

[a] $p < .05$.
[b] Premature rupture of membranes.
[c] Positive obstetrical history.

naires were administered monthly to further determine drug usage. We know that the quality of parenting and maternal attitudes play an important role in the outcome of the child from our previous studies[15,16] To measure these variables, two personality questionnaires, Coopersmith Self Esteem Scale and the Depression Adjective check list, were administered and data collected on family, housing, environment, welfare, etc., by the project social worker.

After birth the neonate had a physical and neurological examination. While in the hospital, daily observations were made for withdrawal-like symptoms (irritability, tremors, tone abnormalities, feeding problems, temperature instability) and scored as mild, moderate, and severe using a previously devised scoring system.[17]

A Brazelton Neonatal Behavioral Assessment was performed using the subscales of habituation to light and rattle, auditory and visual interaction, and consolability.[18]

At discharge we reviewed both maternal and neonatal charts for pertinent information.

If the neonate was full term and free of serious neonatal complications such as Apgar score of < 3 at 1 minute and <5 at 5 minutes, sepsis, moderate-to-severe respiratory distress, exchange transfusions, and seizures he/she was enrolled in a follow-up program after obtaining a second written consent.

In follow-up the infant was seen at 2 weeks and then at 2, 4, 6, and 12 months of age. A physical examination and various behavioral evaluations were performed at each visit. At 6 and 12 months the infants also had a neurological examination and the Bayley Scales of Infant Development. Social service updates were obtained at each follow-up visit. Well baby and emergency medical and social service assistance were also provided.

RESULTS

TABLE 1 is a summary of the maternal characteristics of the three groups. The groups include the following pregnant women: Group I, 25 on methadone maintenance; Group II, 42 on multi substance abuse; and Group III, 44 on no drugs of abuse. Group I women were older but within child-bearing age and had a higher rate of pregnancy and number of children. The rate of obstetrical complications was similar in all groups but groups I and II had more frequent admissions for premature labor and a higher incidence of fetal heart rate abnormalities. Cigarette smoking of greater than one pack per day was significantly more frequent in groups I and II. Group I mothers were taking a mean dose of 51.9±4 mg of methadone per day during the first trimester and 49.1±4 mg during the third trimester of gestation. However, 12% used only methadone. The other 88% were using cocaine, marijuana, and alcohol in various combinations. In Group II, 70% were using cocaine in combination with marijuana and/or mild-to-moderate intake of alcohol and 30% were using marijuana with or without alcohol. The quantity of substance abuse decreased between the first and third trimester in both groups. All three groups were of similar socioeconomic class with the majority being on welfare or with no income. Many lived in substandard housing or welfare hotels. The Depression Adjective Check List administered during pregnancy demonstrated a more depressed score in the drug-free mothers (Group III) ($p <$ .05). This unexpected difference in the depression scale may be related to the drug intake of the mother. The scores on the self-esteem scale, however, showed that the mothers in groups I and II had lower self esteem ($p <$ .05). Low self esteem is associated with drug abuse.[3]

TABLE 2 is a summary of the neonatal data. The infants of mothers on methadone maintenance seemed to be most affected. The rate of prematurity was higher, birth weight lower, with a higher incidence of small size for gestational age and a mean head circumference significantly less than in Group III infants. These findings have been reported by others also. Group II infants fell between Group I and Group III. Symptoms of abstinence syndrome were also more frequent and severe in Group I infants. This also has been reported previously.[17]

The Brazelton assessments revealed significantly depressed responses to the interactive items in group I ($p <$ .05) infants but no significant differences were noted between the group II and group III infants. At discharge, those infants who were full term and without serious neonatal complications except abstinence syndrome were enrolled in the follow-up project.

During follow-up, one infant in Group I and three in Group II expired from the sudden

TABLE 2. Neonatal Characteristics

	Group I Methadone (N = 24)	Group II Multidrug (N = 41)	Group III Control (N = 44)
Gestational age (wk)[a]	38.2 ± 0.5[b]	39.3 ± 0.3[b]	40 ± 0.2
Premature rate (%)	25%	7%	2%
Apgar (5 min)[a]	8.7 ± 0.1	8.9 ± 0.0	8.6 ± 0.1
Sex			
Male (N)	16	22	15
Female (N)	8	19	26
Birthweight (g)[a]	2830 ± 92[b]	3174 ± 67[b]	3438 ± 75
Small for gestational age	25%	10%	5%
Head circumferenc (P)[a,c]	20.9 ± 5.4[b]	32.6 ± 4.5	46.7 ± 3.9
Withdrawal			
None	38%	82%	
Mild	29%	15%	
Moderate	33%[b]	3%	
Severe	0%	0%	
Abnormal neurological exam	42%[b]	10%	8%
Neonatal complications	29%	29%	34%
Prolonged hospitalization	38%[b]	15%	5%

[a]Expressed as M ± SE.
[b]$p <$ .05.
[c]P, percentile.

infant death syndrome. The autopsies were performed by the Medical Examiners Office in Manhattan, N.Y. All four infants were full term and with no history of serious neonatal complications. They died between 6 and 10 weeks of life. The infant in Group I was born to a mother who was using cocaine in addition to her methadone, the two infants in Group II were born to mothers on cocaine and marijuana and the third infant was born to a mother with heavy marijuana and mild alcohol abuse. No infant expired in Group III.

The follow-up data are presented in TABLES 3 and 4. The infants in Group I are shorter and continue to have significantly smaller head circumferences, which have been described by others. The frequency of otitis media is consistently higher in Groups I and II through the first 12 months of life. Anemia was more common in Group I children. These findings may be associated with developmental problems in childhood.[19,20] TABLE 5 summarizes the neurobehavioral data at 6 and 12 months. Neurological abnormalities of tone, coordination, irritability, and delays in developmental milestones were more common in Groups I and II at 6 months and more common in Group I at 12 months. The Bayley MDI scores were also significantly lower in the Group I infants at both 6 and 12 months of age but in the low average range, which also has been previously reported.[17]

TABLE 3. Six Months Data

	Group I Methadone ($N = 16$)	Group II Multidrug ($N = 29$)	Group III Control ($N = 31$)
Weight $(P)^{a,c}$	43.9 ± 8.8	63.5 ± 5.8	52.0 ± 5.5
Height $(P)^{a,c}$	34.3 ± 6.8	63.4 ± 5.1	65.0 ± 4.1
Head circumference $(P)^{a,c}$	14.1 ± 3.7^b	49.0 ± 4.5	40.6 ± 3.9
Blood pressure (systolic)^a	90.4 ± 1.3	92.6 ± 2.2	88.0 ± 1.4
Visits to clinic^a	1.5 ± 0.6	1.4 ± 0.2	0.8 ± 0.2
Incidence of infections (%)			
Otitis media	38^b	34	16
Respiratory	6	3	10
Monilial rash	25	10	13
Thrush	6	3	10

^{a}Expressed as M ± SE.
$^b p < .05$.
$^c P$, percentile.

DISCUSSION

As can be seen, the infants born to mothers on methadone maintenance for their heroin addiction are at higher risk for problems in the neonatal period (prematurity, low birth weight, decreased head circumference and length, and moderate-to-severe abstinence syndrome) and for neurobehavioral problems in infancy and early childhood.[21-24] The infants born to the mothers with multidrug abuse fall in between the other two groups, as far as outcome measures are concerned, with no significant differences from controls.

Reports on the effects of maternal cocaine use have revealed effects on birthweight and length and head circumference. The numbers in this study were small and perhaps the quality and route of cocaine intake in 1982 were different. Comparing the group I infants in this study to our previous study of infants born to mothers on methadone maintenance, they appear to be more affected in the neonatal period as far as birthweight, length and head circumference, and head circumference and Bayley MDI scores at 6 and 12 months of age. The incidence of other substance abuse, especially of cocaine and marijuana, was

TABLE 4. Twelve Months Data

	Group I Methadone ($N = 12$)	Group II Multidrug ($N = 18$)	Group III Control ($N = 28$)
Weight $(P)^a$	50.2 ± 4.9	48.8 ± 7.4	49.6 ± 5.1
Height $(P)^a$	48.8 ± 9.8	61.4 ± 5.1	68.9 ± 4.5
Head circumference $(P)^a$	17.4 ± 4.9^b	29.4 ± 5.0	33.0 ± 3.4
BP systolic (mm Hg)^a	93.6 ± 3.7	98.1 ± 4.7	99.3 ± 2.7
Visits to clinic	1.4 ± 0.5	1.2 ± 0.3	1.2 ± 0.3
Incidence of infections (%)			
Otitis media	50^b	50^b	25
Respiratory	7	6	8
Rash (impetigo, monilial)	17	28	11
Anemia (%)	33^c	6	6

^{a}Expressed as Mean $\pm$ SE.
$^b p < .05$.
$^c p < .09$.

significantly higher in the second study. A higher incidence of fetal alcohol syndrome has been reported in infants born to mothers on marijuana and alcohol.[25]

The incidence of SIDS has been consistently higher in infants of substance-abusing mothers. During 1970 to 1980, the incidence of SIDS in infants of mothers on methadone maintenace was reported to be in the 2–3% range (20–30/1,000 live births versus 2–3/1,000 live births in the general population.[26–30] Recently a 1–17% incidence of SIDS has been described in infants of multidrug abusers including those abusing cocaine.[13,14] The mechanisms and causes for this high incidence of SIDS are not known. It has been difficult to make any association between a specific substance abuse and SIDS as most of these mothers are multidrug users.[14]

SIDS has a usual peak incidence at 3 and 4 months of age. Most of the infants of substance-abusing mothers expired somewhat earlier, during the first 2–3 months of life. Abnormalities in the regulation of respiratory pattern have been described. Infants born to mothers on methadone maintenance showed a depressed response to carbon dioxide.[31] Chasnoff and Davidson found abnormal pneumograms more frequently in infants of mothers who used cocaine or multiple drugs.[13,14] They described greater duration of apneas and more periodic breathing. In addition, the mean respiratory rate was higher and

TABLE 5. Neurobehavioral Data at 6 and 12 Months of Age

	Group I Methodone	Group II Multidrug	Group III Control
6 Months	$N = 16$	$N = 29$	$N = 31$
Neuro S→Abnl.	$44\%^b$	21%	16%
Bayley MDI^a	91.5 ± 2.2^b	104.7 ± 2.9	100.9 ± 2.8
PDI^a	96.7 ± 4.0	104.3 ± 0.8	100.2 ± 2.7
12 Months	$N = 12$	$N = 18$	$N = 28$
Neuro S→Abnl.	$42\%^b$	6%	4%
Bayley PDI^a	93.8 ± 3.7 ^{b}	105.4 ± 2.8	105.0 ± 3.2
MDI^a	101.8 ± 4.7	107.2 ± 3.0	106.4 ± 2.8

^{a}Expressed as Mean $\pm$ SE.
$^b p < .05$.
Neuro S→Abnl = Neurological examination: suspect to abnormal.

the mean heart rate was lower than in controls.[14] The frequency of abnormalities was higher in those infants less than 2 months of age.[14] In addition 4/22 had apnea of prematurity.[13] The authors suggested that these findings place these infants at higher risk for SIDS. However, none of the infants with abnormal pneumograms died of SIDS, and recently the value of the pneumogram[32,33] in predicting SIDS has been questioned as has the apnea hypothesis. Another possible mechanism related to SIDS is autonomic dysfunction with developmental abnormalities of the cardiac sympathetic system. This may manifest itself as an imbalance in the development of the right and left cardiac sympathetic nerves or as an imbalance in the sympathetic versus parasympathetic activity making the heart more susceptible to arrhythmias and cardiac death.[29] These abnormalities may be secondary to drug exposure *in utero*. For example, cocaine may interfere with the development or function of the sympathetic nervous system because of its blocking effect on the uptake of norepinephrine at the adrenergic nerve end terminals. This would make infants more susceptible to arrhythmias during the adjustment period and predispose them to SIDS.

Other abnormalities are present that may be related to autonomic nervous system imbalance in infants of methadone-maintained mothers, such as transient hypertension between two and twelve weeks of age, abstinence syndrome, and abnormal response to noise.[21,23] Another possibility is hypoxic changes in the neonatal heart sustained during episodes of maternal cocaine "high," which is accompanied by decreased uteroplacental perfusion.[34,35] Other risk factors in this group include low socioeconomic status, young mothers, heavy cigarette smoking, and the majority being black.[36-38]

In summary, these infants are at higher risk for multiple problems that include both growth and neurodevelopmental problems and sudden infant death syndrome. Much more research is needed to assess the etiology of these findings and then to arrive at appropriate intervention programs.

REFERENCES

1. NIDA Statistics. August, 1984.
2. PARKER, S., B. ZUCKERMAN, D. FRANK, R. VINCI, M. BAUCHNER et al. 1987. The prevalence of in utero exposure to cocaine and marijuana. Pediatr. Res. 21: 401A (abst. 1364).
3. DEREN, S. 1986. Children of substance abusers: A review of the literature. J. Substance Abuse Treat. 3: 77.
4. ACKER, D., B.P. SACHS, K.J. TRACEY & W.E. WISE. 1984. Abruptio placentae associated with cocaine use. Am. J. Obstet. Gynecol. 146: 220.
5. CHASNOFF, I.J., W.J. BURNS, S.H. SCHNOLL & K.A. BURNS. 1985. Cocaine use in pregnancy. N. Eng. J. Med. 313: 666.
6. LIFSCHITZ, M.H., F. WALTERS & G.S. WILSON. 1986. Perinatal effects of cocaine abuse. Pediatr. Res. 21: 206A (Abst. 322).
7. LINESAY, S., S. EHRLICH & L.P. FINNEGAN. 1987. Cocaine and pregnancy and maternal and infant outcome. Pediatr. Res. 21: 238A (Abst. 387).
8. CHASNOFF, I. & G. CHISURN. 1987. Genitourinary tract dysmorphology and maternal cocaine use. Pediatr. Res. 21: 225A (Abst. 317).
9. CHASNOFF, I.J., M.E. BUSSEY, R. SAVICH & C.M. STACK. 1986. Perinatal cerebral infarction and maternal cocaine use. J. Pediatr. 108: 456.
10. DOBERZAK, T.M., S. SHANZER & S.R. KANDALL. 1987. Neonatal effects of cocaine abuse in pregnancy. Pediatr. Res. 21: 359A (Abst. 1114).
11. DIXON, S.D., R.W. COEN & S. HUTCHFIELD. 1987. Visual dysfunction in cocaine-exposed infants. Pediatr. Res. 21: 359A (Abst. 1112).
12. CHASNOFF, I.J., R. HATCHER & W.J. BURNS. 1982. Polydrug- and methadone-addicted newborns: A continuum of impairment. Pediatrics 70: 210.
13. CHASNOFF, I., C. HUNT, R. KLETTER & D. KAPLAN. 1986. Increased risk of SIDS and

respiratory pattern abnormalities in cocaine exposed infants. Pediatr. Res. **20:** 425A (Abst. 1589).

14. DAVIDSON, S.L., S. SCHULTZ, V. KIRSHNA, X. BEAN, W. WINGERT, L. WACHSMAN & T.G. KEENS. 1986. Abnormal sleeping ventilatory pattern in infants of substance-abusing mothers. Am. J. Dis. Child. **140:** 1015.

15. FIKS, K.B., H.L. JOHNSON & T.S. ROSEN. 1985. Methadone-maintained mothers: 3–year follow-up of parental functioning. Intl. J. Add. **20:** 651.

16. ELARDO, R., R. BRADLEY & B.M. CALDWELL. 1975. The relation of infants' home environments to mental test performance from six to thirty-six months: A longitudinal analysis. Child. Develop. **46:** 71.

17. ROSEN, T.S. & H.L. JOHNSON. 1982. Children of methadone-maintained mothers: Follow-up to 18 months. J. Pediatr. **101:** 192.

18. BRAZELTON, B.T. 1976. Neonatal behavioral assessment scale. Clin. Dev. Med. No. 50.

19. TEELE, D.W., J.O. KLEIN & B.A. ROSNER. 1984. The Greater Boston Otitis Media Group, Otitis media with effusion during the first 3 years of life and development of speech and hearing. Pediatrics **74:** 282.

20. LOZOFF, B., G.M. BRILLENHAM, F.E. VITORI, A.W. WOLF & J.J. UNUTIA. 1982. Developmental deficits in iron deficient infants: Effects of age and severity of iron lack, J. Pediatr. **101:** 948.

21. STRAUSS, M.E., J.K. LESSEN-FIRESTONE, C.J. CHAVEZ & J.C. STRYKER. 1979. Children of methadone-treated women at five years of age. Pharm. Biochem. Behav. **2:** 3 (Suppl.).

22. LIFSHITZ, M.H., G.S. WILSON, E.O. SMITH & M.M. DESMOND. 1983. Fetal and postnatal growth of children born to narcotic dependent women. J. Pediatr. **102:** 686.

23. ROSEN, T.S. & H.L. JOHNSON. 1985. Longterm effects of prenatal methadone maintenance, NIDA Research Monograph. Series 59. DHHS Pub. No: (ADM) **85.**

24. KALTENBACH, K. & L.P. FINNEGAN. 1984. Developmental outcome of children born to methadone maintained women: A review of longitudinal studies. Neurobehav. Toxicol. Teratol. **6:** 271.

25. HINGSON, R., J.J. ALPERT, N. DAY, E. DOOLING, H. KAYNE, S. MORELOCK, E. OPPENHEIMER & B. ZUCKERMAN. 1982. Effects of maternal drinking and marijuana use in fetal growth and development. Pediatrics **70:** 539.

26. CHAVEZ, C.J., E.M. OSTREA, JR., J.C. STRYKER & Z. SMIALEK. 1979. SIDS among infants of drug dependent mothers. J. Pediatr. **95:** 407.

27. FINNEGAN, L.P. 1979. In utero opiate dependence and SIDS. Clin. Perinat. **6:** 163.

28. RAJEGOWDA, B.K., S.R. KANDALL & L. FALCIGERIA. 1978. Sudden unexpected death in infants of narcotic-dependent mothers. Early Hum. Dev. **2:** 219.

29. HUNT, C.E. & R.T. BROUILETTE. 1987. Sudden infant death syndrome. J Pediatr. **110:** 669.

30. SCHWARTZ, P.J. 1987. The quest for the mechanism of the sudden infant death syndrome: doubts and progress. Circulation **75:** 677.

31. OLSEN, G.O. & M.H. LEES. 1980. Ventilatory response to carbon dioxide of infants following chronic prenatal methadone exposure. J. Pediatr. **96:** 983.

32. Infantile Apnea and Home Monitoring in NIH Consensus Development Conference Statement v6. Oct. 1986.

33. WAGGENER, T.B., D.P. SOUTHALL & L.A. SCOTT. 1987. Analysis of breathing patterns in a prospective populations does not predict susceptibility to SIDS. Ped. Res. **22:** 506A. (Abst. 1998).

34. MOORE, T.R., J. SORG, L. MILLER, T.C. KAY & R. RESNIK. 1986. Hemodynamic effects of intravenous cocaine on the pregnant ewe and fetus. Am. J. Obstet. Gynecol. **155:** 883.

35. FERRIS, J.A.J. 1973. Hypoxic changes in conducting tissue of the heart in sudden death in infancy syndrome. Brit. Med. J. **2:** 23.

36. BLACK, L., R.J. DAVID, R.T. BROUILETTE & C. HUNT. 1986. Effects of birthweight and ethnicity on incidence of SIDS. J. Pediatr. **108:** 209.

37. BABSON, S.G. & N.G. CLARKE. 1983. Relationship between infant death and maternal age. J. Pediatr. **103:** 391.

38. TOUBAS, P.L., J.C. DUKE, A. McCAFFREE, C. MALLION, D. BENDALL & W.C. ORR. 1986. Effects of maternal smoking and caffeine habits on infantile apnea: A retrospective study. Pediatrics **78:** 159.

Prevention of Unexpected Infant Death

A Review of Risk-Related Intervention in Six Centers[a]

R. G. CARPENTER,[b] A. GARDNER,[b] J. HARRIS,[c]
M. JUDD,[d] J. LEWRY,[e] C. R. MADDOCK,[f] J. POWELL,[g]
AND E. M. TAYLOR[h]

[b]London School of Hygiene and Tropical Medicine
London, England

[c]Cornwall and Isles of Scilly Health Authority

[d]North and West Hertfordshire Health Authority

[e]Southampton General Hospital
Southampton, England

[f]King's Mill Hospital
Mansfield, England

[g]Portsmouth and South East Hampshire Health Authority

[h]Department of Paediatrics
University of Sheffield
Sheffield, England

INTRODUCTION

Unexpected infant mortality fell abruptly in Sheffield following the set-up of a risk-related intervention study.[1] A high-risk group was identified at birth by the Birth Score, a discriminant score calculated from eight risk factors. For the first two years of the study, half, and subsequently all, of the high-risk infants received extra primary health care for the first six months in the form of five extra home visits by health visitors, highly trained community health nurses. The discriminant score was designed to identify both explained and unexplained unexpected infant deaths, designated "possibly preventable deaths."[2] Sunderland et al.[3] have shown that unexpected deaths due to known causes fell dramatically but that unexpected and unexplained deaths were also reduced during the course of this study. In consequence, the team responsible for the Sheffield Project has been invited to assist in setting up similar schemes in five other areas. The work is continuing in Sheffield and three of these five areas. For this report the areas are labeled A to F, Sheffield being area D. Two studies took place in area B and are referred to as study B1 and B2.

[a]Supported by a series of grants from the Foundation for the Study of Infant Deaths.

PRINCIPLES OF RISK-RELATED INTERVENTION

The principle of risk-related intervention is that those at increased risk should receive more preventive care than those at lower risk. Optimal allocation of preventive resources is achieved when, as a result of the redistribution of resources, the risk is the same for everyone.[4]

The potential advantage of optimizing allocation of resources is illustrated as follows. Suppose the high-risk group is identified by a discriminant score and that scores of cases and controls are normally distributed with the same variance, s^2, but with means m_1 and m_2, respectively. Let

$$d = (m_1 - m_2)/s.$$

If the score is used to divide the population into high and low risk groups for optimal allocation of resources, the best point to choose is approximately at the score

$$x = (3m_1 + m_2)/4.$$

TABLE 1. Specificity and Sensitivity of a High-Risk Group Identified Using a Discriminant Score

d^a	Specificity % Controls Low-Risk	Sensitivity % Cases High-Risk	% Reduction in Case Rate by Optimum Allocation of Care[b]
0.75	71	57	15
1.0	77	60	27
1.25	81	64	39
1.5	84	69	48
2.0	89	77	68
2.5	93	84	81
3.0	96	89	89

[a]d, the difference between mean scores of cases and controls in SD units.
[b]The potential percentage reduction in case rate achievable by optimum allocation of resources.

TABLE 1 shows the specificity and sensitivity of this division of the population in relation to d. TABLE 1 also shows the potential reduction of the overall case rate obtained by optimal allocation of fixed total resources to these two groups, as a percentage of the case rate when the same resources are uniformly allocated to all members of the population regardless of risk.

From TABLE 1 it is seen that, even when cases and control mean scores are only one standard deviation apart, a 27% reduction in case rate can be achieved simply by optimal allocation of resources. At this level of d, the specificity of the high-risk group is only 77% and sensitivity 60%, i.e. the high-risk group will comprise 23% of the population and only 60% of the cases.

METHODS

In the present studies, data are collected at birth on all infants in a defined population. The necessary form is usually tagged to the birth notification form so that coverage is virtually complete. Birth scores were calculated from these data (APPENDIX 1). In four areas, a second questionnaire was completed by the health visitors at four weeks, enabling the Sheffield month score to be calculated (APPENDIX 2).

Because infants with birth scores of less than 400 are very seldom high-risk at one month, in two areas (A and C) only infants scoring 400 or more at birth were scored at one month. In these areas, data additionally collected on a 10% sample of infants with scores below 400 were used to estimate the month scores of the infants who were only scored at birth.

In all the areas, as soon as the forms were returned, the data were processed using a microcomputer, a DEC PDP 11 VO3 in Sheffield and a Commodore 8032 in each of the other areas. The computer generated the necessary slips for notification of high-risk infants and in some areas provided additional data on health visitors' case loads to ensure that they were manageable.

Intervention varied from study to study. In the first two years in Sheffield (study D), infants were weighed and measured at each visit and a questionnaire was completed on the health of the child and family since the last visit. Four extra staff were used. Subsequently, no additional health visitors were allocated to the Study. Existing staff were notified of risk status and encouraged to follow the protocol described in the introduction.

In study A, health visitors were informed and encouraged to maintain regular contact with the family. In studies B1 and C, the community health staff were informed of the procedure in Sheffield and urged to follow it. In studies B2, E, and F, the health visitors were required to weigh infants naked at five extra visits and to determine whether weight gain was satisfactory by plotting the weights on the Sheffield Weight Charts which had been constructed from data assembled in the first two years of the Sheffield project.[5] In addition, in studies E and F a very high risk group comprising the 1% of infants with month scores of 1,000 or more were weighed at weekly intervals to three months of age and every two weeks to six months of age, which amounted to ten extra visits. In areas other than Sheffield, data were obtained on the number of home visits made to high- and low-risk infants.

EVALUATION

Ultimately, the effect of any intervention program will be determined by its impact on mortality. However, short-term changes in mortality rates may be due to a number of causes. Postperinatal mortality may be inflated by increasing short-term survival of very low birth-weight infants. The previous evaluation of the Sheffield intervention project suggested that increased awareness engendered by the project may have been the largest single factor. However, a direct effect of the extra care on the mortality in the high risk group was also demonstrated by the method of logistic analysis of covariance, as described in detail by Carpenter.[4] A similar method, described as regression-discontinuity analysis, has been discussed by Rubin[6,7] and has been used to evaluate a program to prevent recidivism.[8]

The model for the analysis is illustrated in FIGURE 1. The top line shows the relation between risk and score if there were no intervention. (This relation will seldom, if ever, be observed.) A reasonable model for intervention is that each visit by the health visitor produced a small proportional reduction in the child's risk. On a logistic scale, a proportional reduction in risk is represented by subtracting a constant. If all low-risk infants received the same basic care, the relation between risk and score will have the same slope as the first line but will be moved down. This will be the observed relation between risk and score in the low-risk group. If high-risk infants were also given this basic level of care, the line for the low-risk group would be expected to continue all the way up. If infants in the high-risk group all received the same extra care, then the relation between risk and score for high risk infants will again be parallel to the relation in the absence of intervention but at an even lower level. The step at the dividing line between low-risk and high-risk groups corresponds to the effect of the extra care given to high-risk infants. Thus, the relation between risk and score makes it possible to use the low-risk group as a contemporary control group for the high-risk group. This paper focuses primarily on the effect of intervention on the mortality of high-risk infants.

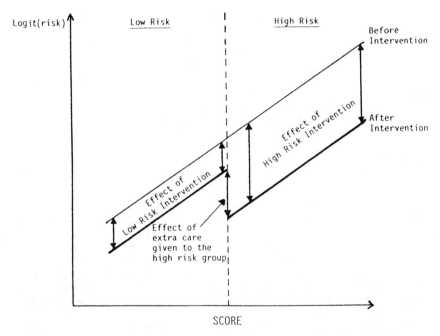

FIGURE 1. The effect of intervention on the relation of logit risk to score in high- and low-risk groups.

RESULTS

In all, more than 85,000 infants have been scored at birth and one month of age in the six areas. In addition, in Areas A and C, 13,559 infants were scored at birth but were not rescored at one month as described above.

TABLE 2 shows the estimated increase of risk of unexpected infant death per 100 points of month score. In Areas A and C, where most of the low risk scores were estimated from the birth score, the relationship is not as strong as in the other studies. For studies B, D, E, and F the logistic regression coefficients are very similar and the average of these four coefficients corresponds to a mean proportional increase of risk of 2.03 per hundred points of score with 95% confidence intervals (2.02; 2.04).

TABLE 2. The Increase of Risk per 100 Points of Score Observed in Six Areas

Area	Logistic Scale		Proportional Increase per 100 Points
	Estimate	SE	
A[a]	0.540	0.158	
C[a]	0.427	0.120	
B	0.684	0.160 ⎫	
D	0.743	0.143 ⎪	2.03
E	0.675	0.169 ⎬	
F	0.740	0.277 ⎭	

[a]Modified score system (see text)

The practical implications of this relationship are illustrated in FIGURE 2. Scores range from below 400 to over 800 points, and the fitted data suggest that, in the absence of intervention, there would be a 16-fold increase in risk over this range of scores.

TABLE 3 summarizes the effect of intervention on mortality of high-risk infants. For studies A, B1, and C, where intervention was minimal, the fitted model shows a step up at the critical point. In area D, Sheffield, there is a significant step down at this point corresponding to a fairly vigorous intervention program. When the extra home visits include stripping and weighing the infants and charting of all weights, a substantial reduction in mortality of high-risk infants is observed.

DISCUSSION

There are two components to risk related intervention, the identification of a high-risk group and the implementation of an effective intervention procedure. TABLE 2 shows that the Sheffield month score system is a powerful predictor of risk and is remarkably consistent in widely different areas of the United Kingdom. Since no effective intervention program was in operation in study B1, and complete data on month scores are available for this study, the data may be used to estimate the effectiveness of the score in identifying high-risk infants. In this study, 10.5% of the population were high-risk and 56.5% of the deaths were in this group, giving a specificity of 89.5% and a sensitivity of 56.5%.

The birth scoring system systematically passes minimum essential data plus a systematic evaluation of it from the maternity hospital to the health visitor. The month score requires the health visitor to assess the infant's progress at one month and to examine certain aspects of the home. These data are again systematically evaluated, and she and the family doctor are advised of the result.

It has been suggested that health visitors, as trained community health professionals, are competent to identify high-risk infants and to organize their care without the aid of a scoring system. In fact, health visitors have seldom personally encountered cases of SIDS, and a study revealed a wide variation in their perception of factors indicative of risk (J. Powell, personal communication). Data collected in Area E showed that health visitors are certainly no better than the score system in identifying risk. Studies by Rawaf[9] found that even when infants are thought to be at risk, left to themselves, health visitors generally do little about it.

One advantage of the score system devised is that the primary health care staff receives a written reminder of the risk status of individual infants. By using a computer for scoring, data were automatically checked for consistency and completeness, notification slips were generated in the required format, and case load data were tabulated for management of the health visitors' case loads. In addition, data were available for subsequent evaluation and analysis, including the possibility of up-dating the score system.

Problems arise with up-dating a score system while it is being used for intervention. These have been discussed by Carpenter.[4] The possibility of constructing a system of continuous up-dating has been discussed by Alexander-Watts.[10] Recent data from Sheffield suggest that maternal smoking and a maternal history of psychological or serious emotional disturbance may be important additional risk factors which should be included in any revised score system.

In TABLE 3, a reduction in high-risk mortality only occurred when an effective intervention program was implemented.

At Child Health Clinics, infants are often weighed in their clothes. Two-week weight gain estimated from such data are uncorrelated with two-week weight gain calculated from naked weights obtained at home. (Westland, B., personal communication). Weighing babies naked also ensures that the mother is seen handling the child and that the

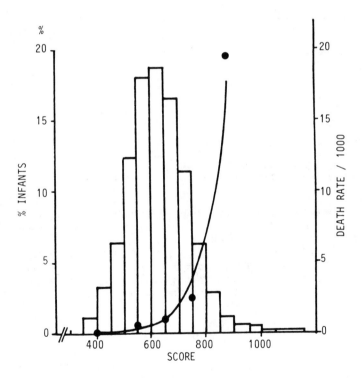

FIGURE 2. The distribution of month scores and the observed and fitted relation of "possibly preventable" infant mortality to score. Data from Study B1.

child is seen. Otherwise, the health visitor will often only see the top of the baby's head. The Sheffield weight charts,[5] unlike any others, are designed to detect deviations in weight gain over a two-week or eight-week period. Analysis of data from Area E showed that significant failure of weight gain very rarely occurred in the absence of illness. Plotting the weights has thus led to the identification of a variety of conditions.

The advantage of seeing the child at home is that the mother is more likely to express her concerns and to seek advice than in a busy health clinic. In addition, the health visitor is better placed to identify real problems, to offer relevant advice, and, occasionally, to rush a baby to the hospital.

An analysis of the first 33 of the recent series of Sheffield cases using Emery's[11] classification of deaths appeared to suggest that the score was predicting only those deaths in which there was a significant level of infection and not those which were completely unexplained. The alternative hypothesis was that completely unexplained deaths of high-risk infants were being prevented. The analysis of the last six-and-a-half-year series of Sheffield cases shows that the latter explanation is much more likely. This observation is compatible with the hypothesis that SIDS comprises a variety of conditions and that death arises from a combination of adverse congenital, developmental, social, and

TABLE 3. The Effect of Extra Care on Mortality of High-Risk Infants in Six Areas

Extra Care for High-Risk Infants	Area	Proportional Change in Mortality
None	A	1.57
None	B1	1.21
1 home visit	C	1.73
5 home visits	D	0.79[a]
5 home visits with weighing & charting[b]	B2	0.56
	E	0.20[a]
	F	0.43[a]

[a]Significantly less than 1, $p < 0.05$.
[b]Infants were weighed naked; weights were plotted on Sheffield weight charts.

environmental factors. An improved level of health care, resulting from home visits by health professionals and the careful monitoring of weight gain, is likely to mitigate some of these adverse factors and so reduce mortality.

These studies show that a high-risk group, comprising 11% of the population, can be identified at birth and that without intervention more than 50% of unexpected infant deaths will occur in this group. Mortality in the high-risk group can be more than halved by intervention, and total "possibly preventable" infant mortality reduced by 25%.

SUMMARY

Over seventy percent of unexpected infant deaths are registered as SIDS. Over 85,000 infants have been screened at birth and one month of age for risk of unexpected death using the Sheffield Score system. Scores range from below 400 to over 800 points. Infants with scores over 800 are at more than 16 times greater risk than infants with scores below 400. Family doctors and health visitors were alerted to high-risk infants, who were examined at home and weighed naked at home five times in the first six months. Mortality in the high-risk group was reduced by more than 50% ($p<0.02$ in one area and $p<0.05$ in another). It is concluded that with few extra resources unexpected infant mortality can be reduced by 25% by this approach.

ACKNOWLEDGMENTS

The paper summarizes the work of many doctors, health visitors, and others involved in the studies. Without their willing cooperation and dedicated work nothing would have been achieved.

REFERENCES

1. CARPENTER, R.G., A. GARDNER, M. JEPSON, E.M. TAYLOR, A. SALVIN, R. SUNDERLAND & J.L. EMERY. 1983. Evaluation of seven years of birth scoring and increased visiting of high risk infants to prevent unexpected infant deaths in Sheffield. Lancet **i:** 723–7.
2. CARPENTER, R.G., A. GARDNER, P.M. MCWEENY & J.L. EMERY. 1977. Multistage scoring system for identification of infants at risk of unexpected death. Arch. Dis. Child. **52:** 606–612.
3. SUNDERLAND, R., A. GARDNER & R.R. GORDON. 1986. Why did postperinatal mortality rates fall in the 1970's. J. Epidemiol. Community Health **40:** 228–231.
4. CARPENTER, R.G. 1983. Scoring to provide risk-related primary health care: Evaluation and up-dating during use (with discussion). J. R. Stat. Soc. Ser. A **146:** 1–32.
5. CARPENTER, R.G. & A. GARDNER. 1985. Sheffield Weight Charts. Foundation for the Study of Infant Deaths. London.
6. RUBIN, D.B. 1977. Assignment to treatment groups on the basis of a covariate. J. Educ. Stat. **2:** 1–26.
7. RUBIN, D.B. 1978. Bayesian inference for causal effects: The role of randomization. Ann. Stat. **6:** 34–58.
8. BERK, R.A. & D. RAUMA. 1983. Capitalizing on non-random assignment to treatment: A regression-discontinuity evaluation of a crime-control program. J. Am. Stat. Assoc. **78:** 21–27.
9. AL-RAWAF, S. 1982. Infant's Health Care in Camden and Islington. Ph.D. thesis, University of London.
10. ALEXANDER-WATTS, F. 1983. Discussion of Dr. Carpenter's paper. J. R. Stat. Soc. Ser. A. **146:** 26.
11. TAYLOR, E.M. & J.L. EMERY. 1982. A study of the causes of postperinatal deaths classified in terms of preventability. Arch. Dis. Child. **57:** 668–73.
12. TAYLOR, E.M., J.L. EMERY & R.G. CARPENTER. 1983. Identification of children at risk of unexpected death. Lancet **ii:** 1033–4.

APPENDIX 1.
The Calculation of the Sheffield Birth Score

Indicant	Facet	Score
Mother's age	$10 \times (50 -$ age in years)	
Previous pregnancies	0	0
	1	21
	2	43
	3	64
	4	85
	5	107
	6	128
	7	149
	8	171
	9 or more	192
Duration of 2nd stage of labor	< 5min	127
	5–14 min	100
	15–29 min	72
	30 min –2 hr	45
	> 2 hr	18
	NA	76
	Unknown	76
Mother's blood group[a]	O, B, AB	44
	A	0
Birthweight (g)	< 2000 g	93
	2000–2499 g	78
	2500–2999 g	62
	3000–3499 g	47
	3500–3999 g	31
	4000–4499 g	16
	4500–5500 g	0
Twin	Yes	103
	No	0
Feeding intention	Breast only	0
	Bottle or both	38
Urinary infection during pregnancy	Yes	54
	No	0
	?	5
Cut-point for total score		500
	High-risk	500 and over
	Low-risk	499 and under

[a]Replaced in Areas E and F by "Mother smokes," scored: No = 0, 1–10 cigarettes/day = 20, 11+/day = 40.

APPENDIX 2.
The Calculation of the Sheffield Month Score

Indicant	Facet	Score
Birth score	(APPENDIX 1)	
Cyanotic or apneic attacks in	Yes	237
hospital before initial discharge	No	0
Difficulty establishing feeds	Yes	83
	No	0
	Not known	36
State of repair of home	Excellent	9
	Good	43
	Average	78
	Fair	112
	Poor	147
	Not seen	73
Interval to last live birth	$2 \times (100 - \text{number of months})$	
	1st live birth	128
	100 months or more	0
Hospital admission	Yes	154
	No	0
Cut-point for total score		754
	High-risk	754 and over
	Low-risk	753 and under

Evaluation of the Nottingham Birth Scoring System

RICHARD J. MADELEY,[a] DAVID HULL,[b] AND
J. MARK ELWOOD[a]

[a]Department of Community Medicine and Epidemiology
University of Nottingham Medical School
Queen's Medical Centre
Clifton Boulevard
Nottingham, NG7 2UH England

[b]Department of Child Health
University of Nottingham Medical School
Queen's Medical Centre
Clifton Boulevard
Nottingham, NG7 2UH England

INTRODUCTION

The Nottingham Health Authority serves a population of 600,000, with, on average, 6,500 live births per year. Three hundred thousand of these poeple live within the city of Nottingham, which is the regional capital of the East Midlands, and the remainder in three suburban districts which entirely surround the city. These suburban districts, which have a combined population of 300,000, are significantly better-off in economic terms than the city itself.

In 1976, the health authority set up a multidisciplinary team with the duties of reviewing the standard of services provided for mothers and young children, and recommending any improvements that might be needed. The senior author (R. J. M.) was the epidemiologist/community physician on the team and the second author (D. H.) the chairman. At a very early meeting, routine data relating to Nottingham, supplied by the Office of Population Censuses and Surveys (OPCS) in London, were reviewed. These showed an increase in the postneonatal mortality rate in the city of Nottingham in 1974 compared with the previous year. Also, over a ten-year period the rate in the city had been consistently higher than that in the suburban districts.

It was decided to undertake an epidemiological analysis of postneonatal death in the city, and the senior author was asked to undertake a rapid survey, using available data, and to report to the next meeting of the team. An analysis was carried out of death notifications for the years 1974–1976 which had been received by the health authority from registrars of deaths. This analysis showed that most deaths were attributable to respiratory infections and the sudden infant death syndrome (SIDS), and that they were likelier to occur at home, in the winter, and in the less well-off parts of the city.

Because of the interest evoked by these data, it was decided to carry out a case-control study whose objective was to contrast those infants dying in the postneonatal period with those who did not. This was done by comparing data from the birth notification of the dead infant with data from two notifications chosen at random from those of liveborn children who had been born on the same day and had survived the postneonatal period. A comparison of the two groups showed that those who subsequently died were significantly likelier to be of low birthweight (<2,500 g), bottle-fed, born in a household

106

the head of which was a partly-skilled or unskilled manual worker, and born in an election ward classified by the Nottinghamshire County Council as socially deprived.[1] When the health visitors' records of the dead infants were compared with those of the control group, the analysis showed that those infants who subsequently died were significantly likelier not to have attended a child health clinic by six weeks of age and not to have established a set feeding pattern by four weeks of age (either breast or bottle).

A major debate then took place within the team about whether any further research was needed. The main debate centered on whether we should further analyze the data so that we might be able to set up a birth scoring system of the type already operating in Sheffield. Early reports from Sheffield had claimed that such an approach was beneficial,[2-4] although scepticism had also been expressed.[5] The results so far obtained were in any case widely disseminated among health workers in Nottingham, and presented at regional and national meetings.

The majority of the team, including the authors, felt that an approach like that used

TABLE 1. The Nottingham Birth Scoring System

Effect of Risk Factors on Score	
Risk Factor	Change in Score[a]
1 January 1978–31 March 1985	
Born in deprived polling district	+200
Birthweight <2,000 g	+425
2,000–2,499 g	+215
2,500–2,999 g	0
3,000–3,499 g	−215
>3,500 g	−425
Age of mother	−30 (× age in years)
1 January 1978–31 December 1979	
Breast-fed baby	−400
Second stage of labor 15 min or less	+400
1 January 1980–31 March 1985	
Legitimate birth	−400
Delivery less than 18 months after birth of previous child	+400

[a]Starting score is 1,000.

in Sheffield was justified. Using the technique of step-wise discriminant analysis, the team devised a birth scoring system which identified a high-risk group consisting of 9% of the infant population in whom 53% of postneonatal deaths would be expected to occur (odds ratio = 11.6, 95% confidence limits 21.90 and 5.79). The factors used in the birth scoring system are shown in TABLE 1. Babies scoring +500 points or higher were assigned to the high-risk category.[6,7]

From January 1, 1978, each liveborn infant in Nottingham was scored by a midwife. Those infants designated as being at high-risk were to receive ten home visits from their health visitor, who also had the responsibility of establishing liaison with the infant's general practitioner. Infants designated as low-risk would continue to receive the standard four visits. During the course of these extra visits, the health visitor would advise the mother on feeding matters, early recognition of symptoms, and general matters relating to the care of the infant. In 1980, two important changes were made to the system by the addition of two new risk factors, "illegitimate birth" and "delivery less than 18 months

TABLE 2. Causes of Death Recorded on Death Certificates for Postneonatal Deaths in the City of Nottingham for 1974–1976 and 1978–1981

	1974–1976		1978–1981	
Cause of Death	n	%	n	%
Respiratory infections	26	28.3	25	43.9
Sudden infant death syndrome	37	40.2	14	24.6
Congenital abnormalities	14	15.2	9	15.8
Gastroenteritis	5	5.4	3	5.3
Meningitis	3	3.3	2	3.5
Cardiomyopathy	2	2.2	0	0
Epiglottitis	2	2.2	0	0
Trauma	2	2.2	2	3.5
Otitis media	1	1.1	0	0
Septicemia	0	0	1	1.8
Intussusception	0	0	1	1.8
Total	92	100	57	100
Postneonatal death rate per 1,000 live births	7.4		4.7	

after the birth of the previous child.'' Most ''illegitimate births'' in Nottingham are to teenagers or women in their very early twenties who have never been married. These changes reduced the size of the high-risk group in 1978–1979 from 11.9% to 8.6%. It remained at or around this level until the system was stopped in March 1985.

From 1980, there was great pressure to publish articles on the results of the scheme because of both local interest and the positive results being claimed by the Sheffield group. Apart from one interim report,[8] this pressure was resisted until such a time that adequate data existed. A detailed analysis of the years 1978–1981 was commenced in late 1982. The remainder of this paper presents the most important results of this analysis, and their implications for policy development.

RESULTS

A comparison of causes of postneonatal death in the years 1974–1976 and 1978–1981 (TABLE 2) showed an apparently large reduction in the number of deaths attributed to SIDS, but this reduction can be explained by a local change in the criteria for recording SIDS. During the later period, these criteria were very considerably tightened, and there was a greater tendency to relate inflammatory disease in the lungs to respiratory disease rather than to SIDS. Thus, as shown in TABLE 2, the sum of the percentage of deaths attributable to respiratory infections plus the percentage attributable to SIDS remained remarkably constant, at 68%, for both 1974–1976 and 1978–1981.

More infants died at home or were dead on arrival at the hospital during the years 1978–1981 (43 of 57, i.e. 75%) than during the earlier period of 1974–1976 (61 of 92, i.e. 66%), but the difference is not significant. In both periods, three-quarters of postneonatal deaths occurred before the end of the child's fifth month of life. In both periods postneonatal deaths showed a strong seasonal relationship, with more deaths occuring in the winter months.

Analysis of the data for 1974–1976 had showed that the home addresses of the families in which a postneonatal death had occurred were markedly clustered in less well-off parts of the city (FIG. 1). Although this effect was still present in the 1978–1981 period, it was less pronounced (FIG. 1), because the public housing policy of the Nottingham City Council (involving slum clearance programs) had the effect of moving population from central wards to the periphery of the city.

Analysis of trends in OPCS data for the period of 1972–1982 was undertaken. The resulting graph (FIG. 2) gives the impression that the postneonatal mortality rate for the city of Nottingham underwent a steady downward trend throughout this period, from a rate well above that for England and Wales to one closely resembling it. There is no suggestion of a trend in the combined data for the three suburban districts (Broxtowe, Gedling, and Rushcliffe) throughout this period (FIG. 2). For England and Wales there seems to be a slow downward trend in the rate during the first part of the period, but the rate then during appears to remain constant 1978–1982.

Crucially, in the data relating to the city of Nottingham (FIG. 2), there seems to be little suggestion of a faster fall in the postneonatal mortality rate after the introduction of the birth scoring system in 1978. This conclusion was confirmed by the use of regression analysis,[9] and the Mantel-Haenszel extension test for trend.[10] As indicated in TABLE 3, the value of the regression coefficient (b) for the 1978–1984 period fell within the 95% confidence limits of the 1972–1977 period. Therefore the results obtained in the second period could easily be explained as merely the continuation of a trend from the earlier period. The Mantel-Haenszel extension test, applied to the rates during the years 1973–1982, gave a figure of 17.60 for the global χ^2 value (9 degrees of freedom), which is almost identical to the χ^2 value of 13.16 (1 degree of freedom) obtained from the test for trend. This means that during the years 1973–1982 there was almost no departure from a steady trend, and certainly no significant departure (17.60 − 13.16 = 4.44, 8 degrees of freedom, NS).

By means of a second case-control study, covering the period of 1978–1981 and using four liveborn controls for each death, it was possible to compare the relative risks for

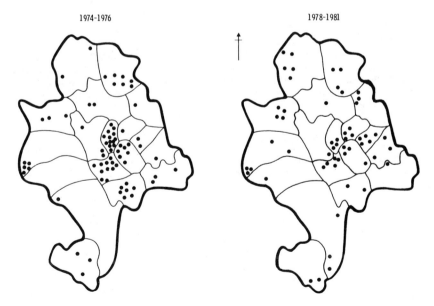

FIGURE 1. The location of home addresses for children dying in the postneonatal period in Nottingham, England.

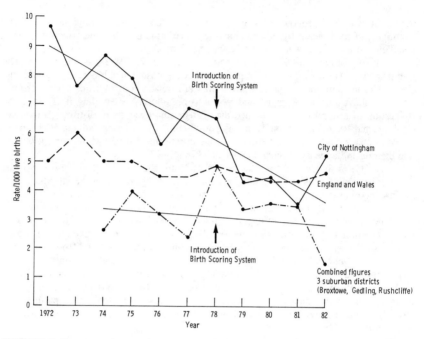

FIGURE 2. Postneonatal mortality rates for the city of Nottingham, three suburban districts combined, and England and Wales.

different risk factors in the two periods. If the high-risk intervention is completely successful, the outcome for the children designated as high-risk should be the same as that for those not so designated; and the relative risk should fall to 1. It has been suggested by Carpenter[11] that if the intervention in the form of extra health visiting has been successful, there should be a fall in the percentage of deaths in the high-risk group. TABLE 4 compares the relative risks and the percentages of deaths in the high-risk groups for the 1974–1976 and 1978–1981 time periods.

There was a substantially lower relative risk for the group analyzed in 1978–1981 than for the original 1974–1976 high-risk group (TABLE 4). At first glance, this result provides support for the hypothesis that a successful intervention by health visitors, doctors and parents has had a beneficial effect, thereby reducing the size of the difference between the relative risks of the high-risk and control groups. However, this would be a very

TABLE 3. Regression Analysis of Postneonatal Mortality Rates in the City of Nottingham for 1972–1984

Period	a	b	SE (b)	95% Conf. Limits of b	Test of $b = 0$[a]	p
1972–1984	39.82	−0.431	0.0793	−0.59, −0.27	−5.43 (11 df)	<0.001
1972–1977	53.19	−0.609	0.2611	−1.13, −0.09	−2.33 (4 df)	NS
1978–1984	16.39	−0.143	0.1843	−1.51, +0.23	−0.77 (5 df)	NS

[a] t value.

superficial conclusion. Firstly, the reduction in the risk of the high-risk group could be due to an entirely different effect or combination of effects.

As regards the actual figures, a number of factors may be at work which would tend to reduce the difference between the two groups over a period even if no intervention of any kind had been undertaken. For example, the phenonemon of "shrinkage" described by Hills[12] and Lachenbruch[13] ensures that when the discrimination between the high-risk group and the rest of the population is applied in a prospective fashion, it will be less in practice than in the case-control data from which it is derived. This phenonemon arises partly from fluctuations in the frequency of a variable in the general population, and partly because those variables chosen for inclusion in a scoring system may well have been chosen because they were enjoying a period of unusually sharp discrimination at the time of the original survey.

Another important factor is that during the period of 1978–1979, the size of the high-risk group in the city of Nottingham was, at 17% of the infant population, considerably higher in practice than had been predicted from the original case-control study. Even if the intervention itself were totally ineffective, this increase in the size of the high-risk group would have had the effect of lowering its relative risk, because such an increase would raise the sensitivity of the scoring system, but reduce both the

TABLE 4. Postneonatal Death and Risk Status in the City of Nottingham for 1974–1976 and 1978–1981

	1974–1976			1978–1981		
	High-Risk	Low-Risk	Total	High-Risk	Low-Risk	Total
No. of deaths	38	34	72	16	33	49
No. of controls	13	131	144	39	188	227
Relative risk	11.3			2.3		
(95% conf. limits)	(21.9, 5.8)			(4.6, 1.2)		
χ^2 value	48.5			5.1		
p value	<0.0001			<0.05		

specificity of the system and the relative risk of the high-risk group. Over the period of 1974–1981, the importance of some of the risk factors may have changed. For example, because of the significant movement of population away from inner-city wards, as already described above, "area of residence" did not mean the same thing at the end of the period as at the beginning.

The data arising from the two case-control studies of data for the periods of 1974–1976 and 1978–1981 were analyzed by logistic regression using the GLIM programme.[14] This process gives the independent contribution of each variable, as well as the amount of the total variance explained by these variables. The results of this analysis (TABLE 5) showed that only a very small amount of the total variance is explained by the variables used in the birth scoring system, and commonly used in studies of postneonatal mortality. These results resemble those of Carpenter,[11] in describing the Sheffield system, and of Pharoah and Morris,[15] who found that only 25% of the improvement in postneonatal mortality in England and Wales in the 1970s could be attributed to changes in maternal age, parity, and social class.

The fact that most of the variance is not explained by conventional risk factors is not surprising since many of the key factors, e.g. the degree of "wantedness" of the child, the relationship between the child and the mother, the coping ability of the mother (and

TABLE 5. Logistic Regression Analysis (GLIM Program) of the Independent Contributions of Key Variables to Postneonatal Mortality in the City of Nottingham for 1974–1976 and 1978–1981

	1974–1976	1978–1981
Variable	*Contribution*	
Birthweight	<0.001	<0.01
Feeding intention	<0.01	<0.05
Social class	<0.02	NS
Legal status	NS	<0.01
Parity	NS	NS
Born in deprived area	NS	NS
Age of mother	NS	NS
Total variance	242.50	269.80
Change in variance due to above variables	64.10	46.30
Percentage of total variance explained by above variables	26.43	17.16

in particular her ability to recognize illness), the mental state of the mother, and the standard of living in the family, are all very difficult, if not impossible, to measure.

DISCUSSION

The evaluation of birth scoring systems is not an easy exercise. A major problem is that in no case known to the authors has it been possible to mount for any length of time a randomized prospective trial of a scoring system. The possibility of such a trial in Nottingham was fully discussed, but it was clear that the opposition of significant numbers of midwives, health visitors and doctors to such a proposed course of action made it an impractical proposition. Because of this problem, it is impossible to conclude that the fall in mortality during the period of 1978–1981 is in any way due to the setting up of the birth scoring system. This is a frequent difficulty for practitioners of health services research. As Williams[16] has pointed out:

> It is obvious that assessing the impact of health services research will be a complicated task. Various approaches to evaluation that are available in biomedical and clinical research cannot be used. Rarely is there an opportunity to carry out an evaluation with a rigid experimental design, and the relationship of cause and effect has usually to be assessed inductively from observations of the course of events. At the same time there are formidable methodological problems inherent in an historical enquiry that tries to relate research findings to changes of policy, strategy or practice.

The results presented here suggest there is little evidence that the birth scoring system caused the decline in mortality to speed up during the period of 1978–1981. An important point, however, is that, because postneonatal death is in fact a quite rare event, an intervention which was actually effective would be unlikely to show a statistically significant improvement during a realistic time scale.

A number of other trends taking place during the period 1974–1981 are very likely to have had some effect on the situation. For example, the rate of breast feeding in the city of Nottingham increased from a figure of 48% during the earlier period to 58.5% during the latter, reflecting a national trend. This change affected both the high-risk and low-risk groups. Bottle feeding, which exerted a significant independent effect in both time periods of the study, has also been mentioned as an important etiological factor in a number of other studies.[17-21] At the same time, it seems likely that there may well have been an absolute improvement in the postneonatal mortality rate in bottle-fed infants as the result of better health education in general, and of the publicity surrounding the controversy in the mid-1970s about the dangers of hypernatremia caused by the feeding of over-strength cow's milk to babies.[22,23]

There was also a marked change in the parity distribution, with significantly fewer births to mothers already having three or more living children ($p<0.001$). High parity carries a high relative risk of postneonatal death. During the period 1968–1981, there was a significant correlation between the birth rate and the postneonatal mortality rate in the city of Nottingham ($r = 0.51$, $p<0.05$).

Important changes in the environmental and economic circumstances of Nottingham occurred during the study period.[24] At the time of the 1971 census, 28% of all houses in the city were without exclusive use of hot water, a fixed bath, or an inside toilet. By the time of the 1981 census, this figure had fallen to 4%. While it would be naive to suggest that there is a direct causal relationship between better housing and a fall in the postneonatal mortality rate, it seems equally improbable that such a dramatic improvement in the environment of the less well-off sectors of the community has not had some effect, however small. If it is accepted that the standard of care given to a baby by its mother, or the strength of a mother-child relationship, is relevant to the health of the child, then it does not seem far-fetched to suggest that the provision of hot water, a fixed bath, and an inside toilet where none existed previously will help the situation by making life easier for the mother. She can then commit more of herself to the infant, increasing the chance of correctly diagnosing respiratory infections at an earlier stage, and of taking the appropriate action, e.g., seeking medical help.

The birth scoring system was not the only policy development affecting services for children in Nottingham at that time. An important difference between the health care systems of the United States and the United Kingdom is that, in the latter, approximately 90% of doctor-patient contacts occur solely in the primary care sector, i.e., outside the hospital and with the general practitioner with whom the patient is registered. During the period of the study not only was there a documented increase in the number of general practitioners operating in this sector, but these doctors were also, in general, better trained at both the undergraduate and postgraduate level. Hospital pediatric services were further developed with an increase in the number of all grades of medical staff and of nurses.

All of these groups of health professionals were exposed to the impact of the birth scoring system, the research on which it was based, and other research from other centers being undertaken and published during the period. Of importance during this period was the work arising from the so-called "Multicenter Study"[25] based upon interviews with the parents of infants who had died between one week and two years of age in several towns in England. These showed that many of these infants, even many of those for whom the death was attributed to SIDS, had had some symptoms, often of a non-specific nature, in the period leading up to death.

The implications of these important findings were much discussed at professional meetings, and a consensus emerged. If a general practitioner requested the admission to the hospital of an infant with non-specific symptoms, because he felt that something was "not right" with the child, then the consensus was that this action would be regarded by the hospital staff as legitimate. Similarly, if a mother telephoned the general practitioner to request an immediate appointment at the doctor's office or a home visit by the doctor, then this request should be taken very seriously. During the period of 1975–1985, admissions of children to the hospital in the first year of life increased threefold in Nottingham, mostly from admissions for respiratory tract infections.[26] This increase represents a significant lowering of the threshold for hospital admission, and is quite plausibly a factor in the lowering of the postneonatal mortality rate.

What reasons explain the apparent failure of birth scoring systems to work as well in practice, as they might perhaps in theory? We think that the key factor is that the very low percentage of the total variance explained by conventional risk factors has implications for the credibility of these schemes in the eyes of health workers.

In the opinion of health visitors in Nottingham, babies fell into one of four categories:

(A) Babies that they thought were high-risk, and were so classified by the system.
(B) Babies they thought were low-risk, and were so classified by the system (the great majority).
(C) Babies classified as high-risk by the system, but as low risk by the health visitor.
(D) Babies classified as low-risk by the system, but as high-risk by the health visitor.

An early management problem arose from categories C and D, i.e., how to handle the situation where a health visitor felt strongly about what she saw as the misclassification of a particular baby. A typical example of the type of case in category C would be one in which a premature baby born to a youngish middle-class mother had required artificial feeding. The typical reaction of the health visitor would be that an initially high-risk baby who had survived the dangerous period of the first few days and was doing very well at two months should be considered low-risk. A typical case in category D would be one in which the mother had developed significant psychological problems after returning home with the baby, or in which there was severe marital stress, affecting the care of the infant. The key point is that in circumstances of this type, because the risk factors explain such a low percentage of the variance, the health visitor's opinion, often based on years of experience, may well be as valid as the risk score. It is thus understandable that health visitors are likely to become resentful if their views are over-ridden by numerical scores.

Another key point arises from the fact that the absolute risk of postneonatal death, either from SIDS or from any other cause, is very low. Because this risk is so low, a baby who possesses a very adverse combination of risk factors and who happens to contract a respiratory infection in the winter months is actually very unlikely to come to any harm, with or without medical treatment. Data arising from the previously mentioned Department of Health and Social Security (DHSS) "Multicentre Study"[25] show that for every child having "major" symptoms who died, 163 had such symptoms and did not die. "Major" symptoms, defined as "those needing a medical opinion the same day," included wheezing, noisy or altered cough, unusual drowsiness, altered cry, and feeding difficulties. The implications of this observation for birth scoring systems are very considerable. In practice, if a health visitor thinks that a baby has been wrongly classified as high-risk and does not visit it so frequently or/and so carefully, no harm is likely to come to it. A further point often raised by the health visitors themselves was that a baby designated as being at high-risk by the birth scoring system usually could have in any case been so designated without the presence of the score.

What are the costs of birth scoring systems? On the face of it, the absolute costs are small. In Nottingham, it was necessary to print and distribute to the maternity units 6,500 forms per year. Once there, they had to be filled in and added up by the midwives, attached to the birth notification, and transferred to the health visitors, with a copy to the child health unit headquarters of the health authority. The health visitor would check the arithmetic and, in practice, assess how the risk score measured up to her judgement. Although no extra staff were taken on as a direct result of the scheme, it is clear that such a process must have taken up a considerable amount of staff time over the seven years and three months of its operation. The opportunity costs of the scheme, i.e., what else these health workers could have been doing with their time, must have been very considerable.

During 1984, these factors were much discussed in Nottingham, with a view to determining future policy developments, including whether or not the birth scoring system should continue. In addition to the evaluation of the Nottingham scheme just presented, it was necessary to examine the major claims made on behalf of the Sheffield system, because other health authorities in the United Kingdom and further afield, for example in the Irish Republic, were asking us about the advisability of birth scoring systems in general as well as about our own experience in particular. We therefore examined in detail new publications concerning the Sheffield scheme,[11,27] the correspondence arising from them,[11,28] and other relevant work, in particular the final report of the DHSS Multicenter Study.[29] It was very clear that the results from Sheffield were controversial. We also carried out an analysis of routinely available OPCS data relating to Sheffield (FIG. 3), which demonstrated two striking features. Firstly it showed that the postneonatal mortality

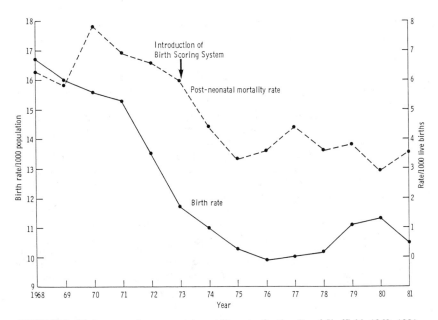

FIGURE 3. Birth rates and postneonatal mortality rates for the city of Sheffield, 1968–1981.

rate was falling rapidly before the introduction of the birth scoring system in 1973 and that from 1976 the rate leveled off. Secondly, the postneonatal mortality rate showed a remarkable correlation with the birth rate ($r = 0.83$, $p<0.001$). In the late 1960s and early 1970s in England, a large number of the women in those groups whose infants were likely to experience postneonatal death started taking the contraceptive pill. FIGURE 3 provides strong support for the hypothesis that the smaller numbers of better planned-for babies were better looked after by health workers and, above all, by their parents. This greater degree of care would lower the mortality rate, especially from respiratory infections and those cases of SIDS where symptoms were present for some hours before death.

The final consideration in deciding to discontinue the Nottingham scheme were the data contained in TABLE 5, which showed that by 1981 the only significant risk factors were low birthweight, bottle feeding, and being born to a single mother. All of these would be known to the health visitor in any case. Therefore, since there was no need for an extra piece of paper and an additional system, birth scoring was discontinued as of March 31, 1985. Additionally, the whole question of risk-related visiting was de-emphasized, with the health visitor being encouraged to allocate her time as determined by her clinical judgement and experience.

RECOMMENDATIONS

On the basis of our experience, we would not advise the setting up of birth scoring systems. We think that some cases of SIDS are probably not preventable by health service or parental action, given our current level of knowledge. Those that possibly are preventable are likelier to be saved by a system that responds quickly and effectively to suspicious symptoms in *any* baby. Thus the most effective use of the health visitor's time may well be to carry out visits in such circumstances, or to carry out follow-up visits at home for babies with respiratory infections, rather than to carry out extra, prospective visits for infants who, even if correctly classified as high-risk, are, in absolute terms, highly unlikely to come to any harm. In the English context, this approach means a higher consultation rate at the general practitioner's office, a larger number of home visits, and a higher admission rate to the hospital.

An increase in the rate of breast feeding would probably reduce the incidence of SIDS slightly. In no study known to the authors has it been claimed that breast feeding increases the death rate, while some suggest a beneficial effect.[30,31,32] Decisions taken by the agencies outside the health service may well be relevant. For example, the fact that deaths from SIDS and respiratory infections are so much commoner in the winter may be related to the ambient temperature at which houses are kept, and to the cost of heating them. Government policy in the United Kingdom has been to increase the costs of fuel faster than the general rate of inflation, in order to encourage economy of use. This policy affects most adversely the less well-off sectors of the community, which are precisely those most at-risk of postneonatal death.

In conclusion, we would say that some cases of SIDS are theoretically and philosophically potentially preventable. However, the mechanisms for prevention are complex and multifactorial, and no one single solution is likely to provide the answer on its own.

SUMMARY

A case-control study of postneonatal deaths occurring in 1974–1976 in the City of Nottingham, England, revealed that most were attributable to respiratory infections and SIDS, and primarily occurred in wintertime, at home, in the less well-off parts of Nottingham. By means of a step-wise discriminant analysis, 9% of the infant population was identified as a high-risk group in whom 53% of postneonatal deaths could be expected to occur. From January 1, 1978, this group of infants was followed up more intensively by health visitors and general practitioners, who gave advice on the early recognition of respiratory symptoms. Although the postneonatal mortality rate fell from 6.5 per 1,000 live births in 1977 to 5.2 per 1,000 in 1983, it is not possible to show that the rate of improvement was any faster after the introduction of the system. The system was discontinued on March 31, 1985. Birth scoring systems are not recommended; instead, resources should be concentrated on general improvements in services and symptom recognition, and basic research into the causes of SIDS.

ACKNOWLEDGMENTS

Thanks are due to Miss Ruth Buxton for typing several drafts.

REFERENCES

1. NOTTINGHAMSHIRE COUNTY COUNCIL. 1975. County Deprived Area Study. Planning Department, Nottinghamshire County Council. Nottingham.
2. CARPENTER, R. G. & J. L. EMERY. 1974. Identification and follow-up of infants at risk or sudden infant death in infancy. Nature **250:** 729.
3. CARPENTER, R. G. & J. L. EMERY. 1977. Final results of study of infants at risk of sudden death. Nature **268:** 724–725.
4. CARPENTER, R. G., A. GARDNER, P. M. MCWEENY, J. L. EMERY. 1977. Multistage scoring system for identifying infants at risk of unexpected death. Arch. Dis. Child. **52:** 606–612.
5. MAGURA, S. 1975. Sudden infant death in infancy. Nature **256:** 519.
6. MADELEY, R. J. 1978. Relating health services to needs by the use of simple epidemiology. Public Health **92:** 224–230.
7. MADELEY, R. J. & A. LATHAM. 1979. Management aspects of high-risk strategies in child health. Community Medicine **1:** 36–39.
8. MADELEY, R. J. 1982. Positive discrimination in child health : An interim report from Nottingham. Public Health **96:** 358–364.
9. HILL, A. B. 1971. In Principles of Medical Statistics, 9th ed.: 180–192. Lancet Ltd. London.
10. MANTEL, N. 1963. Chi-square tests with one degree of freedom : Extensions of the Mantel-Haenszel procedure. J. Am. Stat. Assoc. **58:** 690–700.
11. CARPENTER, R. G. 1983. Scoring to provide risk-related primary health care : Evaluation and up-dating during use. J. R. Stat. Soc. A. **146:** 1–34.
12. HILLS, M. 1967. Discrimination and allocation with discrete data. Appl. Stat. **16:**237–250.
13. LACHENBRUCH, P. A. 1968. On experimental probabilities of misclassification in discriminant analysis, necessary sample size and a relation with the multiple correlation coefficient. Biometrics **24:** 823–834.
14. BAKER, R. J. & J. A. NELDER. 1978. The GLIM System Release 3 Manual. Numerical Algorithm Group. Oxford.
15. PHAROAH, P. O. D. & J. N. MORRIS. 1979. Postneonatal Mortality. Epidemiol. Rev. **1:** 170–183.
16. WILLIAMS, B. T. 1983. Health systems research : What does it accomplish? World Health Forum **4:** 336–339.
17. MINISTRY OF HEALTH. 1965. Enquiry into Sudden Death in Infancy : Reports on Public Health and Medical Subjects No. 113. HMSO, London.
18. PARISH, W. E., A. M. BARRETT & R. R. A. COOMBS. 1960. Inhalation of cows milk by sensitised guinea pigs in the conscious and anaesthetised state. Immunology **3:** 307–324.
19. PARISH, W. E., C. B. RICHARDS, N. E. FRANCE & R. R. A. COOMBS. 1964. Further investigation on the hypothesis that some cases of cot-death are due to a modified anaphylactic reaction to cows milk. Int. Arch. Allergy **24,** 4 : 205–243.
20. DOWNHAM, M. A. P. S. 1976. Breast feeding protects against respiratory syncytial virus infections. Br. Med. J. **2:** 274–276.
21. PULLAN, C. R., G. L. TOMS, A. J. MARTIN, J. K. G. WEBB & D. R. APPLETON. 1980. Infant health and breast feeding during the first 16 weeks of life. Br. Med. J. **2:** 1034–1036.
22. SMITH, B. A. M. 1974. Feeding over-strength cows milk to babies. Br. Med. J. **4:** 741–742.
23. SUNDERLAND, R. & J. L. EMERY. 1979. Apparent disappearance of hypernatraemic dehydration from infant deaths in Sheffield. Br. Med. J. **2:** 575–576.
24. NOTTINGHAMSHIRE COUNTY COUNCIL. 1983. Disadvantage in Nottinghamshire. Planning Department, Nottinghamshire County Council. Nottingham.
25. STANTON, A. N., M. A. P. S. DOWNHAM, J. R. OAKLEY, J. L. EMERY & J. KNOWELDEN. 1978. Terminal symptoms in children dying suddenly and unexpectedly at home. Br. Med. J. **2:** 1249–1251.
26. DUROJAIYE, L. I. A. 1986. Acute medical paediatric admissions to University Hospital

Nottingham. Bachelor of Medical Sciences Honours Dissertation, Department of Community Medicine and Epidemiology, University of Nottingham.

27. CARPENTER, R. G., A. GARDNER, M. JEPSON, E. M. TAYLOR, A. SALVIA, R. SUNDERLAND, J. L. EMERY, E. PURSALL, J. ROE & THE HEALTH VISITORS OF SHEFFIELD. 1983. Prevention of unexpected infant death—evaluation of the first seven years of the Sheffield intervention programme. Lancet 1: 723–727.

28. GEDALLA, B. 1983. Sheffield cot deaths project. Lancet 2: 48–49.

29. KNOWELDEN, J., J. KEELING & J. P. NICHOLL. 1984. A Multicentre Study of Postneonatal Mortality. University of Sheffield. Sheffield.

30. CUNNINGHAM, A. S. 1979. Morbidity in breastfed and artificially fed infants 1. J Pediatr. 90: 726–729.

31. CUNNINGHAM, A. S. 1979. Morbidity in breastfed and artificially fed infants 2. J. Pediatr. 95: 685–689.

32. WATKINS, C. J., S. R. LEEDER & R. T. CORKHILL. 1979. The relationship between breast and bottle feeding and respiratory illness in the first year of life. J. Epidemiol. Community Health 13: 180–182.

Methylxanthine Treatment in Infants at Risk for Sudden Infant Death Syndrome

CARL E. HUNT AND ROBERT T. BROUILLETTE

Department of Pediatrics
The Children's Memorial Hospital
Northwestern University Medical School
Chicago, Illinois 60614

INTRODUCTION

The efficacy of theophylline treatment in reducing apnea and periodic breathing and in increasing minute volume has been well documented in apnea of prematurity.[1,2] Kelly and Shannon previously reported that theophylline also reduces apnea and periodic breathing in infants with unexplained apnea.[3] We performed a study to evaluate whether theophylline treatment would significantly reduce apnea and periodic breathing in infants at risk for Sudden Infant Death Syndrome (SIDS). Our results[4] confirmed that, as in apnea of prematurity, theophylline is quite effective in significantly decreasing the frequency of episodes of periodic breathing and of brief or prolonged apnea in infants at risk for SIDS. Theophylline treatment improved the respiratory pattern in almost all these infants and completely normalized the findings in more than 80% of them. In addition, theophylline-related normalization of the pneumogram was associated with an absence of recurrent episodes of apnea in the group which had initially been symptomatic for apnea of infancy, and with an absence of any episodes in the asymptomatic siblings of prior SIDS victims.

One of the major limitations in previous reports of theophylline administration to infants at increased risk for SIDS has been the small number of infants evaluated. The purpose of this report is to summarize the results of theophylline treatment in 300 infants considered to be at increased risk for SIDS.

METHODS

Infants with apparent life-threatening events or asymptomatic infants at increased epidemiologic risk for SIDS comprise the study population. The groups at epidemiologic risk included preterm infants, siblings of prior SIDS victims, and infants with intrauterine drug exposure. Pneumograms were performed and analyzed as previously reported.[4,5] For each pneumogram, the following parameters were measured: apnea density (A_6/D%), episodes of periodic breathing, and longest apnea. A_6/D% was calculated by determining the total duration of all respiratory pauses ≥ 6.0 sec in duration and expressing this total as a percentage of total sleep time. The total number of periodic breathing episodes/100 min of sleep was calculated; an episode, defined as at least three respiratory pauses of ≥ 3 sec, was considered to have ended when a normal respiratory pattern had been present for ≥ 20 sec. The duration of each respiratory pause was measured as the interval between end-expiration and the beginning of the next inspiration. Pneumograms were considered abnormal if the values for A_6/D% and periodic breathing exceeded the 95th percentile for normal infants (0.9% and 2.9 episodes/100 min, respectively) or exceeded 20 sec for longest apnea.[5]

Treatment with theophylline was recommended for all infants with an abnormal pneumogram. A home monitor was also recommended if the respiratory pattern did not normalize with theophylline. Despite normalization of clinical systems and respiratory pattern with theophylline, a home monitor was also utilized whenever requested by the referring physician and/or family. Peak blood levels of theophylline were checked at least monthly and maintained in the 7–10 mg/ml range. Pneumograms were performed at home at 3–4 month intervals and theophylline treatment was discontinued as soon as the respiratory pattern without theophylline had become normal. To perform these home follow-up pneumograms, theophylline treatment was suspended two days prior to beginning the pneumogram, and the infant was on a home monitor while not receiving theophylline. Theophylline treatment was then reinstituted immediately upon completion of the pneumogram, pending its analysis. Depending on the reason for beginning the use of a home monitor, its use was generally discontinued concurrently with, or prior to, discontinuing theophylline treatment. The infants included in this report comprise all those for whom theophylline treatment was recommended in 1982–1986 who have returned for follow-up evaluations and who have subsequently exhibited normalized respiratory patterns and have been discontinued from all treatment. Group values are expressed as the mean ± SEM.

RESULTS

For 300 infants evaluated at Children's Memorial Hospital in 1982–1986 and for whom theophylline treatment was recommended, treatment has now been completed, and the infants have been discharged from our follow-up clinic. In 148 of these patients (TABLE 1), an initial pneumogram was performed due to unexplained apparent life-threatening cardiorespiratory symptoms during sleep. It was also performed in 152 infants (TABLE 1) who were asymptomatic but thought to be at increased risk for SIDS (4 of these latter infants had two reasons for increased risk).

In 198 of the 300 infants (66%) in whom theophylline treatment was initiated prior to six months of age, the effects of theophylline on the respiratory pattern were analyzed by performing a repeat pneumogram within two weeks of beginning theophylline treatment. In these 198 infants, the postnatal age at the time of the first pneumogram was 29.7 ± 1.6 days (range 3–153 days). The peak blood level of theophylline was 10.2 ± 0.2 mg/ml

TABLE 1. Indications for the Initial Pneumogram in 300 Infants

Indication	No. of Infants
Symptomatic:[a]	
Apnea of infancy	109
Preterm infants	39
Total	148
Asymptomatic:	
Preterm infants	77
Family history of SIDS	53
Other	26
Total	156[b]

[a]Unexplained apparent life-threatening cardiorespiratory symptoms during sleep.
[b]Four of the infants in this group each had 2 indications present.

TABLE 2. Effects of Theophylline on Respiratory Pattern in 198 Infants

Parameter	Mean ± SEM	Range
Apnea density (%)		
Initial	2.3 ± 0.2	0.03–14.8
Theophylline[a]	0.4 ± 0.04[b]	0–5.0
Periodic breathing (episodes/100 min)		
Initial	4.2 ± 0.2	0–15.0
Theophylline[a]	0.3 ± 0.04[b]	0–4.2
Longest apnea (sec)		
Initial	13.6 ± 0.5	7–85
Theophylline[a]	10.5 ± 0.3[b]	5–32

[a]The repeat pneumogram in the presence of theophylline was performed within 14 days of the initiation of theophylline treatment.
[b]$p < 0.005$.

(range 4.5–20.7 mg/ml), and the repeat pneumogram in the presence of theophylline was performed an average of 6.7 ± 0.2 days after the first pneumogram (range 1–14 days). The effects of theophylline on the respiratory pattern are summarized in TABLE 2 and FIGURE 1.

In virtually all instances, the respiratory pattern improved significantly with theophylline treatment. The repeat pneumogram in the presence of theophylline was considered to be normal if $A_6/D\%$ was $\leq 0.9\%$, periodic breathing was ≤ 2.9 episodes/100 min and longest apnea was ≤ 20 sec. Using these criteria, the repeat pneumogram was normal in 186 of 198 infants (93.9%). $A_6/D\%$, which failed to normalize in 12/144 infants (8.3%) with an initially abnormal value ($> 0.9\%$), was somewhat less likely to normalize when the initial value was in the higher portion of the abnormal range. Thus, it failed to normalize in 9/74 infants (12.2%) with an initial value $\geq 2.0\%$. Periodic breathing failed to normalize in 4/131 infants (3%) with an initial value > 2.9 episodes/100 min. It was less likely to normalize ($p \leq 0.1$) when the initial value was most markedly abnormal, thus failing to normalize in 4/40 infants with an initial value ≥ 6.0 episodes/100 min. Longest apnea failed to normalize in 9/43 infants (20.9%) with an initial value ≥ 15 sec and also failed to normalize in 3/15 (20%) of infants with an initial value > 20 sec.

A home monitor was prescribed for a total of 107 of the 300 infants (35.7%). We recommended a home monitor in 7/148 symptomatic infants (4.7%) because their clinical symptoms failed to be eliminated, and in 18/300 infants (6.0%) because their pneumogram failed to normalize completely. In addition to these 25 infants, a home monitor was also utilized in 82/300 infants (27.3%) because of the preference of the referring physician and/or family. In total, a home monitor was utilized in 69/148 symptomatic infants (46.6%) but only in 38/152 asymptomatic infants (25%), a difference which is statistically significant ($p \leq .001$).

Subsequent clinical symptoms were determined by family reports of sleep-related episodes of color change and/or observed episodes of bradycardia or apnea requiring stimulation. No apparent life-threatening events occurred following initiation of intervention in the 152 asymptomatic infants, whether treated with theophylline alone or also on a home monitor. Among the symptomatic group, at least one subsequent apparent life-threatening event occurred in 8/148 infants (5.4%), all of whom were also on a home monitor. The repeat pneumogram in the presence of theophylline had normalized in three of these infants, had not normalized in three others, and was not performed in the remaining two patients.

Twenty-two infants (7.3%) did not continue to receive theophylline until the

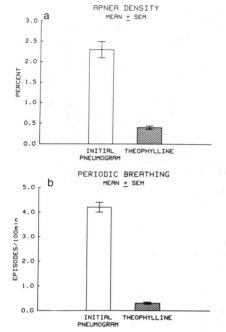

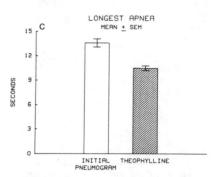

FIGURE 1. Effects of theophylline on respiratory pattern in 198 infants. At the time of the repeat pneumogram, the peak blood level of theophylline was 10.2 ± 0.2 µg/ml. (**a**) Apnea density (A_6/D%); (**b**) periodic breathing; (**c**) longest apnea. For each comparison, the decrease with theophylline is statistically significant ($p < 0.005$).

respiratory pattern was normal without theophylline. Parents elected to discontinue or not to begin theophylline treatment in 10/148 symptomatic infants (6.8%) and 12/152 asymptomatic infants (7.9%). Among these 22 infants, three families (14%) refused to initiate theophylline treatment and 19 families (86%) prematurely discontinued theophylline. In all instances in which theophylline treatment was prematurely discontinued, a home monitor had been included as part of the initial intervention program.

A total of 6 infants, 4 of whom were preterm, have died of SIDS since we began our theophylline treatment program in 1977. As summarized in TABLE 3, in none of these cases was theophylline treatment being monitored optimally. For 4 of these 6 infants, a home monitor had also been prescribed.

DISCUSSION

This retrospective review of our clinical experience with theophylline treatment summarizes our results in 148 infants with apnea-related symptoms and 152 asymptomatic infants considered to be at increased epidemiologic risk for SIDS. As previously reported,[4] theophylline was quite effective in significantly improving the respiratory pattern (TABLE 2, FIGURE 1). Indeed, theophylline treatment improved the pneumogram in virtually all instances and normalized the pneumogram in 93.9% of the 198 infants so evaluated. Although a substantial number of families also elected to utilize a home monitor (35.7%), theophylline-related normalization of the respiratory pattern was associated with an absence of recurrent life-threatening events in the symptomatic group and with a failure to develop life-threatening events in the asymptomatic group. Most infants were able to tolerate theophylline treatment, and it was prematurely discontinued only in 19 infants (6.3%). Six SIDS deaths have occurred in our total experience with theophylline (TABLE 3), but in none of these instances was treatment being appropriately monitored.

The mechanisms by which theophylline improves the respiratory pattern and reduces the potential for life-threatening events are not well understood. The possible mechanisms include enhanced chemical drive, improved asphyxic arousal responsiveness, other beneficial effects on brainstem cardiorespiratory regulation, or nonspecific effects unrelated to cardiorespiratory control. Both hypercarbic and hypoxic ventilatory sensitivity have been reported to be deficient in infants at risk for SIDS.[6] Although there are no reports of theophylline-related improvements in ventilatory sensitivity in at-risk infants, theophylline has been shown to improve CO_2 sensitivity in apnea of prematurity[7-9] and to increase hypoxic ventilatory drive in adults.[10] Eldridge et al. have suggested that theophylline enhances ventilatory drive by competitive antagonism of adenosine at neuronal receptor sites.[11] Although deficient arousal responsiveness, especially to hypoxia, has been reported in infants at increased risk for SIDS,[12] the effect of theophylline on arousal responsiveness has not been studied. In fetal lambs, however,

TABLE 3. Summary of all SIDS Deaths Occurring in Infants Treated with Theophylline

Case	Treatment	Brief Clinical Summary[a]
1	Theophylline	Birthweight 1,810 g. Symptomatic prior to NICU discharge, with abnormal pneumogram. Pneumogram normalized with theophylline and clinical symptoms resolved. Was also discharged on a home monitor, which was discontinued three weeks later (no alarms). Died five weeks later, with no intervening blood level determinations or dose adjustments.
2	Theophylline	Asymptomatic, sibling of three previous SIDS victims. Died at 13 months of age, six months after the last blood level determination and dose adjustment.
3	Theophylline plus monitor	Birthweight 1,130 g. Abnormal pneumogram prior to NICU discharge, normalized with theophylline. Neither the theophylline nor the monitor was continued, and death occurred two months later.
4	Theophylline plus monitor	Sibling of five prior SIDS victims. At the time of death at three months of age, both the theophylline and monitor were being used, but the theophylline peak blood level three days previously was only 4.1 μg/ml.
5	Theophylline plus monitor	Birthweight 1,360 g. Abnormal pneumogram prior to NICU discharge, normalized with theophylline. Died three months later, with no intervening blood level determinations or dose adjustments.
6	Theophylline plus monitor	Birthweight 1,450 g. Admitted to hospital six weeks after NICU discharge with history of apparent life-threatening event at home. Was treated with theophylline despite two normal pneumograms. Died six weeks later, with no apparent monitoring of theophylline blood levels and failure to respond to 10-minute monitor alarm.

[a]The first death occurred in 1977, the first year of the theophylline treatment program, and the last death in 1987. In all 6 infants, autopsy confirmed the absence of any identifiable cause of death.

enhancement of arousal responses by theophylline has been observed.[13] Theophylline might also improve one or more of the other abnormalities in brainstem cardiorespiratory control which potentially contribute to the development of SIDS.[14] As a nonspecific benefit, the known effects of theophylline on improving respiratory muscle contractility and recovery from fatigue[15-18] may also contribute to the presumed clinical benefits in infants at increased risk of SIDS. Administration of theophylline in apnea of prematurity does result in increased wakefulness and increased REM compared to non-REM sleep,[19] but it is unknown what state changes may occur in older infants or what effect such changes might have on cardiorespiratory control.

All of our evaluations of methylxanthine efficacy in apnea of infancy and in asymptomatic infants at increased epidemiologic risk for SIDS have been performed exclusively with theophylline. We have not yet utilized caffeine in these infants because of the lack of routine availability of an appropriate assay measurement and the lack of a commercially available liquid preparation. Caffeine, however, appears to have the same effect on respiratory pattern as theophylline, and the same relationship between improvement in respiratory pattern and in clinical symptoms.[20] In addition, for the same degree of respiratory stimulation, caffeine may have fewer behavioral side effects. Although not yet prospectively compared in older infants, in apnea of prematurity caffeine treatment resulted in significantly fewer problems with tachycardia, arousal, and gastrointestinal intolerance.[21]

There are several limitations to this retrospective analysis of theophylline efficacy in infants at increased risk for SIDS. Since all infants with an abnormal pneumogram received intervention, we do not know what the actual rate for SIDS or subsequent life-threatening events would have been had these 300 infants not received theophylline. In addition, we cannot assess the relative efficacy of available interventions since there was no prospective random assignment to theophylline or home monitor alone, or theophylline plus monitor. The extent to which we can extrapolate our observations to all infants at risk is limited by the inclusion of only those infants who returned for follow-up until clinically normal and were eventually discharged from our follow-up clinic. Consequently, although we think that we have identified all SIDS deaths in our infants treated with theophylline, we have no systematic information regarding efficacy or side effects in infants other than the 300 reported herein. Since the families experiencing greater difficulties with side effects might have been less likely to continue theophylline treatment and to return for follow-up, our retrospective review may underestimate the frequency of behavioral side effects leading to premature discontinuation of theophylline treatment. It is unlikely, however, that we have underestimated the frequency of apparent life-threatening events with theophylline treatment since these families would be more likely to return for ongoing clinical management. Finally, considering the low risk for SIDS even in the symptomatic apnea group ($\leq 5\%$), and the even lower risk in the asymptomatic groups at increased epidemiologic risk ($\leq 2\%$), with just 300 infants it would not have been possible to reach any conclusion regarding possible effects of our treatment program on risk of SIDS, even if treatment had been prospectively and randomly assigned.

In summary, theophylline treatment appears to be effective in significantly improving the respiratory pattern, in preventing recurrent symptoms in apnea of infancy, and in preventing life-threatening events in asymptomatic at-risk infants. To resolve the question of whether methylxanthine treatment is an effective alternative to a home monitor in apnea of infancy, a prospective study, in which patients are randomly assigned to drug treatment or a home monitor, is necessary. Although our report does not resolve this question, the results do indicate that such a study is ethically justified and potentially beneficial to patients with apnea of infancy. To determine whether theophylline can in fact reduce the incidence of SIDS, prospective studies in which asymptomatic infants at increased epidemiological risk are randomly assigned to theophylline treatment or no treatment are necessary. Since the pneumogram may not be the most appropriate test to document the theophylline-related effects on cardiorespiratory control or on other factors pertinent to the risk of SIDS,[14] subsequent studies are needed to determine the most representative clinical test for quantitating the extent to which methylxanthines favorably affect sleep-related cardiorespiratory control. Realistically, however, it may not be possible to resolve any of the questions regarding effects of methylxanthines on the risk of life-threatening events or of SIDS until the controversies regarding the pathophysiology of SIDS and the prospective identification of future SIDS victims are at least in part resolved.

ACKNOWLEDGMENT

To Donna Hanson, B.S.N., and Linda Klemka, M.S., for their assistance in data preparation and analysis, and to Susan Seidler, M.B.A., and Mary Pat Cusentino for their assistance in preparation of this manuscript.

REFERENCES

1. ARANDA, J. V. & T. TURMEN. 1979. Methylxanthines in apnea of prematurity. Clin. Perinatol. **6:** 87–108.
2. MARTIN, R. J., M. J. MILLER & W. A. CARLO. 1986. Pathogenesis of apnea in preterm infants. J. Pediatr. **109:** 733–741.
3. KELLY, D. H. & D. C. SHANNON. 1981. Treatment of apnea and excessive periodic breathing in full-term infant. Pediatrics **68:** 183–186.
4. HUNT, C. E., R. T. BROUILLETTE & D. HANSON. 1983. Theophylline improves pneumogram abnormalities in infants at risk for sudden infant death syndrome. J. Pediatr. **103(6):** 969–974.
5. HUNT, C. E., R. T. BROUILLETTE, D. HANSON, R. J. DAVID, I. M. STEIN & M. WEISSBLUTH. 1985. Home pneumograms in normal infants. J. Pediatr. **106(4):** 551–555.
6. HUNT, C. E., K. MCCULLOCH & R. T. BROUILLETTE. 1981. Diminished hypoxic ventilatory responses in near-miss sudden infant death syndrome. J. Appl. Physiol. **50:** 1313–1317.
7. RIGATTO, H., U. DESAI, F. LEAHY, Z. KALAPESI & D. CATES. 1981. The effect of 2% CO_2, 100% O_2, theophylline and 15% O_2 on "inspiratory drive" and "effective" timing in preterm infants. Early Hum. Dev. **5:** 63–70.
8. DAVI, M. J., K. SANKARAN, K. J. SIMONS, F. E. R. SIMONS, M. M. SESHIA & H. RIGATTO. 1978. Physiologic changes induced by theophylline in the treatment of apnea in preterm infants. J. Pediatr. **92:** 91–95.
9. GERHARDT, T., J. MCCARTHY & E. BANCALARI. 1979. Effect of aminophylline on respiratory center activity and metabolic rate in premature infants with idiopathic apnea. Pediatrics **63:** 537–542.
10. SANDERS, J. S., T. M. BERMAN, M. M. BARTLETT & R. S. KRONENBERG. 1980. Increased hypoxic ventilatory drive due to administration of aminophylline in normal men. Chest **78:** 279–282.
11. ELDRIDGE, F. L., D. E. MILLHORN & J. P. KILEY. 1985. Antagonism by theophylline of respiratory inhibition induced by adenosine. J. Appl. Physiol. **59(5):** 1428–1433.
12. MCCULLOCH, K., R. T. BROUILLETTE, A. J. GUZZETTA & C. E. HUNT. 1982. Arousal responses in near-miss SIDS infants and normal infants. J. Pediatr. **101:** 911–917.
13. MOSS, I. R. & E. M. SCRAPELLI. 1981. Stimulatory effect of theophylline on regulation of fetal breathing movements. Pediatr. Res. **15:** 870–873.
14. HUNT, C. E. & R. T. BROUILLETTE. 1987. Sudden infant death syndrome: 1987 perspective. J. Pediatr. **110(5):** 669–678.
15. AUBIER, M. A. DETROYER, M. SAMPSON, P. T. MACKLEM & C. ROUSSOS. 1981. Aminophylline improves diaphragmatic contractility. N. Engl. J. Med. **305:** 249–252.

16. SIGRIST, S., D. THOMAS, S. HOWELL & C. H. ROUSSOS. 1982. The effect of aminophylline on inspiratory muscle contractility. Am. Rev. Respir. Dis. **126:** 46–50.
17. HOWELL, S., R. S. FITZGERALD & C. H. ROUSSOS. 1985. Effects of aminophylline, isoproterenol, and neostigmine on hypercapnic depression of diaphragmatic contractility. Am. Rev. Respir. Dis. **132:** 241–247.
18. VIIRES, N., M. AUBIER, D. MURCIANO, C. MARTY & R. PARIENTE. 1986. Effects of theophylline on isolated diaphragmatic fibers. Am. Rev. Respir. Dis. **133:** 1060–1064.
19. DIETRICH, J., A. N. KRAUSS, M. REIDENBERG, D. E. DRAYER & P. A. M. AULD. 1978. Alterations in state in apneic pre-term infants receiving theophylline. Clin. Pharmacol. Ther. **24:** 474–478.
20. ANWAR, M., H. MONDESTIN, N. MOJICA, R. NOVO, M. GRAFF, M. HIATT & T. HEGYI. 1986. Effect of caffeine on pneumogram and apnoea of infancy. Arch. Dis. Child. **61:** 891–895.
21. BAIRAM, A., M. J. BOUTROY, Y. BADONNEL & P. VERT. 1987. Theophylline versus caffeine: Comparative effects in treatment of idiopathic apnea in the preterm infant. J. Pediatr. **110(4):** 636–639.

Chairman's Remarks

GAVIN C. ARNEIL

Scottish Cot Death Trust
Royal Hospital for Sick Children
Yorkhill, Glasgow, G3 8SJ
Scotland

The first essential in coping with a bereavement involving SIDS is to grasp the fact that one is dealing not only with a dead baby but with a damaged family. Three generations are often involved, grandparents, parents and siblings. Each generation has differing problems. Grandparents grieve for their affected child and dead grandchild. Parents grieve for their lost child. Siblings, usually young, miss and grieve for their sib and are overwhelmed by the surrounding atmosphere of gloom and despair. They are fearful that they too may "die in their sleep" and often feel guilty lest their "hostile" thoughts may have caused the incomprehensible tragedy to "their baby."

Maternal aspects are relevant to the problem in a number of ways. Hormonal, emotional and psychological disequilibrium following the birth still complicate the mother's problems of deep personal involvement with part of herself, "her" baby. The mother may be terrified of another SID occurring and may already be pregnant. If not, she may seek advice on whether, and when, to have a "new" baby—not, it is hoped, to be regarded as a "replacement" for the lost one, but as a person in his or her own right. Proper grieving, a period of questioning and acceptance of the cot death, are desirable antecedents to beginning the next pregnancy. Professional support begun early and continued at a number of levels is vital for optimal care. Initially, police, family doctors, pathologists, pediatricians, clerics and health visitors are involved. They should be trained not only to cope with the emergency but also to continue to care for the family throughout the periods of shock, grief, questioning, anger and acceptance which follow seriatim. Continuous professional support is needed for many months, certainly during subsequent pregnancies and during the infancy of all subsequent sibs. Support by a "befriender" who herself has experienced a cot death is beneficial to some bereaved parents but is not desired by all.

Befriending can present problems if it results in unsuitable advice or projection of another person's problems or controversial views. Parent befriending seems less necessary when a good professional, cooperative "package deal" supports parents over a period of years from the death. Certainly close cooperation between professional counseling and amateur befriending is desirable in each locality. No family which has suffered a cot death will ever be the same again; but while many are damaged, and some may break up, paradoxically, some are strengthened.

Apnea monitoring is a hotly contested subject. On the one hand we have the ultrascientific, cardiorespiratory, academic approach, demanding perfection in function with perfect detection of all forms of central and obstructive apnea. It also seeks statistically irrefutable proof or disproof under controlled conditions of the efficacy or otherwise of apnea monitors in preventing cot deaths. On the other hand we now have a plethora of doctors with genuine first hand knowledge of apnea monitoring, of its use in hundreds of families with sibs of SIDS cases. They understand the enormous benefits which can be brought to such families in the form of sleep, confidence, relaxation, and improved chances of continuing marital harmony. Such good results are only obtained when appropriate training, support, and encouragement are given to the families. Indisputably, monitoring is the only possible chance of survival for a sibling actually affected by apnea which will be lethal unless treated, or for when progressively more severe, intermittent apnea occurs (as found in some respiratory disease) and predicts that death may occur within hours. So far, no meaningful or acceptable controlled trial has proved possible, and probably none will ever be possible.

It is relatively easy to devalue the effects of apnea monitoring by undermining parents' confidence in it, thus reducing its reassurance value to that of alternatives which give no warning of apnea and no possibility of resuscitation. But this is manipulation of statistics rather than a controlled trial. Properly informed of its benefits and shortcomings, those parents wishing to monitor rarely fail to benefit and are often reluctant to give up; most insist on a monitor for subsequent siblings.

How then can one resolve the problem of the demand for 100%, statistically certain proof and the obviously great, 95% benefit to the majority of families whose monitor (provided free of cost in Scotland) completely changes the pattern of life for the parents and gives them the only hope of resuscitation for *their* baby if potentially lethal apnea occurs?

It is perhaps easier to square the circle.

The Sudden Infant Death Syndrome

Siblings and Their Place in the Family

FREDERICK MANDELL, MARY McCLAIN

AND ROBERT REECE

Children's Hospital
Boston, Massachusetts 02115

The sudden and unexpected death of an infant deeply affects the entire family.[1] Family relationships are immediately changed,[2] and surviving children not only mourn, but also assume new roles.[3]

We prepare children for older-sibling roles. That place of the big brother or big sister in the family is crystallized with the birth of a new infant.[4] When crib death occurs in such a family, new big-brother and big-sister roles are suddenly terminated, often in a catastrophic manner. Death has entered the confines of the family; it has disrupted family security and safety. Death has taken another child close in age. Often children do not understand that other children can die. The role of the older sibling is lost. There is a void of developmental opportunity, and, as a survivor, the child immediately comes to possess some new characteristics as a result of the loss.[5]

METHODS

In the present study, continued from a previous study,[3] 36 families who had sustained the sudden and unexpected death of an infant and who had surviving children were interviewed at least two months following the loss to obtain data about surviving siblings. Among the 36 families there were 45 surviving siblings. These siblings ranged in age from 16 months to 6 years. The interview sought information relevant to changes in patterns of sleep, toilet training, feeding habits, peer relationships and parent-child interactions.

RESULTS

These parents reported that all but 1 of the 45 surviving children had responses to the death which the parents perceived as notable. Eighty percent of the mothers perceived changes in their child's interaction with them after the loss. Most parents in our previously reported study described their own needs for being physically closer to their surviving children. One mother in that study stated, "We wanted and needed to hold him more. . . . I don't know who needed the hugging more, he or us." Some parents commented that they had wanted to retain infant behavior in a surviving child. This desire seemed to imply the parents' need for the intimacy of parent-infant bonding, as well as their fears for the safety of surviving children. Only a few mothers were able to express their own needs to have some distance from their surviving children. There were many instances of children attempting to comfort their parents in the time of distress, but for most of the surviving children, the sight of crying and confused parents was perplexing and frightening.[3]

The newly-acquired situation in the family often also included newly-acquired separation anxiety. Some of the children expressed the fear that their parents would also disappear. Some parents also talked about the tendency of surviving children to test the limits of discipline for several months after their sibling died.

Almost 70% of the children in the study demonstrated changes in sleep patterns following the baby's death. Although several children did not have sleep problems until several months after the death, in most instances this new manner of behaving emerged within a few days. Most sleep-related difficulties were in the form of resistance to going to bed and to sleep. Some children expressed fears about not waking up. Other sleep disturbances were accompanied by fitful dreams or nightmares. Older children who were able to describe the content of the nightmare often talked about the frequent theme of being chased by monsters. One parent related how her three-year-old fought sleep night after night because of her fear that a monster would take her because she had killed her brother. Parents associated these nighttime experiences to the baby's death, especially those present when the baby was found. Most children experiencing nightmares were able to respond to comforting and parental assurance and were able to settle back to sleep. Some families began to allow their children to sleep with them. In some instances this seemed to reassure the children who expressed fear that all those close to them were vulnerable.[3]

Different behavior was also noticed in reactions with peers. These behavioral changes ranged from becoming quiet and withdrawn to showing increased aggression, which included hitting other children. Many of the children evidenced for the first time an unwillingness to go to school, and others became so aggressive toward other siblings and friends that parents interpreted this behavior as mean.

DISCUSSION

The loss of an infant in a family is particularly frightening for siblings in the home because of the unexpected nature of the death and because of the children's inability to understand its meaning and its influence on the family. The abrupt loss of a healthy-appearing infant, without a clear cause, intensifies family grief. In this family setting, surviving siblings experience loss and fear.

The behavioral issues of surviving children are of significant concern to parents of SIDS victims. However, many parents are so overwhelmed by the loss, or prefer to deny additional problems, that they do not bring up these problems with health professionals.

It is important for professionals to know that children's ideas about death are quite different at different age levels. To the preschooler, death is a going away, temporary, but probably reversible. He is unable to accept it as final. To the five- to nine-year-olders, death happens, but it happens to other people. After this age, children understand death and its finality and that it happens to everybody.

In the world of television, children often think that death can be prevented and controlled. In a way this impression gives a child a sense of power over death. In our society we experience a taboo against talking about the death of children. It is a confusing time for surviving siblings.

Health professionals encourage adult patients to talk about crises. Children also need to express their interpretation of what happened. Children respond differently to loss. Some children have many questions, and they question the death just as they question other things they do not understand. Other children may have fears that this will happen to them or their parents.[4] Children think magically, and in some way they may have wished that their new brother or sister would go away. These children need to be reassured that they are not responsible for the events which have transpired and that the same thing will not happen to them. Children readily participate in silence surrounding infant death, and they quickly understand that the silence is a cover for something awful. Children's fantasies of death can be as frightening as the tragedy itself.

During the time following the sibling death, children can feel especially vulnerable. Interactions between the husband and wife have changed and parental behavior toward the surviving child is significantly modified. Parents recognize their overprotectiveness and permissiveness; however, their own intimate grief often forestalls the spontaneous expression of concern around surviving children. Behavioral responses of aggression or quietude in young surviving children may be misinterpreted by parents and health professionals; the consequences of the sibling death can become a source of distraction, dismay and fright for the surviving child.

We have also observed that this kind of unexpected death deeply affects the professional who is in a position to provide guidance for a surviving sibling—the infant's pediatrician. Forty-one of the forty-seven physicians indicated by questionnaire that they had discussed the death with the family. However, pediatricians are often uncomfortable following a sudden unexpected death in their practice. Many pediatricians found that they were able to provide only limited support for SIDS families. Eleven respondents said they purposely avoided discussions of parental feelings; six others indicated these discussions were brief. Eleven percent of these pediatricians completely avoided follow-up contacts with families after the death. Thus, the physician's own anxiety often prevents him/her from using a most basic grief counseling skill, namely that of listening empathetically as a family, parents and siblings, begins its grief work.

Children may avoid thinking about death. They may blame themselves. Children need to know that it is all right to cry, to question, and to express feelings. A time is a time, a place is a place; they come together only once. This is a time when professionals can help children whose intimate world has suddenly become insecure.

REFERENCES

1. ZEBAL B. & S. WOOLSEY. 1984. SIDS and the family: The pediatrician's role. Pediatr. Ann. **13(3):** 237–261.
2. MANDELL, F., E. MCANULTY & R. REECE. 1980. Observations of paternal response to sudden unanticipated infant death. Pediatrics **65:** 221–225.
3. MANDELL, F., E. MCANULTY & A. CARLSON. 1983. Unexpected death of an infant sibling. Pediatrics **72(5):** 252–257.
4. WESTON, D.L. & R.C. IRWIN. 1963. Preschool child's response to death of an infant sibling. Am. J. Dis. Child. **106:** 564.
5. KRELL, R. & L. RABKIN. 1979. The effects of sibling death on the surviving child: A family perspective. Fam. Process **18:** 471.

The Origin of Maternal Feelings of Guilt in SIDS

Relationship with the Normal Psychological Reactions of Maternity[a]

LUISELLA ZERBI SCHWARTZ[b]

Centro SIDS
Università di Milano
Milan, Italy

INTRODUCTION

To anyone who has dealt with the psychological aftermath of the sudden infant death syndrome (SIDS), one aspect is very familiar, the guilty feelings present among the mothers of the SIDS victims. At times these feelings are overt and manifest; at other times, they are not so obvious at a superficial level. What is the source of this guilty feeling? Is it based on some reality? Or is it an expression of something else, of something buried at a deeper level?

In this paper I will briefly review some aspects of the emotional consequences of having an infant victim of SIDS in comparison with those of other infantile deaths. I will then attempt to provide, within the framework of psychoanalytical theory and on the basis of interviews, projective tests, and dream interpretation, a key for considering these reactions as part of the "normal" emotional correlates of maternity.

During the last 6 years I have been involved, as a part of a team with pediatricians at the SIDS Center of the University of Milan, in a series of meetings—that in some cases have continued for a couple of years—with families of SIDS victims.[1,2] The issues which emerged during interviews with 49 families constitute the material on which I have based the present analysis.

THE PSYCHOSOCIAL IMPACT OF SIDS

Some of the emotional consequences of a SIDS event are similar to those found in other cases of neonatal or infantile death. Among these are a sense of inability to generate an infant who can survive, guilty feelings related to events and/or fantasies which occurred during the pregnancy, a tendency to idealize the dead infant, and difficulties in accomplishing a successful process of mourning, largely due to the paucity of memories directly related to the dead infant.[3-5]

[a]This work was supported in part by CNR, Consiglio Nazionale delle Ricerche Grant no. '82-'87. 01943.56, Progetto finalizzato Medicina Preventiva e Riabilitativa: Patologia Perinatale e sue Sequele.

[b]Address for correspondence: Centro SIDS, Clinica Pediatrica I, Università di Milano, Via Commenda 9, 20122 Milan, Italy.

However, there are also emotional reactions characteristic of SIDS and dependent on the following issues:

1. Death is sudden and unexpected, without warning signs.
2. Death almost always occurs during sleep and often at night, when the infant is out of parental control.
3. Parents do not receive from the physicians (pediatricians, coroners, pathologists) definite answers about the cause of death; mostly, answers are by exclusion, e.g., "Your infant did not die because of . . . nor because of. . . . "
4. For all cases of SIDS, in most countries there is a mandatory autopsy and a police investigation to rule out child abuse and infanticide.

The sudden infant death syndrome has more than one aspect; besides the infants who die, there are the parents and the older siblings who remain and who have to face and overcome this traumatic and often unexplained event. The available experience has indicated that several problems exist, common to most affected families.[6,7] Knowledge and understanding of these problems are necessary to provide effective support and to prevent further consequences of the SIDS event at both the psychological and the social level. Accordingly, I will list some of these problems, with brief comments included when necessary.

Emotional difficulties in the parental couple

1. Increased divorce frequency.[8]
2. Increased mobility. This largely reflects the difficulty in facing the neighbors' suspicious and unfriendly attitude;[9] after SIDS there is a "need to escape."
3. Inability to cope with the partner's reaction. The individual grief modality is often different for each parent and not always easy to understand. Fathers of SIDS victims often increase their work involvement, thereby reducing their presence at home.[10]
4. Exchange of reciprocal accusations. The circumstances of the SIDS event encourage questions and accusations: "Did you place his head properly on the pillow?" "You were watching the television and couldn't hear him crying." "You went to chat with the neighbour while our baby died." "Why did you change his formula?" "Why didn't you take him to the doc last week, as supposed?" "You overslept this morning, that's why you didn't see that he was sick and dying."

Psychosocial effects of SIDS

1. Guilty feelings (mostly on the mother's side). This aspect will be discussed in depth below.
2. Increased rate of abortions.[11]
3. Difficulties with the next pregnancy and child. Throughout the pregnancy and after delivery the mother fears that SIDS will recur; this leads to major anxiety and to the need for medical reassurance on the health of the new infant.[12]
4. Discomfort and embarrassment about the police investigation.
5. Difficulties with neighbors. This includes unspoken suspicions and malevolent gossip. This phenomenon is inversely correlated with the amount and depth of knowledge about SIDS in the general population.[13]
6. Deterioration of the patient-physician relationship. There is a loss of confidence and often the appearance of aggressiveness toward the physicians who are unable to provide a precise diagnosis, or an adequate explanation, and who have often seen the infant a few days before his death without noticing anything abnormal.[14]

Effects of SIDS on siblings

1. Need to elaborate the concept of death. Most siblings of a SIDS victim, usually 3–5 years old, never before had a close contact with death, with "gone forever." They are for the first time forced to grasp the concept that "the loved ones" may go and never return, that they may die. This is a painful moment which will carry a significant burden.

2. Guilty feelings. The jealousy of older siblings toward the new baby who competes for the mother's time and love is a well-known phenomenon. This jealousy often results in the desire for the "disappearance" of the intruder, and one day the intruder disappears for real, he dies. A young child distinguishes poorly between fantasy and reality; he wanted the young brother to go away, to disappear, and now it has really happened, the young brother is dead. The older sibling often views this event as the realization, the unwanted realization, of his unexpressed wishes; he has but one option, to feel guilty.

3. Behavioral problems:

   a. Sleep difficulties and nightmares. The older sibling is often told that the baby died while asleep. Presented with the association of sleep with death, he begins to regard sleep as a moment of danger and to fear that during sleep he himself might die. The old saying "Sleep is a small death" may seem quite true to him.

   b. Changes in social interaction. These children behave differently with their parents and with their peers; the behavior can range from withdrawn and excessively quiet to aggressive.

   c. Regression in developmental stages. This includes bed-wetting, regression in toilet training, and requests to be fed from a bottle. This has been viewed as representing a major disruption or the unconscious attempt to substitute for the dead infant by assuming his behavior.[15,16]

WHEN SIDS OCCURS

Generalized categorizations, as those just made in the preceding section, are necessary for an overview of the problem and for outlining ground rules for intervention or for prevention of some aspects of the psychosocial impact of SIDS. However, if one listens to the actual tale of the events as made by the parents and then analyzes the overall family picture in which SIDS has occurred, together with the various events as they took place after the infant's death, it becomes evident that there is something else : that there is something that goes beyond the mourning for the lost infant, beyond the social problems, beyond the superficial mechanisms generating guilty feelings. It is for this reason that I will now present in some detail 4 distinct case histories, chosen from among the entire group of 49, not because of any exceptional aspect, but because they are representative of what it seems to me is a component of SIDS important for understanding some of the psychological reactions. These case histories will be followed by a few considerations.

Case 1

A healthy, 6-month-old infant, M., was found in her crib already cyanotic and rigid by the mother, whose scream awakened a 3-year-old sister of the infant, who was sleeping in the same room.

The father's first reaction was to destroy the crib, viewed as responsible (he had instantly remembered his own fears of suffocation, experienced as a young child when he was playing and hiding under the blankets of his parents' bed). In the emergency room the father had a violent reaction to the police questioning ("they were looking for the killer") and to the autopsy ("I knew that it was the crib's fault, why torture her body?").

The parental couple, wealthy middle class, had their first contact with the SIDS Center 3 months after the event, when the mother was already 2 months pregnant (the day of M.'s death she wanted another child; later she thought, "It is not right to want to have a son for such an egotistical reason").

During the first interview, the mother talked extensively about her menstrual difficulties, of a diagnosis of sterility (related to a closed Fallopian tube), and of the 4 pregnancies and 2 abortions which proved the contrary. She seemed to need reassurance about her own generative power. At this time the mother was in a serious state of anxiety and described the occurrence of frequent nightmares.

The couple had been well informed and had regular contacts with private physicians. Nonetheless, there was a clear lack of confidence and of esteem toward medicine in general and toward the current knowledge on SIDS in particular.

Since the beginning, and repeatedly afterwards for several months, the mother told of a special attitude toward M. "She was the fourth, but I did not know how to treat her. It was as if I didn't know anymore how to grow up a child; she was an anarchist, never following the rules, and I had to call the pediatrician at home every week to reassure me that everything was fine."

Case 2

R. was a 25-year-old unwed mother, with a teenage appearance. She did not have a regular job or family relations. She was receiving financial support for herself and for her son from the boy's father, who had not made a legal statement of paternity.

The 8-month-old boy had been brought, already dead, to the emergency room of the Department of Pediatrics, where the SIDS Center is located. He was found to be well nourished, well cared for, and without any sign of careless treatment (there were not even the rather common lower back reddening).

R. was desperate, frightened, and totally lost. She immediately developed an important emotional relationship of total dependence with the senior pediatrician of the SIDS Center. During the first formal meeting, which took place a week after the SIDS event, the major and more pressing problems were represented by the doubts on the cause of death, which were continuously reconsidered by R. in the attempt to find a sign of her own guilt for something done or omitted. The last evening, the child had hit a table with his head while crawling on the floor ("I couldn't keep him anymore in my arms all the time"). It had been one of the first times that she had added special spaghetti for infants (routinely used in Italy) to the soup of meat and vegetables ("The pediatrician had told me that it was the right time to start but, perhaps, I should have waited"). The infant had cried during the night but she had not responded ("He was doing it every night, I had learned that he just wanted to be taken in my arms and he was calming down by himself").

In the subsequent encounters, there was the progressive emergence of an attempt to find a culprit outside of herself: the ambulance which took too much time to arrive, the physicians who perhaps had not done all that was possible, the autopsy which left ugly traces on the infant's body without providing safe answers about why he died.

She reported also a very negative and psychologically aggressive attitude by the neighbors, her growing discomfort for the situation, the need to change her residence to escape this difficult condition. She was spending much time with a friend who had a small daughter and who had in the past kept her own son, if needed.

As time progressed, she started to ask questions about the risk for a second son and expressed the desire for another pregnancy, which she then carried out uneventfully. For the entire first year, the SIDS Center continued to provide support and guidance for any, even minor, problem of the new child, who was simultaneously and regularly followed by another, private physician.

Case 3

S., a 2-month-old infant still breast-fed by the mother, was found dead at 7:40 A.M. He was still almost warm; only the extremities were cold. The father went immediately to see his own mother who, learning what had happened, felt sick. The mother went alone to the emergency room where her hopes were revived when the medical personnel "jumped on the baby" in a desperate and useless attempt to revive it. As the infant was recognized as dead, a policeman began to question her rudely, hinting at her responsibility and trying to make her feel guilty. In that hospital, where no one was taking care of her, the mother felt totally alone, desperate, and without any help.

The parents of S., a couple of middle-class professionals, showed since the first meeting an extreme interest for the information available on SIDS. This interest was clearly shared by both of them, and they were both efficient in providing all documents related to S. However, they had difficulties in living together with their different reactions to their son's death. The father prepared designs for a new model of monitor with an effective alarm system. This son who had died had been wanted and planned for by the parents, with the unexpressed hope of overcoming difficulties in their relationship which a few years of marriage had unmasked.

As the meetings progressed, reciprocal accusations became evident (a fall during the pregnancy, allergies of doubtful significance, the sudden cardiac death of an uncle). One year later they divorced.

Case 4

P. died of SIDS when he was two and one-half months old. He had been conceived outside the marriage by the mother, who had another son, 11 years old, and who was still living with the husband. P. was never brought home and had been given full-time to a paid baby-sitter, who was fully responsible for him, while the mother was trying to decide whether to leave her husband and create a family with her lover.

Despite living in the parental home, the older son grew up under the responsibility of the maternal grandmother who was also living under the same roof and who opposed the second pregnancy and the possibility of a divorce.

P. had been found dead at 11:00 A.M. by the baby-sitter, who first tried cardiopulmonary resuscitation and then called an ambulance. The parents were informed when the infant was already in the hospital. The baby-sitter was quite shocked and wanted to be informed in detail about SIDS by the physicians. The mother refused any contact with the physicians and with the baby-sitter, whom she stubbornly thought to be the culprit, and did not want to see the dead infant. The police investigation raised no reaction, and there was no opposition to the autopsy, which was viewed as necessary to definitively prove the baby-sitter's guilt.

All relatives and friends, with one exception, were excluded from the event ("No one wanted him besides us, they'll be happy now") and no one attended the funeral. The mother never went to the cemetery. On the other hand, the father of the dead infant wanted to dress him prior to the funeral, went every day to the cemetery, and showed depressive signs.

The older sibling had only vague information about both P.'s birth and death. He had never seen him. The mother noticed that he became closer to her and wanted to do more things with her. He also asked for one of P.'s teddy bears, but the mother refused and kept it for herself.

Considerations

In these 4 case histories there were many of the events typical of SIDS, as clearly described in the literature: lack of information about the existence of SIDS among the parents, as well as among the general population, the brutality of some of the police investigations, the neighbors' malevolence, the involvement of the sibling, the accusations, etc. All of these elements tend to augment the guilty feeling and to interfere with successful mourning.

However, there were also other important elements simultaneously present. In each of these 4 cases the infant who subsequently died of SIDS had been desired because of some motives beyond its natural meaning (the accomplishment of a natural instinct). Each one of those infants had an emotional and social meaning that was transcendental to its own being and that was more closely related to the individual personal or social history of the mother or of the parental couple. In these 4 cases the infants were representing for their mothers one or more of the following: a sign of her own normality and feminine potency, a sign of her own value and desirability, the justification for the sexual pleasure otherwise viewed as merely selfish, and a means for the strengthening and healing of an endangered relationship. Accordingly, the death of these infants represented also the loss of all these different and quite meaningful attributes of the maternal self, of which these infants were of course unaware carriers.[17–21]

MATERNITY, GUILTY FEELINGS, AND SIDS

Before proceeding with the events related to SIDS, it is necessary to briefly summarize the psychiatric and psychoanalytical theories on the deep emotional dynamics of maternity. This overview is largely based on the work by Deutsch[22] and Benedeck.[23]

Pregnancy and maternity represent the highest point, the acme of feminine psychosexual achievement, and they put again to test all the preceding developmental steps for the acquisition of a full feminine identity (infancy, Oedipal period, adolescence). During pregnancy and childbirth, the psychic economy is affected by the stress secondary to the physical effects (hormonal changes, pain) as well as the psychosocial events involved in changing from the role of daughter to that of a mother responsible for the raising of a child.

These significant difficulties may be overcome by the use, as "internal resources," of good maternal relations and of positive identifications with a "good mother." On the other hand, there is a deep emotional stress due to the sudden reappearance of the hostile, unconscious, latent, or unresolved emotions directed against her own mother and against the infantile figure (the infantile self, or the younger siblings).

These psychological conflictual ramifications, and the reactions to them, tend to form patterns exhibiting a sort of psychological unity. The following is an outline of the most important patterns, as very clearly described by Normand.[24]

Problems and Conflicts Related to the Feminine Sexual Identity

Deutsch[22] and Bosselman[25] described a masculine-aggressive type, who has never accepted the feminine role. Some such women are overtly homosexual and never become pregnant or, if they do, get abortions; others are compelled to try to deny the problem by having children. Some women fitting in the latter group find pregnancy pleasant because of an increased sense of power and prestige, which is in part the result of the unconscious equation, baby = penis. However, they may break down when delivery makes them feel painfully feminine. With the regression that occurs, old conflicts emerge involving hostility toward their own mother, and the baby is hated as a sign of their despised feminine role.

Unresolved Emotional Oedipal Forces

Another major type of dynamic pattern that may lead a woman to reject her baby involves unresolved Oedipal forces. The child is the concrete symbol of her success in achieving the childhood fantasy of displacing her mother, winning her father's love, and having a baby by him. This leads to anxiety and the urge to be rid of the incriminating evidence. Guilt appears and results in pathological behavior.

Rejection of the Infant

Rejection of the baby can result also from the woman's wish to be a baby herself, dependent on her own mother. Jealousy of her child relates to the woman's own childhood, her wish to enjoy her mother's exclusive attention, and her hatred of sibling rivals. Identification with the baby leads her to fear the same angry, greedy attitude from it that she herself feels toward her mother.

General Comments

It is essential to recognize that these unconscious emotional dynamics are present and active, with different degrees and configurations, in *every woman* who faces pregnancy and maternity. These emotional forces may give rise to several obstetric problems, including psychological sterility, spontaneous abortions, excessive gravidic nausea, and premature delivery,[26] as well as postpartum blues, infrequently leading to severe postpartum mental disorders.[24,27] A decisive factor for the outcome is in the ego, which, in emotionally mature women, makes use of the parturition experience to resolve old conflicts and to strengthen the feminine position.

What is the link between these emotional dynamics—forceful, but still within the boundaries of normality—and what happens to so many mothers of SIDS victims? Most of the time SIDS occurs during the very first postpartum months. These mothers had quite recently gone through the emotional processes of maternity, some of them successfully or on their way to solving their problems in a positive manner. And then, all of a sudden, there was the unexpected and extremely painful event: the infant had died, often during the night, without preceding illnesses or warning signs of impending danger; and the physicians' "mumbo-jumbo"[28] did not help to understand what really happened to the baby. It is almost as if the unconscious emotional ambivalences had suddenly and powerfully materialized as happens in a dream, where the hostile and aggressive wishes escape censorship and removal and appear intermingled and confused with reality. The special facts that so characteristically surround a SIDS event are probably a major determinant for its psychological sequelae. Indeed, even in the absence of specific comparative studies, there is a consensus that other infantile deaths occurring with different modalities, particularly when due to well-known diseases or preceded by a serious illness, do not lead to guilty feelings or to difficulties in mourning successfully. By contrast, with SIDS the guilty feelings are almost omnipresent, regardless of whether they are experienced directly or projected on others.

The presence of this phenomenon, noted by all the SIDS investigators,[6,7,11,14,29] has almost unavoidably led some to question if many of these guilty feelings are not just simple reflections of "true guilt." In a paper like this one, it is not possible to ignore entirely the sensitive issue of infanticide as one possible cause of guilty feelings. Extreme positions, such as the one proposed by Asch[30] ("A large percentage of crib deaths are actually infanticides occurring as part of a post-partum depression unknown to or disguised by the family and/or the family physician"), have not only been rejected as repugnant[31] but have also been dismissed on more solid scientific grounds.[31] However, on a more well-founded basis, even if more cautiously than Asch, Emery[32] has proposed a similar concept and has also proposed the involvement of postpartum depression.

While it would certainly be inappropriate to review here the data pro and con the role of infanticide in cases diagnosed as SIDS, it seems fair to comment on the proposed role of postpartum depression. Postpartum psychoses (including postpartum depression) are rare conditions in which the intensity of the emotional dynamics overwhelms an ego which is quite fragile and could sometimes be truly endangered. These are major mental disorders with important symptoms, such as delusions, obsessions and hallucinations; they cannot be ignored by the relatives nor by the physicians. Normand[24] has proposed that these disorders may actually represent a desperate attempt by the mother to save her child: "She rejects the child actually or symbolically. A protective motive, the desire to save the baby from her hostility, may also play a part in the turning away" (developing a postpartum disorder). Thus, the mother attacks herself instead of the child.

Under these conditions, isolated cases of attempted or successful infanticide may infrequently occur. Nonetheless, one has to remember that mothers of SIDS victims, as a group, are not known to have a significant incidence of major postpartum disorders.

The proponents of the theory that infanticide is a somewhat frequent occurrence in SIDS invoke the presence of a mental crisis. But it is difficult to accept the idea that mothers from different cultural backgrounds, in different countries, in different periods have always—during such a mental crisis—chosen the same modality for killing their infant: silent, nighttime, without external signs. It just does not fit. As suicides differ widely for their modalities, the same should occur for infanticides induced by a "mental crisis."

SURFACING OF DEEP AMBIVALENCES

As mentioned above, unspecific guilty feelings are amost always reported by or found in SIDS mothers. The true origin of these guilty feelings is, however, usually hidden— and with reason. The unconscious and scarring aggressive dynamics that have generated these deep guilty feelings cannot be accepted by the ego and therefore cannot be expressed at this conscious level. But they can be expressed in specific and appropriate forms, as elicited by projective tests or by a dream (in which we can say what we don't want to hear).

I will now describe and analyze some representative personality configurations and dreams that can be interpreted within the 3 dynamic frameworks depicted in the preceding section.

Problems and Conflicts Related to the Feminine Sexual Identity

F., a 27-year-old woman, strong-willed and respected in her profession, had moved to Milan by herself when she was 18 years old and had improved her professional level by studying in the evenings with great drive. She was born into a large family, the first girl after 4 boys, with whom she had repeatedly identified in her infantile and adolescent behavior. She had suffered from nocturnal enuresis since the beginning of the menstrual cycles which she had initially viewed as an unpleasant obstacle to her games. The oldest brother, who was at the top of his class and went to a university, had always been a sort of idealized figure to her. The father had been viewed as good, sweet, but not involved in the family management, which was fully controlled by her mother, a rather cold but efficient and respected woman.

When she was 16 years old, the level of conflicts with her mother heightened ("She wanted me to help her and to behave as a woman") and culminated in her departure from home with the alibi of finding a job. She had been married for a few years without major sexual problems, except for a mismatch between desire and fulfillment, which were both present but usually not together. The pregnancy of the infant who later became a SIDS victim had been planned and without difficulties ("I was feeling very well; I didn't even quit jogging"). After the infant's death, acute episodes of anxiety had appeared and required pharmacological treatment; however, in a lesser way they had been present since the child's birth. She felt extremely guilty for his death, despite being, because of her own profession, quite knowledgeable about the management and care of infants.

She was able to verbalize by herself that perhaps she was feeling guilty because she had not totally wanted this infant (". . . . as if he had known"). The birth of the infant had made it more difficult for her to continue her studies. Just after the delivery, she thought a lot about this. All her friends and relatives had been telling her that she couldn't continue her studies, because to do so would also have implied that she was neglecting her husband.

The Rorschach test showed the presence of conflicts related to the feminine identification (confirmed by the personal history) and of deteriorated maternal images.

Unresolved Emotional Oedipal Forces

D., a 32-year-old woman whose second son died of SIDS at 3 months of age, told this dream : "I was walking on the street and I had the sensation of being followed. I turned and saw the devil. One is always told to fear the devil but I turned again in all quiet, as if I were stronger than him. Now I have no more fear, but when I was a little girl I was in awe of the devil, because that is what they teach you. I woke up in great distress".

During the year following the SIDS event, the sexual desire for her husband disappeared completely; together with this there appeared a state of depression and a sort of emotional indifference toward the first son. At the same time, she developed aggressiveness toward her sisters, her mother, and her mother-in-law ("It was as if they had been all thinking 'what have you done?' "). Massive and continuous psychological support allowed this woman to have another pregnancy, and the subsequent maternity was accompanied by extreme anxiety, insomnia, and the inability to leave the child alone.

In her dream, it is possible to identify in the devil who follows her the persecution of the infantile guilty feelings secondary to the sexual desire for her father and the wish to eliminate her mother. The suppression of the evidence of her fault, by the infant's death, is represented by the seeming tranquillity with which she turns toward the devil (I am not guilty. There is not even any longer the baby to prove it!). She also has to suppress the other incriminating evidence, and this she achieves by eliminating the sexual desire for her husband. Finally, the women of the family reactivate the original hostile emotions.

G. was in a relationship strongly opposed by her partner's family, to whom he was totally tied because of a complete financial dependence related to his work. The infant who died of SIDS was the second-born and had somehow sanctioned the creation of a new and more solid family and the permanent tie with the partner.

Almost immediately after the SIDS event, G. had another pregnancy, which was made very difficult by major anxiety, insomnia, and nightmares; she came with 2 dreams. "I was opening a drawer and, inside, there was an infant and I showed it to the lady-warden [of the house], like that!" This was followed by, "I was walking in the street and I was carrying a baby girl in my arms, I encountered the lady-warden who told me accusingly 'Where did you get it?'; as I put her down on the ground, the baby divided herself, becoming two twin little girls."

In the personal history of this woman there are important events, such as the separation of her parents when she was an adolescent, a beautiful mother with whom G. was in a very conflictual relationship, and the strong figure of the maternal grandfather, with whom she had a special relationship of extremely intense affection. On this basis, it is possible to attempt an interpretation of those 2 dreams.

If one realizes the Oedipal wishes to have a child with a paternal figure, it then becomes unavoidable that one will confront a superegoic mother (the lady-warden) who can see the infant in uterus (the drawer) and, by accusing her of stealing ("Where did you get it?"), forces her to give up the child. However, there is the possibility to realize the much-desired revenge through an immediate and substitutive pregnancy (the girl becomes a pair of twins).

Rejection of the Infant

Z., a 33-year-old woman married for 10 years, had wanted and planned the first pregnancy; she easily became pregnant as soon as she gave up the IUD; during pregnancy she often had nausea and insomnia. Z. was the only daughter of parents to whom she was closely related in a dependent relationship; the decision to have the pregnancy had come after the death of her parents.

The Rorschach test showed evidence of strong signs of free anxiety and of a very regressive and symbiotic relationship with a maternal figure.

Z., after the SIDS event, reported the two following, brief dreams: "I was ready to the moment of delivery, but a cesarean section became necessary and I died," and "I was going to breast-feed C. [the infant who died of SIDS] in her room and I found her dead." This latter dream recurred a number of times, always associated with feelings of anguish.

A possible interpretation here lies in the deep feeling that to become a mother and an adult means seeing the violent death of her wishes to take the place of the new child and return in a dependent position with her own mother. The wish to depend on her mother is tightly related to oral and exclusive desires; this helps to understand the second dream, where the competitor for the maternal breast is eliminated (". . . I found her dead").

Considerations

In all the above cases, the women involved had no major psychological disturbances requiring treatment; rather, they were persons with a rich emotional and affective life, with a good capability to relate and to adapt. It is evident that, beyond the terrible pain for the loss of the infant, the SIDS event triggered in these, as well as in most cases, a major emotional suffering related to the intolerable and unacceptable deep aggressive emotions directed against the infant. For the necessary removal of these unacceptable wishes, these women pay a huge emotional price, which further increases the sharpness of their suffering and which, in some cases, makes extremely difficult successful mourning and the normal emotional detachment from the dead infant.

One last dream, reported by a young mother who lost her second son because of SIDS, expresses well the presence of emotional ambivalences that cause so much pain and difficulties to the mothers of SIDS infants (anxiety, insomnia, and intractable aggressiveness): "There were many prams all in line and they contained plastic bags with dead infants inside. I went closer and did look in all of them to see in which one there was my baby." This dream occurred the night after she heard in the news that a newborn was found alive after having been abandoned in a plastic bag by his own mother, an unmarried youngster who had tried to hide her pregnancy and maternity from her parents. Thus, this mother of a SIDS victim identified herself, because of her own aggressive feelings, with the infanticidal mother. It has to be noted that the circumstances of this SIDS event were such to completely exclude any responsibility on her part. On the other hand, the fact that in the broadcasted information the abandoned infant had survived, points to the simultaneous presence in this mother of a SIDS victim of a strong desire for her beloved infant, the desire to have him still alive.

CONCLUSIONS

Even a nonprofessional observer is impressed by the efforts made by the mothers to carefully, painstakingly reanalyze every detail of the last moments and actions, in an almost desperate attempt to identify what went wrong, what each of them did wrong. Even her own sleep is perceived as not free from guilt. Then, the analysis goes backwards again, to the type of feeding, to the adherence to the golden rules; and then it goes further back, to the pregnancy, and to her habits: did she smoke, did she take some prescription drugs that might have caused harm; and, more important and painful: was the pregnancy a desired one, or one just accepted, or one meant to pursue other goals, in the relationship with either the husband or other persons. These questions, we all know, come back over and over again.

Despite the well-recognized presence of the maternal feelings of guilt in the mothers of SIDS victims, there have been few attempts to investigate this problem in detail. Some relatively superficial and obvious reasons for guilty feelings include the following: (1) failure to have insured her own survival through her child, as an expression of continuation of herself; (2) an inferiority feeling in comparison to the other women; (3) fear of forgetting the infant because of the few memories—often there is not even a picture; and so on.

There is, however, a deeper level at which the guilty feelings are related to the development of the feminine identity and to the beginning of the desire to become a mother. Within a psychoanalytical approach, it is accepted that this desire does not depend only on instinct, or on hormonal release, or on the learning of a social role, but that it is also the end-product of the emotional events and fantasies originated by the conflict with the mother, the ambivalent desire and fear of making a child with her own father (what is called the resolution of the Oedipal complex). It is worth noting that it is in conjunction with these infantile fantasies that there is the development of the superego, the internal judge and censor that condemns these wishes.

There is an abundance of studies, within psychological research, on maternity and on the consequences of these unsolved conflicts. As an example, the classic study by Maria

Langer,[26] based on data collected from a large population of women who were either in departments of obstetrics or undergoing individual psychotherapy, shows that many somatic disturbances, including obstacles to the reproductive process, depend on persisting fears of being punished by an interiorized and vindictive mother who will make her daughter pay for those infantile wishes. She also showed that the resolution, during therapy, of these fears eliminates the physical symptoms as well.

Does this relate to SIDS? The mystery still surrounding the SIDS event, the related lack of adequate explanations, the circumstances (often nighttime), the occurrence during the neonatal period—all this can well elicit the same problem. The study by Mandel on mothers of SIDS victims, showing the many difficulties with their subsequent pregnancies,[11] seems to fit well with this concept.

The material collected in this work, the dreams of the mothers of SIDS victims and the Rorschach tests, points to the presence of deep fears of persecution and of feelings that parts of oneself are damaged and destructive. *This is true even in mothers for whom the sequence of events was such as to completely rule out any, even minor, responsibility for the infant's death.*

It is important to note that guilty feelings and defense mechanisms against aggressive impulses are normal mechanisms that, in varying degrees, can be found in every man and woman. The SIDS event brings to the surface something which is already there.

It is essential to distinguish between reality and the world of emotions and aggressive fantasies that can easily produce guilty feelings preceived as real. This concept could be of practical use for the professionals involved in SIDS. The physician who deals with the mothers of SIDS victims should not be frightened by being exposed to the latent emotional dynamics, even if he is working only at the ego level, i.e., giving information, answering questions, and so on. Because of his respected position, of his knowledge on what has to be done, the physician has a special power and role. He could tell the mother ''I have heard your doubts, your fears, I know where are they coming from, and I know that you are not really guilty.'' For once, the physician could become the good and loving mother.

ACKNOWLEDGMENTS

I wish to express my gratitude to Drs. P. Rusinenti, P. Salice, and A. Segantini, the pediatricians who shared with me many of the meetings with the families of SIDS victims; to Dr. G. Giaconia for help in overcoming my own difficulties in facing exposure to these disquieting emotions; to Peter, my husband, for his encouragement, continuous feedback, participation in the preparation of this manuscript, and, particularly, for having translated my psychoanalytical jargon into more straightforward language.

REFERENCES

1. SEGANTINI, A., V. CARNELLI, D. PORTALEONE, L. ZERBI-SCHWARTZ, G. FALZI, P. SALICE, P.J. SCHWARTZ & P. CAREDDU. 1983. The sudden infant death syndrome in Italy. A multidisciplinary approach. Pediatr. Med. Chir. 5 (Suppl. III):57–60.
2. ZERBI SCHWARTZ, L., A. SEGANTINI, P. SALICE & D. PORTALEONE. 1983. Psychological approach to the families of victims of ''sudden infant death syndrome''. *In* Second European Congress of Obstetric Anaesthesia and Analgesia, Rome, Italy: 100.
3. LEWIS, E. 1979. Mourning by the family after a stillbirth or neonatal death. Arch. Dis. Child. **54:** 303–306.
4. ELLIOTT, B.A. 1978. Neonatal death: Reflections for parents. Pediatrics **62:** 100–102.
5. BENFIELD, D.G., S.A. LEIB & J.H. VOLLMAN. 1978. Grief response of parents to neonatal death and parent participation in deciding care. Pediatrics **62:** 171–177.

6. FRIEDMAN, S.B. 1974. Psychological aspects of sudden unexpected death in infants and children. Pediatr. Clin. North Am. **21:** 103–111.
7. BUGLASS, K. 1981. Psychological aspects of the sudden infant death syndrome ("cot death"). J. Child Psychol. Psychiatry **22:** 411–421.
8. CORNWELL, J., B. NURCOMBE & L. STEVENS. 1977. Family response to loss of a child by sudden infant death syndrome. Med. J. Aust. **1:** 656–658.
9. DEFRAIN, J.D. & L. ERNST. 1978. The psychological effect of sudden infant death syndrome on surviving family members. J. Fam. Practice **6:** 985–989.
10. MANDELL, F., E. MCANULTY & R.M. REECE. 1980. Observations of paternal response to sudden unanticipated infant death. Pediatrics **65:** 221–225.
11. MANDELL, F. & L.C. WOLFE. 1975. Sudden infant death syndrome and subsequent pregnancy. Pediatrics **56:** 774–776.
12. SZYBIST, C. 1973. The Subsequent Child. National Foundation for Sudden Infant Death. New York.
13. WATSON, E. 1981. An epidemiologic and sociological study of unexpected death in infancy in nine areas of Southern England. Med. Sci. Law **21:** 99–104.
14. BERGMAN, A.B. 1974. Psychological aspects of sudden unexpected death in infants and children. Pediatr. Clin. North Am. **21:** 115–121.
15. WILLIAMS, M.L. 1981. Sibling reaction to cot death. Med. J. Aust. **2:** 227–231.
16. MANDELL, F., E. MCANULTY & A. CARLSON. 1983. Unexpected death of an infant sibling. Pediatrics **72:** 652–657.
17. MEAD, M. 1949. Human reproduction. *In* Male and Female. M. Mead, Ed. William Morrow & Co. New York.
18. MACINTYRE, S. 1976. Who wants babies? The social construction of instincts. *In* Sexual Divisions and Society: Process and Change. D.R. Baker & S. Allen, Eds. Tavistock. London.
19. WYATT, F. 1967. Clinical notes on the motives of reproduction. J. Soc. Issues **23:** 29–56.
20. FLAPAN, M. 1969. A paradigm for the analysis of child bearing motivations of married women prior to birth of the first child. Am. J. Orthopsychiatry **39:** 402–417.
21. PASINI, W. 1974. Désir d'enfant et contraception. Casterman. Paris.
22. DEUTSCH, H. 1945. The Psychology of Women. Grune & Stratton. New York.
23. BENEDEK, T.F. 1959. Sexual functions in women and their disturbance. *In* American Handbook of Psychiatry. S. Arieti, Ed. Vol 1: 727. Basic Books. New York.
24. NORMAND, W.C. 1967. Post partum disorders *In* Comprehensive Textbook of Psychiatry. A.M. Freedman & H.I. Kaplan, Eds. The Williams & Wilkins Co. Baltimore.
25. BOSSELMAN, B.C. 1964. Neurosis and Psychosis. Charles C. Thomas. Springfield, Ill.
26. LANGER, M. 1951. Maternidad y sexo. Paidos. Buenos Aires.
27. ZILBOORG, G. 1931. Depressive reactions related to parenthood. Am. J. Psychiatry **87:** 927.
28. BERGMAN, A.B. 1974. Humanizing society. *In* SIDS 1974. R.R. Robinson, Ed.: 303. The Canadian Foundation for the Study of Infant Deaths. Toronto.
29. BERGMAN, A.B. 1986. The "Discovery" of Sudden Infant Death Syndrome. Praeger. New York.
30. ASCH, S.W. 1968. Crib deaths: Their possible relation to postpartum depression and infanticide. Mt. Sinai J. Med. N.Y. **35:** 214–220.
31. KUKULL, W.A. & D.R. PETERSON. 1977. Sudden infant death and infanticide. Am. J. Epidemiol. **106:** 485–487.
32. EMERY, J.L. 1985. Infanticide, filicide, and cot death. Arch. Dis. Child. **60:** 505–507.

Family and Health-Professional Interactions

SYLVIA LIMERICK

The Foundation for the Study of Infant Deaths
15 Belgrave Square
London SWIX 8PS
England

We were shopping in town—myself, my mum, my 16 month-old boy and the baby Sarah. I looked into the pram to check on Sarah. Her face was blue, there was blood coming from her nose and what looked like a bruise over her left eye. I ran the ten minutes to the Health Centre. Luckily all the doctors were there and they rushed into a surgery with her. It was half an hour before they told me she was dead.
(SIDS, 9-week-old infant)

My baby started to cry for her feed, I picked her up and she immediately stopped crying, closed her eyes and seemed to go unconscious. She gave three strange little sighs and a gurgling noise came from her throat and I knew she was dead.
(SIDS, 5-week-old infant)

Crispin woke about 7 A.M. He wasn't crying but he appeared unhappy and miserable. He had a pressure mark on his head where he had obviously not moved his head all night. I heated his bottle and changed his nappy. He only took about 1/2 oz milk. He was listless and lethargic. I called the doctor but sadly he did not arrive in time. About 9:30 A.M. I noticed Crispin wasn't breathing. I tried artificial respiration and called an ambulance but he was confirmed dead. The autopsy revealed no cause of death.
(SIDS, 10-week-old infant)

These descriptions of babies dying unexpectedly in their parents' presence illustrate the traumatic nature of the bereavement and how varied the immediate histories may be. Sudden and unexpected deaths are now the most common kind of death in infants after the first month of life. The incidence is greater in households living in a difficult socio-economic environment, but many occur in families living in the most favorable circumstances.

Although reactions vary widely according to an individual's social, emotional, cultural and spiritual resources and previous life-experience, grief tends to follow a pattern in which disbelief gives way to unbearable sorrow, irrational feelings, guilt and anger—later alternating with depression and apathy—before there is acceptance of the death.

Expression of grief is necessary before recovery and growth can occur. Although most parents look to their relatives and friends for comfort and help, they need informed support and kind explanation from health professionals to help them resolve many anxieties and feelings of self-reproach. This support is especially important for emotionally isolated parents and unmarried mothers without extended families. Professional parents often find a bereavement due to sudden infant death particularly difficult to accept.

The organization of health care and the system for investigating deaths vary from country to country. My recommendations are based on experiences in Britain, where the Foundation for the Study of Infant Deaths has given support to over 6,000 bereaved families, and I have surveyed in detail the managment of 713 sudden infant deaths.[a] The suggestions which I will present can be adapted to the circumstances in other countries.

PROBLEMS POSED BY SUDDEN INFANT DEATH

Unlike stillbirths and early neonatal deaths, which occur mostly in the hospital, the vast majority of sudden infant deaths occur at home or in the community, where the parents feel wholly responsible. The babies have survived birth and the first, more hazardous week of life; symptoms of illness, if any, were seldom considered very serious, so the parents are emotionally unprepared. The most distressing aspects of the death, the unexpectedness and the absence of a convincing cause, make the feelings of shock, guilt and bewilderment likely to be more severe and long-lasting than after a death which is anticipated or understood.

Furthermore, in Britain there follows a coroner's (procurator fiscal in Scotland) inquiry to rule out unnatural death and to provide the registrar of deaths with a certified medical cause of death. This procedure often includes the visit of a coroner's officer or, more often, of uniformed police to inspect the crib and room where the baby died and to ask questions, this at a time when the distraught parents are searching in their own minds for a reason for the death. This visit is followed by a wait of up to a week to hear the findings of the necropsy arranged by the coroner and also, occasionally, by an inquest. The procedure ends with the issuance of a death certificate which parents often do not understand.

The uncertain reaction of neighbors and friends, who may be embarrassed by an untimely death or perhaps scared for their own children, can increase the parents' sense of isolation. "Neighbours keep the children away from our house, afraid that the sight of them will upset me. Friends avoided the subject when I needed to talk about it." And, "it was particularly distressing to hear people say we must forget the baby." Those who hardly knew the baby easily underestimate the extent of parental grief over the loss of an infant.

When the reason for the death is obscure, public doubt and malicious gossip are easily aroused by confusion with nonaccidental injury. Many do not realize that unexpected infant deaths from natural causes each year greatly outnumber deaths in the same age group due to nonaccidental injury.

THE IMPACT OF SUDDEN INFANT DEATH

Impact on the Family

The *mother* is emotionally vulnerable. Often still recovering from pregnancy and postnatal adjustment, and exhausted by the early weeks of a new pregnancy, her self-confidence in her mothering ability may be shattered, especially if the death took her

---

[a]References 1–12 have also been useful in formulating these recommendations for health-professional interactions with families bereaved by a sudden infant death.

first child—and a quarter of sudden infant deaths are first children. "As his mother, I feel totally useless. I cannot even think of having another baby when I don't know why my first one, so perfect in every way, died." Or, "I tortured myself saying when and where did I go wrong." Very occasionally a mother is so consumed with self blame that she imagines and falsely claims she "killed" her child.

A *father,* too, may experience a sense of bitterness and futility that a life which held so much joy and hope is cut off before it has been given a chance. Or, he may be worried lest some paternal genetic factor was involved or whether the baby had adequate care. "My husband took it all inwardly: he carried, and still does, a terrible guilt complex." And, "my husband refuses to talk about the tragedy."

With good communication, many couples grow closer together and more mature through sharing and overcoming what is often the first disaster in their life together. For others, however, despair and feelings of inadequacy can lead to recrimination which threatens marital harmony, disrupts family relationships, including those with grandparents and surviving and subsequent children, and sometimes undermines confidence in the medical and nursing profession, especially if a doctor or child health clinic had recently been consulted about the baby's health.

Grandparents feel the loss of a grandchild acutely. While they probably have previous experience of bereavement which can be a help to the younger generation, in their own grief and search for an explanation, they sometimes comment on the way the baby was cared for. Such comments can be very hurtful to the bereaved parents and may exacerbate a difficult in-law relationship. Sometimes they protect the mother from discussing the tragedy further, not understanding her need to talk it through.

Surviving children are affected by a death in the family. Their reactions may be influenced by their temperament, their relationship to the baby and to their parents, and their perception of death, which varies with age. Children may express their grief in a variety of ways. Some may be very distressed, others may appear unconcerned, and some may be naughty or difficult.

Very young children may be frightened that they, too, will disappear or that their jealous thoughts were responsible for the death. They may be disturbed by their parents' emotional state and show their grief and insecurity in infantile behavior. They need to be assured they are loved. Older children may need to talk to someone other than their parents, whom they are afraid of upsetting, someone who can then help the family to share their grief.

Impact on Health Professionals

Doctors and other health-care professionals may also feel shocked and very distressed by a baby's death. Some find this comparatively rare tragedy a very difficult one in which to counsel the bereaved family. Some do not feel capable of helping because of their own fear of death or sense of failure, especially if they had recently reassured the parents about the baby's health.

The key to effective support, both immediate and longer term, is speedy communication between those initially concerned, accident and emergency department staff, coroner (or medical examiner), the family doctor, community or public health services, the pediatrician, and the pathologist, in order to exchange relevant information and decide who will counsel the family. This *counselor's* role is to be the *compassionate listener* who is sufficiently knowledgeable about babies and likely reactions to bereavement to be able to answer questions about the cause of death, to give reassurance on many aspects of infant care, and to help the family to share their grief.

IMMEDIATE MANAGEMENT OF SUDDEN INFANT DEATH

Discovery of the Dead Baby

Discovery of the child dying or dead is the most horrifying trauma. To scream for help is a common reaction of mothers, some of whom become hysterical. Many parents attempt mouth-to-mouth-and-nose resuscitation themselves or summon a professional neighbor to try resuscitation. Such attempts are likely to disturb the baby's stomach contents and may cause bruising. It is important that the doctor who certifies death informs the police or coroner if such resuscitation has been done so that any resulting disfigurement is not misinterpreted.

The police are often called by the parents or by neighbors, or they come because an ambulance has been summoned. Although parents may be stunned and disbelieving, they are acutely sensitive to a manner implying suspicion; therefore, officials need to act with tact, sympathy and kindness. The baby may be rushed to a doctor's surgery or a doctor called to the home. More often, however, the baby is taken by ambulance directly to a hospital accident and emergency department, and the first, most painful phase of supporting the family falls to the accident and emergency staff.

Ambulance staff should always remember the need for considerate handling of the dead baby in the parents' presence; there should be flexibility in applying rules concerning the carrying of dead bodies. Parents, if they wish, should be encouraged to accompany the baby to the hospital.

Accident and Emergency staff in hospitals need training about sudden infant deaths as well as nonaccidental injury. A very few unexpected infant deaths are the result of accidents or nonaccidental injury. Exceedingly rarely, an unexpected death due to nonaccidental injury initially present as a sudden death without apparent cause.

Guidelines on the management of unexpected infant deaths should be available and should include the following recommendations, many of which (2,7,8–11) apply also to certification of death by a doctor at home.

1. Verification of death should be made in the hospital accident and emergency department, rather than in the ambulance.
2. If resuscitation is attempted and/or while the baby's physical condition is being evaluated, a member of the staff should stay with the parent (or parents) in an area of privacy, should ask sympathetically for details of the baby's health, of family illness, and of recent events, and should obtain the name of the family's doctor. If possible, a pediatrician should be called.
3. If only one parent is present and agrees, the other parent or relative should be contacted.
4. A suitable person should look after any siblings.
5. The hospital chaplain, if available, may be wanted to baptize a dying baby or give support to the parents.
6. All information should be reviewed briefly by professional staff before breaking the news to the parents that the child is dead.
7. Unless there is a history of diagnosed illness, obvious signs of injury or, a parental attitude which arouses suspicion, tell parents that the death appears to be a sudden infant death, but emphasize the importance of a postmortem examination, which the coroner will arrange, to establish the cause of death.
8. Explain to parents that it is the coroner's duty to investigate all sudden deaths of unknown cause and advise parents that they will be asked to make a statement to the coroner's officer or the police, who may visit them at home.
9. To assist the pathologist, clinical information about the baby and family which is relevant to the case should be transmitted to the coroner.

10. Clothe the infant and make him as presentable as possible. Offer parents the opportunity to see and hold their baby for as long as they wish before the baby is taken to the mortuary. This helps parents to acknowledge the reality of the death and, very simply, enables them to say good-bye.
11. Offer parents written information about sudden unexpected infant deaths and subsequent procedures, such as the leaflet, *Information for Parents Following the Sudden and Unexpected Death of Their Baby* (see APPENDIX).
12. If identification of the body to the coroner's officer or police is required, a member of the staff or the hospital chaplain should accompany the parents to the mortuary.
13. A member of the staff or the hospital chaplain or social worker should give support to the parents and any accompanying children until satisfactory transport is ready to take the family home.
14. Before the parents leave the accident and emergency department, the doctor or a member of the hospital staff should telephone the family's doctor and/or pediatrician, and the health visitor or midwife, and should discuss with the parents the arrangements for immediate, continued support.

Role of the Family's Doctor and Health Visitor (Child Health Community Nurse)

The speedy arrival of the family's doctor or pediatrician and of the health visitor is of great consolation to the parents and prevents later misunderstanding.

The doctor may consider offering parents a *drug* to alleviate the initial shock. Many parents are realistic about the need to grieve and do not want to suppress or postpone their reactions but are grateful for something to induce sleep which gives them strength to cope.

If the mother was *breastfeeding,* she will need advice on the suppression of lactation. "The continued milk supply caused great physical pain as well as heartache."

The doctor will want to take note of *siblings* and remember that twin babies carry extra risk of sudden death. A surviving twin should be under close medical observation. However, parents need great reassurance that older children are not at risk.

It is helpful to advise parents of likely *grief reactions* such as fantasizing about the baby, distressing dreams, and strong positive or negative sexual feelings, and to reassure them that these and other symptoms are normal and temporary. "The most useful advice and comfort was from our general practititioner about normal feelings of guilt and imagining hearing the baby cry. This happened on numerous occasions and knowing it was normal has reduced the distress and fear it causes."

The doctor can discuss with the parents and give to them further copies of the leaflet mentioned above, *Information for Parents Following the Sudden and Unexpected Death of Their Baby* (see APPENDIX). This leaflet explains what the postmortem may show and tries to answer the most usual questions about it, and also gives the address and telephone number of the Foundation for the Study of Infant Deaths, through which parents can contact other parents. Most parents are grateful for advice on the procedure for registering the death and making funeral arrangements. "I often turn to your leaflet for comfort and reassurance, without the information I would always have blamed myself for her death. It helped immensely to explain the facts to relatives who know nothing about sudden infant deaths."

The doctor will want to make sure that the parents have a *relative or close friend* very near them during the 48 hours after death, and to offer an explanation to them and to the minister of religion if he is supporting the family. "It is terrible being alone for the first night after such a shock."

Parents often want to talk to their *health visitor* (child health community nurse) or *midwife,* whoever knew their baby best. The nurse or midwife can give immediate practical help and can arrange in advance a mutually convenient time to meet with the parents in their home when the findings of the postmortem become available. If the father is absent, it may indicate he is not supporting the mother. Sometimes these visits are made in the week following the funeral, which is a particularly harrowing time. Relatives have departed, the father has to return to work; in this period of anticlimax a mother can feel utterly bereft and both parents often grieve deeply.

EARLY EXPLANATION TO THE FAMILY

The family doctor will need to arrange a subsequent meeting with the parents to discuss the *registered cause of death.* In the early stages of their reaction, the reason for death appears very important to the parents as they search through all they did or failed to do, trying to find a cause for the death. Many do not understand the medical terminology and need an explanation, not only for themselves, but also for relatives and friends.

There can be many reasons for unexpected infant deaths. The *postmortem examination* may explain why the baby died by revealing evidence of an unsuspected congenital abnormality or rare disease or evidence of rapid, overwhelming infection. In the great majority of cases, however, the cause of death is obscure and the death is registered as sudden infant death syndrome. Postmortem evidence of minor infection which may have contributed to the death is sometimes found and mentioned on the death certificate together with SIDS.

If a severe infection is found at postmortem, some parents are relieved to learn there was a recognized cause of death, while others may reproach themselves or their doctor for failing to notice their child's fatal condition. Doctors need to be informed by the coroner of the initial (macroscopic) and final (bacteriological, histological) necropsy findings, and they should consult with the pathologist if any clarification is needed.

Many parents either decide for themselves what caused the death or have a deep fear that they allowed the baby to suffocate; they may have had theories suggested by friends or press reports. By being asked to describe all that happened, a mother can express her fears and have her *misconceptions* dispelled.

Reassurance concerning blame and guilt needs to be given in the presence of both parents and anyone else who had cared for the baby; a babysitter, childminder or grandparents may need separate counseling as well. It may be helpful to mention to them that parents often blame themselves and sometimes each other; this will give the family a chance to reveal or deny such feelings. The doctor should be prepared for expressions of anger or bitterness directed towards the medical profession and should recognize these as signs of normal grieving, not necessarily calling his competence into question.

Doctors may need to give guidance on the emotional needs of *siblings,* whom the parents in their grief may overprotect, neglect, or use as scapegoats. "I withdrew emotionally from my three-year-old—afraid to love her too much." Or, "is there anyone who could help as the doctors and health visitors have stopped coming and I now feel aggressive towards my older two children and would hate to do anything to them that I would regret?" It is important for parents to observe and listen to their children and to give them the opportunity to express their feelings vocally or in play or behavior. Parents should be helped to avoid idealizing the baby that has died and to avoid explanations which they do not believe or which may create more fear and confusion.

Many parents are frightened by the intensity of their *emotions* and have unrealistic expectations of how soon they will recover. While people need privacy and time to grieve on their own, most mothers sooner or later feel an urge to talk repeatedly about the baby and to work through their grief, long after other members of the family have come to terms with the death. A father often tries to repress his emotions, sometimes to the extent of refusing to talk about the baby. He can become frustrated at his inability to console the mother, who may be upset at his apparent lack of caring. The doctor can help parents to understand that people grieve in different ways and reach different stages at different times.

Abnormal grief may show itself in avoidance of mourning, prolonged grief, or a delayed reaction. Bereavement may revive memories of previous loss or of emotional crises which were inadequately resolved. The help of a clergyman, social worker or psychiatrist may be necessary.

CONTINUED SUPPORT FOR THE FAMILY

The *doctor* should ensure that a *counselor* continues support to the family to the extent that the parents and siblings need it. The doctor should maintain a liason with this counselor, who may be the health visitor, a minister of religion, a social worker, or a bereavement counselor. The doctor can also offer the support available through organizations like the Foundation for the Study of Infant Deaths in the United Kingdom, or the Scottish Cot Death Trust. Similar organizations exist in the United States, Canada, Australia, New Zealand, Ireland, and several other European countries.

Support from Parents' Organizations

Each year, between six and seven hundred families who have suffered the sudden death of an infant make their initial contact with the Foundation for the Study of Infant Deaths in the United Kingdom. Newly bereaved parents telephone, write to, or visit the office or the representative parent in their locality. Sometimes they telephone within hours of finding the baby dead; more usually contact is made days or weeks later. A few are so stunned or distressed they cannot talk but want someone to talk to them; others are desperate or grateful for a sympathetic listener. Many want to know about sudden infant deaths and research, while a few express feelings of anger at their baby's death.

The Foundation's role is to respond to each individual's need; to be prepared to listen; to ask about the baby and what happened; and to be able to give explanation, reassurance, counsel or advice in answer to a wide variety of questions. The Foundation personally writes to all parents, enclosing further copies (if needed) of the *Information for Parents* leaflet (see APPENDIX) and copies of the twice-yearly newsletter which comments on research findings. Those who want further, detailed information are referred to appropriate articles or books. Many parents are eager to give information to help research, and the Foundation invites them to complete a medical/epidemiological questionnaire inquiring into both the history of the pregnancy and the health of the baby and family.

The Foundation also offers to put parents in touch with formerly bereaved parents or with support groups, Friends of the Foundation, who offer an individual befriending service. Over half accept this offer either at once or a few months later. *Befrienders* provide empathy, credibility, unlimited time, an opportunity to share tumultuous emotions, reassurance that reactions are "normal", and hope for recovery. The Foundation takes care in selection and matching of befrienders and would hesitate to ask any parent to befriend others until at least a year had elapsed since his or her own tragedy. The befriender has to be a source of emotional strength. Many Friends of the Foundation are also active in disseminating information locally about sudden infant deaths and in raising funds for the Foundation's research program. Such constructive outlets can help mothers and fathers overcome their frustration by doing something positive in memory of their child, and taking part in community activities again can break down the sense of isolation that surrounds many bereaved people.

The Foundation also sometimes assists parents in obtaining *further professional help* from a pediatrician, psychiatrist or child psychologist. An increasing proportion of time is spent in giving reassurance and advice to parents expecting or caring for a subsequent baby. To evaluate different methods of giving support to such parents, the Foundation has sponsored a research project comparing the use of apnea monitors and weighing scales.

LATER COUNSELING

The family doctor should offer parents a later interview with a pediatrician. Obtaining independent opinion is mutually beneficial to parents and family doctor; it restores parental confidence in their health-professional advisers and shares some of the load of counseling. Even if a doctor has given support and explanation early on, the opportunity should also be available for later consultation when the parents will be less shocked and better able to comprehend, and because they may want to discuss future children and consider genetic counseling.

Future Children

All parents fear the tragedy of sudden infant death will recur in their future children. Some studies have shown a slightly increased risk, which, with careful explanation, can be accepted by some parents but causes excessive anxiety in others. Where possible, it is helpful to reassure the parents that the postmortem findings did not reveal any hereditary cause of death but that the mother will be given special attention during the next pregnancy and when caring for the future child.

Since the next baby needs to be regarded as a new personality and not a replacement, the parents should be advised to complete mourning the child that has died before embarking on another pregnancy. Some parents want another baby straight away; others fear they are going to be advised not to have any more children; and some, sadly, are too frightened to try. The topic can be helpfully discussed, and guidance can be given; then the timing of future children is left to parental choice unless there are medical considerations. Special help will be needed for parents who have been voluntarily sterilized and for those few mothers who are already pregnant and whose grieving may be suspended until after the subsequent baby's birth.

The Foundation's leaflet, *Your Next Child,* describes some commonly felt anxieties, and *When to Consult a Doctor About Your Baby,* designed to help parents identify potentially serious symptoms of illness, is welcomed by many as practical advice which any new mother is reassured to have. (see APPENDIX for information about obtaining leaflets from the Foundation.)

With their subsequent children, parents who have lost a baby unexpectedly will need extra attention, understanding and support from their obstetrician, pediatrician, family doctor and health visitor. This is especially important if they have not come to terms with their previous loss and have unresolved guilt feelings. "So many things regarding my baby's death play on my mind since the recent birth of another son". While it is natural for a mother to be extra anxious and somewhat overprotective, a few mothers are unable to cope and seek substitute care; "I love the new baby very much, but I just can't have the responsibility of looking after him." Panic often overwhelms the mother for trivial reasons and is especially likely until the new baby has survived the age at which the previous child died.

The Goals of Counseling

Intense grieving after the death of a baby is likely to last several months and may recur throughout the first year, especially at anniversaries of the baby's birth and death. The aim of counseling is to help parents understand their baby's death, identify their fears and misconceptions, and share and work through their grief until they can accept their loss and again face the future with confidence. Health professionals can help parents to reach the stage when, as one mother wrote, "We can't forget but it no longer hurts to remember."

SUMMARY

Sudden infant deaths are the most common kind of death in infants aged between one month and one year. The unexpectedness, the legal investigation, and the absence of a convincing cause all have a devastating impact on bereaved parents, who look to health professionals for reassurance and explanation. Doctors and nurses may feel inadequate. As a result of the author's 17 years experience helping families and surveying procedures, recommendations on management are made which can be adapted to different health-care and legal systems in other countries. Recommendations include speedy notification of the death to the family's normal health-care advisers, and guidelines for immediate management by hospital accident and emergency staff. Parents need written information and the opportunity to talk with someone compassionate and informed about sudden infant deaths. Suggestions for doctors and nurses stress the importance of immediate support, early explanation of the postmortem report, and continued befriending by other suitable parents. Later counseling should be offered to discuss the care of future children and rebuild parental confidence.

REFERENCES

1. BLUGLASS, K. 1981. J. Child Psychol. Psychiatry 22: 411–421.
2. CORNWELL, J., B. NURCOMBE & L. STEVENS. 1977. Med. J. Aust. 1: 656–658.
3. DEFRAIN, J. & L. ERNST. 1978. J. Fam. Practice 6: 985–989.
4. DEFRAIN, J., J. TAYLOR & L. ERNST. 1982. Coping with Sudden Infant Death. Lexington Books. Toronto.
5. EMERY, J. L. 1972. Br. Med. J. 1: 612.
6. LEWIS, S. 1981. The Health Visitor 54(8): 322–325.
7. STEELE, R. 1980. Understanding Crib Death: 50. The Canadian Public Health Association. Canada.
8. GORER, G. 1965. Death, Grief and Mourning in Contemporary Britain. Doubleday. Garden City, New York.
9. WATSON, E. 1975. Public Health 89: 153–155.
10. WATSON, E. 1981. Med. Sci. Law 21: 99–104.
11. GOLDING, J., S. R. LIMERICK & A. MACFARLANE. 1985. Sudden Infant Death-Patterns, Puzzles and Problems. Open Books. Wells, U.K.
12. LIMERICK, S. R. & M. A. P. S. DOWNHAM. 1978. Br. Med. J. 1: 1527–1529.

APPENDIX

Leaflets
Information for Parents Following the Sudden and Unexpected Death of Their Baby
Your Next Child
When to Consult a Doctor about Your Baby
Guidelines for Accident and Emergency Departments
Checklist for General Practitioners

Available from
The Foundation for the Study of Infant Deaths
15 Belgrave Square
London SW1X 8PS, United Kingdom

The Federal SIDS Support Network in Perspective

JEHU C. HUNTER

National Center for the Prevention of Sudden Infant Death Syndrome
Suite 203, 330 North Charles Street
Baltimore, Maryland 21201

There are two major components of the sudden infant death syndrome (SIDS): SIDS as a medical enigma that is considered in terms of epidemiologic characteristics, pathological findings, risk factors, and approaches to prevention; and SIDS as a human problem with tremendous psychological ramifications which affect the parents, siblings, relatives, and the community. Historically, caregivers have been held responsible for *any* untoward event that affected infants in their care. For example, the passage in 1 Kings, third chapter, nineteenth verse, states, "and this woman's child died in the night; because she overlaid it." This passage may be one of the earliest references to the phenomenon that is now recognized as SIDS.

In its initial response in 1971 to the insistence by parents of SIDS victims that the federal government "do something" about the problem of SIDS, the Department of Health, Education and Welfare (DHEW, now the Department of Health and Human Services) encouraged a coordinated research-service approach to this complex problem. An historical perspective on SIDS research by HASSELMEYER and HUNTER is presented elsewhere in these proceedings. This paper will outline the development of a national SIDS support network that was directed and coordinated by the Office of Maternal and Child Health (OMCH), DHEW. In a classic example of a productive collaborative effort, the National Institute of Child Health and Human Development (NICHD; Hasselmeyer and Hunter) and OMCH (Geraldine Norris-Funke) were in frequent contact. An important goal of the federal effort was to transfer to the public, by way of the community health services arm of the U.S. Public Health Service, new knowledge developed through NIH research. The targets of information garnered and distributed by OMCH were parents of SIDS victims, emergency first-responders, coroners and medical examiners, and state departments of public health. In state departments of public health, public health nurses responsible for the delivery of maternal and child health services were a prime target. These health professionals would have the major responsibility for the education and support of bereaved parents and their families. The OMCH also sought to include in its support network privately organized groups for parents of SIDS victims, who had served and would continue to serve those families of SIDS victims who felt the need and desire to discuss their plight with someone who had suffered a SIDS loss.

Through the collaboration of NICHD, OMCH and the National Center for Health Statistics (NCHS), a certifiable code for SIDS, 798.0, was incorporated into the *International Classification of Diseases,* 9th edition, 1975. For primary mortality tabulations, this action made it possible, under the nosology guidelines published by the NCHS,[1] to classify sudden infant deaths of unknown cause occurring under one year of age as SIDS. The SIDS code made it possible for the first time to gather accurate mortality statistics pertaining to this phenomenon and, just as important, helped bereaved parents to accept the death of their infant as a bona fide medical event.

In 1974, Public Law 93–270 provided fiscal support for the establishment of the SIDS Counseling and Information Service Program. Between 1974 and 1981, SIDS counseling and information service projects were established in practically every state in the United States. In 1981, this program was consolidated in the Maternal and Child Health Block Grant to states. Under the MCH Block Grant, each state agency administering programs under Title V of the Social Security Act assumed the responsibility for developing its own SIDS support programs in the context of determining and establishing priorities for maternal and child health problems within its jurisdiction and allocating fiscal resources accordingly. Currently, some form of information and counseling support is available in each of the fifty states, the District of Columbia, Puerto Rico and the U.S. Virgin Islands.

Efforts of OMCH have not been limited to the development of counseling and information centers. Before Public Law 93–270, OMCH directed the development of three films. Two of these were directed primarily to bereaved parents and their families: *You Are Not Alone* and *After Our Baby Died.* The third, *A Call for Help,* was directed to emergency first-responders. All of these films have been highly regarded by their audiences.

On November 20–21, 1975, under a grant from OMCH, the Office of the Medical Investigator, School of Medicine, University of New Mexico, conducted a conference of pathologists to develop minimal protocols for investigative and autopsy examinations. Pathologists associated with the SIDS counseling and information projects discussed earlier were invited to participate. In addition, representatives of the National Association of Medical Examiners and the Pathology and Biology Section of the American Academy of Forensic Sciences were invited to attend, with the expectation that they would report the conclusions and recommendations of the conference to their organizations. The aim of the conference was to standardize investigative and autopsy procedures in order to assure uniformity in the mode of reporting data pertaining to SIDS from the 24 counseling and information projects that were then being supported by OMCH. An important result of this conference was the recommendation that a copy of the report of any initial scene investigation conducted by a law enforcement agency or medical examiner be included with the investigation protocol.[2] It was further recommended that the follow-up detailed inquiry into the circumstances of death be conducted by an individual, preferably someone not identified with a punitive agency, who is thoroughly acquainted with all the nuances of SIDS and that the inquiry not be carried out in a manner that was punitive or threatening. It was suggested that the inquiry be conducted no earlier than two weeks following the SIDS event. The full report of the conference suggested forms for organizing and collecting anatomic, microscopic, investigative, familial, and socio-economic data. A considerable portion of the recommended format for collecting SIDS postmortem information was used by the study centers which participated in the NICHD Cooperative Epidemiologic Study of SIDS Risk Factors.

The Sudden Infant Death Syndrome Program in the Office of Maternal and Child Health currently supports the National SIDS Clearinghouse. The SIDS Clearinghouse publishes a newsletter, the SIDS Fact Sheet. This publication has provided current information about grief management, the relationship of infantile apnea to SIDS, current research activity pertaining to SIDS, SIDS vital statistics, and reports on federal, state and privately supported SIDS programs. In 1986, the SIDS Clearinghouse published the *Directory of Sudden Infant Death Syndrome Programs and Resources.* Copies of the directory may be obtained from the National SIDS Clearinghouse at 8201 Greensboro Drive, Suite 600, McLean, Virginia 22102.

How have these varied efforts by the Office of Maternal and Child Health provided a support network for SIDS parents? In knowledge there is power. For SIDS parents, knowledge about the syndrome, about the grief process, and about the impact of such a death on the parents, siblings, and other family members helps them to cope with the immediate impact of the death and, in the long term, helps them to accept the loss and get on with their lives. State SIDS programs and local and national groups for parents of SIDS victims offer choices for parents seeking information and counseling. The Office of Maternal and Child Health, through its Sudden Infant Death Syndrome Program, has fostered the development of local, state and national networks that combine information and counseling efforts in a productive way so that emergency first-responders, health-care professionals, and parents operate from a shared knowledge and appreciation of the SIDS tragedy. This network approach has sharply reduced the number and frequency of criminal charges against the parents of SIDS victims, and has led to the evolution of a more knowledgeable approach to the management of grief both by emergency and health-care professionals and by those who receive support.

REFERENCES

1. U.S., DEPARTMENT OF HEALTH, EDUCATION AND WELFARE, NATIONAL CENTER FOR HEALTH STATISTICS. April 1975. Nosology Guidelines, Sudden Infant Death Syndrome.
2. JONES, A.M. & J.T. WESTON. 1976. The examination of the sudden infant death syndrome infant: Investigative and autopsy protocols. J. Forensic Sci. 21(4): 833–841.

Home Monitoring for the Sudden Infant Death Syndrome

The Case For

DOROTHY H. KELLY[a]

Children's Service
Massachusetts General Hospital
Boston, Massachusetts

INTRODUCTION

Many infants are referred to medical centers for evaluation of their cardiopulmonary status because they have a family history of SIDS or apnea or because they have had a frightening episode of apnea and/or severe choking with color and tone change. In our country, many of these infants are monitored at home,[1,2] despite the lack of any study which demonstrates the efficacy of this treatment modality or documents which infants should be monitored. To address the questions of selection criteria and efficacy of home monitoring, I will describe in this paper the protocol of our program and the outcome of the infants referred to us.

PATIENTS AND METHODS

Evaluation of Infants

Since January 1973, we have evaluated full term and preterm infants who have had a frightening episode of apnea and/or severe choking (an *event*) as well as infants who had one or more siblings with SIDS and/or apnea. In the former group (symptomatic infants) routine evaluation,[3] which included a careful history (FIG. 1) from all observers of the event, was performed in an attempt to determine the cause of the episode. In addition, all infants were recorded for twelve hours at night by pneumogram technique[4] to determine if they had an increase in frequency or duration of apnea or bradycardia or an increase in periodic breathing, as compared to normal infants.[5] Further testing of the infant's control of breathing was done as indicated using polysomnography, ventilatory response to hypoxia, hyperoxia and hypercarbia, and/or arousal responses.

The asymptomatic infants, who were referred for evaluation because of a family history of SIDS and/or apnea, routinely had a complete personal and family history taken and a twelve-hour nocturnal pneumogram at approximately 2 weeks of age. In addition, a daytime nap polygraph and a physical and neurologic examination by a program physician were offered.

[a]Address correspondence to: Pediatric Pulmonary Laboratory, Massachusetts General Hospital, Boston, MA 02114.

Massachusetts General Hospital History Form For AOI or AOP
Name _____

HISTORY OF EVENT (leading to evaluation): Please circle features and complete as needed.

Date: _____; Age: _____; # hours after feed: _____

Last Immunization (specify date / type): _____; Medications: _____

Recent illness: _____

OBSERVER	LOCATION	INFANT POSITION	STATE	COLOR	COLOR CHANGE
Parent	Holding infant	Prone	Asleep	Cyanotic	Entire body
MD	Same room	Supine	Awake	Grey	Extremities
RN	Audible distance	Upright	Drowsy	Pale	Face
Other _____	In car	Infant seat	Feeding	Red	Perioral
	Other _____	Other _____	Other _____	Purple	Lips
				Normal	Other _____

BREATHING	TONE	EYES	NOISE	FLUID	HEART RATE
No effort	Limp	Closed	Cough	Milk	Bradycardia @ ___bpm
Shallow	Stiff	Dazed	Choke	Vomitus	Tachycardia @ ___bpm
Struggling	Tonic/clonic	Scared	Stridor	Mucus	Normal
Rapid	Normal	Rolled	Gasp	Blood	Unknown
Normal	Other _____	Staring	Cry	None	
Other _____		Normal	None	Other _____	
		Other _____	Other _____		

STIMULATION	DURATION OF EVENT	ABNORMALITIES FOLLOWING EVENT
None	_____ sec / min	Abnormal breathing x _____ min / hrs
Gentle		Color change x _____ min / hrs
Vigorous		Behavior _____
MTM: # breaths _____		None
CPR: duration _____		

EMT/ER Observations:

Please describe event briefly, noting chronology of signs/symptoms:

PREVIOUS SYMPTOMS: If any present, please elaborate.
Apnea _____; Color changes _____; Stridor _____; Seizure _____; Other _____

FIGURE 1. Form used to obtain history on referred patients from all observers of the event.

Management of Infants

From January 1973 through April 1986, 13,401 infants were referred for evaluation (TABLE 1). No treatment was recommended for 34% of these infants (including both symptomatic infants with a benign history of the event and infants with a positive family history). All of their test results were normal. A treatable cause (gastroesophageal reflux, sepsis, pneumonia, seizure disorder, alkalosis, anemia, respiratory syncytial virus infection, meningitis, etc.) was found in 31% of the infants. Since these infants had no

TABLE 1. Results of Evaluation of Referred Infants

Category	% of Total Referrals
Normal infant (minor event or positive family history with no symptoms and a normal evaluation)	34%
Treatable cause (gastroesophageal reflux, infections, seizures etc.)	31%
Idiopathic apnea of prematurity or of infancy	
treated with methylxanthines	24%
monitored at home	11%

further events and exhibited a normal pneumogram after they received specific treatment for the diagnosed cause, no additional treatment was recommended. Finally, 35% of the referrals were diagnosed as having idiopathic apnea of prematurity (AOP) or idiopathic apnea of infancy (AOI). Sixty-nine percent of the patients with AOP or AOI (24% of the total referrals) were treated with theophylline. The criteria for treatment were (1) postconceptional age $\leq$ 44 weeks, (2) abnormal pneumogram, (3) no pneumogram or no clinical abnormalities with theophylline, and (4) no serious side effects from the medication. The remainder of the patients with AOP or AOI (11% of the total referrals) were treated with a monitor at home according to our protocol[6] (TABLE 1). Theophylline was added in the last group if the infant had repeated symptoms, a markedly abnormal end tidal CO_2 (average $\geq$ 50 mm Hg), or repeated episodes of hypoxia.

RESULTS

Outcome of the Nonmonitored Population

There were 19 SIDS deaths among the 11,943 referred infants for whom home monitoring was not recommended (TABLE 2). Fifteen (79%) of these 19 deaths occurred when there was noncompliance with recommended therapy by the caretakers or by the physicians (mortality rate 1.3/1,000) (TABLE 2). The remaining 4 deaths (21%) were associated with compliance with treatment recommendations. The mortality rate (0.3/1,000) in the compliant nonmonitored population was one-third of the rate in the noncompliant nonmonitored population. Thus, failure of triage, using our protocol, resulted in four deaths, three of whom were preterm infants.

TABLE 2. Association of Compliance and Noncompliance with Deaths among Referred Infants

Category	Monitored Infants (1,445)		Nonmonitored Infants (11,943)		Total Population (13,401)	
	No. of Deaths	Mortality Rate[a]	No. of Deaths	Mortality Rate[a]	No. of Deaths	Mortality Rate[a]
Compliance	6	4.2	4	0.3	10	0.7
Noncompliance	12	8.3	15	1.3	27	2.1
Others[b]	3	2.1			3	0.2
Total	21	14.5	19	1.6	40	3.0

[a]Mortality rate/1,000 infants
[b]see text

Outcome of the Monitored Population

There were 21 deaths among the 1,445 infants who were monitored and had completed monitoring by April 1987 (mortality rate 14.5/1,000; TABLE 2). Two of these deaths occurred 3 and 13 months, respectively, after monitoring had been discontinued according to our protocol. Both occurred in patients with a seizure disorder. Of the remaining deaths, 1 parent refused to be interviewed regarding the circumstances surrounding the death, and 12 parents acknowledged a delay in properly assisting the infant. The delay generally occurred because they did not hear the alarm or did not have the infant on the monitor (11/12). The remaining 6 deaths that occurred during monitoring are unexplained. Two of these 6 infants were preterm whereas only 2/12 of the monitored infants in the noncompliant group were preterm. Thus, the mortality rate for unexplained deaths during monitoring was 4.2/1,000 and for infants whose caretakers were noncompliant was 8.3/1,000 (TABLE 2).

Outcome in Compliant and in Noncompliant Populations

For the total population of infants, the mortality rate associated with noncompliance was greater than with compliance (2.1/1,000 vs. 0.7/1,000; TABLE 2). In fact, 69% of all the deaths whose circumstances were known after caretaker interview occurred with noncompliance, whereas only 31% of deaths occurred with compliance. (This value for

TABLE 3. Characteristics of Presenting Episode and Family History in 21 Monitored Infants who Died

Characteristics of Presenting Episode	No. of Infants	% of Total Deaths
Sleep onset requiring		
Resuscitation	13[a]	61.9
Vigorous stimulation	6[b]	28.6
Awake onset	0	0
No presenting episode	2[c]	9.5
Total	21	100

[a]Includes 1 infant who had 1 previous sibling die of SIDS and 2 infants who each had 2 previous siblings die of SIDS.
[b]Includes 1 infant who had 2 previous siblings die of SIDS.
[c]Includes 2 infants who each had 2 previous siblings die of SIDS.

the compliance category includes the two infants who died 3 and 13 months, respectively, after monitoring was discontinued.)

The characteristics of the presenting episode or family history in the monitored infants who died are listed in TABLE 3. The majority (13/19) of the infants who were symptomatic on presentation had an initial episode characterized by sleep onset apnea requiring resuscitation (TABLE 3). Thus, in our program, infants who presented with such an episode were at high risk of dying (13.2% of the infants in this category have died[7]). A second high-risk category in our program has been identified. Of the 27 infants who had 2 or more previous siblings die of SIDS, 18.5% have died and an additional 29.6% have had a severe episode of sleep apnea successfully resolved by their caretakers' use of vigorous stimulation or resuscitation.[8]

Overall, in the high-risk infants who were monitored, approximately 30% had subsequent significant episodes of apnea during sleep. These events were successfully terminated by resuscitation or vigorous stimulation of the infant by the caretaker.

DISCUSSION

The data presented demonstrated that, using the current protocol, the death rate in nonmonitored patients in the noncompliant group was 4.3 times the death rate of the nonmonitored patients in the compliant group. Those infants who were managed with home monitoring using our criteria had an overall mortality rate which was 10-fold increased over the background SIDS rate. However, of those deaths whose circumstances are known, the majority (67%) were coincident with noncompliance. Finally, in those high-risk monitored infants, the rate of successful intervention for subsequent severe sleep apnea events is 20 times the mortality rate of the monitored population.

Thus, based on these data, we believe that (1) most infants who are referred do not require monitoring, (2) most resuscitations can be successful with proper monitoring of those infants who meet our monitoring criteria, and (3) most infants who are monitored will survive. We have identified several characteristics of infants that place them in categories of higher mortality rate than most monitored infants. We suggest that the management of these infants should be changed in an attempt to decrease this mortality rate. For these infants, we recommend that (1) parents be informed of the high risk status of their infant and, if they choose to continue to care for their infant at home, they be made to understand that proper monitoring and CPR techniques must be used at all times, (2) long term hospitalization be an available alternative to home care and, (3) for any infant in whom repeated resuscitations (≥2) have occurred continuous recording of events should be instituted in an attempt to understand the pathophysiology of the event so that more sophisticated resuscitative measures as well as possibly more correct treatment can be provided.

Finally, for those few infants whose deaths were a failure of our triage (4/13,401; 3 premature infants) we must continue to develop more sophisticated methods of physiological study and of analysis of the physiological data in an attempt to identify pathophysiological mechanisms so that such deaths may be avoided in the future.

REFERENCES

1. KELLY, D. H., D. C. SHANNON & K. O'CONNELL. 1978. The care of infants with near-miss sudden infant death syndrome. Pediatrics **61**: 511–514.
2. WARD, S. L., T. G. KEENS, L. S. CHAN, B. E. CHIPPS, S. H. CARSON, D. D. DEMING, V. KRISHNA, H. M. MACDONALD, G. I. MARTIN, K. S. MEREDITH, T. A. MERRITT, B. G. NICKERSON, R. A. STODDARD & A. L. VAN DER HAL. 1986. Sudden infant death syndrome in infants evaluated by apnea programs in California. Pediatrics **77(4)**: 451–458.
3. GUILLEMINAULT, C. & R. KOROBKIN. 1979. Sudden infant death: Near miss events and sleep research: Some recommendations to improve comparability of results among investigators. Sleep **1**: 423–433.
4. STEIN, I. M. & D. C. SHANNON. 1975. The pediatric pneumogram: A new method for detecting and quantitating apnea in infants. Pediatrics **55**: 599–603.
5. KELLY, D. H., L. M. STELLWAGEN, E. KAITZ & D. C. SHANNON. 1985. Apnea and periodic breathing in normal full term infants during the first twelve months. Pediatr. Pulmonol. **1**: 215–219.
6. KELLY, D. H. & D. C. SHANNON. Medical management of cardiorespiratory monitoring in infantile apnea. *In* SIDS: Medical Aspects and Psychological Management. J. L. Culbertson, H. Krous & R. Bendell, Eds. Johns Hopkins University Press. In press.

7. OREN, J., D. H. KELLY & D. C. SHANNON. 1986. Identification of a high-risk group for sudden infant death syndrome among infants who were resuscitated for sleep apnea. Pediatrics **77:** 495–499.
8. OREN, J., D. H. KELLY & D. C. SHANNON. 1987. Familial occurrence of sudden infant death syndrome and apnea of infancy. Pediatrics **80:** 355–358.

Home Monitoring for the Sudden Infant Death Syndrome

The Case Against[a]

JOAN E. HODGMAN[b] AND TOKE HOPPENBROUWERS

Department of Pediatrics
University of Southern California School of Medicine
and Los Angeles County-USC Medical Center
Los Angeles, California 90089

Home monitoring has become popular for management of infants who are perceived to be at increased risk for the Sudden Infant Death Syndrome (SIDS). It is frequently recommended for infants with unexplained apnea of infancy, for subsequent siblings of SIDS, and for premature infants with apnea. This paper will explore the appropriateness, the effectiveness, and the risk of home monitoring for these infants. A discussion of home monitoring for infants with bronchopulmonary dysplasia (BPD), neurologic disorders, and other pathology is beyond the scope of this paper.

The American Academy of Pediatrics has issued two statements concerning SIDS and home monitoring. The first, which responded to over-the-counter sales of monitors, discouraged their use except as a research tool.[1] The second, a response to the growing clinical use of home monitors for infants with apnea, made no firm recommendations but did advocate 24 hour surveillance for infants who had had one or more episodes of prolonged apnea.[2] Prolonged apnea was defined as "cessation of breathing for 20 seconds or longer, or as a briefer episode associated with bradycardia, cyanosis, or pallor." Unfortunately, the abnormality of brief apneic episodes associated with bradycardia was neither then nor later established. This definition has resulted in attributing pathological significance to entirely normal patterns. Recently, the National Institutes of Health sponsored a "Consensus Statement on Infantile Apnea and Home Monitoring."[3] Both the advocates for and against monitoring were sensibly excluded from the conference which produced this consensus statement. The statement, which is long and carefully thought out, covers types of infants at risk, safety of monitors, evidence for their effectiveness and recommendations for their use, and avenues for further research. It concluded that the infant who had an apparent life-threatening event (ALTE) should benefit from home monitoring but that there is insufficient evidence to recommend monitoring in other groups for which it has been advocated. It stated, "The effectiveness of home monitoring in reducing infant mortality and morbidity is not yet established."

[a]These studies were supported by funds from NIHCHD (Contracts N01-HD-2-2777 and HD4-2810, Grant HD 13689-03); the National Foundation for SIDS, Los Angeles Chapter; the Guild for Infant Survival, San Gabriel Valley and Orange County Chapters; and the Aurthur Zimtbaum Foundation of New York.
[b]To whom correspondence should be addressed at Womens Hospital, 1240 Mission Road, Los Angeles, CA 90033.

EVIDENCE FOR EFFECTIVENESS OF HOME MONITORING

The only truly convincing evidence for effectiveness of home monitoring in preventing SIDS would be a controlled clinical trial. Unfortunately, no such study has been done. In the absence of a controlled study, less compelling evidence for effectiveness has been advanced. A decline in the rate of SIDS following the introduction of monitoring is one such line of evidence. However, rates fluctuate spontaneously from year to year with no discernable cause. Changes in incidence can vary as much as 300% in the same population over time. Three reports of annual rates may serve as examples (TABLE 1). These studies, reporting rates prior to 1973, were specifically chosen to avoid contamination of the figures by home monitoring. Borhani and coauthors[4] reported rates varying from 0.9 to 2.2 deaths from SIDS per 1,000 live births in California during 1964–1970. Strimer et al.,[5] reporting on total SIDS deaths in the greater Cleveland area for 1956–1965, found annual rates between 2.58 and 3.54. In Philadelphia for 1960–1972, Valdes-Dapena et al.[6] reported a variation of 0.61–1.85 in whites and 3.53–5.60 in blacks. Consequently, with this magnitude of spontaneous background variation it is difficult to attribute a small decrease to a specific intervention. At present, a decrease in the rate of SIDS paralleling the growing use of monitors cannot be attributed to the increase in this form of management.

TABLE 1. Spontaneous Variability in SIDS Rates

Author[a]	Years	Rates[b] (range)	Subjects
Strimer et al.[5]	1956–1965	1.98–2.95	White
		3.88–8.20	Non-white
Valdes-Dapena et al.[6]	1960–1972	0.61–1.85	White
		3.53–5.60	Black
Borhani et al.[4]	1964–1970	0.9–2.2	Total

[a]Numbers refer to citations in REFERENCES.
[b]SIDS/1,000 live births.

For reasons which are not entirely clear, the incidence of SIDS tends to parallel perinatal mortality (FIG. 1). Perinatal mortality itself has been dropping worldwide for the last 10 years. One possible explanation for this decline in both rates is improved maternal and infant care. There are other examples where improvement in mortality accompanied general public health measures before specific therapy was available. For instance, mortality from tuberculosis decreased significantly, before the advent of antibiotics. It is well known that identification of a problem may change it by observation alone without specific intervention. Years ago in our own hospital we became concerned about the high mortality in infants born to diabetic mothers. When we segregated these infants in one nursery for closer observation, the mortality decreased by 30% in the next year. It was a shame that at the time we segregated these infants we did not have any specific therapy to offer them, because any new management we might have tried would have been considered a dramatic success. A specific example of this effect in relation to SIDS was provided by Carpenter,[7] who reported a decrease in incidence of SIDS in patients who were provided improvements in well-baby care. It is more plausible to attribute the decline in SIDS rates to nonspecific improvement in infant care rather than to claim a causal relationship between monitoring and the incidence of SIDS.

The second line of evidence advanced for the effectiveness of home monitors is the number of alarms registered and the nature of intervention by the parents. There are two

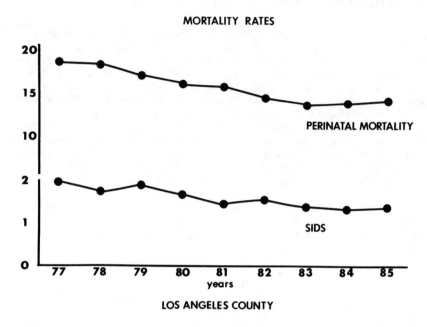

FIGURE 1. Comparison of perinatal mortality rates (deaths/1,000 total births) with deaths from SIDS (deaths/1,000 live births) in Los Angeles County, 1977–1985.

problems with such evidence. First, the impedance respiratory monitor has a proclivity for false alarms when the infant is breathing shallowly but normally.[8] Second, normal physiological phenomena such as brief cardiac decelerations will trigger alarms. This negates the validity of equating alarms with risk. Parents are under great stress when responding to an alarm in their infant and should not be expected to make scientifically accurate observations during such periods of intense anxiety. Wasserman[9] observed a correlation between the level of anxiety in the parents and their perception of the severity of the event causing the alarm. The more anxious parent felt the infant was in greater trouble than did the less anxious parent. While parents report that the alarms signaled serious problems requiring stimulation or resuscitation, it is not wise to depend on such observations as justification for the use of home monitors.

GROUPS AT RISK FOR SIDS

Infants who have been resuscitated from an episode of unexplained prolonged apnea (ALTE) are considered at risk to subsequently die of SIDS, and these situations have been referred to as near miss for SIDS or aborted SIDS deaths. The magnitude of their risk for subsequent death is not well defined. The best data from a series of unmonitored infants is that reported by Bergman *et al.*,[10] which indicated that one of forty infants later succumbed, an incidence of 2.5%. The highest incidence, reported by Kelly *et al.*,[11] was four deaths in a series of 84 monitored patients, a rate of 4.8%. In this series, deaths occurred only among the 27 infants who required more than one resuscitation. In spite of uncertainties about the exact magnitude of the risk, most experts agree that infants are indeed at increased risk of subsequent death following an ALTE. Although the risk for this group is real and monitoring is frequently recommended for these infants, there is no study to demonstrate its effectiveness. We should not lose sight of the fact that apnea preceeding death from SIDS is a relatively unusual occurrence. Froggatt et al.,[12] in a study covering all SIDS cases in Northern Ireland, found only a few with a history of preceding apneic spells; this low percentage has been confirmed by more recent reports.[13] The vast majority of infants dying of SIDS did not have documented prolonged apnea before death.

The subsequent sibling born into a family with a death from SIDS is also considered at increased risk for SIDS. The magnitude of this risk is not large, with reports varying between 2 and 5 times that for the normal population.[12,14] The lower value was obtained when maternal age and birth order were controlled, but it appears that subsequent siblings from families with lower socioeconomic status were underrepresented in this study.[14] Since no objective criteria for home monitoring have been identified for this group, it is an inappropriate intervention, unless monitoring is to be predicated on family anxiety.

The premature infant is clearly at increased risk of SIDS, and the risk increases with decreasing gestational age.[15] SIDS is the most common cause of death in premature infants following discharge from the nursery. In our own follow-up program, 1% of surviving infants who weighed less than 1,500 g at birth (very low birthweight, VLBW) died of SIDS. This is over 6 times the background rate in our county.

Although in one study the premature infant with BPD has been reported at particular risk, even when compared to other premature infants, other investigators have not confirmed this special risk.[16] When infants needing active treatment with oxygen and diuretics were excluded from the comparison, stable infants with BPD were not found to be at increased risk.[17] This study draws attention to the problem of including as SIDS those infants who die suddenly from other causes. With the general acceptance of SIDS as a cause of death, there is currently a tendency to attribute to SIDS any death in which there are no clear-cut pathological findings, even when the death is not unexpected by history.

The question of risk in the case of multiple births is confounded by the lower birthweights involved. When birthweight is controlled, the risk for the twin of less than 2,500 g is approximately twice that for the singleton, while for larger infants the risk is not increased.[18] The risk for the surviving twin, moreover, is very low, in the order of 3.6 per 1,000,000 live births.

The increased risk of 5-fold magnitude for the infant born to the drug abusing mother has been recognized most recently.[19] In the original reports the drugs were narcotics, but later reports have implicated cocaine as well.[20]

Epidemiological factors will identify groups of infants who are at increased risk to die of SIDS. In two groups, the ALTE and the preterm VLBW, the risk is well documented and of significant magnitude. In other groups, such as the drug abusing mother, the risk is not yet well defined. In subsequent siblings and surviving twins of an infant who died of SIDS, the risk appears to be much less than previously considered.

PHYSIOLOGICAL CRITERIA USED TO RECOMMEND MONITORING

In addition to the epidemiological criteria discussed above, various physiological phenomena have been used in an effort to identify infants at increased risk and, hence, potential candidates for monitoring. To date, none of these physiological criteria have been reliable predictors for SIDS. Episodes of prolonged apnea, defined as pauses of 20 sec or longer, are most frequently incriminated. Apnea of this duration are rare in the normal infant born at full-term.[21] While some infants exhibit clustered episodes of prolonged apnea, this alone does not predict death from SIDS.[13,22] The risk is increased by the history of an ALTE, not by the presence of apnea on subsequent polygraphic recordings. Shorter apnea of between 10 and 20 sec are seen in otherwise healthy infants on the average of 7–8 times per night, and apnea of 9 sec or less are even more common (FIGS. 2 and 3).[21] Frequently, the brief apnea reported in the literature represent pauses between normal breaths (FIG. 4). Our own studies demonstrated that infants had no increase in the incidence of apnea following an ALTE while subsequent siblings had fewer episodes of short apnea and no more episodes of longer apnea than did normal, control infants.[23,24]

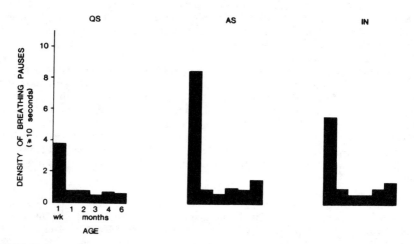

FIGURE 2. Density of breathing pauses equal to or longer than 10 sec in quiet sleep (QS), active sleep (AS), and intermediate sleep (IS) as a function of age (*abscissa*). An elevated number of these apnea characterized the first week of life.

In the nursery, premature infants with prolonged apnea have been considered at greater risk for SIDS than premature infants without apnea. Monitoring after discharge from the nursery is being recommended for the former group. Apnea longer than 20 sec are very common in the infant born after a short gestation, but the incidence decreases sharply after the first week of life. In our nursery, apnea of 20-sec duration or longer occurred in 15% of infants studied after the first week of life, when they were between 32 and 36 postconceptual weeks of age.[25] The incidence of recurrent apnea was less frequent, occurring in 4.5% of these infants, a figure similar to that reported by others.[26,27] We compared a group of these infants at 40 weeks postconception and at 1 and 3 months postnatal age with healthy premature infants of the same gestational age who had not exhibited apnea during their nursery stay.[28] We found no differences between these two groups in either cardiac and respiratory behavior or transcutaneous gases. These results

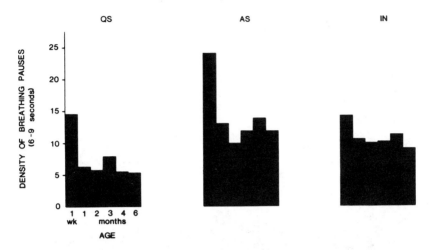

FIGURE 3. Density of breathing pauses between 6 and 9 sec as a function of age (*abscissa*). At one week of age, only the density in AS was significantly elevated compared to later ages. Abbreviations as in FIGURE 2.

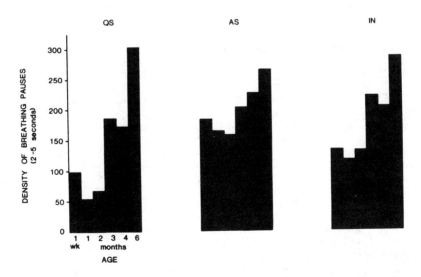

FIGURE 4. Density of breathing pauses between 2 and 5 sec as a function of age (*abscissa*). Profound increase of such pauses at 3 months of age, especially in QS. Abbreviations as in FIGURE 2.

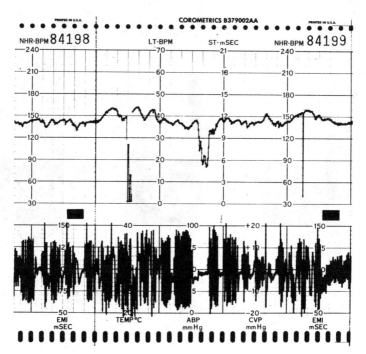

FIGURE 5. Cardiorespiratory tracing (Corometrics) of a premature infant of 34-weeks gestation at 2 weeks of age. Each small square = 10 sec. Apena of less than 20 sec is accompanied by a brief cardiac deceleration to below 90 beats per minute.

are congruent with the finding that apnea in the premature nursery does not predispose to SIDS.[29]

Brief drops in heart rate to levels below 90–100 beats per min (BPM) have been called bradycardia and implicated as a risk factor, particularly when associated with apneic pauses. Such drops should more properly be designated as cardiac decelerations because of their short duration (FIG. 5). This pattern should be distinguished from true bradycardia, where the drop in heart rate is sustained for at least 1 min. In spite of reports in the literature by some investigators that cardiac decelerations are rare or are never seen without apnea in full-term infants,[30,31] others report that this pattern is found in over 30% of infants studied.[32,33] In studies of full-term and preterm infants from our service, cardiac decelerations of less than 30-sec duration were frequent. We found one or more of these occurring in two-thirds of the healthy full-term infants at 1 month of age. In 33% of these infants, the cardiac deceleration was accompanied by a brief apnea of less than 12-sec duration. In 8-hr recordings of healthy preterm infants studied at 32–36 weeks postconception, 210 cardiac decelerations to below 90 BPM could be identified in 45 of the 66 infants.[25] Sixty-eight percent of these decelerations were not associated with any significant changes in respiratory tracings. Most of the apnea of 15–20 sec were accompanied by a cardiac deceleration in these healthy preterm infants. Since these drops are reflexes in response to vagal stimulation, their presence is reassuring rather than alarming. These patterns cannot be considered abnormal, and the term *short apnea with "bradycardia"* should be dropped from the definition of abnormal apnea.

Periodic breathing is another cardiorespiratory pattern that has been implicated as a factor for increased risk of SIDS. Kelly and Shannon[34] have reported an increased incidence of periodic breathing in infants with ALTE. This finding has not been confirmed by others.[35–37] In our studies, the incidence of periodic breathing was the same for our full-term control and at-risk groups.[23] FIGURE 6 shows the considerable density of periodic breathing in the normal infant born at full-term. Interestingly, both our groups had an incidence similar to that of the at-risk groups studied by Kelly and Shannon,[34] but their control group had surprisingly low levels. Although there is general agreement that periodic breathing increases with decreasing gestational age, there have been few studies quantifying periodic breathing in the healthy preterm infant. An incidence of 94% was

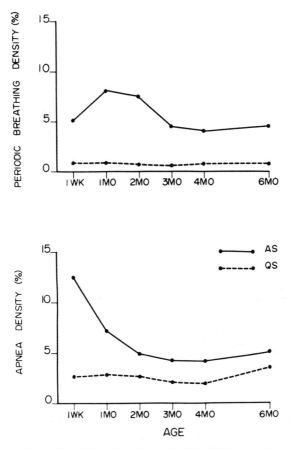

FIGURE 6. *Upper Panel:* Periodic breathing density in AS and QS as function of age in normal infants born at full-term. Increase in density at 1 and 2 months was not statistically significant. Also, note the very low incidence of periodic breathing during QS. *Lower Panel:* Apnea density is plotted as function of age and sleep state. Approximately 2.5 out of every 100 min in QS contain an apnea. In contrast, approximately 1 out of every 8 min in AS contains an apnea in the newborn period. This figure decreases to 1 out of 20 min at other ages examined. Abbreviations as in FIGURE 2.

found in preterm and 36% in full-term infants studied during the first 2–11 weeks of life.[38] We found 57 of 66 premature infants had a mean of 47.5 min of periodic breathing during an 8 hr tracing, with a very wide range from 2 to 195 min.[25]

In summary, we can conclude that many apnea previously considered abnormal are in fact normal. The presence of prolonged apnea, while not common in normal infants beyond the neonatal period, does not predict SIDS. Premature infants with apnea in the nursery are at no greater risk than premature infants without such apnea. Cardiac decelerations are an entirely normal response to physiological stimuli. And, finally, the incidence of periodic breathing documented in at-risk infants also does not deviate from normal. In other words, the typical criteria used to recommend home monitoring in infants at increased statistical risk for SIDS are inappropriate. The infant who will die cannot be identified by physiological characteristics. Extensive experience with polysomnography has not provided justification for its use to identify infants at risk by current criteria. The use of the pneumogram to identify infants for subsequent monitoring and to dictate management appears particularly ill-advised.

RESULTS OF HOME MONITORING

The use of home monitors is predicated on the belief that apnea is the final common pathway to death and, most importantly, that the apnea can be interrupted. This belief is

TABLE 2. Deaths in Monitored Infants

Author[a]	Infants Studied Only	Infants Monitored	Deaths	
			Off	On
Guilleminault et al.[35]	22	156	1	0
Duffty & Bryan[41]		124	—	1
Kahn & Blum[42]	261	58	1	0
Kelly et al.[11]		84	—	4
Rosen et al.[45]		26	1	1
Southall et al.[44]	200[b]	4[b]	2[b]	0[b]
Ward et al.[46]	1565	1841	4	7
Total, all studies	2048	2293	9	13

[a]Numbers refer to citations in REFERENCES.

[b]Values for cases managed by Southall et al.; data in text refer to summary of both these and some cases reported by other investigators.

speculative because the mechanism of death is still unknown. Moreover, infants have died while being monitored. On some occassions the failure has been due to mechanical defects in the monitor, or the monitor was detached from the infant. There is a tendency not to count these as monitor failures, yet they are certainly due to defects in a monitoring program. More disturbing are deaths occurring when the infants could not be resuscitated after a monitor alarm. There has been only one report of a monitored death in a hospitalized infant and, unfortunately, no written record of the events preceding death was available. The infant was limp and not breathing, with a dusky but not blue color, and with no heart beat. Despite expert cardiorespiratory resuscitation, neither heart beat nor respiration could be revived. Other instances of death during monitoring are limited to anecdotal accounts.[40] One infant was found pallid rather than dusky; in two, an airway could not be established even though in one case a pediatric anesthesiologist tried. These cases, while providing little useful information, suggest that cardiac as well as respiratory mechanisms may be involved in the final pathway.

Reliable figures on the number of infants monitored and the results of monitoring are difficult to obtain (TABLE 2). The most extensive series followed by a single group was reported by Kelley et al.,[11] who observed four deaths among 84 monitored infants. Duffty and Bryant[41] reported one death of a subsequent sibling among 52 monitored in their program, an incidence comparable to that expected without monitoring. Deaths following dicontinuance of the monitor have been reported in one instance each by Kahn and Blum[42] and by Guilleminault et al.[43] These cases were summarized in 1983 by Southall et al.,[44] who included, along with their own cases, the experience of a number of the other investigators studying infants with ALTE. They found 7 deaths in 176 monitored infants compared to 5 deaths in 455 infants who were studied but not monitored. It is impossible to draw firm conclusions from this report because the monitored and nonmonitored groups were comparable only in having a history of an ALTE. Two further deaths were reported by Rosen et al.[45] from a group of 26 infants with ALTE. One of these deaths occurred in an infant managed by drugs alone and the other in an infant on only a respiratory monitor. The largest number of cases of monitored infants was collected by Ward et al.,[46] who canvassed monitoring programs in California in 1986. For infants referred to these programs, they compared the results on those for whom monitoring was recommended with the results on those for whom monitoring was not recommended and showed no decrease in mortality in the former group. Although these were uncontrolled series of cases, this is the best information available to date. The evidence does not permit the conclusion that home monitoring is effective in preventing SIDS.

RISKS OF HOME MONITORING

Safety of the monitor is always important, but it is especially so when it is to be used in the home. Accidents have been reported, including 2 deaths that appeared due to electrocution.[47] This is particularly disturbing as it is easy to see how such deaths could be attributed to SIDS.

Information about the impact of the monitor on the family, obtained by questionnaires and by interviews of families from monitoring programs,[48,49] first came from teams enthusiastic about the benefits of monitoring; their conclusions were mostly favorable. A subsequent report by a psychiatrist not directly involved in the monitoring program appears to offer a more judicious approach.[9] The majority of the families found the monitor both produced and assuaged anxiety. The willingness to accommodate to the demands of monitoring was directly related to the perceived risk for the infant. Most families completed the monitoring program in spite of the associated pressures. The major acute problems centered on difficulty in obtaining relief from constant surveillance with its attendant fatigue, the mechanical problems with the monitor of frequent false alarms and lead breakage, and differences between the father's and mother's acceptance of the need for monitoring. In one study, 14% of the couples felt that their relationship worsened during the experience, and 2 of the 74 couples separated.[49] Without controls, it is not possible to know how much of the family friction could be blamed on the presence of the monitor. Although most families felt the monitor had little influence on their older children, psychiatric interviews uncovered a different picture.[9] Twelve of 16 siblings had psychological problems reported at the first follow-up interview, although these appeared to have largely resolved by the second follow-up. The monitored infants were reported as spoiled by one-half of the parents at the first interview. At the second follow-up, when they were starting school, an apparently startling 9 of 13 previously monitored infants exhibited neurologic soft signs such as gross and fine motor problems, short attention span, and speech problems. There were neither control data nor standards presented to put these findings into context. All of the authors attempted to link these problems to the need for resuscitation, although not all affected infants were resuscitated. No mention was made of the possibility that monitoring may have affected the infants' development.

One of the most discouraging aspects of home monitoring is that, although the number of infants who have been monitored is large it has not advanced our knowledge of the causation or mechanism of SIDS. Even in cases where infants have died while being monitored, the final, common pathway to death has not been established.

CONCLUSIONS

In the absence of controlled studies, there is no compelling evidence that monitoring is effective in preventing deaths from SIDS. In many instances monitoring is not appropriate, either because the risk is not sufficiently enhanced or the physiological criteria used to identify infants are not valid. The data available do not show any advantage for monitored infants.

More than 10 years of widespread home monitoring of infants has not advanced our knowledge of either the cause or the mechanism of death from SIDS. Rates have declined, but it is unlikely that the decline can be attributed to monitoring. SIDS remains the number one medical cause of death during the first year of life after the neonatal period.

Home monitoring is expensive, and evaluation and management of monitored children has diverted financial resources from other lines of endeavor which could be more fruitful.

Bergman, Beckwith and Ray[50] voiced their concerns in 1975 regarding the lack of conclusive proof that SIDS is related to sleep apnea, the absence of supporting scientific evidence that home monitors can prevent SIDS, and the potential adverse effects on the emotional health of the family. These concerns are as valid in 1987 as they were in 1975.

ACKNOWLEDGMENT

We wish to express our deep appreciation for support from NIHCHD; the National Foundation for SIDS, Los Angeles Chapter; the Guild for Infant Survival, San Gabriel Valley Chapter and Orange County Chapter; and the Arthur Zimtbaum Foundation of New York.

REFERENCES

1. AMERICAN ACADEMY OF PEDIATRICS COMMITTEE ON INFANT AND PRESCHOOL CHILD. 1975. Pediatrics 55: 144.
2. AMERICAN ACADEMY OF PEDIATRICS, TASK FORCE ON PROLONGED APNEA. 1978. Pediatrics 61: 651–652.
3. NATIONAL INSTITUTES OF HEALTH. 1987. Pediatrics 79: 292–299.
4. BORHANI, N. O., P. A. ROONEY & J. F. KRAUS. 1973. Calif. Med. 118: 12–16.
5. STRIMER, R., L. ADELSON & R. OSEASOHN. 1969. J. Am. Med. Assoc. 209: 1493–1497.
6. VALDES-DAPENA, M., J. A. McGOVERN, L. J. BIRLE et al. 1974. J. Pediatr. 84: 776–777.
7. CARPENTER, R. G. 1983. In Sudden Infant Death Syndrome. J. T. Tildon, L. M. Roeder & A. Steinschneider, Eds.: 705–718. Academic Press. New York.
8. JEFFERY, H., R. A. CUNNINGHAM, A. CUBIS et al. 1981. Aust. N.Z. J. Med. 11: 406–411.

9. WASSERMAN, A. L. 1984. Pediatrics **74:** 323–329.
10. BERGMAN, A. B., J. B. BECKWITH & C. G. RAY. 1970. Sudden Infant Death Syndrome. University of Washington Press. Seattle, Washington.
11. KELLY, D. H., D. C. SHANNON & K. O'CONNELL. 1978. Pediatrics **61:** 511–513.
12. FROGGATT, P., M. A. LYNAS & G. MACKENZIE. 1971. J. Prev. Soc. Med.**25:** 119–134.
13. SOUTHALL, D. P., J. M. RICHARDS, V. STEBBENS, et al. 1986. Pediatrics **78:** 787–796.
14. PETERSON, D. R., E. E. SABOTTA & J. R. DALING. 1986. J. Pediatr.**108:** 911–914.
15. KULKARNI, P., R. T. HALL, P. G. RHODES, et al. 1978. Pediatrics **62:** 178–183.
16. WERTHAMMER, J. BROWN, E. R., R. K. NEFF & H. W. TAEUSCH, JR. 1982. Pediatrics **6:** 301–308.
17. PIECUCH, R., R. CLYMAN & R. BALLARD. 1987. Pediatr. Res. **21:** 373A.
18. KRAUS, J. F. 1983. *In* Sudden Infant Death Syndrome. J. T. Tildon, L. M. Roeder & A. Steinschneider, Eds.: 43–58. Academic Press. New York.
19. CHAVEZ, C. J., E. M. OSTREA, JR. & Z. SMIALEK. 1979. J. Pediatr. **95:** 407–409.
20. I. J. CHASNOFF, Ed. 1986. Drug Use in Pregnancy:Mother & Child.:60. MTP Press Limited. Lancaster/Boston/The Hague/Dordrecht.
21. HOPPENBROUWERS, T., J. E. HODGMAN, D. MCGINTY et al. 1980. Pediatr. Res. **14:** 1230.
22. MONOD, N., P. PLOUIN, B. STERNBERG et al. 1986. Biol. Neonate **50:** 147–153.
23. HODGMAN, J. E., T. HOPPENBROUWERS, S. GEIDEL et al. 1982. Pediatrics **69:** 785–792.
24. HOPPENBROUWERS, T., J. E. HODGMAN, D. MCGINTY et al. 1980. Pediatrics **66:** 205–214.
25. HODGMAN, J. E., T. HOPPENBROUWERS, L. A. CABAL et al. 1982. Clin. Res. **30:** 143A.
26. HENDERSON-SMART, D. J. 1981. Aust. Paediatr. J. **17:** 273–276.
27. ROSEN, C. L., D. G. GLAZE & J. D. FROST. 1986. Am. J. Dis. Child. **40:** 547–550.
28. HOPPENBROUWERS, T., J. E. HODGMAN, D. ARAKAWA et al. 1985. Pediatr. Res. **18:** 346A.
29. SOUTHALL, D. P., J. M. RICHARDS, K. J. RHODEN et al. 1982. Pediatrics **70:** 844–851.
30. MORGAN, B. C. & W. G. GUNTHEROTH. 1965. J. Pediatr. **67:** 1199.
31. DEUEL, R. K. 1973. Arch. Neurol. **28:** 71–76.
32. VALIMAKI, I., & P. A. TARLO. 1971. Am. J. Obstet. Gynecol. **110:** 343–349.
33. STEIN, I. M., M. FALLON, R. L. MERISALO et al. 1983. Neuropediatrics **14:** 73–75.
34. KELLY, D. H. & D. C. SHANNON. 1979. Pediatrics **63:** 355–360.
35. GUILLEMINAULT, C., R. ARIAGNO, R. KOROBKIN et al. 1979. Pediatrics **64:** 882.
36. FLORES-GUEVARA, R., B. STERNBERG, P. PEIRANO et al. 1986. Neuropediatrics **17:** 59–62.
37. FRANKS, C. I., J. B. G. WATSON, B. H. BROWN et al. 1980. Arch. Dis. Child. **55:** 595–599.
38. FENNER, A., U. SCHALK, H. HOENICKE et al. 1973. Pediatr. Res. **7:** 174–183.
39. LEWAK, N. 1975. Pediatrics **56:** 296–298.
40. PERSONAL COMMUNICATION.
41. DUFFTY, P. & M. H. BRYAN. 1982. Pediatrics **70:** 69–74.
42. KAHN, A. D. BLUM. 1982. Eur. J. Pediatr. **139:** 94–100.
43. GUILLEMINAULT, C., R. L. ARIAGNO, L. S. FORNO, et al. 1979. Pediatrics **63:** 837–843.
44. SOUTHALL, D. P. 1983. Pediatrics **72:** 133–138.
45. ROSEN, C. L., J. D. FROST & G. M. HARRISON. 1983. Pediatrics **71:** 731–736.
46. WARD S. L., T. G. KEENS, L. S. CHAN, B. E. CHIPPS, S. H. CARSON, D. D. DEMING, V. KRISHNA, H. M. MACDONALD, G. I. MARTIN, K. S. MEREDITH, T. A. MERRITT, B. G. NICKERSON, R. A. STODDARD & A. L. VAN DER HAL. 1986. Pediatrics **77:** 451–458.
47. KATCHER, M. L., M. M. SHAPIRO & C. GUIST. 1986. Pediatrics **78:** 775–779.
48. BLACK, L., L. HERSHER & A. STEINSCHNEIDER. 1978. Pediatrics **62:** 681–685.
49. CAIN, L. P., D. H. KELLY & D. C. SHANNON. 1980. Pediatrics **66:** 37–4.
50. BERGMAN, A. B., J. B. BECKWITH & C. G. RAY. 1975. Pediatrics **56:** 1–3.

Conduction Tissue and SIDS[a]

SIEW YEN HO AND ROBERT H. ANDERSON[b]

Department of Paediatrics
Cardiothoracic Institute
Fulham Road
London SW3 6HP
United Kingdom

INTRODUCTION

Many theories have been invoked to explain sudden infant death. Several of these involve the heart, focusing particularly on the conduction tissues. Among these may be cited the possibility of cartilaginous change, of increased fibrosis, of "molding" of archipelagoes of conduction fibers extending into the central fibrous body, of stenosis of the penetrating atrioventricular bundle, of lesions of the arterial supply to the cardiac nodes, of the presence of the branching atrioventricular bundle at a location to the left of the septal crest, and of the presence of accessory pathways for atrioventricular conduction. It is exceedingly difficult to "prove" any of these concepts. Of necessity, morphological studies are conducted after the event of death, and hardly ever is there documented evidence detailing the cardiac rhythm at death. Furthermore, the majority of the changes described can, with careful study, also be found in the hearts of infants dying from known causes, thus raising the possibility that their presence in hearts from SIDS victims is simply coincidental. In this review, we will examine the evidence underscoring these various concepts, supplementing it with our own findings in hearts from the United Kingdom Multicenter Perinatal Death Study.

THE MULTICENTER PERINATAL DEATH STUDY

The Multicenter Study of Postneonatal Mortality was set up in Sheffield, United Kingdom, in 1975 in order to determine whether there is a pathological basis for sudden infant death. Participating centers had pediatric pathologists who were able to perform detailed necropsies.[1] Some organ systems were sent to specialist units for further investigation. Our unit, which has histological facilities to study the cardiac conduction system, received 49 hearts for investigation between 1976 and 1979. All the hearts received had only a reference number attached. The hearts were checked grossly for structural normality and absence of congenital malformations before being processed by established procedures.[2] One in 25 of the sections was mounted and stained with a modified Masson's technique, enabling easy distinction between fibrous tissue and myocardium. Furthermore, specialized myocardium usually stained slightly paler than working myocardium. Additional sections were mounted and stained with Hematoxylin and eosin where necessary. All the sections examined had only the coded specimen number as a reference: the cause of death of each patient was unknown to us. The code

[a]These studies were supported by the British Heart Foundation and the Joseph Levy Foundation.
[b]Author to whom correspondence should be addressed.

was finally broken this year (1987) when the cause of death was revealed by the referring centers. This information gave us the opportunity to assess our findings in the group with explained deaths (19 hearts) and compare them with the group where death was sudden and unexplained (30 hearts). The former group, which acted as a control, included five patients who were in category B of the Sheffield score, that is, infants for whom a potentially treatable condition was a major cause or contributing factor of death. The latter group, the sudden, unexplained deaths, included 11 hearts from infants who had died during the course of minor, not normally fatal, conditions. The age range of the group with explained deaths was 1 day to 1 year and 7 months. The range for the sudden infant death group was 5 weeks to 1 year and 3 months.

THE NORMAL CONDUCTION SYSTEM

Before delving into the various proposed cardiac substrates for sudden infant death, it is helpful to review the "normal" anatomy of the cardiac conduction system as we understand it. The components of the specialized system are the sinus node and the atrioventricular conduction axis. The latter, in turn, comprises the atrioventricular node, the penetrating atrioventricular bundle (bundle of His), the branching bundle, and the ventricular bundle branches. Conduction between the cardiac nodes is mediated through ordinary working atrial myocardium which has no histologically specialized characteristics sufficient to support the concept of "specialized tracts."[3] It is true that the internodal myocardium is organized into broad bands such as the terminal crest and the anterosuperior rim of the oval fossa. In no way do these broad pathways constitute specialized tracts insulated or histologically distinct from the remainder of the atrial myocardium. The preferential atrial conduction, which certainly occurs, does so because of the geometric arrangement of the working atrial myocardial fibers.[4]

The sinus node is a cigar-shaped structure which, in infants, measures approximately 4 to 6 mm in length. It is located subepicardially in the terminal groove, lateral to the junction of the superior caval vein with the right atrium (FIG. 1). Occasionally, it has a horse-shoe shape and is draped across the cavo-atrial junction, just behind the atrial crest. The origin and course of arterial supply to the node is highly variable. A recent study of 50 normal hearts showed the nodal artery arising from the right coronary artery in 33 hearts and from the left coronary artery in the remaining hearts.[5] The course of the artery in the cavo-arterial junction was precaval in 29, and retrocaval in 18; it formed an arterial circle in 3 hearts. Although the nodal cells are usually arranged around a prominent artery, the artery may branch within the nodal substance or the main artery may be located alongside the node.[6] The node itself is a histologically discrete structure. It is made up of small, densely packed nodal cells set in a fibrous tissue matrix. The transition between nodal and atrial myocardium at the nodal periphery is brief (FIG. 2), and the clear demarcation is occasionally interrupted by tongues of nodal cells which, extending beyond it, then merge imperceptibly with the atrial musculature. The "tail" of the node (the cauda) may extend a fair distance intramyocardially along the terminal crest, lateral to the orifice of the inferior caval vein.

The atrioventricular node is also an atrial structure. Although right atrial structures are the best landmarks to its location, it is an interatrial structure, rather than being exclusively right atrial.[7] Transitional fibers extend between the compact node and atrial myocardium. These fibers stream in from the atrial septum, along the length of the node, and cascade down into the attachment of the septal leaflet of the tricuspid valve. Seen in cross section, the node has the appearance of a half-oval set against the central fibrous body (FIG. 3). The compact node extends forward into the central fibrous body to become

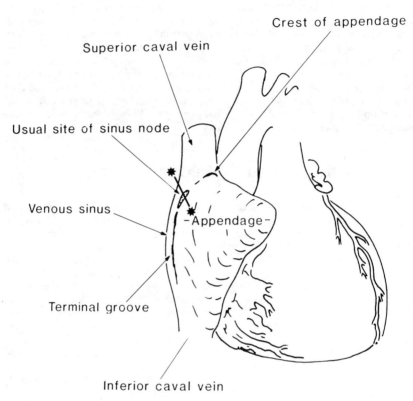

FIGURE 1. Diagram showing the usual location of the sinus node. *—* indicates the plane of section for FIGURE 2.

the penetrating bundle. The point of penetration is the apex of the nodal triangle bordered by the tendon of Todaro and the annular attachment of the tricuspid valve (FIG. 4). Although the penetrating bundle is a direct continuation of the axis of cells making up the compact node, a distinction is made between it and the compact node at the point where atrial transitional cells cease to make contact with the axis[8] (FIG. 3). Irregular groups of specialized cells are frequently found in the central fibrous body at this region of the nodal-bundle axis (FIG. 5). Their implicated role in sudden infant death is discussed later. In the normal heart, the atrioventricular conduction axis is the only muscular connection between atrial and ventricular musculature. Throughout the remaining atrioventricular junction, atrial and ventricular tissues are in contiguity but are separated by the tissue of the atrioventricular groove (including the annular attachments of the atrioventricular valves). While nodelike remnants of specialized "ring tissue" are present, particularly at the insertion of atrial myocardium into the tricuspid valve, these do not make contact with the ventricular myocardium.[9]

The conduction axis usually becomes the branching ventricular system immediately after penetration. A nonbranching bundle interposes between the penetrating and branching portions in some hearts. In its proximal segments, the ventricular system is isolated from the septal myocardium by connective tissue sheaths. From the branching bundle, the left bundle branch descends in subendocardial position on the left aspect of the ventricular septum, forming an extensive fanlike sheet of cells. There are usually three major divisions of the left bundle branch, which have numerous interconnecting fascicles as they approach the apical extent of the septum.

Unlike the fan-shaped left bundle branch, the right bundle branch is a discrete cord of cells in its proximal course. It traverses the septomarginal trabeculation before ramifying in the ventricular apex. It is often described as the direct continuation of the conduction axis, but there are variations.[10] When it is present in the form of a branch of the conduction axis, the remaining axis continues as a dead-end tract into the ventricular outlet musculature.[11]

PROPOSED CARDIAC SUBSTRATES FOR SUDDEN INFANT DEATH

Increased Fibrosis

One anatomical aspect of the cardiac conduction system is its intimate relationship with fibrous tissue. For this reason, a fibrous tissue stain gives optimal histological differentiation. It is the fibrous framework of the sinus nodal cells which renders the node so easily recognizable. Therefore, unless the whole nodal structure becomes densely fibrotic, an increase in fibrous tissue content is difficult to demonstrate without quantification. In our study of hearts from the multicenter study, we encountered one fibrotic sinus node in each group. The remaining sinus nodes did not show structural abnormalities, except that one heart in each group had a node less then half the anticipated normal size (TABLE 1).

Increased fibrosis in the atrioventricular node and penetrating bundle is a subject of contention. As discussed above, the node is adjacent to the central fibrous body, while the

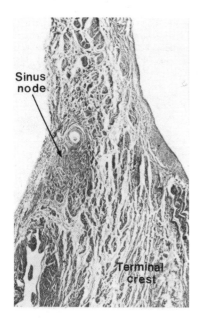

FIGURE 2. Histological section through the right cavo-atrial junction showing the sinus node and its accompanying artery. Magnification: 40×, reproduced at 75%.

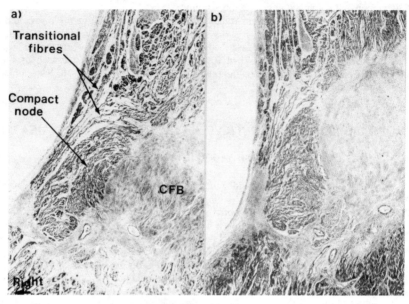

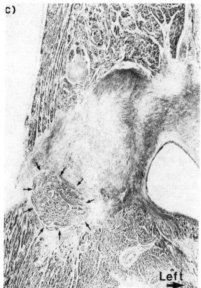

FIGURE 3. A series of histological sections through the atrioventricular junctional area showing the transition from the compact atrioventricular node (**a**) to the penetrating bundle, indicated by the *arrows* (**c**). (**b**) The atrial myocardium is still in contact with the nodal bundle axis. CFB = central fibrous body. Magnification: 25×, reproduced at 75%.

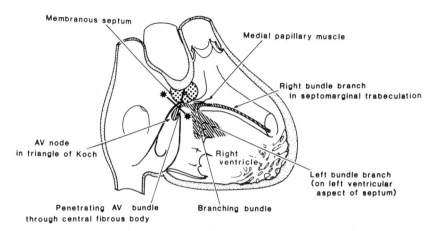

FIGURE 4. Diagram showing the disposition of the atrioventricular conduction axis as viewed from the right side of the heart. *—* indicates the plane of histologic sections shown in FIGURE 3.

penetrating bundle is completely surrounded by the fibrous skeleton. Also as discussed above, it is a normal finding in almost all child and adult hearts to find archipelagoes of specialized tissue extending from the conduction axis into the central fibrous body. These interdigitations between conduction axis and central fibrous body have been described variously as "fronds", "loops", "spurious blind end branches" and "fragments of atrioventricular node tissue."[12–14] According to Ferris,[15] the conduction tissue is normal

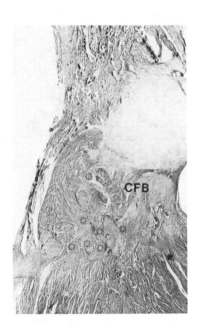

FIGURE 5. Histological section through the atrioventricular node region of a heart from the control group showing the extensions of specialized tissue (✿) into the central fibrous body. CFB = central fibrous body. Magnification: 25×, reproduced at 75%.

at birth, but the atrioventricular node and bundle subsequently undergo remodeling. The change in morphology is achieved through a progressive increase in and maturation of fibrous tissue in the region but is not associated with any inflammatory reaction. The corresponding reduction in size of the penetrating bundle by atrophy is thought to be a response to changes of vascular supply in the area. Whether these archipelagoes represent an incursion of specialized tissue into the fibrous body or a fibrotic invasion of the nodal bundle axis is a moot point. Thus, Kendeel and Ferris[16] claimed to have demonstrated in a quantitative study that hearts from the sudden infant death group showed a significant increase in fibrous tissue in the atrioventricular junctional area. Interestingly, their single photomicrographic illustration showed multiple archipelagoes at the distal part of the compact node. It would appear that their interpretation of fibrotic encroachment upon the nodal-bundle region is inextricably related to the process described by others as "molding". Without performing quantitation, we have been unable to distinguish between the extent of archipelagoes in control hearts and the extent in hearts from infants dying suddenly.

TABLE 1. Structural Analysis of Sinus Nodes in Hearts from SIDS Victims and Controls

Feature	SIDS $(n)^a$	Controls $(n)^b$
Fibrotic node	1	1
Hypoplastic node	1	1
Medial hypertrophy SNA^c	1	1
Intimal hyperplasia SNA^c	1	0
Totals (% of total in category)	4 (17%)	3 (20%)

^{a}Twenty-four hearts from SIDS victims were analyzed.
^{b}Fifteen control hearts were analyzed.
^{c}SNA = sinus node artery.

"Molding" of Archipelagoes of Conduction Fibers

It is known that the conduction axis is larger in fetuses and neonates than in adults when considered in relation to heart size. "Molding" describes an apparent transformation of the atrioventricular node and penetrating bundle from the supposed shaggy contours of the fetal stage to the smoothly outlined adult configuration. This shaping is said to be achieved by a degenerative process with necrosis and macrophage infiltration.[12,17] It was proposed that these histopathological changes could trigger lethal conduction disturbances during this period of postulated electrical instability.[12] That the process is one of "active resorption" is disputed by other workers.[18,19] Histological investigations of this sort can only provide "still frames" of developmental processes. Action replays compiled from diverse stills by cutting room experts are therefore open to interpretation. Be that as it may, the archipelagoes of conduction tissue within the central fibrous body certainly form loops and sinuate structures which are thought to potentiate electrical instability.[12] These structures are found with equal frequency in hearts from infants dying from known causes and infants dying suddenly.[12,18-20] Moreover, although seen most frequently in infant hearts, archipelagoes are also found in normal adult hearts.[21] Thus, our observations question the very premise that the "shaggy" fetal system becomes smooth during infancy.

Moderate to marked presence of the so-called molding of the atrioventricular node was seen in 9 and 14 hearts in the sudden death and the explained death (control) groups, respectively (TABLE 2). Extensive archipelagoes forming potential and actual nodo-

TABLE 2. Structural Analysis of Archipelagoes in Hearts from SIDS Victims and Controls

	SIDS[a]		Controls[b]	
Feature	n	% of Total	n	% of Total
Molding	9	30	14	74
Potential nodo-ventricular connection	1	3	3	16
Actual nodo-ventricular connection	1	3	2	11

[a]A total of 30 hearts.
[b]A total of 19 hearts.

ventricular connections and fasciculo-ventricular connections were present in each group (TABLE 2 and FIG. 6). Fibrous separation of the penetrating bundle, giving a dispersed cross-sectional appearance, was observed in 4 hearts in each group.

Maturation of the Central Fibrous Body

Proceeding hand-in-hand with the shaping of the nodal-bundle axis is the maturation of the central fibrous body. It is thought that this maturation serves to divide the extensive networks of archipelagoes which extend between the conduction axis and the crest of the ventricular septum.[22] In this setting, prior to their division, these structures represent pathways for nodo-ventricular and fasciculo-ventricular ("Mahaim") conduction. The

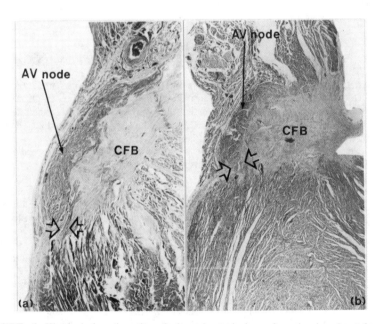

FIGURE. 6. Histological sections through the atrioventricular node region in a heart from the control group (**a**) and one from the sudden infant death group (**b**) showing an accessory nodo-ventricular connection (between *open arrows*) in each. CFB = central fibrous body. Magnification: 20×, reproduced at 75%.

elimination of these short-circuiting tracts could theoretically enhance electrical stability. If the ventricular fragments of these tracts persist, they could serve as parasystolic focuses,[23] providing a substrate for ventricular fibrillation. Occasionally, islands of conduction tissue are seen on the left side of the central fibrous body, a finding which may be interpreted as incomplete maturation. Excesses in the developmental process can result in dispersion of the nodal-bundle axis and, in extreme circumstances, sever nodal-bundle continuity. James and Marshall,[14] in reviewing delayed completion of the normal molding of the atrioventricular node and penetrating bundle, espoused the proposal that some fibroblasts may be genetically programmed to misbehave. We have no evidence to prove or disprove this graphic postulation. As mentioned previously, potential and actual accessory connections were seen in hearts from both our explained death (control) and sudden death groups.

The central fibrous body in the infant has a myxoid appearance characteristic of young connective tissue. Employing special stains, Lie et al.[19] were unable to demonstrate cartilage in any of their hearts from infants who were victims of sudden death or of an explained death. With maturation, the central fibrous body becomes more compact and collagenous. While cartilage or even bone is present in the central fibrous body of some animal hearts, such as the beef heart, cartilaginous transformation within the human heart is exceedingly rare. Ferris and Aherne[24] reported the presence of cartilage in the central fibrous body in 2 children who died suddenly and unexpectedly. Its observed location was similar to that of the fibrous interdigitation which they had seen in other infants who had died of the cot death syndrome. In a family of dogs associated with sudden death, metamorphosis of collagen to cartilage and bone within the central fibrous system has been ascribed to ischemic changes consequential to hereditary focal stenoses of small arteries in the atrioventricular junctional area.[23] None of the hearts in our study contained cartilage or bone in the central fibrous body.

Pathology and Abnormality of the Atrioventricular Bundle

In a detailed and elegantly illustrated investigation, Keith and Flack[25] in 1906 charted the course of the atrioventricular bundle in calf and human hearts. They emphasized the anatomical relationship between the bundle, the central fibrous body (including the membranous septum), and the aortic valve. Since the bundle is located in a active part of the heart which bears the brunt of left ventricular ejection, Keith and Flack reasoned that it is also particularly vulnerable to disease processes of the valves. They cited His for proposing in 1899 that a lesion of the atrioventricular bundle could be a cause of rhythm irregularity between atria and ventricles.

Studying sudden death in a breed of dogs, James and Drake[26] found degenerative lesions with fatty replacement in the bundle in 10 out of 11 dogs. Eight of the dogs were 3 to 10.5 years old. As cartilage was found in the adjacent central fibrous body, together with focal narrowing of the nutrient arteries, they postulated a chronic ischemic cause for the degenerative lesions. Small areas of necrosis in the atrioventricular bundle in 3 sudden death infants were described by Jankus.[27] These appeared to be related to an inflammatory process and in turn produced lethal arrhythmias.

In the absence of anatomico-electrophysiological correlations, speculations abound on the association between pathological changes of the bundle and sudden death. While it is known that mechanical severance of the bundle disrupts the continuity of cardiac conduction, the precise effect of pathological damage is unclear. Even more obscure is the effect, if any, of bundle stenosis. James and his colleagues[28] proposed stenosis of the His bundle as a substrate for sudden death in a breed of pug dogs. Such stenosis was observed in an infant who died suddenly[29] but also had bacterial bronchopneumonia. Our present study yielded a stenotic penetrating bundle in one heart, which was from the explained death (control) group (TABLE 3).

Lesions of the Arterial Supply to the Cardiac Nodes

These lesions can produce ischemia or infarction of the specialized myocardium. Lesions producing marked reduction in luminal cross-sectional area of the intranodal sinus node artery were found in three infants diagnosed with sudden infant death syndrome.[30] Recent or remote injury to the nodal cells was not present. The possibility of a fatal outcome due to temporary nodal dysfunction was considered. Along similar lines, vascular alterations in the supply to the atrioventricular system may be implicated in some cases of sudden death.[31] Arterial lesions were found in both of our groups of hearts. In the sudden death group, the sinus node artery was seen to be affected by focal wall thickening in 1 heart, the atrioventricular node artery in 2 hearts, and both arteries in 1 heart (TABLE 1). One heart in the "control" group showed medial hypertrophy of the sinus node artery (TABLE 1).

TABLE 3. Structural Analysis of the Atrioventricular Bundle in Hearts from SIDS Victims and Controls

Feature	SIDS[a]		Controls[b]	
	n	% of Total	n	% of Total
Dispersion	5	17	4	21
Stenosis	0	0	1	5
Hypoplasia	1	3	1	5
Fasciculo-ventricular connection	2	7	1	5

[a]A total of 30 hearts.
[b]A total of 19 hearts.

Location of the Branching Atrioventricular Bundle

In a recent study, Bharati and her colleagues[32] stated that there was a more common occurrence of left-sided atrioventricular bundle in hearts from infants with sudden infant death syndrome than in those from infants with known causes of death. They hypothesized that a bundle located to the left of the septal crest was more prone to arrhythmogenic forces in the transition from neonatal to adult circulation. Massing and James,[10] however, considered a course to the left of the septal crest to be a minor variation from normal, in contrast to right-sided locations, which were associated with a slender origin for the left bundle branch. They contended that very small lesions in such a region would be sufficient to cause marked conduction disturbance and sudden unexpected death.[10,33]

Our own studies do not substantiate the proposition of Bharati and her colleagues.[32] A branching bundle situated on the left and beneath the septal crest (FIG. 7) was less common in the hearts from the sudden infant death group (4 out of 30 hearts) than in those from the control group (4 out of 19 hearts; TABLE 4). The right bundle branch was tiny in 2 of the hearts showing this pattern in the sudden death group and in 1 from the control group, while the left bundle branch had a narrow origin in 1 other heart in the latter group. The branching bundle was located slightly to the right of the septal crest in 1 heart in the control group; the left bundle branch had a slender origin in this heart. In the entire

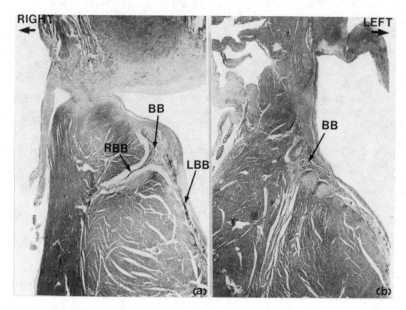

FIGURE 7. Histological sections showing the left sided position of the branching bundle in a heart from the control group (**a**) and a heart from the sudden infant death group (**b**). Note the hypoplastic right bundle branch in (**a**). BB = branching bundle; LBB = left bundle branch; RBB = right bundle branch. Magnification: 20×, reproduced at 75%.

combined series of hearts examined, there were also a total of 6 others, with the branch point astride the septal crest, in which narrow origins of the left bundle branch were seen.

The morphology of the bundle branches is highly variable. While, to our knowledge, abnormalities in this region of the conduction system have not been implicated in sudden death in infants, they have been described in older people. Our sections showed a variation in right bundle branch morphology in both groups studied. This branch was tiny in a total of 6 hearts (TABLE 4) and had a platelike origin in 2 hearts. The morphology of the left bundle branch showed greater diversity, which was concentrated in the unexplained (SIDS) death group (TABLE 4). In this group, a loop of left bundle branch

TABLE 4. Structural Analysis of the Bundle Branches in Hearts from SIDS Victims and Controls

Feature	SIDS[a]		Controls[b]	
	n	% of Total	n	% of Total
Branching bundle to left Left Bundle Branch	4	13	4	21
Loop	2	7	0	0
Accessory branch	6	20	3	16
Fibrosis	1	3	0	0
Slender origin	2	7	5	26
Hypoplastic right bundle branch	3	10	3	16

[a]A total of 30 hearts.
[b]A total of 19 hearts.

tissue (FIG. 8) was found in 2 hearts (TABLE 4). Another 2 hearts from this group had narrow origins of the bundle branch, while 1 other had its origin nearly interrupted by fibrous tissue (TABLE 4). It was interesting to observe an intramyocardial strand (accessory branch) arising from the proximal portion of the left bundle in 6 hearts in the sudden death group (TABLE 4). In 1 of these the strand was closely related to the septal crest.

Petechial Hemorrhages

Ferris[34] reported petechial hemorrhages in the region of the sinus node and internodal tissue tracts in 11 of 50 hearts studied. He attached much significance to these hemorrhages in the mechanism of sudden death. It should be noted that Ferris's study had

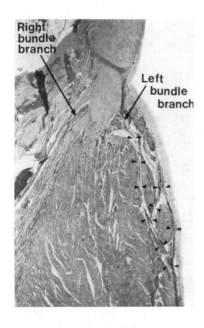

FIGURE 8. Histological section showing the strands of left bundle branch tissue which form intramyocardial loops (*arrowheads*) in a heart from the sudden infant death group. Magnification: 25×, reproduced at 75%.

no designated controls and the diagnosis of sudden death in infancy in his cohort was made on gross necropsy appearances only. Other workers, including ourselves, were unable to verify Ferris' findings, since petechial hemorrhages were found with equal frequency in both control and sudden infant death groups.[18,19] These hemorrhages may well be the outcome rather than the cause of a terminal event.

Accessory Pathways for Atrioventricular Conduction

Apart from the previously described nodo-ventricular and fasciculo-ventricular connections, other accessory pathways can short-circuit the atrioventricular junctional area and produce pre-excitation.[35] Particularly well correlated with sudden cardiac death are those accessory pathways producing the classical Wolff-Parkinson-White syndrome.

These are the accessory atrioventricular connections, which can exist at any point around the atrioventricular junction. It is plausible that the presence of these fibers could result in atrial fibrillation culminating in sudden death in some infants. The current state of knowledge on pre-excitation of the Wolff-Parkinson-White type in infancy indicates the rhythm problems to be due mostly to left-sided connections. The arrhythmia tends to have a relatively benign course, resolving spontaneously with increasing age.[36,37] Accessory pathways were found in 2 of 7 hearts from infants whose deaths were diagnosed as sudden infant death syndrome.[38] In our previous study of 15 children who died suddenly, there was 1 heart with an accessory connection. One heart from the sudden infant death group in our current study had a potential accessory connection in the posterior septal junctional area, where a gap in the atrioventricular groove tissue gave the possibility of an atrioventricular connection. In the absence of previous documentation of arrhythmia in these children, however, the link between a functioning re-entry circuit and sudden death cannot be established.

CONCLUSIONS

The conduction system of the heart is one of the major conundrums in the investigation into sudden death, be it in the adult or infant. Headlines such as "Cot Deaths—Why Not the Heart?"[15] and "Are Some Crib Deaths Sudden Cardiac Deaths?"[39] are both eyecatching and provocative. Indeed, we muse, why the heart?—or, more specifically, the cardiac conduction system. The logic behind incriminating the conduction system is entirely dependent upon the idea that sudden death is the result of a lethal arrhythmic episode which is an expression of an abnormality in the conduction system. Investigations following this trend of thought should ideally be conducted in such a way that anatomico-electrophysiological material is available for examination in tandem. In reality, joint studies are rarely possible. Most studies into sudden infant death in this respect are, of necessity, based entirely on postmortem material. The conclusions expressed are then distilled through the alembic of the investigators' minds. Our own studies have shown a very wide range of morphological findings within the groups of hearts studied from infants dying of known causes or of SIDS. When the sudden infant death group is compared with the explained death group, similar findings are seen in both (TABLES 1–4). We cannot prove any of the manifold published concepts. A tangible relationship between anatomical lesions of the conduction system and sudden, unexpected death in infancy therefore remains elusive. Any connection between the two is speculative and, at best, circumstantial. Further extensive studies, not only of hearts from infants dying suddenly but also from those with known causes of death, are still required in order to establish the range of abnormalities that can be found in the "normal" heart. These studies may then set the scene for proving or disproving the involvement of the conduction system in sudden infant death.

REFERENCES

1. KNOWELDEN, J., J. KEELING & J. P. NICHOLL. 1984. Post Neonatal Mortality: A Multicentre Study. Her Majesty's Stationary Office. London.
2. SMITH, A., S. Y. HO & R. H. ANDERSON. 1977. Histologic study of the cardiac conducting system as a routine procedure. Med. Lab. Sci. **34:** 223–229.
3. JAMES, T. N. 1963. The connecting pathways between the sinus node and the A-V node and between the right and left atrium in the human heart. Am. Heart J. **66:** 498.

4. ANDERSON, R. H., S. Y. HO, A. SMITH & A. E. BECKER. 1981. The internodal atrial myocardium. Anat. Rec. **201:** 75–82.
5. BUSQUET, J., F. FONTAN, R. H. ANDERSON, S. Y. HO & M. J. DAVIES. 1984. The surgical significance of the atrial branches of the coronary arteries. Int. J. Cardiol. **6:** 223–234.
6. ANDERSON, K. R., S. Y. HO & R. H. ANDERSON. 1979. The location and vascular supply of the sinus node in the human heart. Br. Heart J. **41:** 28–32.
7. SCHERF, D. & J. COHEN. 1964. The Atrioventricular Node and Selected Cardiac Arrhythmias. Grune & Stratton. New York.
8. ANDERSON, R. H., A. E. BECKER, C. BRECHENMACHER, M. J. DAVIES & L. ROSSI. 1975. The human atrioventricular junctional area. A morphological study of the AV node and bundle. Eur. J. Cardiol. **3:** 11–25.
9. ANDERSON, R. H., M. J. DAVIES & A. E. BECKER. 1974. Atrioventricular ring specialized tissue in the normal heart. Eur. J. Cardiol. **2:** 219–230.
10. MASSING, G. K. & T. N. JAMES. 1976. Anatomical configuration of the His bundle and bundle branches in the human heart. Circulation **53:** 609–621.
11. KUROSAWA, H., A. E. BECKER. 1985. Dead-end tract of the conduction axis. Int. J. Cardiol. **7:** 13–18.
12. JAMES, T. N. 1968. Sudden death in babies. New observations in the heart. Am. J. Cardiol. **22:** 479–506.
13. GREEN, J. R., M. H. KOROVETZ, D. R. SHANKLIN, J. J. DEVITO & W. J. TAYLOR. 1969. Sudden unexpected death in three generations. Arch. Intern. Med. **124:** 359–363.
14. JAMES, T. N. & M. L. MARSHALL. 1976. Persistent foetal dispersion of the atrioventricular node and His bundle within the central fibrous body. Circulation **53:** 1026–1034.
15. FERRIS, J. A. J. 1972. Cot deaths—why not the heart? Med. Sci. Law **12:** 173–177.
16. KENDEEL, S. R. & J. A. J. FERRIS. 1975. Fibrosis of the conducting tissue in infancy. J. Pathol. **117:** 123–131.
17. ANDERSON, W. R., J. F. EDLAND & E. A SCHENK. 1970. Conduction system changes in the sudden infant death syndrome. Am. J. Pathol. **59:** 35a.
18. ANDERSON, R. H., J. BOULTON, C. BURROW & A. SMITH. 1974. Sudden death in infancy, a study of the cardiac specialized tissue. Br. Med. J. **2:** 135–139.
19. LIE, J. T., H. S. ROSENBERG & E. E. ERICKSON. 1976. Histopathology of the conduction system in the sudden infant death syndrome. Circulation **53:** 3–8.
20. VALDES-DAPENA, M. A., M. GREEN, N. BASAVARAND, C. CATHERMAN & R. C. TRUEX. 1973. The myocardial conduction system in sudden death in infancy. New Engl. J. Med. **289:** 1179–1180.
21. ANDERSON, R. H., K. R. ANDERSON, S. Y. HO & A. E. BECKER. 1979. Anatomy of arrhythmias. *In* Paediatric Cardiology, Heart Disease in the Newborn. M. J. Godman & R. M. Marguis, Eds. Vol. 2: 367–386. Churchill Livingstone. Edinburgh.
22. JANSE, M. J., R. H. ANDERSON, F. J. L. VAN CAPELLE & D. DURRER. 1976. A combined electrophysiological and anatomical study of the human fetal heart. Am. Heart J. **91:** 556–562.
23. JAMES, T. N. 1985. Normal variations and pathologic changes in structures of the cardiac conduction system and their functional significance. J. Am. Coll. Cardiol. **5:** 71B–78B.
24. FERRIS, J. A. J. & W. A. AHERNE. 1971. Cartilage in relation to the conducting tissue of the heart in sudden death. Lancet **1:** 64–66.
25. KEITH, A. & M. W. FLACK. 1906. The auriculoventricular bundle of the human heart. Lancet **2:** 359–364.
26. JAMES, T. N. & E. H. DRAKE. 1968. Sudden death in Doberman pinschers. Ann. Intern. Med. **68:** 821–829.
27. JANKUS, A. 1976. The cardiac conduction system in sudden infant death syndrome: A report on three cases. Pathol. **8:** 275–280.
28. JAMES, T. N., B. T. ROBERTSON, A. L. WALDO & C. E BRANCH. 1975. Hereditary stenosis of the His bundle in pug dogs. Circulation **52:** 1152–1160.
29. SOUTHALL, D. P., W. A. ARROWSMITH, J. R. OAKLEY, G. MCENERGY, R. H. ANDERSON & E. A. SHINEBOURNE. 1979. Prolonged QT intervals and cardiac arrhythmias in two neonates: Sudden infant death in one case. Arch. Dis. Child. **54:** 776–779.
30. KOZAKEWICH, H. P. W., B. M. MCMANUS & G. G. VAWTER. 1982. The sinus node in sudden infant death syndrome. Circulation **65:** 1242–1246.

31. ANDERSON, K. R. & R. W. HILL. 1982. Occlusive lesions of cardiac conducting tissue arteries in sudden infant death syndrome. Pediatrics **69:** 50–52.
32. BHARATI, S., E. KRONGAD & M. LEV. 1985. Study of the conduction system in a population of patients with sudden infant death syndrome. Pediatr. Cardiol. **6:**29–40.
33. JAMES, T. N., R. C. SCHLANT & T. K. MARSHALL. 1978. Randomly distributed focal myocardial lesions causing destruction in the His bundle or a narrow-origin left bundle branch. Circulation **57:** 816–823.
34. FERRIS, J. A. J. 1973. Hypoxic changes in conducting tissue of the heart in sudden death in infancy syndrome. Br. Med. J. **2:** 23–25.
35. BECKER, A. E., R. H. ANDERSON, D. DURRER & H. J. J. WELLENS. 1978. The anatomical substrates of Wolff-Parkinson-White syndrome. A clinicopathologic correlation in seven patients. Circulation **57:** 870–879
36. LUBBERS, W. J., T. G. LOSEKOOT, R. H. ANDERSON & H. J. J. WELLENS. 1974. Paroxysmal supraventricular tachycardia in infancy and childhood. Eur. J. Cardiol. **2:** 91–99.
37. SOUTHALL, D. P. 1983. A new look at the normal range of heart rate and rhythm patterns in childhood. *In* Paediatric Cardiology. R. H. Anderson, R. J. Macartney, E. A. Shinebourne & M. Tynan, Eds. Vol. 5:3–21. Churchill Livingstone. Edinburgh.
38. MARINO, T. A. & B. M. KANE. 1985. Cardiac atrioventricular junctional tissues in hearts from infants that died suddenly. J. Am. Coll. Cardiol. **5:** 1178–1184.
39. VALDES-DAPENA, M. 1985. Are some crib deaths sudden cardiac deaths? J. Am. Coll. Cardiol. **5:** 113B–117B.

Problems in the Interpretation of Cardiac Pathology in Reference to SIDS[a]

G. THIENE[b]

Institute of Pathologic Anatomy
University of Padua
Padua, Italy

INTRODUCTION

Unlike cases of sudden death in youths and adults, where an organic substrate accounting for the catastrophic event is usually found at routine postmortem study,[1] sudden infant death syndrome (SIDS) does not present at autopsy significant evidence concerning the cause of death. Thus, most theories advanced to explain SIDS are based on alleged physiological mechanisms (fear-paralysis reflex, imbalance of heart innervation, apnea, anaphylaxis, etc.).[2–5] Traditional procedures of pathological investigation have failed to furnish a contribution that might resolve this puzzle and, indeed, the role of the pathologist consists in formulating the diagnosis of SIDS by merely excluding other causes of death. This frustrating feeling of impotence, however, should not discourage a search for an organic substrate in each case, especially in the study of the heart. In fact, an abrupt event like SIDS is most likely due to a primary or secondary cardiac arrest by acute electrical instability (asystole or ventricular fibrillation). It is for this reason that attention is still addressed to the heart in order to discover concealed physiopathological mechanisms.[6]

I am aware that SIDS usually does not present overt cardiac pathology, but my task here is to treat problems of methodology concerning the postmortem examination, in the absence of antemortem clinical data, of the heart of the infant who dies suddenly.

GROSS ANATOMICAL EXAMINATION

The first recommendation is that a single expert pathologist perform the autopsy, and that all organs, including the brain, be inspected. Before considering a primary cardiac arrest, and thus concentrating attention on the heart, any extracardiac cause of death should be ruled out.

The traditional procedure of measuring heart size and weight should not be omitted, and the figures obtained should be compared with normal values for infants of the appropriate age and length.[7] An increase in heart weight is, of course, the first hint of a

[a]This work was supported by the National Council for Research Target Project, Perinatal Pathology and its Sequelae (Rome, Italy), and by the Veneto Region Research Program, Juvenile Sudden Death (Venice, Italy).
[b]Address for correspondence: Istituto di Anatomia Patologica, Via Gabelli 61, Padova, Italy.

191

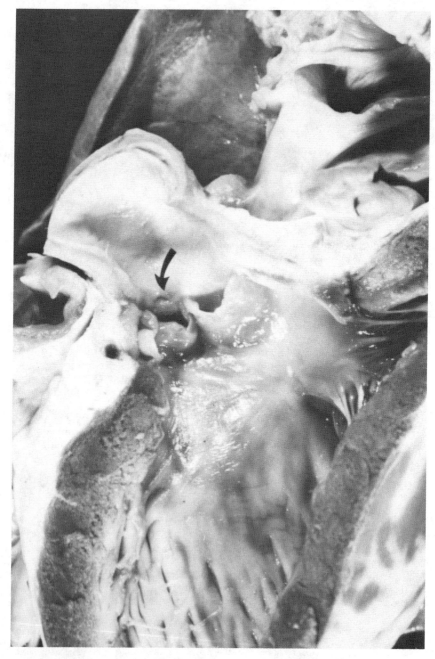

FIGURE 1. Gross view of the aortic root from a 7-month-old infant with dysplastic great arteries who died suddenly. The coronary ostia (*arrow*) are stenotic due to hyperplasia of elastic tunica media of the aorta.

myocardial arrest. After the presence of gross cardiac malformations has been excluded, the origin of the coronary arteries should be carefully inspected. Minor anomalies are a well-recognized cause of sudden death in youth.[8] In infancy, an anomalous origin of the left coronary artery from the pulmonary trunk presents with overt clinical signs. Due to the difficulty in assessing the coronary ostia in the small heart of an infant, minor anomalies may escape notice. Dysplastic great arteries present as hyperplasia of the elastic fibers of the tunica media,[9] which may obstruct the coronary ostia (FIG. 1). Aortic valvelike ridges, located in front of the coronary ostia, may also interfere with coronary perfusion and thus account for ischemia and the possibility of cardiac arrest.[10]

In hypertrophic cardiomyopathy,[11] inspection of the ventricular free walls may disclose a disproportionate thickening, whose precise nature will be better defined upon histological examination. A thin, parchmentlike free wall of the right ventricle is a typical feature of Uhl's disease. Unlike arrhythmogenic right ventricular cardiomyopathy, which is a leading cause of sudden death in youths or adults,[12] Uhl's disease in infants, which presents with signs and symptoms of congestive right ventricular failure,[13] is not associated with cardiac electrical instability at risk for life-threatening arrhythmias.

HISTOLOGICAL EXAMINATION OF THE ORDINARY MYOCARDIUM

Histological examination of atrial and ventricular walls and septa is imperative, even in apparently normal hearts. Hyperacute viral myocarditis may occur in infancy and is only detected by microscopy. Primary hypertrophic cardiomyopathy exhibits histologically the features of myocardial disarray, a disorder which is geometrically prone to electrical impulse re-entry, with consequent onset of malignant arrhythmias.[1] It is noteworthy that myocardial disarray is neither specific for nor pathognomonic of hypertrophic cardiomyopathy and may be observed even in small areas of the myocardium in normal hearts.[14] Moreover, it is the histological substrate of other primary cardiomyopathies, such as restrictive cardiomyopathy, which is characterized by ventricular free wall stiffness with impaired diastolic relaxation.[15] Unlike hypertrophic cardiomyopathy, restrictive cardiomyopathy does not necessarily imply cardiomegaly; heart size and weight may be normal, and only the atrial chambers may appear dilatated, due to impaired ventricular filling.

A heart judged pale and hypertrophic by the naked eye may reveal upon histological examination a storage condition, such as Pompe's disease, which should be considered a secondary form of hypertrophic cardiomyopathy.[16] With conventional staining techniques, the myocytes appear thick and empty because of glycogen storage, and the myocardium shows a "honeycomb" pattern in cross sections or a "bamboo" appearance in longitudinal sections.

Since even minimal endocardial fibroelastosis may account for some otherwise unexplained forms of cardiomegaly,[17] a search for fibroelastosis should be correctly performed by using special stains for elastic tissue (FIG. 2).

Myocardial contraction bands are a frequent observation in cardiac pathology and are currently considered a sign of early myocardial ischemia or hyperadrenergic action.[18] Such necrosis is not a rarity in infant victims of sudden death; whether the lesion in SIDS is primary, thus accounting for malignant arrhythmias and sudden death, or secondary to cardiac arrest is controversial. Reperfusion is a well-recognized mechanism of contraction band necrosis.[19] The lesion might be produced by a prolonged terminal episode or by the reanimation procedures which follow cardiac arrest.

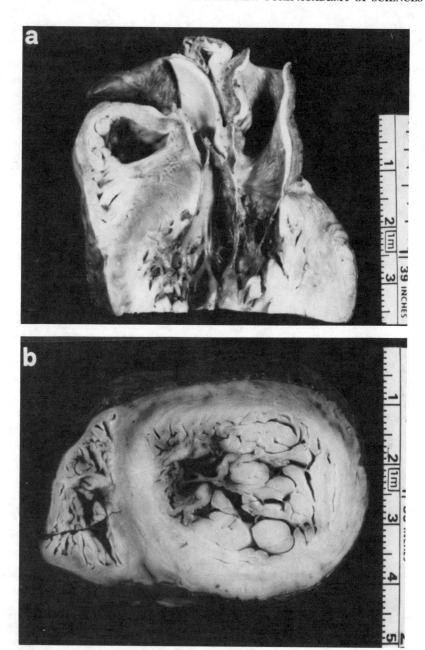

FIGURE 2. Sudden death in a 6-month-old infant with cardiomegaly. Long axis (**a**) and cross section (**b**) views of the heart (*above*) disclose striking hypertrophy. Histological examination (**c**, *facing page*) ruled out myocardial disarray or storage disease and detected endocardial fibroelastosis; Weigert-Von Gieson stain, ×48.

HISTOLOGICAL EXAMINATION OF THE CONDUCTION SYSTEM

The question of the involvement of the conduction system is the most controversial issue of cardiac pathology in SIDS. In fact, the vast majority of SIDS cases do not present any gross or histological abnormality of the ordinary myocardium, and deaths are usually dismissed with the term *mors sine materia* to stress the absence of organic substrates. Thus, an insight into the *core* of the heart, where cardiac rhythm takes origin and spreads, represents the last chance to achieve a solution to the problem. In fact, pacemaker and impulse transmission are intrinsic to the heart and delegated to the specialized myocardium. This does not mean that specialized conduction is totally independent from innervation, but it does play a primary, fundamental role in the electric order (or disorder) of the heart. This role has probably been overrated in the past, and minimal (or simply variants of normal?) alterations have been considered a potential source of life-threatening arrhythmias (FIG. 3). Dispersion of specialized tissue within the central fibrous body, with degenerative and resorptive changes due to postnatal molding,[20] as well as accessory atrioventricular pathways[21,22] have been cited as possible substrates of lethal arrhythmias or conduction disturbances (FIGS. 4 and 5). However, the finding of anatomical substrates for malignant cardiac arrhythmias does not mean that such arrhythmias ever existed. In this regard, conduction system studies in babies with SIDS and in age-matched controls did not discern any significant differences.[23] Moreover, major findings, such as sinus or atrioventricular node agenesis, or lack of conduction axis continuity, have never been described in SIDS cases.

In reference to accessory pathways, the existence of pre-excitation anatomical

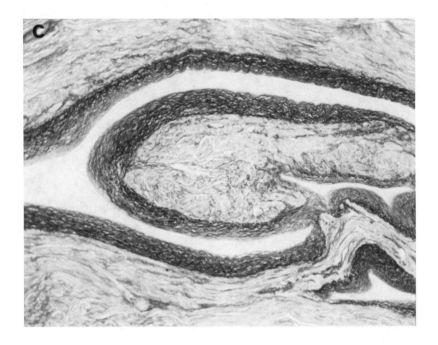

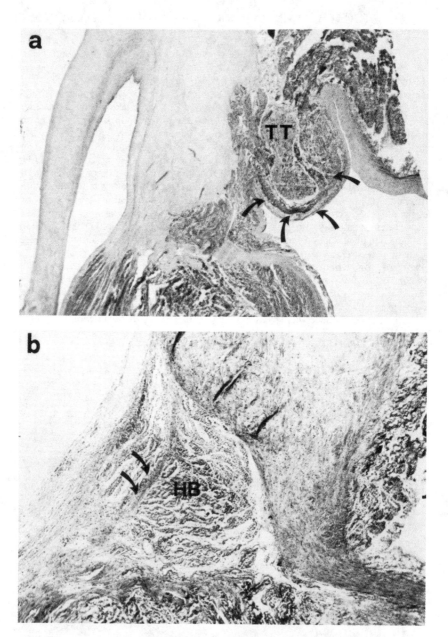

FIGURE 3. Histology of the atrioventricular specialized junction in a case of familial infant sudden death. The atrial ordinary myocardium (**a**), which approaches the atrioventricular node, creates a circuit (*arrows*) around the tendon of Todaro (TT). The His bundle (HB) (**b**) is split into 2 parts by a collagen bundle (*arrows*). Hematoxylin and eosin stain: (**a**), ×15; (**b**), ×48.

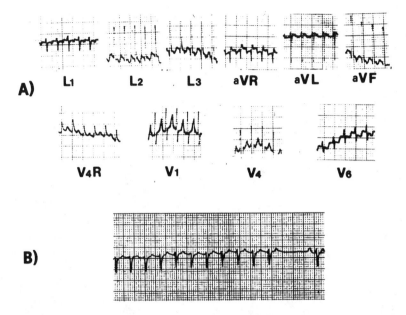

FIGURE 4. Infant sudden death after a prolonged period of supraventricular tachycardia with heart rate of 320 beats/min (**A**). Reversion to sinus rhythm after rate slowed down to 210 beats/min (**B**). The baby died 48 hr later due to irreversible acidosis and anuria.

substrates cannot be excluded without the study of all the lateral rings, an investigation which requires thousands of histologic sections for each heart. At the septum, a minor variety of Ebstein's anomaly with a gap in the central fibrous ring brings about a septal bypass of the atrioventricular node.[24]

In conclusion, three objections may be cited when considering the results of conduction system studies in hearts from infants with SIDS:

(1) There are no clinicopathological correlations because of missing ECG recordings. Thus, a functional significance cannot be attributed to minor conduction system abnormalities in the absence of documentation of malignant arrythmias by ECG.

(2) Control studies to assess whether the alleged lesions are really pathological, or simply variants of normal, have not been consistently performed.

(3) Only sino-atrial and atrioventricular specialized junctions have been examined by serial histological sections. When present, atrioventricular accessory pathways are most frequently localized in the lateral rings, not in the atrioventricular septum.

Therefore, the search continues for a better definition of what is normal or abnormal in the cardiac conduction system of the infant heart.

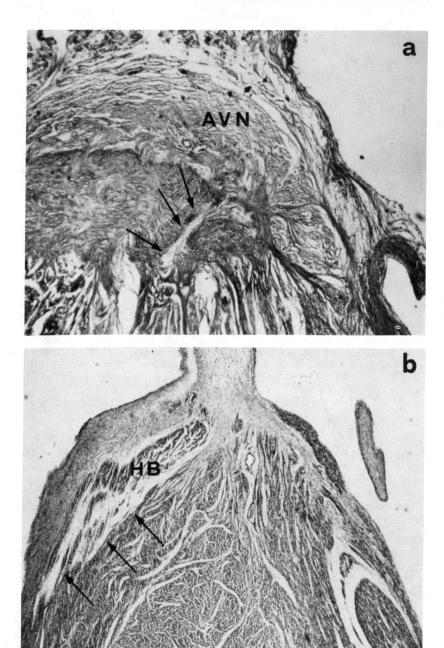

FIGURE 5. Histology of specialized atrioventricular junction from the case described in FIGURE 4: *arrows* indicate nodoventricular (**a**) and fasciculoventricular (**b**) bypass fibers. AVN = atrioventricular node; HB = His bundle. (**a**) Azan stain, ×48; (**b**) hematoxylin and eosin stain, ×19.

REFERENCES

1. ROSSI, L. & G. THIENE. 1983. Arrhythmologic Pathology of Sudden Cardiac Death. Casa Editrice Ambrosiana. Milan.
2. KAADA, B. 1986. Sudden Infant Death Syndrome: The Possible Role of "the Fear Paralysis Reflex." Norwegian University Press. Oslo.
3. SCHWARTZ, P. J., M. MONTEMERLO, M. FACCHINI, et al. 1982. The QT interval throughout the first 6 months of life: A prospective study. Circulation 66: 496.
4. GUNTHEROTH, W. G. 1982. The Sudden Infant Death Syndrome. Futura Publishing Company. New York.
5. GUNTHER, M. 1966. Cot death: Anaphylactic reaction after uterine infection as another potential cause. Lancet 1: 912.
6. JAMES, T. M. 1968. Sudden death in babies: New observation in the heart. Am. J. Cardiol. 22: 479.
7. ROWLATT, U. F., H. J. A. RIMOLDI & M. LEV. 1963. The quantitative anatomy of the normal child's heart. Arch. Pathol. 10: 499.
8. ROBERTS, W. C. 1986. Congenital coronary arterial anomalies unassociated with major anomalies of the heart or great vessels. In Congenital Heart Disease in Adults. W. C. Roberts, Ed. F. A. Davis Company. Philadelphia.
9. DONALD, A. H., L. M. GERLIS & J. SOMMERVILLE. 1969. Familial arteriopathy with associated pulmonary and systemic arterial stenoses. Br. Heart J. 31: 375.
10. VIRMANI, R., P. K. C. CHUM, R. E. GOLDSTEIN, et al. 1984. Acute take-off of the coronary arteries along the aortic wall and congenital coronary ostial valve-like ridges: Association with sudden death. J. Am. Coll. Cardiol. 3: 766.
11. MARON, B. J., W. C. ROBERTS, H. A. McALLISTER, et al. 1980. Sudden death in young athletes. Circulation 62: 218.
12. THIENE, G., A. NAVA, D. CORRADO, et al. 1988. Right ventricular cardiomyopathy and sudden death in young people. New Engl. J. Med. 318: 129.
13. UHL, H. S. 1952. A previously undescribed congenital malformation of the heart: Almost total absence of the myocardium of the right ventricle. Bull. John Hopkins Hosp. 91: 197.
14. BECKER, A. E. & G. CARUSO. 1982. Myocardial disarray. A critical review. Br. Heart J. 47: 527.
15. BOFFA, G. M., O. MILANESI, R. RAZZOLINI, et al. 1983. Cardiomiopatia restrittiva primaria. Rev. Lat. Cardiol. 4: 263.
16. EHLERS, K. H. & M. A. ENGLE. 1963. Glycogen storage disease of the myocardium. Am. Heart J. 65: 145.
17. HARRIS, L. C. & Q. X. NGHIEM. 1972. Cardiomyopathies in infants and children. Prog. Cardiovasc. Dis. 15: 255.
18. ROSSI, L. & L. MATTURRI. 1985. Bande di contrazione nel miocardio infartuale: un problema istopatologico-clinico da rivisitare. G. Ital. Cardiol. 15: 359.
19. SHAPER, W. 1983. Reperfusion of ischemic myocardium: Ultrastructural and histochemical aspects. J. Am. Coll. Cardiol. 1: 1037.
20. BUJA, G. F., D. CORRADO, P. A. PELLEGRINO, et al. 1986. Fatal paroxysmal supraventricular tachycardia in an infant. Chest 89: 145.
21. ANDERSON, R. H., J. BOUTON, C. T. BURROW, et al. 1986. Sudden death in infancy: A study of cardiac specialized tissue. Br. Med. J. 20: 135.
22. MARINO, T. A. & B. A. KANE. 1985. Cardiac atrioventricular junctional tissues in hearts from infants who died suddenly. J. Am. Coll. Cardiol. 5: 1178.
23. KOZAKEWICH, H. P. W., B. M. McMANUS & G. F. VAWTER. 1982. The sinus node in sudden infant death syndrome. Circulation 65: 1242.
24. ROSSI, L. & G. THIENE. 1984. Mild Ebstein's anomaly associated with supraventricular tachycardia and sudden death: Clinico-morphological features in 3 patients. Am. J. Cardiol. 53: 322.

Sympathetic Neural and α-Adrenergic Modulation of Arrhythmias[a]

MICHAEL R. ROSEN,[b] PETER DANILO, Jr.,
RICHARD B. ROBINSON, ANURADHA SHAH, AND
SUSAN F. STEINBERG

*Departments of Pharmacology, Pediatrics and Medicine
and Division of Developmental Pharmacology
Columbia University
College of Physicans and Surgeons
New York, New York
and
Department of Physiology and Biophysics
State University of New York at Stony Brook
Stony Brook, New York*

The sympathetic nervous system is an important contributor to the modulation of cardiac rhythm. In addition, its role in the genesis of cardiac arrhythmias has been demonstrated in experimental models such as digitalis toxicity (e.g., see Refs. 1 and 2) and myocardial ischemia and infarction (e.g., see Refs. 3 and 4). All the arrhythmogenic mechanisms identified to date, including automaticity, triggered activity, and reentry, are modulated importantly by catecholamines, whose role in producing experimental ventricular tachycardia and fibrillation has been well documented (e.g., see Refs. 5 and 6). Studies in human subjects, too, have suggested a role for catecholamines and for abnormalities in sympathetic innervation in the genesis of arrhythmias and/or sudden death (e.g., see Refs. 7 and 8). To be sure, some of this information does less to prove that sympathetic input is the cause of the arrhythmogenic event than it does to show that removal of sympathetic influence reduces the frequency of the event. Hence, the proof is not one that demonstrates invariable cause and effect, but rather, one that demonstrates an important association.

The subject of this volume is the sudden infant death syndrome, and one of the causes of sudden infant death is believed to be lethal arrhythmias (e.g., see Ref. 9). Our research in the past few years has centered on the role of sympathetic innervation in the modulation of the postjunctional effects of autonomic agonists on the heart. In this presentation we will use the α_1-adrenergic receptor system as a model to demonstrate how innervation can control cardiac rhythm and contribute to the occurrence of arrhythmias.

[a]This work was supported by USPHS-NHLBI Grant HL-28958.
[b]To whom correspondence should be addressed at: Department of Pharmacology, College of Physicians and Surgeons, Columbia University, 630 West 168th Street, New York, New York 10032.

THE HYPOTHESIS

The general hypothesis we have been testing is that immature pathways determine receptor-effector coupling in the fetal and neonatal heart, and that the act of sympathetic innervation of the cardiac cell induces changes in either the efficiency of receptor-effector coupling or in the actual effector to which the receptor is coupled. As shall be demonstrated in the review of our studies, below, in considering α_1-adrenergic effects on the heart, this leads to the following: in the immature heart that is not innervated by sympathetic nerves, α_1-adrenergic stimulation induces an increase in automaticity of ventricular specialized conducting fibers, a response that can be viewed as arrhythmogenic. In the adult, α_1-adrenergic stimulation induces a decrease in automaticity in the same type of fibers, a response that can be viewed as antiarrhythmic. Based on the above reasoning, our experiments have required that we use animal models in which we can study the changes that occur in the electrophysiological response to α_1-adrenergic receptor stimulation, as well as the biochemical and ionic links between the receptor and the ultimate physiological response.

THE EXPERIMENTAL MODEL

Our studies are performed using two experimental models of growth and development in early life: the dog and the rat. Canine studies are conducted on isolated Purkinje fiber bundles and ventricles obtained from fetal hearts in the mid- and late trimesters of pregnancy, from neonatal hearts in the first month of life, and from adult hearts. The procedures for performing hysterotomies on pentobarbital-anesthetized pregnant dogs and for obtaining the hearts from anesthetized neonatal and adult dogs have been described by us previously.[10,11]

Neonatal rat hearts are obtained in the first 24 hr of life, are dissociated into single cells, and are plated into tissue culture using previously described techniques.[12] Cultures are made either of pure myocytes or of myocytes in coculture with sympathetic ganglion cells, which subsequently innervate the myocytes.[13] The reason for using the tissue culture model is that it permits a more precise manipulation of the relationship between nerve and muscle than is possible in the intact heart.

Other studies are performed using isolated Purkinje myocytes that have been obtained from the canine heart using enzymatic disaggregation techniques.[14] These myocytes are used for the biophysical analysis of specific ionic currents involved in the response to receptor stimulation. The advantage of this preparation is that the confounding effects of the geometric inhomogeneity of intact cardiac tissues do not occur in the single myocyte.

The methods used by us for microelectrode study of isolated Purkinje fiber bundles,[11] for optoelectrical recording from cells in tissue culture,[15] for voltage clamp analysis of ionic currents,[16] and for biochemical identification of GTP regulatory proteins[17] have been detailed by us previously and will not be repeated here.

RESULTS

Our earliest results that implicated the sympathetic nervous system in the modulation of α_1-adrenergic effects on the heart came from studies performed in the canine heart. We found that adult canine Purkinje fibers responded to the effects of low concentrations of epinephrine or phenylephrine with a decrease in automatic rate,[11] a response that was

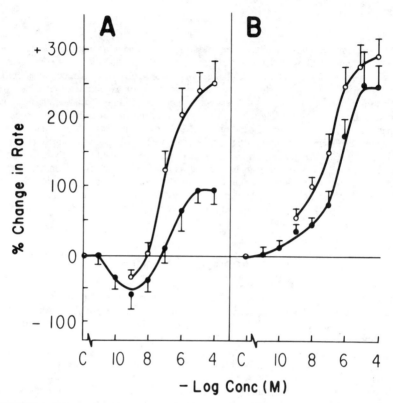

FIGURE 1. Effects of epinephrine on automaticity of neonatal (*white circles*) and adult (*black circles*) canine Purkinje fiber bundles. Control automatic rate did not differ among groups, and is expressed as 0. Rate is expressed as % change from control (mean ± SE). In panel **A** are data from 10 adult and 9 neonatal fibers; in panel **B**, 5 adult and 10 neonatal fibers. Panel **A** shows a biphasic concentration-response curve to epinephrine, with rate decreasing at low concentrations and increasing at high concentrations. In panel **B**, a monophasic curve is seen, with rate increasing at all concentrations. The biphasic response was characteristic of 2/3 of adult preparations and 1/2 of the neonates. (Modified after ref. 11.)

blocked by phentolamine and by prazosin, but not by yohimbine (FIG. 1A).[11,18] Studies by Posner *et al.*[19], using epinephrine, came to the same conclusion and demonstrated as well an increase in K^+ flux across the membrane associated with the decrease in automatic rate. This action of α_1 stimulation to reduce automaticity was not unique to the canine Purkinje system but occurred in isolated human atrium, as well.[20] Moreover, it was not merely a phenomenon observed in isolated cardiac fibers but was also demonstrable in the ventricle of the intact dog.[21]

In contrast to the actions of phenylephrine to reduce automaticity of isolated Purkinje fibers in the adult heart, we found that in early neonates, especially in the first few hours of life, phenylephrine induced an increase in automaticity (FIG. 1B). This effect occurred in over 90% of canine neonates in the first 24 hr of life, and was still seen in 50% of neonates at one month of age.[11,22] In contrast, in the experiments on adult animals referred to above, phenylephrine reduced automaticity in two-thirds to three-fourths of the population. The increase in automaticity in the neonates was blocked by phentolamine, but not by propranolol, and was interpreted as α-adrenergic.[22]

Hence, we were confronted with a developmental change in the response to α_1-adrenergic stimulation, from an increase in automaticity, which might be viewed as potentially arrhythmogenic in the neonate, to a decrease in automaticity in the adult. In interpreting our data, we envisioned a likely association between the transition in the α response and the occurrence of sympathetic innervation. This idea was based on the demonstration of rapidly increasing tissue catecholamine levels in the postnatal period in the neonate, an event consistent with rapidly developing sympathetic innervation.[23]

Given this association, we decided to study the relationship between innervation and the α_1-adrenergic response in a setting that permitted precise control and evaluation of the extent of sympathetic innervation. To do this, we used rat myocytes in pure tissue culture or in coculture with sympathetic neurons. The change in species from dog to rat was justified by the demonstration that intact neonatal rat ventricles uniformly responded to α-adrenergic stimulation with an increase in automaticity, whereas 100% of adult rats showed a decrease in automaticity.[15] The results of the studies of cells in tissue culture are summarized in FIGURE 2. Note that in the absence of innervation, all neonatal rat preparations in tissue culture showed an increase in automaticity; whereas once innervation occurred, automaticity decreased in about two-thirds of the preparations. Moreover, both the increase in automaticity in the noninnervated preparations and the decrease in automaticity in innervated preparations were blocked by prazosin. No effect of atropine, of propranolol, or of adenosine deaminase was demonstrable, thereby ruling out vagal, β-adrenergic, or purinergic effects.[15]

Given the association of sympathetic innervation with the qualitative change in the α_1-adrenergic response, it was natural to question what the intermediate steps were. We had studied developmental changes in the α_1 receptor, per se, in canine ventricle and had noted age-related changes in a low affinity binding site ($K_D = 1.2 \pm 0.43$ nM, adult, and 1.9 ± 0.67 nM, neonate; B_{max} 510 $\pm$ 155 fmol/mg, adult, and 1,710 $\pm$ 440 fmol/mg,

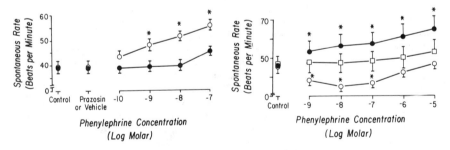

FIGURE 2. Chronotropic response of non-innervated and innervated newborn rat myocardial cultures to the α-adrenergic agonist, phenylephrine. * indicates a significant difference ($p<0.05$) in rate in response to phenylephrine, compared to control. **Left:** Chronotropic response of non-innervated muscle cells in the absence (*white circles*) and presence (*black circles*) of the α_1-antagonist, prazosin (1×10^{-6} M). In the absence of antagonist, all cultures responded to phenylephrine with an increase in spontaneous rate. **Right:** Chronotropic responses of innervated muscle cells. All experiments were conducted in the presence of the cholinergic antagonist, atropine (1×10^{-7} M), and the β-adrenergic antagonist, propranolol (1×10^{-7} M). Cultures were divided into positive- and negative-responding groups by their response to phenylephrine, 1×10^{-8} M. 37% of the cultures exhibited an increase in rate (*black circles*), whereas the remaining 63% exhibited a decrease in rate (*white circles*). In the presence of prazosin (*squares*), none of the innervated cultures exhibited any change in rate in response to phenylephrine. (Modified after ref. 15.)

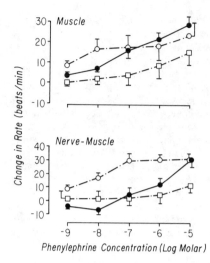

FIGURE 3. Effect of pretreatment with pertussis toxin on the α_1-adrenergic-mediated chronotropic response in non-innervated and innervated newborn rat myocardial cultures. **Upper Panel:** Non-innervated muscle cells. **Lower Panel:** Innervated muscle cells. In both panels, *black circles* represent the control data; *white circles* represent the dose-response relation in cultures pretreated with 0.5 μg/ml pertussis toxin for 16–20 hr; *squares* represent the dose-response relation in the presence of the α_1-selective blocker, prazosin (1×10^{-7} *M*) in pertussis toxin-pretreated cultures. (Modified after ref. 17.)

neonate).[24] However, such a change did not seem to explain the phenomenon we were seeing with respect to automaticity.

An area that showed more promise was the investigation of developmental changes in the GTP regulatory proteins which couple receptors to effector mechanisms. At the time our studies commenced, we were aware of the important role played by such N proteins in the coupling of autonomic receptor-effector systems (e.g., see Ref. 25). With this as background, we commenced to study the possible relationship between a GTP regulatory protein and the α_1-adrenergic response. We initially found that a particular 41-kD regulatory protein which was ADP-ribosylatable by pertussis toxin was present in only small quantities in rat myocytes in tissue culture. However, in the innervated cocultures, the level of this protein detected increased by two- to threefold.[17] The presence of only small amounts of detectable protein in the noninnervated cells (which showed an increase in automaticity in response to phenylephrine) and large amounts of protein in the innervated cultures (which showed a negative chronotropic response to phenylephrine) implied a possible cause-and-effect relationship between this regulatory protein and the type of α-adrenergic response that was seen. What made the association even more likely was the demonstration that functional "removal" of the regulatory protein, by ADP-ribosylating it with pertussis toxin, resulted in conversion of the α-adrenergic response in innervated cocultures from inhibition to excitation of automaticity (FIG. 3).

Having demonstrated this association between a 41-kD pertussis toxin-sensitive protein and the type of α-adrenergic response seen in tissue culture, we believed it necessary to test whether this finding held true in intact tissues, and in the canine heart, as well. We therefore studied the relationship between the regulatory protein, age, and sympathetic innervation in the canine heart. FIGURE 4 shows the pertussis toxin-sensitive substrate levels in ventricular myocardium from a group of fetal and neonatal dogs. Note that prior to delivery the level of detectable pertussis toxin-sensitive substrate is low. Following delivery, the level increases rapidly. Moreover, in studies of tissue norepinephrine levels, we have found that at day 2 postpartum the level is about 100 ng/g tissue. This increases to over 1,400 ng/g by day 4.[23] This result is consistent with rapid development of sympathetic innervation and suggests there may be an association between innervation and the level of detectable pertussis toxin-sensitive substrate.

To test whether this pertussis toxin-sensitive substrate is important to the type of α-adrenergic response seen in the dog, as is the case in the rat myocyte in tissue culture, we performed a series of experiments in which adult canine Purkinje tissues were incubated in pertussis toxin for 24 hr and then superfused with phenylephrine[26] (FIG. 5). We found that all fibers exposed to a concentration of pertussis toxin (0.5 μg/ml) sufficient to completely ADP-ribosylate the protein, and thus render it inactive, demonstrated an increase in automaticity in response to phenylephrine. This response was blocked by prazosin, but not by propranolol. In contrast, we found high levels of functional substrate and a predominantly negative chronotropic response to phenylephrine in adult tissues not exposed to toxin. Using intermediate concentrations of pertussis toxin between 0.1 and 0.5 μg/ml, we demonstrated a smooth concentration-response relationship between the amount of functional regulatory protein and the proportion of fibers showing a decrease in automaticity. Hence in the adult animal, with presumably complete sympathetic innervation, we could demonstrate a close association between the automatic response and the level of detectable protein.

Given that the transducer for the α_1-adrenergic inhibition of automaticity appeared to be a specific pertussis toxin-sensitive substrate, the next question we asked concerned the mechanism responsible for the decrease in automaticity induced by α-adrenergic stimulation. These experiments were done using single-cell voltage clamp of canine Purkinje myocytes.[16] It was found that phenylephrine induced an increase in electrogenic Na^+/K^+ pump current that could be blocked by prazosin. Moreover, in myocytes that had been pretreated with pertussis toxin, this increase in pump current did not occur. Hence, it appeared reasonable to state that, following the maturation of innervation, a particular GTP regulatory protein induced an increase in the Na^+/K^+ pump function of the heart (whether due to a direct or an indirect effect on the Na^+/K^+ pump), thereby accounting for the decrease in automaticity. These experiments showed an additional result, that is, a potassium conductance that is decreased by α_1-adrenergic stimulation, via the linkage of a pertussis toxin-sensitive protein. Such an effect would tend to increase automaticity. Hence, the two effects of α_1-adrenergic stimulation run counter to one another. One would anticipate that, in any innervated tissue, the determinant of whether or not a decrease in automaticity will appear is whether, in that particular preparation, the effect on Na^+/K^+ pumping or on potassium conductance is predominant.

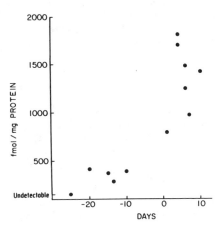

FIGURE 4. Pertussis toxin-sensitive substrate (expressed as fmol/mg crude protein) in fetal and neonatal dogs. "0" is day of birth; values to the left are fetal age; to the right, neonatal age. Each data point is the result obtained from one canine ventricle. Note the marked increase in substrate levels postnatally. See text for discussion.

DISCUSSION

Our results may be summarized as follows: in the more immature state, that is, in the heart that is not sympathetically innervated or is minimally innervated, there is a link between the α_1-adrenergic receptor and an effector that increases automaticity. This entire pathway, which either operates through a GTP regulatory protein that is not pertussis toxin-sensitive, or may not require a regulatory protein at all, remains a mystery to us and is the subject of current, intensive investigation. However, we have learned a fair amount about what happens as sympathetic innervation occurs; that is, a 41-kD pertussis toxin-sensitive substrate is rapidly identifiable in increasing quantities that correlate well with the extent of innervation (reflected by tissue catecholamine levels). Moreover, in the

Fibers showing a positive (+) and negative (−) chronotropic response

	Pertussis Toxin (μg/ml)				
	0	0.1	0.25	0.3	0.5
+	6(37%)	2(33%)	4(57%)	4(67%)	6(100%)
−	10(63%)	4(67%)	3(43%)	2(33%)	0(0%)

FIGURE 5. Results from a group of Purkinje fibers, either untreated (control fibers: **column 0**) or exposed to 0.1–0.5 μg/ml of pertussis toxin for 24 hr, which were superfused with phenylephrine (5×10^{-9} M, then 5×10^{-8} M) and then assayed for pertussis toxin-sensitive substrate. Fibers showing a positive (+) or a negative (−) chronotropic response to phenylephrine are indicated. Of the control fibers, 6 showed an increase in automaticity in response to phenylephrine and 10 a decrease (37% and 63% respectively). The SDS-PAGE patterns (**gray panels;** only region surrounding position of 41 kD band is shown) showed a dense band at 41 kD for fibers having a negative response, consistent with a high level of pertussis toxin substrate. In the positive responders only minimal activity at 41 kD was detectable. Of the 6 fibers that received 0.1 μg/ml of toxin, the proportion showing, respectively, increased or decreased automaticity was identical to that of the controls. At 0.25 μg/ml, 57% of fibers showed increased automaticity and only 43% a decrease. No 41 kD substrate was detectable electrophoretically among the former, and only a faint band among the latter. At 0.3 μg/ml of toxin, the proportion showing increased automaticity had increased to 67%; and at 0.5 μg/ml, 100‘% of fibers showed increased automaticity. At this latter concentration no 41 kD band was detectable on the gel. Gels are not presented for 0.1 and 0.3 μg/ml toxin, but the dose-response relationship between automaticity and the 41 kD protein was a smooth one.

adult, this substrate (labeled N_2 in FIGURE 6) is linked, directly or indirectly, to the Na^+/K^+ pump; and either the same or a different pertussis toxin-sensitive substrate (labeled N_1) is linked to a potassium conductance (presumably a specific ion channel). Where the primary link results in pump stimulation, automaticity will decrease; where the primary link results in a decreased K^+ conductance by the channel, automaticity will increase. It is important to stress that the immature pathway also persists in the adult, in that functional inactivation of the regulatory protein results in a return to the α_1-adrenergic-mediated increase in automaticity characteristic of the neonate.[26]

If we relate these observations to information available on the development of muscarinic and β-adrenergic responsiveness, they permit some speculation on the genesis of arrhythmias in the postnatal period. FIGURE 7 provides a framework for this discussion.

ADULT

$$\alpha_1 \text{ agonist} \longrightarrow \downarrow \text{automaticity}$$

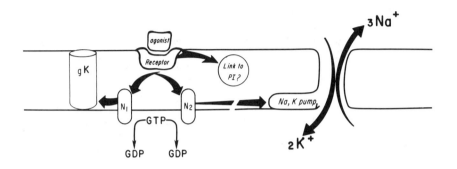

N_I and N_2 = pertussis toxin sensitive substrate

N_I and N_2 = may or may not be identical

FIGURE 6. Schematic summarizing experimental results to date. See text for discussion. gK = potassium conductance, presumably by a specific ion channel. PI = phosphatidylinositol, the inclusion of which suggests that a role for the PI system may be incorporated in the α response.

We have demonstrated, above, that in the neonate α_1-adrenergic stimulation increases automaticity; in the adult automaticity tends to decrease. We previously have shown that α_2-adrenergic stimulation has no effect on automaticity in the adult.[18] However, preliminary studies in our laboratories have shown that automaticity is increased by α_2 stimulation in the neonate. We know from prior studies that β-adrenergic stimulation increases automaticity in the adult (e.g., see Ref. 11). In the newborn, the β-adrenergic-induced increase in automaticity is far greater.[11] Finally, we have shown that, whereas muscarinic stimulation uniformly decreases automaticity in the adult, in the neonate it

DEVELOPMENTAL CHANGES ON THE EFFECTS OF AUTONOMIC AGONISTS ON PURKINJE FIBER AUTOMATICITY

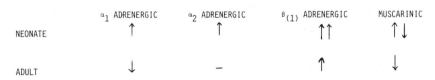

	α_1 ADRENERGIC	α_2 ADRENERGIC	$\beta_{(1)}$ ADRENERGIC	MUSCARINIC
NEONATE	↑	↑	↑↑	↑↓
ADULT	↓	−	↑	↓

FIGURE 7. Summary of the effects of autonomic stimulation on automaticity of neonatal and adult canine Purkinje fibers. See text for discussion.

increases automaticity at higher concentrations.[27] The mechanism for this positive chronotropic response to acetylcholine in the neonate is largely unknown, although in the dog it appears to be muscarinic.[27]

Synthesizing the information in FIGURE 7, it is obvious that, in the absence of significant sympathetic innervation, all four receptor systems can increase automaticity, and only one, the muscarinic, can be counted on to decrease automaticity. In the adult, the α_2 effect no longer occurs, the muscarinic effect is uniformly inhibitory of automaticity, the β-adrenergic effect is less excitatory than in the neonate, and the α_1 effect tends to be inhibitory. Hence, each response changes with development. We believe that the period of developing sympathetic innervation is central to many of the changes described in FIGURE 7. Based on this information, it is reasonable to propose that any event that causes the normal pattern of sympathetic innervation of the heart to deviate can cause imbalances in any one or several of the types of autonomic input described, and, as a result, can favor the occurrence of lethal or nonlethal arrhythmias. Obviously, many steps must be taken before we know the extent to which this supposition accurately reflects reality; nonetheless, such work is underway, and we expect the answers to be forthcoming.

SUMMARY

α_1-Adrenergic stimulation of the neonatal heart may induce either an increase or a decrease in ventricular automaticity, with the latter response predominating as age increases. We used isolated tissues from the hearts of neonatal and adult dogs and rats, as well as rat myocytes in tissue culture alone or in coculture with sympathetic nerves, to study the role of sympathetic innervation in modulating the α-adrenergic response. In the absence of sympathetic innervation, α-adrenergic stimulation uniformly increases automaticity. As the myocyte is innervated, an increased quantity of a GTP regulatory protein is detectable. That this protein is an essential transducer of α-adrenergic inhibition of automaticity is evidenced by the conversion of the α response from excitatory to inhibitory as the protein develops. ADP-ribosylation of the protein with pertussis toxin causes the α response to revert to excitation in both adult canine hearts and innervated myocytes in tissue culture. Hence, we have evidence for sympathetic modulation of cardiac rhythm via a regulatory protein whose function depends on normal neuronal development. Abnormal development of innervation may predispose to arrhythmogenesis via persistence of a primitive response to α stimulation.

REFERENCES

1. ROSEN, M. R. 1981. Interactions of digitalis with the autonomic nervous system and their relationship to cardiac arrhythmias. *In* Disturbances in Neurogenic Control of the Circulation. F. Abboud *et al.*, Eds.:251–263. American Physiological Society. Bethesda, Maryland.
2. GILLIS, R. A. & J. A. QUEST. 1979. The role of the nervous system in the cardiovascular effects of digitalis. Pharmacol. Rev. **31:** 19–97.
3. SHERIDAN, D. J. 1987. Reperfusion-induced arrhythmias: an experimental observation awaiting clinical discovery? *In* Life-Threatening Arrhythmias During Ischemia and Infarction. D. Hearse *et al.*, Eds.:49–62. Raven Press. New York.
4. CORR, P., K. YAMADA & F. WITKOWSKI. 1986. Mechanisms controlling cardiac autonomic function and their relationship to arrhythmogenesis. *In* The Heart and Cardiovascular System. H. Fozzard *et al.*, Eds.:1343–1404. Raven Press. New York.
5. VERRIER, R. L. & S. H. HOHNLOSER. 1987. How is the nervous system implicated in the

genesis of cardiac arrhythmias? *In* Life-Threatening Arrhythmias During Ischemia and Infarction. D. Hearse *et al.*, Eds.:153–168. Raven Press. New York.

6. ROSENFELD, J., M. ROSEN & B. HOFFMAN. 1978. Pharmacologic and behavioral effects on arrhythmias that immediately follow abrupt coronary occlusion: A canine model of sudden coronary death. Am. J. Cardiol. **41:** 1075–1082.

7. CAMPBELL, R. W. F. 1987. Ventricular fibrillation: Facts, fiction, and the future. *In* Life-Threatening Arrhythmias During Ischemia and Infarction. D. Hearse *et al.*, Eds.:1–9. Raven Press. New York.

8. RYDEN, L., R. ARINIEGO, K. ARNMAN, *et al.* 1983. A double blind trial of metoprolol in acute myocardial infarction. Effects on ventricular tachycardia. N. Engl. J. Med. **308:** 614–618.

9. SCHWARTZ, P. J. 1976. Cardiac sympathetic innervation and the sudden infant death syndrome; a possible pathogenetic link. Am. J. Med. **60:** 167–172.

10. DANILO, P., R. REDER, O. BINAH & M. LEGATO. 1984. Fetal canine cardiac Purkinje fibers: Electrophysiology and ultrastructure. Am. J. Physiol. **246:** H250–H260.

11. ROSEN, M. R., A. J. HORDOF, J. P. ILVENTO & P. DANILO, JR. 1977. Effects of adrenergic amines on electrophysiological properties and automaticity of neonatal and adult canine Purkinje fibers: Evidence for alpha- and beta-adrenergic actions. Circ. Res. **40:** 390–400.

12. LAU, Y., R. ROBINSON, M. ROSEN & J. BILEZIKIAN. 1980. Beta-adrenergic receptors in cultured rat cardiac myoblasts and fibroblasts. Circ. Res. **47:** 41–48.

13. ROBINSON, R. B. 1985. Models of cardiac development: Transplants, organ culture, cell dispersion and cell culture. *In* The Developing Heart. M. Legato, Ed.:69–94. Kluwer-Nijhoff. Boston.

14. COHEN, I. S., N. B. DATYNER, G. A. GINTANT, N. K. MULRINE & P. PENNEFATHER. 1987. Properties of an electrogenic sodium-potassium pump in isolated canine Purkinje myocytes. J. Physiol. **383:** 251–267.

15. DRUGGE, E. D., M. R. ROSEN & R. B. ROBINSON. 1985. Neuronal regulation of the development of the cardiac alpha adrenergic chronotropic response. Circ. Res. **57:** 415–423.

16. SHAH, A., I. COHEN & M. ROSEN. Stimulation of cardiac alpha$_1$ receptors increases Na/K pump activity via a pertussis toxin sensitive pathway. Biophys. J. In press.

17. STEINBERG, S. F., E. D. DRUGGE, J. P. BILEZIKIAN & R. B. ROBINSON. 1985. Innervated cardiac myocytes acquire a pertussis toxin-specific regulatory protein functionally linked to the alpha$_1$ receptor. Science **230:** 186–188.

18. ROSEN, M. R., R. M. WEISS & P. DANILO, JR. 1984. Effects of alpha adrenergic agonists and blockers on Purkinje fiber transmembrane potentials and automaticity in the dog. J. Pharmacol. Exp. Ther. **231:** 566–571.

19. POSNER, P., E. FARRAR & C. LAMBERT. 1976. Inhibitory effects of catecholamines in canine cardiac Purkinje fibers. Am. J. Physiol. **231:** 1415–1420.

20. MARY-RABINE, L., A. HORDOF, F. BOWMAN, J. MALM & M. R. ROSEN. 1978. Alpha and beta adrenergic effects on human atrial specialized conducting fibers. Circulation **57:** 84–90.

21. HORDOF, A. J., E. ROSE, P. DANILO, JR. & M. R. ROSEN. 1982. Alpha and beta adrenergic effects of epinephrine on ventricular pacemakers in dogs. Am. J. Physiol. **242:** 677–682.

22. REDER, R. F., P. DANILO, JR. & M. R. ROSEN. 1984. Developmental changes in alpha adrenergic effects on canine Purkinje fiber automaticity. Dev. Pharmacol. Ther. **7:** 94–108.

23. DANILO, P. 1985. Electrophysiology of the fetal and neonatal heart. *In* The Developing Heart. M. Legato, Ed.:21–38. Martinus Nijhoff. Boston.

24. BUCHTHAL, S. D., J. P. BILEZIKIAN & P. DANILO, JR. 1987. Alpha$_1$ adrenergic receptors on the adult, neonatal, and fetal canine heart. Dev. Pharm. Ther. **10:** 90–99.

25. SPIEGEL, A. M. 1987. Signal transduction by guanine nucleotide binding proteins. Mol. Cell. Endocrinol. **49:** 1–16.

26. ROSEN, M. R., S. F. STEINBERG, Y. K. CHOW, J. P. BILEZIKIAN & P. DANILO, JR. 1988. The role of a pertussis toxin-sensitive protein in the modulation of canine Purkinje fiber automaticity. Circ. Res. **62:** 315–323.

27. DANILO, P., JR., M. R. ROSEN & A. J. HORDOF. 1978. Effects of acetylcholine on the ventricular specialized conducting system of neonatal and adult dogs. Circ. Res. **43:** 777–784.

Cardiac Innervation, Neonatal Electrocardiography, and SIDS

A Key for a Novel Preventive Strategy?[a]

PETER J. SCHWARTZ[b] AND ALESSANDRO SEGANTINI

Unità di Studio delle Aritmie
Centro di Fisiologia Clinica e Ipertensione
Istituto Clinica Medica II
Istituto Clinica Pediatrica I
Centro SIDS
Università degli Studi
Milan, Italy

The once-respected theory that diabetes mellitus was a sexually transmitted disease had its own seemingly logical background in the non-infrequent observation that members of a married couple were both affected. It also reflected the lack of knowledge of the actual pathogenetic mechanisms and, especially, the insufficient development of sound epidemiologic concepts coupled with elementary statistics. The latter would have immediately raised the suspicion that, in dealing with a relatively frequent disease, the presence of the same disease in genetically unrelated members of the same household might have been expected on the basis of chance alone. These conceptual and technical limitations, well understandable at the turn of the last century, would seem less justifiable nowadays. Nonetheless, they seem to recur often in the research of another puzzling disease: the Sudden Infant Death Syndrome.

In this paper we will first examine some of the methodological problems that hamper SIDS research, and we will then present and discuss the various aspects and implications of a cardiac mechanism in the genesis of *some* of those unexplained infantile deaths that constitute the Sudden Infant Death Syndrome.[1]

HURDLES AND TRAPS

The uniqueness of SIDS, as a clinical entity, seems to be shared by the SIDS investigators. There is an exceptional diversity of backgrounds among the people involved in SIDS research, who include pathologists, epidemiologists, neonatologists, pediatricians, sleep physiologists, respiratory physiologists, cardiologists, immunologists, psychologists, and so on. This diversity results in something quite damaging for any scientific community, the lack of a common language. As a consequence, all too often, when reading published studies or when listening to oral presentations, the interested audience does not have the expertise necessary to recognize potential weaknesses and to identify

[a]This work was supported in part by CNR: Consiglio Nazionale delle Ricerche Grant no. '82–'87. 01943.56, Progetto finalizzato Medicina Preventiva e Riabilitativa: Patologia Perinatale e sue Sequele.

[b]To whom correspondence and reprint requests should be addressed at Clinica Medica II—Pad. Sacco, Via F. Sforza 35, 20122 Milan, Italy.

wrong conclusions. It is not possible to touch this issue without quoting the incredibly appropriate sentence used so long ago by Peter Froggatt:[2] "The theories of the accredited scientist and of the quack look alike to the eyes of the gullible beholder." In the area of SIDS, we all can easily become the "gullible beholder." For this reason we should all make an extra effort to beware of methodological errors which, although subtle, could nonetheless lead to unwarranted conclusions.

Many of the aspects that make the understanding and the prevention of SIDS such a difficult target for successful research have recently been analyzed.[3] Here, we will specifically examine the implications of the observation that SIDS is a multifactorial disease, the complexities inherent in the definition of infants "at high risk," and the vexed question of the "near-miss" infants.

A Multifactorial Disease

There is a consensus that SIDS is multifactorial, i.e., that different mechanisms and causes are involved, even if they are not all equally important. In other words, while a number of SIDS victims probably die a respiratory or a cardiac death, a probably smaller number die because of any one of a variety of causes such as botulism, accidents of any sort, rapidly lethal infections, and so on. The concept that few mechanisms are operant in the majority of SIDS cases, while a large number of different causes is probably involved in a small percentage of these deaths, is important for the determination of priorities in the areas of research. Furthermore, this concept is critical for the statistical approach used in those studies which aim at determining the significance of a given factor or marker, "marker X," either for the identification of individuals at greater risk or for the acquisition of new insights into the pathogenetic mechanisms.

Let us imagine the most common situation, that of a study aimed at comparing the incidence of marker X in, probably, a large population of normal infants and in, almost certainly, a small population of SIDS victims. *If* SIDS were not multifactorial, but had only one cause, the analysis would be rather straightforward; one would simply compare the mean incidence of marker X in the two populations. In the absence of a statistically significant difference between the mean incidence in the two populations, and provided that a type beta error is excluded, the null hypothesis could not be rejected. It would then be fair to conclude that marker X is not relevant to the occurrence of SIDS and, moreover, that its presence does not modify the probability of a given infant to become a SIDS victim. But, because SIDS *is* multifactorial, this simple method of analysis cannot be applied. The presence, or the excess presence, of marker X would be expected only in that fraction of SIDS cases in which the mechanisms related to marker X are critically involved. In contrast, one would expect its absence, or a "normal" frequency of its distribution, in those cases of SIDS in which the mechanism of death is unrelated to marker X. Therefore, a statistical analysis different from comparison of the means is necessary. If the distribution of marker X in the normal population is known, or if the "control group" is sufficiently large, it becomes possible to calculate in how many of the SIDS victims marker X would have been expected and to compare it with the number in whom it was actually present. This is appropriate if marker X is a discrete variable. If marker X is a continuous variable, it is useful to determine the 90th or 95th percentile of its distribution in the normal population and then to examine how many of the SIDS cases fall into that region, considering that, according to the null hypothesis, only 10% or 5% of the cases, respectively, would be expected to do so.

Later on in this paper we will see some specific examples of this point. It is sufficient here to add that if marker X were of critical importance in 25% of SIDS cases, comparison of the mean incidence of it in the SIDS and non-SIDS populations would almost certainly lead to the conclusion that there was no difference for the two populations and thus *no role at all* for marker X in SIDS: a wrong conclusion that would make more difficult the progressive dissection and understanding of the different mechanisms operant in SIDS.

Infants at "High Risk"

For any disease characterized by a very low incidence, any risk factor examined will yield quite a high number of false positives. In the case of SIDS, with an incidence close to 2 in 1,000, a factor that would increase the risk by even five times would still leave a rate of 99% false positives. This consideration is critically relevant for the many studies performed in so called "high risk" infants, such as siblings of SIDS victims, premature infants, and so on. These groups seem to have an incidence of SIDS below or close to 0.5%[4] which, although double that for normal infants, is relatively low. This implies that, with a 99% or 99.5% rate of false positives, if 1,000 of these infants were studied, only 5 of them would actually become SIDS victims. It follows that conclusions drawn from studies of 30 to 50 such subjects, focusing on the absence of a given variable or marker, are not scientifically sound. While they may effectively persuade an audience, they have only dubious bearing on the SIDS problem. Nonetheless, such studies continue to be published and to muddy the waters of an already difficult area of research.

As analyzed in greater detail elsewhere,[1,5] the several published studies based on negative findings in small populations of infants "at risk" reveal that an alarming degree of confusion surrounds the relative importance of positive and negative findings. The presence of a given factor indicates a potential role for this marker; what remains to be assessed is the degree of correlation with the occurrence of the event under study, e.g., death due to SIDS. The absence of the same marker indicates only that it is not present in the particular population under study, which makes the size of this population absolutely critical. Thus, when the event to be predicted (SIDS death) has a very low incidence even in the subgroup supposedly at high risk, extrapolation to the general population, and particularly to that minute fraction (2/1,000) representing the true SIDS population, becomes difficult. In other words, absence of a given marker would allow ruling out its potential role in SIDS only if the number of SIDS victims in the study were sufficiently high, i.e., several hundred.

The "Near-Miss" Infants

The proposal to broaden the SIDS spectrum to include those living infants who have been resuscitated from what otherwise would have resembled a sudden and unexpected infant death gave origin to the concept of a "near-miss". The reasons, including the less obvious, for including the near-misses in the SIDS group and the pitfalls of this concept have been analyzed in detail elsewhere.[1] The subsequent occurrence of sudden death in some of these infants (1.4% of approximately 800 cases according to a recent review[6] and probably a larger percentage for those infants suffering more than one well-documented episode) has prematurely led to the equation: near-miss equals SIDS.

The infants suffering a near-miss represent a mixed population, only part of which has had a truly unexplained episode of near-death. The label "near-miss" is most of the time applied as the consequence of a judgement made by understandably anxious parents. A careful study[7] recently examined 93 episodes considered to be true alarms by the parents of 20 high risk infants who were under continuous monitoring. All the electrocardiographic tracings recorded during these episodes were normal, indicating that not even apnea of significant duration (which would reduce heart rate) had occurred. Krongrad and

O'Neill[7] conclude: "Our data raise questions regarding parental clinical ability to correctly perceive a true near miss episode in most cases and may explain, in part, the lack of consistency noted in previously published physiologic studies of 'high risk' populations." The mixed origin of the near-miss infants and the presence of spurious cases greatly reduce, by dilution, the chances of pinpointing any relevant alteration present in probably the minority of true cases. As a matter of fact, the studies on near misses represent an easy way to attempt dismissal of the potential role of most biologic markers because, for the reasons just discussed, they are almost bound to end with negative conclusions.

As pointed out years ago,[8] a respiratory death is relatively slow and allows a few minutes to observe apnea, cyanosis, and some sort of struggle or movements. This is in contrast with a cardiac death by ventricular fibrillation, which is instantaneous, peaceful, and silent. It is far more likely that a mother will observe her child dying a respiratory than a cardiac death. This will give her a chance to intervene and to save the infant, thus creating a new "near-miss". It follows that infants suffering a near-miss would more likely be afflicted with a respiratory than a cardiac disorder, and it is not surprising that most studies of near-miss infants reveal some respiratory abnormality. As a matter of fact, with the acceptance of the near-miss as an integral part of SIDS, apnea became the focus of research. The near-miss infants may provide some information highly relevant to the role of respiratory abnormalities in the genesis of SIDS, but they may also constitute a source of quite misleading information if data are uncritically extrapolated to the entire SIDS problem.

The relationship between near-misses, apnea, and SIDS is beyond the scope of this paper. However, it seems fair to keep in mind the existence of very controversial reports and interpretations. For instance, the common knowledge that apneic episodes are or have been frequent among near-miss infants has to be contrasted with the impressive finding of only a 5% incidence of documented apneic episodes among more than 800 victims of certified SIDS.[9]

A CARDIAC MECHANISM FOR SIDS

The historic background of the cardiac theory has been repeatedly reviewed and analyzed (for details and original sources see ref. 1–3, 10–12). This is true also for the possible role of cardiac conduction disorders.[3,13] Here the focus will be kept on that specific aspect of the cardiac theory which has generated more interest and controversy during the past decade: the relationship between SIDS and the autonomic nervous system and, particularly, the relationship between SIDS and cardiac sympathetic innervation.[12]

The Hypothesis of Sympathetic Imbalance

In 1976 it was proposed that *in some cases of SIDS* developmental abnormalities in cardiac sympathetic innervation may favor the onset of lethal arrhythmias and also may become manifest before any symptom, thus allowing early identification of *some* of the infants at risk.[12] These concepts were based in part on the understanding of the pathogenetic mechanism of the idiopathic long Q-T syndrome, probably the most intriguing example of neurally mediated non-coronary sudden death occurring in apparently healthy young individuals with a negative postmortem examination.[14,15] It is relevant to add that the understanding of the pathogenetic mechanisms of the long Q-T syndrome has led to appropriate and specific therapeutic interventions which have resulted in a dramatic fall in the 10-year mortality rate of the affected patients from 70% to approximately 3%.[15]

Based on the firm background of the critical role of sympathetic hyperactivity in the genesis of sudden cardiac death,[16-19] the proposal was made[12] that *some* SIDS deaths might result from ventricular fibrillation induced by a sudden increase in sympathetic activity in a heart with reduced electrical stability. The specific mechanism proposed was an imbalance between right and left cardiac sympathetic nerves, resulting in a left-sided dominance. This type of imbalance is quite arrhythmogenic,[20] facilitates ventricular fibrillation, and often manifests itself by a prolongation of the Q-T interval, which is associated with a particularly high risk for sudden death under a variety of circumstances[21,22] and is viewed as a marker of cardiac electrical instability.

How can such an imbalance occur in infants? It is of course possible that some SIDS victims may simply represent instances of the idiopathic long Q-T syndrome. This is unlikely to account for more than a few cases; nonetheless, it has been almost only in this restricted way that this hypothesis (often referred to as "the Q-T hypothesis") has been discussed in the literature. As originally proposed,[12] there are two other possible mechanisms (below) which are more interesting.

The distribution of right and left cardiac sympathetic nerves is likely to be symmetrical and homogeneous in most infants; however, this distribution will follow the Gaussian or normal curve, as do most biologic phenomena. This implies that a few infants will have to be at the extremes of the curve. Those with the lowest right cardiac sympathetic activity would be the infants at the greatest risk for life-threatening arrhythmias and sudden death. They would be likely to show a constant or paroxysmal prolongation of the Q-T interval.

The sympathetic innervation of the heart develops at different rates in different species and, in man, seems to become functionally complete by approximately the sixth month of life.[23] The right and left sympathetic neural pathways may occasionally develop at different rates, according again to the normal distribution; a delay in the right side or an acceleration in the left may lead to a temporary imbalance of the harmful type described above. A sudden increase in sympathetic activity, elicited by whatever cause (REM sleep, exposure to cold, a sudden noise, apnea leading to a chemoreceptive reflex, and so on) may trigger ventricular tachyarrhythmias in these unstable hearts and precipitate sudden death. The possibility of a *time-limited* imbalance in the cardiac sympathetic innervation implies that these infants would be at high risk for SIDS, but only for a limited period of time. Therefore, if they survive the high risk period, they may have a completely normal life.

If the sympathetic imbalance hypothesis is correct, its markers (Q-T prolongation, heart rate abnormalities) may allow the early identification of some future SIDS victims. The practical implications are self-evident. Since these infants would be at risk of dying because of a sympathetic burst, effective protection could be conferred by administration of a β-adrenergic blocking agent for an 8-to-9-month period.

The sympathetic imbalance hypothesis represents one, specific aspect of a wider concept which invokes a critical role, *in a fraction of the cases of SIDS,* for developmental abnormalities in cardiac innervation that would reduce the electrical stability of the heart and thus predispose some infants to ventricular fibrillation. For example, an insufficient or delayed development of the vagal efferent activity, with the resultant lack of its protective effects,[24,25] accentuates the arrhythmogenic potential of increases in sympathetic activity. The markers of this sympathetic-parasympathetic imbalance would be a higher-than-normal heart rate, reduced heart rate variability, or an impaired baroreflex sensitivity.[24,26] It is worth noting that there is recent and growing evidence pointing to an important relationship between these markers and sudden cardiac death.[26-28]

The value of a scientific hypothesis is that it stimulates research in new directions to allow its confirmation or rejection. As indicated more than 10 years ago,[12] the only way to test the sympathetic imbalance hypothesis is through a large prospective study conducted in an unselected population of infants, with the objective of analyzing the Q-T interval and heart rate during the neonatal period and then following all of these infants for the possible occurrence of SIDS. It should be evident from the initial statistical considerations, and remembering the multifactorial origin of SIDS, that these electrocardiographic abnormalities should be expected only in that unknown fraction of SIDS which is dependent on a cardiac mechanism; they would of course be absent in those infants who encounter SIDS through different mechanisms.

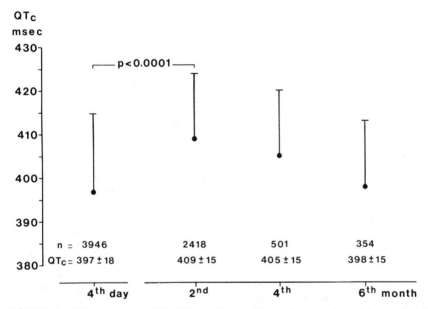

FIGURE 1. Q-T interval in healthy infants. Electrocardiograms were obtained in unselected newborns on the fourth day of life and at the second, fourth, and sixth month of life. QT_c, the Q-T interval corrected for heart rate.

The Milan Prospective Study and the Q-T Controversy

Beginning in the fall of 1975, electrocardiograms were obtained in unselected newborns on the fourth day of life. For a few years, the ECG recordings were repeated at the second, fourth, and sixth month of life. As of May 1987, 14,500 infants have been enrolled and the one-year survival data are available for 10,000 infants. There have been 9 SIDS victims and 6 non-SIDS deaths. Two significant findings have already emerged.

The Q-T interval corrected for heart rate (QT_c) increased from 397 ± 18 msec on the 4th day of life to 409 ± 15 msec ($p<0.0001$) at the second month; it then declined progressively with time, so that by the sixth month it had returned to the same level recorded at birth,[29] as shown in FIGURE 1. While all 6 non-SIDS victims had a QT_c well within the normal limits, 6 of the 9 SIDS victims had a markedly prolonged QT_c (i.e., exceeding the mean by over 2 standard deviations). Four of the SIDS victims actually had a QT_c exceeding the mean by more than 3 SD.[30,31]

What are the legitimate interpretations that can be made from this ongoing study? The difference in QT_c between the fourth day and the second month of life is important, not because of its absolute value, but because it indicates a trend within which a number of individuals (3.6%) have marked QT_c prolongations (changes > 40 msec). This finding is supported by the experimental observation that in puppies there is a sympathetic imbalance with left side predominance at the third week of life,[32] a condition likely to lead to a variable degree of Q-T interval prolongation. The Milan prospective study demonstrated conclusively that the Q-T interval lengthens physiologically and temporarily during the first few months of life. Thus, there is a tendency, which in some infants may become excessive, toward a reduction in cardiac electrical stability during the same time period as the peak incidence of SIDS.

Great care has to be exercised in extrapolating from data on a small number of SIDS victims. However, it would be equally unwise to dismiss the reality of the findings collected *prospectively* in 9 infants who became SIDS victims. The most logical approach suggests taking advantage of another, somewhat similar, large prospective study which, despite some methodologic differences, contributes importantly to the assessment of the relationship between neonatal electrocardiography and SIDS. Southall et al.[33] studied 7,254 infants, 15 of whom subsequently died of SIDS. When comparing data obtained by different investigators in different populations and with different instrumentation, it is wise to avoid the use of absolute measurements and values and instead to rely on the use of the 90th or 95th percentile to define the incidence of the trait (marker X) in the "test" population compared to the 10% or 5%, respectively, which would be expected if there was no difference from the "control" population. Although Southall et al.[33] concluded that there was no difference between the SIDS victims and the control infants, 6 of their 15 SIDS victims had a QT_c greater than the 90th percentile (an incidence 4 times higher than expected and with a risk for SIDS 6 times greater than that of infants with a QT_c below the 90th percentile). FIGURE 2 shows the combined data from these two prospective studies and indicates clearly that, despite differences between the two sets of results, out of 24 subsequent SIDS victims 12 (50%) had a QT_c exceeding the 90th percentile of the normal distribution in the specific populations under study. While more data on SIDS victims are certainly needed, these combined results suggest that, even with a very conservative estimate, probably not less than 25% of the infants who subsequently become SIDS victims can reasonably be expected to have, on the third or fourth day of life, a prolonged Q-T interval.

Given the number of infants with a markedly prolonged QT_c (30/1,000 exceeding the mean by 2 SD and 11/1,000 by 3 SD), our data suggest that the risk of SIDS for these infants would be approximately 22 and 39 times, respectively, that of the normal population. If these findings are confirmed, this would become for SIDS the single most important risk factor identifiable during the first week of life.

A multicenter study has very recently been funded in Italy with the goal of enlarging the data base of the Milan prospective study. By 1990 approximately 50,000 infants will have been studied, and the examination of the electrocardiograms of the SIDS victims should provide a definitive answer on the prognostic significance of QT prolongation during the first week of life.

The sympathetic imbalance hypothesis has rapidly generated an unresolved controversy, which has been repeatedly analyzed in detail.[1,3,5] Here, we will limit ourselves to calling attention once more to methodological traps, as outlined in the first part of this paper. It is indeed somewhat discouraging to observe the relentless sequence of identical oversights by different investigators. In essence, a negative finding (in this specific case, the absence of Q-T interval prolongation) in a population, *not of SIDS victims,* but of "at risk" infants with an average risk of only 1% or even 5% (i.e., 99% to 95% false positives) is of no value whatsoever in assessing any hypothesis.

The small, but definite and so far unavoidable, degree of subjectivity in the measurement of the Q-T interval raises the question of bias in both directions and undeniably contributes to the controversy. This subjectivity is even more important given the fact that clinically important Q-T prolongations may be rather small in absolute values, as exemplified by the many and mostly concordant studies of post-myocardial infarction patients, in whom small Q-T prolongations significantly increase the risk for sudden death.[21]

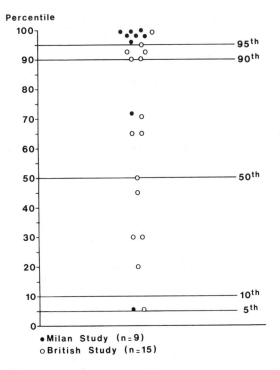

FIGURE 2. Distribution of QT_c among 24 SIDS victims. Combined data from the Milan study (**black circles**) and the British study[33] (**white circles**) are shown.

A very recent study by Valimaki *et al.*[34] seems to contain a potentially exciting finding relevant to the concept of autonomic imbalance in some of the SIDS victims, which was somewhat obscured by the statistical approach chosen for the data analysis. Taking advantage of a clever prospective study designed by Southall, which has provided 24-hr ECG recordings on 29 SIDS victims and on an adequate number of matched control infants, they were able to analyze differences in heart-rate variability (a marker of cardiac vagal efferent activity). They reported that heart-rate variability was reduced in the SIDS victims when compared to the controls, but the difference was not statistically significant. Obtaining no significant difference was the result of comparing the means of the two groups, and it is the obvious consequence to be expected whenever, for instance, some of the "cases" have values at the two opposite extremes of the normal distribution. Their data suggested, however, that there might have been an excess of SIDS victims with a heart-rate variability below the lower limit for normal values as defined by their own control population. This excess might have become evident if they had compared the percentages of SIDS victims and of control infants found to be either in the 90th percentile or below an arbitrary level of heart-rate variability. Should indeed some of the SIDS victims have a lower-than-normal heart-rate variability, a finding already reported to be associated with cardiac deaths (mostly sudden deaths) among post-myocardial infarction patients[35] and pointing to either reduced vagal activity or increased sympathetic activity, there would be important pathophysiological implications for SIDS.

CONCLUSIONS

The present decade is finally witnessing large and controlled prospective studies designed to test specific mechanisms proposed for SIDS.[29,33,36] The respiratory and the cardiac mechanisms are not at all mutually exclusive, as a defect in the control of respiration may trigger a lethal cardiac arrhythmia, given the appropriate substrate (decreased cardiac electrical stability). These two mechanisms seem to be the largest contributors to the whole of SIDS, even if their respective importance still remains to be quantified. It would be logical to concentrate the research efforts on them before extensively investigating other, less likely possibilities.

It is important that the idea of the multifactorial origin of SIDS, with all of its implications, be accepted by the interested investigators. One critical implication is the fact that SIDS will never be completely eliminated, because it will be impossible to deal appropriately with all its potential causes. On the other hand, important and rewarding success may be achieved by progressively removing, after appropriate identification, those factors that produce a substantial number of SIDS deaths.

The concepts and data presented here indicate their indicate that the sympathetic imbalance hypothesis, although not yet proven, has gained plausibility on the basis of current knowledge. The potential for the *early identification of some future SIDS victims* and the likelihood, if the hypothesis is correct, of developing an effective and safe preventive strategy make even more necessary an accurate and unbiased evaluation of the cardiac hypothesis.

REFERENCES

1. SCHWARTZ, P. J. 1981. The sudden infant death syndrome. *In* Reviews in Perinatal Medicine. E. M. Scarpelli & E. V. Cosmi, Eds., Vol. IV: 475–524. Raven Press. NY.
2. FROGGATT, P. 1977. A cardiac cause in cot death: A discarded hypothesis? J. Ir. Med. Assoc. **70:** 408.
3. SCHWARTZ, P. J. 1987. The quest for the mechanisms of the sudden infant death syndrome. Doubts and progress. Circulation **75:** 677–683.
4. PETERSON, D. R., E. E. SABOTTA & J. R. DALING. 1986. Infant mortality among subsequent siblings of infants who died of sudden infant death syndrome. J. Pediatr. **108:** 911.
5. SCHWARTZ, P. J. 1983. Autonomic nervous system, ventricular fibrillation and SIDS. *In* The Sudden Infant Death Syndrome. J. T. Tildon, L. M. Roeder & A. Steinschneider, Eds.: 319–339. Academic Press. NY.
6. SOUTHALL, D. P. 1983. Home monitoring and its role in the sudden infant death syndrome. Pediatrics **72:** 133.
7. KRONGRAD, E. & L. O'NEILL. 1986. Near miss sudden infant death syndrome episodes? A clinical and electrocardiographic correlation. Pediatrics **77:** 811.
8. SCHWARTZ, P. J. 1976. Near-miss sudden infant death. Lancet **2:** 853.

9. VALDES-DAPENA, M. 1985. Are some crib deaths sudden cardiac deaths? J. Am. Coll. Cardiol. **5:** 113B.
10. JAMES, T. N. 1986. Sudden death in babies: New observations in the heart. Am. J. Cardiol. **22:** 479.
11. FROGGATT, P. & T. N. JAMES. 1973. Sudden unexpected death in infants: Evidence of a lethal cardiac arrhythmia. Ulster Med. J. **42:** 136.
12. SCHWARTZ, P. J. 1976. Cardiac sympathetic innervation and the sudden infant death syndrome. A possible pathogenetic link. Am. J. Med. **60:** 167.
13. ROSSI, L. 1984. Anatomopathology of the normal and abnormal A-V conduction system. PACE **7:** 1101–1107.
14. SCHWARTZ, P. J., M. PERITI & A. MALLIANI. 1975. The long QT syndrome. Am. Heart J. **89:** 378.
15. SCHWARTZ, P. J. 1985. The idiopathic long QT syndrome: Progress and questions. Am. Heart J. **129:** 399.
16. SCHWARTZ, P. J. & H. L. STONE. 1982. The role of the autonomic nervous system in sudden coronary death. Ann. N. Y. Acad. Sci. **382:** 162.
17. CORR, P. B., K. A. YAMADA & F. X. WITKOWSKI. 1986. Mechanisms controlling cardiac autonomic function and their relation to arrhythmogenesis *In* The Heart and the Cardiovascular System. H. A. Fozzard, E. Haber, R. B. Jennings & A. M. Katz, Eds.: 1343–1401. Raven Press. New York.
18. SCHWARTZ, P. J. & E. VANOLI. 1981. Cardiac arrhythmias elicited by interaction between acute myocardial ischemia and sympathetic hyperactivity: A new experimental model for the study of antiarrhythmic drugs. J. Cardiovasc. Pharmacol. **3:** 1251–1259.
19. SCHWARTZ, P. J., G. E. BILLMAN & H. L. STONE. 1984. Autonomic mechanisms in ventricular fibrillation induced by myocardial ischemia during exercise in dogs with a healed myocardial infarction. An experimental preparation for sudden cardiac death. Circulation **69:** 780–790.
20. SCHWARTZ, P. J. 1984. Sympathetic imbalance and cardiac arrhythmias. *In* Nervous Control of Cardiovascular Function. W. C. Randall, Ed.: 225–252. Oxford University Press. NY.
21. SCHWARTZ, P. J. & S. WOLF. 1978. QT interval prolongation as predictor of sudden death in patients with myocardial infarction. Circulation **57:** 1074.
22. MOSS, A. J. & P. J. SCHWARTZ. 1982. Delayed repolarization (QT or QTU prolongation) and malignant ventricular arrhythmias. Mod. Concepts Cardiovasc. Med. **51:** 85–90.
23. GOOTMAN, P. M., H. L. COHEN & N. GOOTMAN. 1987. Autonomic nervous system regulation of heart rate in the perinatal period. *In* Pediatric and Fundamental Electrocardiography. J. Liebman, R. Plonsey & Y. Rudy, Eds.: 137–159. Martinus Nijhoff. The Hague.
24. SCHWARTZ, P. J. 1987. Manipulation of the autonomic nervous system in the prevention of sudden cardiac death. *In* Twenty Years of Cardiac Electrophysiology. Where to Go from Here? P. Brugada & H. J. J. Wellens, Eds.: 741. Futura Publishing Co. Mount Kisko, NY.
25. SCHWARTZ, P. J. & M. STRAMBA-BADIALE. 1988. Parasympathetic nervous system and malignant arrhythmias. *In* Neurocardiology. H. E. Kulbertus & M. N. Frank, Eds.: 179. Futura Publishing Co. Mt. Kisko, NY.
26. SCHWARTZ, P. J. & H. L. STONE. 1985. The analysis and modulation of the autonomic reflexes in the prediction and prevention of sudden death. *In* Cardiac Electrophysiology and Arrhythmias. D. P. Zipes & J. Halife, Eds.: 165–176. Grune & Stratton. NY.
27. BILLMAN, G. E., P. J. SCHWARTZ & H. L. STONE. 1982. Baroreceptor reflex control of heart rate: A predictor of sudden cardiac death. Circulation **66:** 874–880.
28. SCHWARTZ, P. J., E. VANOLI, M. STRAMBA-BADIALE, G. M. DE FERRARI, G. E. BILLMAN & R. D. FOREMAN. 1988. Autonomic mechanisms and sudden death. New insights from the analysis of baroreceptor reflexes in conscious dogs with and without a myocardial infarction. Circulation. In press.
29. SCHWARTZ, P. J., M. MONTEMERLO, M. FACCHINI, P. SALICE, D. ROSTI, G. L. POGGIO & R. GIORGETTI. 1982. The QT interval throughout the first six months of life: A prospective study. Circulation **66:** 496.
30. SEGANTINI, A., T. VARISCO, E. MONZA, V. SONGA, M. MONTEMERLO, P. SALICE, G. L. POGGIO, D. ROSTI & P. J. SCHWARTZ. 1986. QT interval and the sudden infant death syndrome: A prospective study. J. Am. Coll. Cardiol. **7:** 118A.

31. SCHWARTZ, P. J., A. SEGANTINI, T. VARISCO, M. MONTEMERLO, D. ROSTI & G. L. POGGIO. Neonatal electrocardiography, autonomic nervous system, and SIDS. Submitted for publication.
32. KRALIOS, F. A. & C. K. MILLAR. 1978. Functional development of cardiac sympathetic nerves in newborn dogs: Evidence for asymmetrical development. Cardiovasc. Res. 12: 547.
33. SOUTHALL, D. P., W. A. ARROWSMITH, V. STEBBENS & J. R. ALEXANDER. 1986. QT interval measurements before sudden infant death syndrome. Arch. Dis. Child. 61: 237.
34. VALIMAKI, I. A. T., T. NIEMINEN, K. J. ANTILA & D. P. SOUTHALL. 1988. Heart-rate variability and SIDS: Examination of heart-rate patterns using an expert system generator. This volume.
35. KLEIGER, R. E., J. P. MILLER, J. T. BIGGER, JR. & A. J. MOSS. 1987. The Multicenter Post-Infarction Research Group: Decreased heart rate variability and its association with increased mortality after acute myocardial infarction. Am. J. Cardiol. 59: 256.
36. HOFFMAN, H. J., K. DAMUS, L. HILLMAN & E. KRONGRAD. 1988. Risk factors for SIDS: Results of the National Institute of Child Health and Human Development SIDS cooperative epidemiological study. This volume.

The Interaction of Chemoreceptors and Baroreceptors with the Central Nervous System

A Critical Role in Early Life[a]

G.G. HADDAD[b,d] AND D.F. DONNELLY[c]

Department of Pediatrics (Pulmonary Division)
Columbia University
College of Physicians and Surgeons
New York, New York 10032

INTRODUCTION

Peripheral chemoreceptor and baroreceptor afferents have been extensively studied in the past 2–3 decades, not only at the sensory level, but also in terms of their interaction with the brainstem and their overall role in regulating cardiovascular and respiratory functions.[1-3] Although most of the studies have been performed in the adult human or animal,[2-14] some have focused on these afferent systems in the fetus and in the newborn postnatally.[15-17] Modest hypoventilation at rest (normoxia) and major diminution of the hypoxic drive have resulted from removal of the carotid bodies or from section of the carotid sinus in the mature subject. Sectioning of the same nerve in the fetus just before birth does not seem to affect the initiation of breathing or its pattern at the time of birth.[18] Additional studies in the newborn have suggested that chemo- and baroreceptor function matures rapidly postnatally (in days), if it is not mature by birth.[19] In the newborn, sectioning of the carotid sinus nerve, for example, induces hypoventilation at rest and a diminished hypoxic drive upon challenge with hypoxic inspired air, much like the response in the adult. Hence, no major differences have been described between the role of the carotid body/sinus in the mature subject and in the newborn. In the past few years, however, data from several laboratories including our own have strongly suggested that this generalization may not be correct.[15-17] These receptors may have a much more critical role to play in the newborn than has previously been appreciated.

It was during an investigation of laryngeal receptors and how hypoxia influences breakthrough breathing subsequent to laryngeal stimulation that we noticed that carotid-denervated piglets have an abnormal breathing pattern with severe apneas. To examine systematically the effect of sinus and/or aortic nerve deafferentation as a function of age postnatally, we undertook examinations of the respiratory and cardiovascular function of young and older piglets after denervation and compared them to controls. We used piglets in this work since they have several advantages over other species. These include: (1) they

[a]This research was supported by NIH Grants HL33783 and HL15736.
[b]Established Investigator of the American Heart Association.
[c]Fellow of the Parker Francis Foundation.
[d]To whom correspondence should be addressed at: Columbia University, College of P. & S., Department of Pediatrics, 630 West 168th Street, New York, NY 10032.

are similar to the newborn human with respect to pre- and postnatal brain development and (2) their body size allows instrumentation for detailed cardiovascular and ventilatory measurements.

MATERIALS AND METHODS

Experiments were performed on 23 piglets. Eighteen were 3–4 days of age ("young") and the other 5 piglets were 1–2 mos of age ("older") at the time of denervation. Eleven young piglets were experimental subjects and the rest served as sham controls. Young animals were bottle-fed by the staff 4–5 times per day until about 4–7 days of age, when piglets started to feed themselves *ad libitum*. The temperature of the housing area was adjusted to the thermoneutral range of piglets at specific ages, i.e., 33–35°C at 3–4 days and 27–29°C at 1–2 mos.

Surgery was performed under halothane/N_2O anesthesia 1–2 days before studies. Denervation was accomplished by section of the carotid sinus nerves, and, in some cases, section of the aortic depressor nerve (ADN). In order to denervate the ADN, the superior laryngeal nerve was first identified and then followed laterally and posteriorly up to the nodose ganglion. The ADN in the piglet takes off from the rest of the vagal fibers just before joining the superior laryngeal nerve. To identify the carotid sinus (CS) nerve, the glossopharyngeal nerve was first identified and followed centrally over the tympanic bulla. The carotid sinus nerve was deafferentated distal to its junction with the glossopharyngeal nerve. This deafferentation was preceded and followed by cyanide injection to check on the completeness of the denervation. In a few animals, we recorded aortic depressor nerve activity to ascertain that it carried baroreceptor afferents. We found that nerve activity was synchronous with heart rate and increased in amplitude with hypertensive agents (e.g., metaraminol). In all piglets studied, we found an ADN only on the left side, but not on the right. Hence, ADN denervation was done only on the left side. Placement of venous and arterial catheters was done at the same time as the denervation.

We examined cardiorespiratory function in these piglets during normoxia and hypoxia. Barometric plethysmography was used to record ventilation and ventilatory pattern.[20] State of consciousness was monitored using EEG and behavioral criteria. ECG and arterial blood pressure were also recorded. During each study, the temperature in the chamber was increased over laboratory temperature in order to have the animal in its thermoneutral range.

RESULTS

Since data from piglets with ADN and CS denervation did not differ from those with CS denervation alone, we have combined the results of these 2 groups, and we refer to these piglets as the denervated group. Data reported here are taken from piglets in a state of quiet wakefulness, with their eyes open or closed but with no twitchings or eye movements. EEG criteria were consistent with a wakeful state or, possibly, drowsiness, but not quiet sleep or REM sleep. Both young and older denervated piglets hypoventilated. Mean Pa_{CO_2} was about 47 mm Hg in the young and 50 mm Hg in the older piglets. Sham controls showed no increase in Pa_{CO_2}. Minute ventilation was diminished in the denervated piglets; this reduction was mostly due to a decrease in respiratory frequency rather than a drop in tidal volume. Both young and older piglets had a diminished hypoxic drive, as shown by their failure to reduce Pa_{CO_2} levels (Fig. 1) when challenged with an inspired fractional concentration of O_2 (FiO_2) of 0.1–0.12. This FiO_2 generally lowered PaO_2 to about 35 Torr.

One striking result was the appearance of prolonged respiratory pauses in the young denervated piglets at rest (normoxia). These were observed repeatedly over the course of a 3–4-hr study, and their duration reached, in some instances, 1–2 min. These prolonged pauses were associated with severe spontaneous desaturation. Blood sampled towards the end of these pauses revealed a PaO_2 of 10–25 Torr. Generally, piglets "aroused" from such pauses briskly and moved about the chamber before quieting down again. To date, we do not have enough data to determine whether such long pauses occurred more in one state of consciousness than another.

Examination of the ventilatory pattern in the older denervated piglets did not show pauses as prolonged as in the young, and the longest pause actually observed was about 15 sec. Although older piglets generally hypoventilated to a similar degree as the young, severe transient hypoventilation did not occur in the older piglets.

Mean heart rate and arterial blood pressure in the denervated piglets were not significantly different from those in sham controls. However, we observed marked oscillations in blood pressure in the young denervated piglets. For example, in some

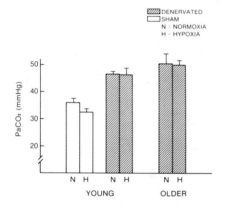

FIGURE 1. Effect of denervation on hypoxic drive in young and older piglets. $PaCO_2$ in the young and older piglets during normoxia (N) and hypoxia (H). Note the higher $PaCO_2$ in the denervated piglets (striped bars) and the lack of their response to hypoxia compared to sham-treated controls (open bars).

piglets systolic pressure dropped to about 50 Torr and increased to more than 150 Torr spontaneously during pauses. Such oscillations were not seen in sham controls.

The most striking and probably most intriguing finding in this study is that the majority of the young piglets (80%) died post-denervation, but none of the young sham or older piglets did. Also remarkable is the consistent time of death of these piglets: all of them died between 4 and 7 days after denervation.

DISCUSSION

There are 2 major findings in this study. First, the response of the young denervated piglet, though similar in direction to that of the older, is more exaggerated. For example, the respiratory pauses we could detect in the young were much more impressive in duration than those of the older piglet. Second, the majority of the young piglets died after denervation while none of the sham or older piglets died. Although the cause of death in these piglets is not yet known, the consistency in the time of death, i.e., 4–7 days post-denervation, indicates to us that the pathophysiology of death in these piglets is probably not heterogeneous and may consist of one chain of events.

There are, however, several possible chains of events that could lead to death post-denervation in the young piglet. First, although we cannot exclude totally the possibility that there was a lack of intake, together with inanition and wasting, over a week's period, we highly doubt that this occurred, since these piglets were seen to feed *ad libitum* and were not grossly dehydrated at the time of death. Second, the repeated apneic attacks we observed led to very low levels of PaO_2 (and consequently to severe lactic acidosis). Attacks such as these could induce, over a relatively short period of time (from minutes to hours), a nonreversible chain of events terminating in cardiorespiratory collapse and death. Another interesting possibility stems from our impression that young piglets do not seem as capable of terminating a respiratory pause as the older piglets. Hence, mechanisms that are responsible for re-initiating breathing may be less operative in the young piglets. One such mechanism is hypoxic arousal. Hypoxic arousal response

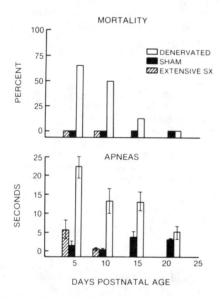

FIGURE 2. Effect of denervation in rats. Percent mortality (%; **upper panel**) and apnea duration (sec.; **lower panel**) plotted against postnatal age (days) for denervated rats (**open bars**), sham-treated controls (**solid bars**), and animals with extensive surgery (SX) (**striped bars**). Note the decreasing mortality rate and duration of apneas with increasing age. (From Hofer.[15] Reprinted with permission from *Life Sciences,* Pergamon Journals.)

can be jeopardized by sleep deprivation, as has previously been reported.[5] We suspect that this may be the case with our young piglets. The gross periodic breathing and prolonged pauses that occurred during rest often led to severe desaturation (as detailed in the RESULTS). This desaturation led to arousal, termination of apnea, and movement of the young piglet about in the chamber before it settled back to a restful position. Such a cycle of rest-apnea-arousal was repeated many times over a study of a few hours. We speculate that this possible sleep deprivation could have increased vulnerability to very prolonged and unterminated apneas. Finally, we cannot exclude the possibility that these piglets died of a cardiac arrhythmia. Such an arrhythmia can arise from heightened sympathetic activity at an age when automatic balance has not been reached.

That young animals die post-denervation is not specific only to this species. In the past few years, data have been gathered on newborn lambs and rats[15-17] (FIG. 2). These studies have shown that denervated rats and lambs not only hypoventilate and have a decrease in the hypoxic drive but also have a high mortality rate as compared to sham controls. We therefore raise the question of whether this is a generalized mammalian phenomenon of early life.

It might be interesting and important to examine our results in the light of data in the literature regarding systems other than respiration. Our current results can be considered from the viewpoint that elimination of a sensory input making its first synapse at the medullary level in the central nervous system causes changes critically detrimental not only to proper functioning of the respiratory neuronal network, but also to survival. Because of the severity of the outcome, we suspect that sublethal or even lethal cellular changes could have taken place in the central nervous system. We do not know yet whether there are such pathological changes in the medulla of denervated piglets. However, pathological changes have certainly been reported in other systems. For example, eye closure in cats and monkeys, with consequent deprivation of visual sensory feedback, can induce marked pathological neuronal changes including rearrangement of synaptic connections, and atrophy or arrest in development of target neurons.[21] Interesting and of relevance to our results is the fact that removal of sensory input may be more critical during development in the young than during adulthood.[22,23]

Another important concept, related to the central integration of afferent information, should be addressed with regard to our findings. Like other neuronal networks in vertebrates or invertebrates, the respiratory network depends on each of the individual components of which it consists.[24,25] The integrative process can be greatly affected if any one of the network's constituents is chemically or structurally altered or ablated. When an important afferent input (carotid chemo- and baroreceptors) to an important integrating area (neurons in the nucleus tractus solitarius, NTS) is eliminated, the integrative process in both the young and the older piglet can certainly be altered. We observed, in both young and older piglets, marked abnormalities in ventilation and the ventilatory pattern. Similarly, the output of the respiratory network can be influenced by alterations in the pattern of maturational changes in the inherent cellular properties of the neurons constituting one or more than one nucleus in the network. We have recently obtained evidence that neurons in the NTS of young rats do not have the "mature" electrophysiological properties of the corresponding neurons in the adult animal.[26] For example, using intracellular techniques, we have shown that neurons in the rat pup NTS have less spike-frequency adaptation to a constant depolarizing current than do adult neurons in the same area.[26] Delayed excitation, a phenomenon that is manifested in the adult as a prolonged delay before the onset of firing following a hyperpolarizing prepulse, is not present in newborn cells. These maturational differences in the repetitive firing patterns may have important implications on the integration of afferent synaptic input and on the shaping of respiratory motor output.

The observations of impaired survival take on added significance in the light of two recent observations on infants dying of the sudden infant death syndrome (SIDS). First, abnormalities in the carotid bodies have been described in SIDS victims.[27,28] For instance, high dopamine (DA) and norepinephrine (NE) levels have been found in carotid bodies of such infants. It is not known if these high levels of catecholamines are due to increased synthesis or decreased release, or if they are primary or secondary, but it is possible that the neurochemical balance in the carotid body is altered in these infants. Although the exact mechanism of sensory transduction is not known, carotid chemoreceptors increase their afferent spiking frequency in response to decreases in PaO_2. Type I cells in the carotid bodies synthesize and store DA and NE, and catecholamines are released during hypoxia.[29,30] When DA is applied in small concentrations to chemoreceptors *in vivo*, spiking discharges are inhibited; antagonists to DA increase resting discharge and sensitivity to hypoxia.[31] In the light of the known effects of catecholamines on the carotid body, it is therefore conceivable that the carotid bodies in these infants have low resting activity or even fail in their response to O_2 deprivation.

The second observation concerns dendritic spine density and SIDS. Recent reports have shown that the brain stem, an area of the central nervous system responsible for integration of vital functions, sleep-waking cycles, arousal, and control of upper airway muscles, has an increase in glial cells and a higher dendritic spine density in SIDS infants compared to controls matched for postconceptional and postnatal age.[32] This increased spine density has been found in several regions of the brain stem, including the nucleus tractus solitarius, the nucleus ambiguus, and the hypoglossus area. Since spine density decreases with age in early life, this higher spine density is suspected to reflect the presence of an immature brain stem in SIDS infants.

REFERENCES

1. COLERIDGE, H. M. & J. C. G. COLERIDGE. 1980. Cardiovascular afferents involved in regulation of peripheral vessels. Annu. Rev. Physiol. **42:** 413–427.
2. EYZAGUIRRE, C. & P. ZAPATA. 1984. Perspectives in carotid body research. J. Appl. Physiol. **57(4):** 931–937.
3. SPYER, K. M. 1981. Neural organization and control of the baroreceptor reflex. Reviews in Physiology and Biochemical Pharmacology. Vol. 88. Springer-Verlag.
4. BISCOE, T. J. & S. R. SAMPSON. 1970. Field potentials evoked in the brain stem of the cat by stimulation of the carotid sinus, glossopharyngeal, aortic and superior laryngeal nerves. J. Physiol. (London) **209:** 341–358.
5. BOWES, G., E. R. TOWNSEND, L. F. KOZAR, S. M. BROMLEY & E. A. PHILLIPSON. 1981. Effect of carotid body denervation on arousal response to hypoxia in sleeping dogs. J. Appl. Physiol. **51:** 40–45.
6. CAVERSON, M. M., J. CIRIELLO & F. R. CALARESU. 1984. Chemoreceptor and baroreceptor inputs to ventrolateral medullary neurons. Am. J. Physiol. **47:** R872–R879.
7. CIRIELLO, J., C. V. ROHLICEK & C. POLOSA. 1983. Aortic baroreceptor reflex pathway: A functional mapping using [^{3}H]2-deoxyglucose autoradiography in the rat. J. Autonom. Nerv. Syst. **8:** 111–128.
8. CRILL, W. E. & D. J. REIS. 1968. Distribution of carotid sinus and depressor nerves in cat brain stem. Am. J. Physiol. **214:** 269–276.
9. DAVIES, R. O. & M. KALIA. 1981. Carotid sinus nerve projections to the brainstem in the cat. Brain Res. Bull. **6:** 531–541.
10. DAVIES, R. O. & M. W. EDWARDS. 1973. Distribution of carotid body chemoreceptor afferents in the medulla of the cat. Brain Res. **64:** 451–454.
11. DAVIES, R. O. & M. W. EDWARDS. 1975. Medullary relay neurons in the carotid body chemoreceptor pathway of cats. Respir. Physiol. **24:** 69–79.
12. DONNELLY, D. F., E. J. SMITH & R. E. DUTTON. 1981. Neural response of carotid chemoreceptors following dopamine blockade. J. Appl. Physiol. **50:** 172–177.
13. DONOGHUE, S., D. JORDAN & K. M. SPYER. 1983. The use of antidromic activation to trace afferent projections in cat and rabbit. J. Physiol. (London) **346:** 8P.
14. DONOGHUE, S., R. B. FELDER, D. JORDAN & K. M. SPYER. 1984. The central projections of carotid baroreceptors and chemoreceptors in the cat: a neurophysiological study. J. Physiol. (London) **347:** 397–409.
15. HOFER, M. A. 1984. Lethal respiratory disturbance in neonatal rats after arterial chemoreceptor denervation. Life Sci. **34:** 489–496.
16. HOFER, M. A. 1985. Sleep-wake organization in infant rats with episodic respiratory disturbance following sinoaortic denervation. Sleep **8:** 40–48.
17. BUREAU, M. A., J. LAMARCHE, P. FOULON & D. DALLE. 1985. Postnatal maturation of respiration in intact and carotid body-chemodenervated lambs. J. Appl. Physiol. **59:** 869–874.
18. JANSEN, A. H., S. IOFFE, B. J. RUSSEL & V. CHERNICK. 1981. Effect of carotid chemoreceptor denervation on breathing *in utero* and after birth. J. Appl. Physiol **51(3):** 630–633.
19. PURVES, M. J. 1966. The effects of hypoxia in the newborn lamb before and after denervation of the carotid chemoreceptors. J. Physiol. (London) **185:** 60–77.

20. HADDAD, G. G., GANDHI, M. R. & R. B. MELLINS. 1982. Maturation of the ventilatory response to hypoxia in puppies during sleep. J. Appl. Physiol. **52:** 309–314.
21. HUBEL, D. H. 1982. Exploration of the primary visual cortex. Nature (London) **299:** 515–524.
22. WIESEL, T. N. 1982. Postnatal development of the visual cortex and the influence of environment. Nature (London) **299:** 583–591.
23. HUBEL, D. H. & T. N. WIESEL. 1970. The period of susceptibility to the physiological effects of unilateral eye closure in kittens. J. Physiol. (London) **206:** 419–436.
24. GETTING, P. A. Comparative analysis of invertebrate control pattern generators. *In* Neural Control of Rhythmic Movements. A. H. Cohen, S. Rossignal & S. Grillner, Eds. Wiley & Sons. New York. In press.
25. GETTING, P. A. & M. S. DEKIN. 1985. Tritonia swimming. A model system for integration within rhythmic motor systems. *In* Model Neural Networks and Behavior. A. I. Selverston, Ed.: 3–20. Plenum Press. New York.
26. HADDAD, G. G. & P. A. GETTING. 1987. Postnatal maturation of electrophysiologic properties of neurons in the ventral region of the nucleus tractus solitarius in the rat. (abstract). Neurosciences **13:** 1585.
27. PERRIN, D. G., L. E. BECKER, A. MADPALLIMATUM, E. CRUTZ, A. C. BRYAN & M. J. SOLE. 1984. Sudden infant death syndrome: Increased carotid-body dopamine and noradrenaline content. Lancet **8(Sept.):** 535–537.
28. PERRIN, D. G., E. CRUTZ, I. E. BECKER & A. C. BRYAN. 1984. Ultrastructure of carotid bodies in sudden infant death syndrome. Pediatrics **73:** 646–651.
29. FIDONE, S., C. GONZALEZ & K. YOSHIZAKI. 1982. Effects of low oxygen on the release of dopamine from the rabbit carotid body in vitro. J. Physiol. (London) **333:** 93–110.
30. FIDONE, S., C. GONZALEZ & K. YOSHIZAKI. 1982. Effects of hypoxia on catecholamine synthesis in rabbit carotid body *in vitro*. J. Physiol. (London) **333:** 81–91.
31. LAHIRI, S., T. NISHINO, A. MOKASHI & E. MULLIGAN. 1980. Interaction of dopamine and haloperidol with O_2 and CO_2 chemoreception in carotid body. J. Appl. Physiol. **49:** 45–51.
32. QUATTROCHI, J. J., P. T. McBRIDE & A. J. YATES. 1985. Brainstem immaturity in sudden infant death syndrome: A quantitative rapid Golgi study of dendritic spines in 95 infants. Brain Res. **325:** 39–48.

Heart-Rate Variability and SIDS

Examination of Heart-Rate Patterns Using an Expert System Generator[a]

I. A. T. VÄLIMÄKI,[b,d,f] T. NIEMINEN,[b] K. J. ANTILA[b]
AND D. P. SOUTHALL[c,e]

[b]Cardiorespiratory Research Unit
University of Turku
Turku, Finland
[c]Cardiothoracic Institute
Brompton Hospital
London, United Kingdom

The sudden infant death syndrome (SIDS) is a major cause of death in infancy after the neonatal period.[1,2] Although the pathophysiological mechanisms leading to SIDS are still obscure, several previous studies support a hypothesis that one etiological factor may be a failure in autonomic cardiorespiratory control.[3] On the other hand, it may be that the etiology of SIDS is multifactorial and therefore complicated to examine. Techniques of artificial intelligence (AI)[g] have appeared helpful in investigating complex medical problems with large sets of clinical and physiological data.[4] The purpose of the project described in this paper was to prospectively collect recordings of cardiorespiratory signals in a large population of infants prior to the occurrence of SIDS and to analyze these data, using advanced signal analysis and AI techniques,[5] after cases of SIDS had been identified.

PATIENTS AND METHODS

A full report on the nature of the data base has already been published.[5] This present project addresses an analysis of the 22 tape recordings made on 16 full-term SIDS cases, 2 recordings on one preterm infant who was a victim of SIDS (subject 17), and a slightly greater number ($n = 23$) of controls matched as closely as possible for sex, birthweight, gestational age, and postnatal age (TABLE 2).[6] One of the 16 full-term SIDS cases (subject 13) had suffered previous episodes of unexplained cyanosis.

Recordings were made using a Medilog 1, 4-channel, miniature, battery-operated tape recorder (Oxford Medical Systems). An electrocardiogram (ECG) was recorded onto channel 1 from a modified transthoracic lead II. The respiratory waveform was recorded

[a]This study was funded by the Academy of Finland, Healthdyne and the Turku University Foundation.

[d]Funded in part by the British Council.

[e]Funded by the British Heart Foundation, the Joseph Levy Foundation, the Waring Scholarship, Healthdyne, Nellcor and the National SIDS Foundation.

[f]To whom correspondence should be addressed at: Cardiorespiratory Research Unit, University of Turku, 20520 Turku, Finland.

[g]A list of the abbreviations used in this paper may be found in TABLE 1.

TABLE 1. List of Abbreviations Used

AI, artificial intelligence
BW, birthweight
CV, coefficient of variation for overall heart-rate variability
CVS, coefficient of variation for beat-to-beat heart-rate variability
ECG, electrocardiogram
HR, heart rate
HRV, heart-rate variability
RMSM, root mean square for differences from the mean, overall HRV
RMSSD, root mean square for successive differences, beat-to-beat HRV
RSA, respiratory sinus arrhythmia

onto channel 2 using a volume-expansion capsule transducer taped firmly to the infants' abdominal wall, midway between the umbilicus and the xiphisternum. In channel 3 there was a device for improving the signal-to-noise ratio of the breathing signal,[6] and a 60-Hz crystal-clock signal was recorded onto channel 4. For further analysis, the cassette recordings from the selected cases were copied onto open-reel magnetic tape using a 1/4 in., high-quality FM tape-recorder (Store 4 DS, Racal Recorders, Ltd.). All tapes were coded so that analysis of the signals was carried out without knowledge of the outcome of the infants.

The ECG and respirogram were plotted onto paper at the speed of 50 mm/min of

TABLE 2. Summary of Clinical Data on SIDS Cases and Controls

SIDS Cases					Controls				
Infant (code no.)	Age at Recording (days)	Gestational Age (weeks)	Birth-weight (kg)	Sex	Infant (code no.)	Age at Recording (days)	Gestational Age (weeks)	Birth-weight (kg)	Sex
1	5, 47[a]	40	2.92	M	18	5	42	2.74	M
					19	48	40	3.35	F
2	6	38	3.49	F	20	6	40	3.30	M
3	2	40	3.74	F	21	2	40	3.40	M
4	8, 52[a]	39	2.81	F	22	7	39	2.64	F
					23	63	37	2.84	F
5	24, 63[a]	40	3.77	F	24	24	40	3.27	F
					25	65	39	3.46	F
6	5, 40[a]	38	3.03	M	26	4	38	2.98	M
					27	56	38	2.98	M
7	3	38	3.01	M	28	3	39	3.20	F
8	2, 41[a]	40	4.79	M	29	3	41	4.58	F
					30	42	40	4.56	F
9	19, 61[a]	40	2.98	F	31	19	39	2.98	F
					32	53	40	3.00	F
10	40	41	3.96	M	33	42	40	3.74	F
11	30	40	2.35	M	34	41	40	2.38	M
12	11	38	1.89	M	35	13	38	1.82	M
13	16	39	2.78	M	36	17	40	2.75	M
14	2	39	2.70	M	37	2	40	2.64	F
15	16	38	2.12	M	38	17	39	2.32	M
16	6	41	2.00	M	39	4	39	2.03	M
17	2, 48[a]	36	2.16	M	40	2, 45[a]	36	2.35	M

[a]Two recordings were made for the same infant at different ages.

original recording time (Mingograf 34, Siemens-Elema). All segments at least 2 min in duration with a respiratory pattern which was regular in amplitude and rate, according to previously defined criteria,[7] were selected from the graphs and included in further analyses ("regular respiratory pattern"). Regular breathing was defined as a pattern of breathing of a minimum duration of 2 min that appeared relatively regular in amplitude and in rate. The first 2 min of each of these segments were analyzed. In 2 SIDS infants (3 recordings) and in 2 controls (2 recordings), no segments with a "regular respiratory pattern" could be located in the recording, and these subjects were omitted from further analysis. For infants younger than 28 days of age at the time of the recording ($n = 15$ in both groups) there was a smaller quantity of regular breathing, and, therefore, the whole record was examined. On records from babies older than 28 days of age at the time of the recording ($n = 9$ in both groups), only the part of the tape from midnight to 6 A.M. was included.

SIGNAL PROCESSING

The ECG and the 60-Hz clock signal from each segment of "regular respiratory pattern" were replayed at 7.5 times real-time into a minicomputer (Nova 3, Data General Corporation). The ECG was preprocessed by an analogue band-pass filter and a voltage threshold trigger. This process utilized an adjustable triggering level, under visual control, to produce a pulse for each R wave. The clock pulses from both the ECG signal and the 60-Hz clock signal recorded on the original analogue tape were fed into the computer, and a special-purpose, 2-channel interval measurement device was used to measure each R–R interval and clock interval, with a resolution of ± 2 ms of the original recording time. The measured duration of the clock intervals falling between each R wave was used to compute an individual calibration coefficient for each R–R interval. This estimation of the duration of the original R–R interval reached the levels of accuracy defined in the report by Abraham et al.[8] The corrected R–R intervals were then stored on disks for further analysis. The respiratory intervals were measured from the same segments as the R–R intervals, using a procedure for computed tape-speed compensation identical to that used for the R–R intervals.

The preprocessed interval vectors were analyzed using a faster computer (Eclipse C/150, Data General Corporation). The indices used to characterize the overall HRV and beat-to-beat variability, RMSM and RMSSD, respectively, were computed as follows:[9]

$$RMSM = \sqrt{\frac{1}{n}\sum_{i=1}^{n}(RR_i - RR_{avg})^2} \quad \text{and} \quad RMSSD = \sqrt{\frac{1}{n-1}\sum_{i=1}^{n-1}(RR_i - RR_{i+1})^2}$$

where RR_i is the ith R–R interval, RR_{avg} is the mean R–R interval and n is the number of R–R intervals.

The corresponding coefficients of variation, CV and CVS were computed as follows:[9]

$$CV = 100 \times RMSM/RR_{avg} \text{ and } CVS = 100 \times RMSSD/RR_{avg}.$$

The power spectrum analysis of the HRV was performed after low-pass filtering and equispaced sampling of the original R–R interval sequence by use of a $\sin(x)/x$ convolution filter. The filtered signal was detrended by computing a 4th order polynomial, least-squares curve fit to the signal and then subtracting the polynomial trend. The power spectrum was then computed for the signal, using a Fast Fourier Transformation algorithm.[10]

The inverse of the median respiratory interval per segment was used to determine the respiratory rate for each segment. In order to quantify the respiratory sinus arrhythmia (RSA, modulation of the heart rate by each respiratory event) the spectral band at the respiratory frequency ± 0.05 Hz in the power spectra was integrated, and the figure was used to represent the respiratory component of the HRV power (quantitative measure of RSA).[11]

The amount of total data processing noise in the R–R interval signal was assessed using a simulation signal. It was 3.8 ms for the RMSM and 5.8 ms for the RMSSD.[11]

STATISTICAL METHODS

The general, two-way mixed model of analysis of variance was used to test the difference between the means in the SIDS cases and in the controls.[12] The random (block) factor in the analysis of variance was the matched pair, and the fixed factor the patient group.

ANALYSIS USING AN EXPERT SYSTEM GENERATOR

For AI analysis, average values of HR, respiratory rate, and indices of HRV and RSA were computed from the data segments with regular respiration for each SIDS and control case. These, together with data on sex, age at the time of recording, and birthweight, were transferred into a microcomputer and utilized as input for an expert system generator program (ExTran, Intelligent Terminals, Edinburgh, UK).[13] This program is an expert system shell capable of inducing diagnostic rules on the basis of "examples" containing attributes (in our case clinical and physiological data) and class identifications (SIDS vs. control). The ExTran program was interactively used to induce a decision tree for SIDS/controls via data files of our example cases.

RESULTS

Recordings of instantaneous heart rate and the corresponding indices of HRV spectra for an infant who subsequently suffered SIDS and a matched control case are shown in FIGURE 1. As a group, the controls had a significantly larger number of regular breathing segments (289 vs. 135, $p = 0.02$, TABLE 3). The average heart rate of the SIDS infants was higher and mean indices of HRV lower than those of the controls infants, but these differences were not statistically significant (TABLE 3). There was no difference between the group averages of the median respiratory rates of the SIDS cases and the controls.

The 21-node decision tree generated by the ExTran program is depicted in FIGURE 2. The program diagnosed 8 cases of SIDS on the basis of respiratory rate < 33/min and CV < 3.46%. Four cases of SIDS were characterized by respiratory rate > 33/min, CVS < 2.18%, and birthweight > 3,520 g and another 4 had, in addition to the respiratory rate and CVS as above, birthweight < 3,520 g, HR > 136/min and CV > 1.89%. Three additional cases of SIDS were classified on the basis of CV < 1.89% and HR between 142 and 155/min.

Interestingly, the program defined a majority cluster of 13 controls on the basis of a respiratory rate between 33 and 47/min, CVS > 2.18%, and RSA < 74.3 units (FIGURE 2). Four of the controls had respiratory rate > 33/min, CVS < 2.18%, birthweight <

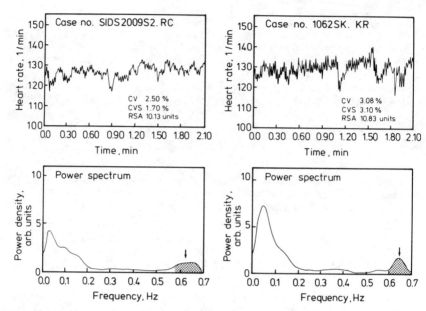

FIGURE 1. Typical heart-rate curves (**upper panels**) from one SIDS case (**left**) and one control case (**right**) with respective indices of HRV and power spectra (**lower panels**). The hatched spectral band is RSA corresponding to the median respiratory rate (*arrow*). See TABLE 1 for definitions of abbreviations.

3,520 g, and HR < 136/min. The remaining 5 controls formed smaller clusters; of these, one infant had exceptionally high heart rate, > 155/min. The program did not make use of data on the sex and age of the infant in making a distinction between the SIDS cases and controls. This indicates reasonable success in matching of cases vs. controls.

TABLE 3. Indices of Heart Rate Variability in Control Infants and Infants who Subsequently Suffered SIDS

Indices	Controls[a]	SIDS[a]	p^b
Regular breathing segments (*n*)	289	135	0.02
Recordings (*n*)	22	22	—
Heart rate (min^{-1})	126.7 ± 15.2	132.2 ± 13.3	0.183 (NS)
Respiratory rate (min^{-1})	38.7 ± 8.2	38.1 ± 9.4	0.270 (NS)
Overall HRV			
RMSM (ms)	15.6 ± 8.5	12.1 ± 6.0	0.183 (NS)
CV (%)	3.14 ± 1.39	2.57 ± 1.08	0.211 (NS)
Beat-to-beat HRV			
RMSSD (ms)	15.3 ± 11.6	10.8 ± 7.6	0.150 (NS)
CVS (%)	3.04 ± 2.02	2.25 ± 1.35	0.147 (NS)
Respiratory HRV[c]	27.0 ± 40.0	24.1 ± 34.6	0.946 (NS)

Note: for explanation of abbreviations, see TABLE 1
[a]Mean ± SD, all cases.
[b]Two-tailed probability from the mixed model analysis of variance (BMDP3V).
[c]Arbitrary units.

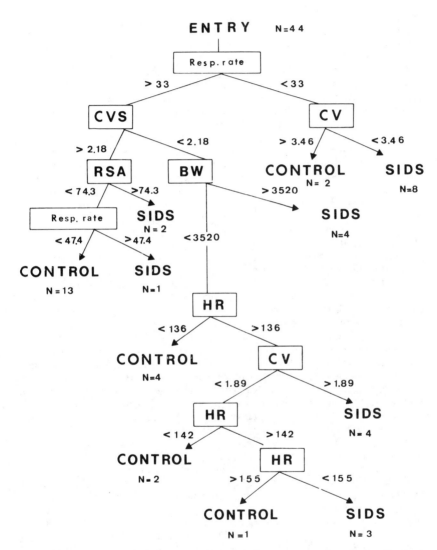

FIGURE 2. Decision tree induced on the basis of clinical and HRV attributes to classify 22 cases of SIDS and 22 controls. See TABLE 1 for definitions of abbreviations. N, no. of cases. Units for attributes: Resp. rate (min^{-1}), CVS (%), CV (%), RSA (arbitrary units), BW (g), HR (min^{-1}).

DISCUSSION

By analysis of variance, we could not differentiate infants destined to suffer SIDS from controls in terms of HR, HRV, or respiratory rate during the state of regular breathing. Nevertheless, the SIDS cases appeared to have lower overall and beat-to-beat HRV and reduced RSA density. This may indicate that chronotropic control of the heart is damped in some SIDS cases, as has been proposed in reports on the heart rate patterns of siblings of SIDS cases.[14,15]

It was interesting to note that there was a significant difference between the SIDS cases and controls in our study in the number of regular breathing segments. This finding suggests that there is a difference in the respiratory control or sleep pattern, resulting in a reduced amount of regular breathing in the SIDS group. With the data available we cannot explain the mechanism of this difference.

Spectral analysis of HRV allows us to quantify the magnitude of the several simultaneous oscillatory components in the HR signal, which result from interaction of control systems mediated by the autonomic nervous system.[16,17,18] In newborn infants the majority of the HRV power lies at the low-frequency range.[16,18,19] Although the magnitude of RSA in relation to the low-frequency HRV is smaller in neonates than in adults, it was possible to identify clear peaks of HRV spectral power at the frequency of respiration because the respiratory rate was sufficiently regular. In the present study there were great intragroup variations in the RSA spectral densities, and no significant difference between the SIDS and control groups was found.

Our filtering and detrending procedures were carried out to avoid the effects of noise and very low frequency changes (slow trends) in the heart rate in the power spectrum analysis. On the basis of numerical estimates and previous studies in neonates with respiratory distress syndrome and infants with SIDS, we have concluded that HRV frequencies >0.05 Hz are accurately reproduced and no physiologically relevant low-frequency activity is filtered out by this technique.[11,19]

Previously, several other investigators have examined HRV in an attempt to identify its possible relationship to SIDS. Harper et al., in a study of siblings of SIDS cases, also found a higher heart rate and lower beat-to-beat HRV during quiet sleep in this group compared with controls.[14,15] They believed that the lower HRV was due to lower respiratory sinus arrhythmia rather than other mechanisms such as motor activity. They postulated a lower vagal tone and chronic hypoxia as background mechanisms in infants at higher risk of SIDS. Leistner et al. detected an increase in heart rate and a lower beat-to-beat and overall HRV in "near-miss SIDS" infants.[20] In view of their additional findings of shorter QT intervals in the near-miss group,[21] they proposed that an increased sympathetic tone or an increase in circulatory catecholamines might explain the difference. Matthews et al.[22] also reported, in one infant who had 3 overnight ECG tape recordings and subsequently suffered SIDS, a lower beat-to-beat HRV and higher heart rate, which was particularly marked in the recording taken at 12 weeks of age. Gordon et al.[23] reported an excess of the low frequency components from spectral analysis of HRV and increased variability of respiratory rate in a group of 8 infants who had previously presented with "near-miss" events or who were siblings of SIDS cases and who subsequently died suddenly and without explanation. The analysis was not performed blind. It is also possible that large quantities of low-frequency HRV were present in the majority of "near-miss" cases, not just those who subsequently died, a suggestion supported by the larger quantities of periodic breathing reported in "near-miss" cases.[23]

Two groups have previously performed analyses of HRV on the same SIDS infants as those studied here. A study by Gordon et al.[25] was confined to 10 postneonatal full-term SIDS cases and a large number of age-matched controls. This analysis was performed blind and showed no significant differences in HRV or breathing patterns between future

SIDS cases and controls. The report by Kitney,[18] on a relatively small proportion of the full-term SIDS cases and non-matched controls, purported to show significantly higher values for the ratio of the low-frequency to the high-frequency densities in the heart-rate spectra of the SIDS cases. This particular analysis was not conducted blind.

Previous investigators have rather seldom utilized sets of several simultaneous clinical or physiological variables to differentiate SIDS cases from controls. Using spectral analysis, Kitney and Ong[24] found that RSA was related to variability of respiration, indicating strong cardiorespiratory synchronization. Respiratory entrainment decreased the spontaneous HRV. However, the SIDS and control groups behaved similarly except in the low-frequency/high-frequency ratio test mentioned above. Gordon *et al.*[25] used multivariate analysis and two-dimensional cluster analysis to investigate low-frequency HRV, variability of respiratory rate, and features of breathing patterns but failed to identify significant differences between SIDS and control groups. In a previous report on our own project, we were unable to find differences between SIDS cases and controls in multiple regression models of HR, HRV, and respiratory rate.[11]

The AI program we used in the present investigation is based on computation of the entropy, i.e., degree of uncertainty of the information, in the attributes of the infant-specific data. The result of the AI analysis supports the impression that if the etiology of SIDS is related to autonomic cardiorespiratory control, there may be several combinations of control failures resulting in this fatal condition. It might be expected that when an expert system shell like this generates a decision tree, the more relevant/important the decisions are, the simpler and more proximal they are in the decision tree, and the larger are the numbers of cases in the clusters formed. It was therefore interesting that, although the average respiratory rates of the test groups were similar, the greatest cluster of SIDS cases could be formed by combining information on respiratory rate and overall HRV. These 8 SIDS cases had respiratory rates clearly lower than the average in TABLE 3, but their CV was fairly normal. There were 11 SIDS cases who had beat-to-beat HRV < 2.18% but 7 controls also belonged to this category further characterized on the basis of birthweight, heart rate and CV (FIGURE 2). However, the majority of controls, 13 normal infants, could be distinguished on the basis of respiratory rate, beat-to-beat HRV and RSA.

In conclusion, infants destined for SIDS did not as a group have significantly higher heart rates or reduced HRV when compared with surviving controls by means of statistical methods. However, we identified a subgroup of SIDS cases with slow respiratory rate and fairly normal overall heart-rate variability, and another cluster of SIDS infants with reduced beat-to-beat HRV, often combined with elevated heart rate, when these variables and birthweight were simultaneously taken into consideration using advanced AI techniques.

SUMMARY

In a prospective, population-based study, HRV was analyzed from 24-hr tape recordings made on 16 full-term and one preterm infant who had subsequently suffered SIDS and compared to similar data on 23 control infants (*n* of recordings, 44). In the SIDS group, heart rate was higher, and overall and beat-to-beat HRV (CV, CVS, respectively) were lower, than in the controls, but not significantly. Respiratory rate and respiratory HRV (by spectral analysis) were similar in both groups. Assuming that cardiorespiratory mechanisms of SIDS are multifactorial, we expected that several subgroups would be detected in both test groups. Therefore, the average data for each recording were subsequently examined by means of an expert system generator (ExTran, Intelligent

Terminals Ltd., Edinburgh, UK). By rules induced with 25 nodes, the following results were obtained: 16/44 recordings were diagnosed as SIDS on the basis of (1) respiratory rate (RR) < 33 and CV $< 3.46\%$ ($n = 8$); (2) RR > 33, CVS $< 2.18\%$, and BW $> 3,520$ g ($n = 4$); and (3) RR > 33, CVS $< 2.18\%$, BW $< 3,520$ g, HR > 136, and CV $> 1.89\%$ ($n = 4$). Seventeen of 44 were considered as non-SIDS when (1) RR was $33-47.4$, CVS $> 2.18\%$, and RSA < 74.3 and (2) RR > 33, CVS $< 2.18\%$, BW $< 3,520$ g, and HR < 142. The remaining 11 cases required more complicated rules in order to be classified. This study shows that although the trend of increased HR and decreased HRV in the SIDS cases was statistically non-significant, an expert system program may be helpful in defining decision rules to identify cases of SIDS on the basis of cardiorespiratory data.

ACKNOWLEDGMENTS

The taped data used in this study were obtained with the help of Drs. E. A. Shinebourne and M. de Swiet and grants from the British Heart Foundation (BHF), the Foundation for the Study of Infant Deaths, and donations from the people of Brighton and Doncaster. We are grateful to Dr. J. Tuominen, D.Pol.Sc., and Mr. J. R. Alexander, M.Sc., for their advice on the statistics, as well as to Mr. R. T. Oja, M.Sc., and Mr. J. Jalonen, M.Sc., for assistance in computer-processing.

REFERENCES

1. GOLDING, J., S. LIMERICK & A. MACFARLANE. 1985. Sudden Infant Death. Patterns, Puzzles and Problems. Open Books Publishing Ltd. England.
2. RINTAHAKA, P. 1985. Sudden infant death syndrome in Finland in 1969–80. Publications of the National Board of Health, Series Original Reports 3/1985. Helsinki.
3. SHANNON, D. C. & D. H. KELLY. 1982. SIDS and near-SIDS. (Second of two parts). New Engl. J. Med. **306:** 1022–1028.
4. CLANCEY, W. J. & E. H. SHORTCLIFFE (Eds.). 1984. Readings in Medical Artificial Intelligence. The First Decade. Addison-Wesley Publishing Company. Reading, MA.
5. SOUTHALL, D. P. *et al.* 1983. Identification of infants destined to die unexpectedly during infancy: Evaluation of predictive importance of prolonged apnoea and disorders of cardiac rhythm or conduction. First report of a multicentered prospective study into the sudden infant death syndrome. Br. Med. J. **286:** 1092–1096.
6. WILSON, A. J., V. STEVENS, C. I. FRANKS, J. ALEXANDER & D. P. SOUTHALL. 1985. Respiratory and heart rate patterns in infants destined to be victims of sudden infant death syndrome: Average rates and their variability measured over 24 hours. Br. Med. J. **290:** 497–501.
7. RICHARDS, J. M., J. R. ALEXANDER, E. A. SHINEBOURNE, M. DE SWIET, A. J. WILSON & D. P. SOUTHALL. 1984. Sequential 22 hour profiles of breathing patterns and heart rate in 110 full term infants during their first six months of life. Pediatrics **74:** 763–777.
8. ABRAHAM, N. G., A. J. WILSON & P. A. CASTLE. 1985. The Oxford Medical Systems Medilog 1 recorder: Extending its application from routine to research. *In* Proceedings of the 5th International Symposium on Ambulatory Monitoring (ISAM): 299–317. CLEUP. Padua.
9. TARLO, P. A., I. VÄLIMÄKI & P. M. RAUTAHARJU. 1971. Quantitative computer analysis of cardiac and respiratory activity in newborn infants. J. Appl. Physiol. **31:** 70–75.
10. JENKINS, G. M. & D. G. WATTS. 1968. Spectral analysis and its applications. Holden-Day. San Francisco.
11. ANTILA, K. J. *et al.* Heart rate variability in infants subsequently suffering sudden infant death syndrome (SIDS). Manuscript submitted.

VÄLIMÄKI et al.: HEART-RATE VARIABILITY 237

VÄLIMÄKI et al.: HEART-RATE VARIABILITY 237

12. DIXON, W. J. (Ed.). 1985. BMDP Statistical Software, 1985 printing: 413–426. University of California Press. Berkeley.
13. A-RAZZAK, M. & T. HASSAN. 1984. Extran 7 Manual. Intelligent Terminals. Edinburgh.
14. HARPER, R. M., B. LEAKE, T. HOPPENBROUWERS, M. B. STERMAN, D. J. MCGINTY & J. HODGMAN. 1978. Polygraphic studies of normal infants and infants at risk for sudden infant death syndrome: Heart rate variability as a function of state. Pediatr. Res. **12:** 778–785.
15. HARPER, R. M., B. LEAKE, J. E. HODGMAN & T. HOPPENBROUWERS. 1982. Developmental patterns of heart rate and heart rate variability during sleep and waking in normal infants and infants at risk for sudden death syndrome. Sleep **5:** 28–38.
16. VÄLIMÄKI, I., H. ANTTILA, K. ANTILA & P. KERO. 1980. Spectral analysis of neonatal heart rate. A preliminary report. *In* Fetal and Neonatal Physiological Measurements. P. Rolfe, Ed.: 104–109. Pitman Medical Ltd. London.
17. AKSELROD, S., D. GORDON, F. A. UBEL, D. C. SHANNON, A. C. BARGER & R. J. COHEN. 1981. Power spectrum analysis of heart rate fluctuation: A quantitative probe of beat-to-beat cardiovascular control. Science **213:** 220–222.
18. KITNEY, R. I. 1984. New findings in the analysis of heart rate variability in infants. Automedica **5:** 289–310.
19. ANTTILA, H., I. VÄLIMÄKI, J. GADZINOWSKI, P. KERO & K. ANTILA. 1986. Power spectrum of heart rate in neonates with respiratory distress. *In* Electronics in Medicine and Biology. K. Copeland, Ed.: 319–324. Institute of Electronic and Radio Engineers. London.
20. LEISTNER, H. L., G. G. HADDAD, R. A. EPSTEIN, T. L. LAI, M. A. EPSTEIN & R. B. MELLINS. 1980. Heart rate and heart rate variability during sleep in aborted sudden infant death syndrome. J. Pediatr. **77:** 51–55.
21. HADDAD, G. G., M. A. EPSTEIN, R. A. EPSTEIN, N. M. MAZZA, R. B. MELLINS & E. KRONGRAD. 1979. The QT interval in aborted sudden infant death syndrome infants. Pediatr. Res. **13:** 136–138.
22. MATTHEWS, T. G. 1984. Is autonomic control a factor in some cases of sudden infant death syndrome? Lancet **i:** 744.
23. GORDON, D., R. J. COHEN, D. KELLY, S. AKSELROD & D. C. SHANNON. 1984. Sudden infant death syndrome: Abnormalities in short term fluctuations in heart rate and respiratory activity. Pediatr. Res. **18:** 921–926.
24. KITNEY, R. I. & H. G. ONG. 1986. An analysis of cardio-respiratory control in babies and its relation to sudden infant death syndrome. Automedica **7:** 105–126.
25. GORDON, D., D. P. SOUTHALL, D. H. KELLY, A. WILSON, S. AKSELROD, J. RICHARDS, B. KENET, R. KENET, R. J. COHEN & D. C. SHANNON. 1986. Analysis of heart rate and respiratory patterns in sudden infant death syndrome victims and control infants. Pediatrics **20:** 680–684.

Sleep and Cardiac Arrhythmias[a]

RICHARD L. VERRIER[b] AND DEBRA A. KIRBY

Cardiovascular Laboratories
Harvard School of Public Health
Boston, Massachusetts

INTRODUCTION

The possibility that sleep-induced arrhythmias may be a factor in the Sudden Infant Death Syndrome (SIDS) is based on two considerations. The first is that death appears to occur during the nocturnal period, when the infants are presumed to be asleep.[1] The second is that there is growing evidence that some of the SIDS events may be cardiac in origin.[2-5] However, since there have been no electrocardiographic records of the infant deaths, discussion of this subject must necessarily be inferential.

Several tacks will be pursued in an attempt to provide insights into the possible mechanisms whereby the sleep/wake cycle can conduce to arrhythmic death in infants. The first will be to discuss the effects of sleep states on cardiac arrhythmogenesis in adults. The second will be to review experimental studies of the effects of the sleep/wake cycle on vulnerability to arrhythmias in animals. The third will be to discuss the potential mechanisms whereby sleep states might conduce to cardiac death in infants.

SLEEP AND ARRHYTHMIAS IN ADULTS

Human studies of the effects of sleep on ventricular arrhythmias have yielded inconsistent results.[6-14] Whereas some investigators have observed that ventricular premature beats (VPBs) were not affected during sleep, others have found that VPBs were suppressed. However, it is noteworthy that those studies which reported a minor effect or an actual increase in arrhythmias during sleep were based on a small number of experimental subjects. Another confounding factor was the use of medication or the fact that the studies were conducted in the hospital setting. In investigations involving larger populations, the results obtained by several investigators indicate that sleep generally ameliorates the incidence of VPBs.[6-14] In particular, Lown and coworkers[8] found, during ambulatory monitoring of 54 subjects in their homes, that VPBs were reduced by at least 50% in 22 subjects during sleep. In 13 subjects, there was a 25% to 35% reduction in arrhythmia rate. The severity and grade of VPBs also decreased from a mean grade of 2.75 in the awake state to 1.78 during sleep. In several subjects, antiarrhythmic agents were notably less effective than sleep in decreasing the grade and frequency of VPBs. In a subsequent study involving 30 patients, DeSilva and coworkers demonstrated that suppression of VPBs occurred in all stages of sleep except for rapid eye movement (REM) sleep (unpublished observations). Stages 3 and 4 of slow wave sleep were most effective

[a]These studies were supported by Grants HL-32905, HL-33567 and HL-35138 from the National Heart, Lung and Blood Institute, NIH, Bethesda, MD.
[b]To whom correspondence should be addressed at: Cardiovascular Laboratories, Harvard School of Public Health, 665 Huntington Avenue, Boston, MA 02115.

238

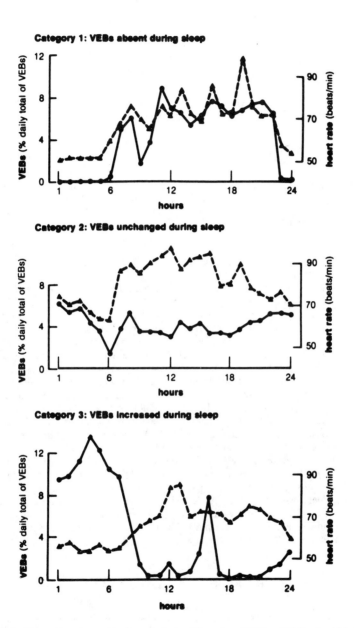

FIGURE 1. Fluctuations in ventricular ectopic beat frequency (VEB, *solid lines*) and heart rate (*dashed lines*) over a 24-hour period in individual subjects. (From Pickering *et al.*[10] Reprinted by permission from *Cardiovascular Medicine.*)

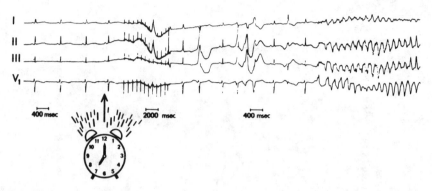

FIGURE 2. The provocation of ventricular fibrillation following an auditory stimulus (alarm clock). QT segment alterations are followed by ventricular premature beats and ventricular fibrillation. The central section of the ECG recording was made at a slower speed than the beginning and end. (From Wellens *et al.*[15] Reprinted by permission from *Circulation.*)

in abating arrhythmias. Pickering and colleagues[10] have reported comparable results. They found that VPBs were almost completely abolished during sleep in 26% of 31 patients, whereas in 71%, the reduction in premature beats was partial. Multiform and repetitive VPBs also decreased during sleep (FIG. 1). Thus, it appears that slow wave sleep exhibits a moderate antiarrhythmic effect in some adult subjects. However, in others there may be no effect on heart rhythm, and in still others, arrhythmias may be exacerbated. With respect to REM sleep, there is evidence that life-threatening arrhythmias may occur. There have been a number of case reports of ventricular tachycardia and fibrillation in association with violent or frightening dreams. It remains speculative, however, whether sudden death occurring during sleep takes place in the REM phase.[7]

Another aspect of the sleep/wake cycle which deserves consideration in relation to cardiac arrhythmogenesis is arousal. Indeed, several investigators have provided evidence that the electrical stability of the heart can be severely compromised during abrupt transitions from sleep to wakefulness.[13,15,16] A particularly striking example was described in a case report by Wellens and coworkers.[15] The patient was a 14-year-old girl who experienced repeated episodes of life-threatening ventricular tachyarrhythmias when awakened from sleep by a loud auditory stimulus (e.g., an alarm clock, falling bedpan, rock-and-roll music, etc.: FIG. 2). The trigger mechanisms appear to be surges in sympathetic nervous system activity, as the syncopal episodes could be prevented by β-adrenergic blockade therapy with propranol. These observations thus suggest that, in certain individuals, arousal from sleep may be highly arrhythmogenic and therefore could be a factor in some SIDS cases.

SLEEP STUDIES IN ANIMALS

Kleitman's[17] pioneering work made evident that prolonged sleep-deprivation in animals led to disorganized aggressive behavior and, eventually, sudden death. Postmortem examination demonstrated no anatomic lesions or chemical imbalance to account for death. A reasonable surmise is that cardiac arrhythmia was the underlying mechanism. Sleep, as a neural event, probably affects cardiac function through the autonomic nervous system. Much evidence suggests that diencephalic areas in the central nervous system serve as focal points of cardiac control[18,19] and that this control is transmitted through peripheral autonomic pathways.[20,21] The same catecholamine neurotransmitters that subserve myocardial function are also associated with specific sleep stages.[22-24] Baust and coworkers[25,26] have shown that denervation of the heart prevents the usual heart-rate responses to various sleep states.

A few studies have been conducted to define the effects of sleep on susceptibility to cardiac arrhythmias. Skinner and coworkers[27] have explored the specific influences of sleep stage on the occurrence of ventricular arrhythmias during left anterior descending coronary artery occlusion in pigs. They found that the period during the early sleep cycle wherein transitional and slow wave sleep alternate was accompanied by an increase in arrhythmias compared to the awake state. This was true both in the acutely infarcted (2 hr.) as well as in the recently infarcted (2 days) pig heart (FIG. 3). The maximum increase in ventricular arrhythmias was observed during sustained periods of slow wave sleep. Later, when REM sleep predominated, the overall incidence of arrhythmia abruptly diminished. Acute coronary artery occlusion performed after the inception of slow wave sleep reduced the latency in onset of ventricular fibrillation compared with that observed during the awake state. Coronary occlusion during REM sleep was associated with the

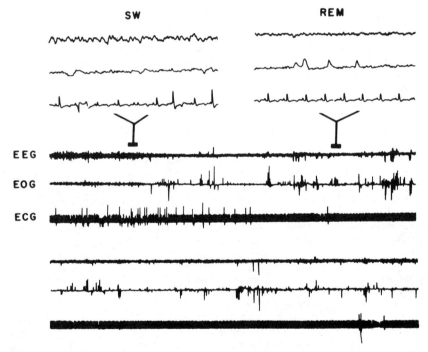

FIGURE 3. REM sleep suppressed ectopic arrhythmias in a pig with a 2-hr-old infarction caused by left anterior descending coronary artery occlusion. The bottom three traces are continuous with the middle three traces; the top three traces are expanded time-scales of the intervals indicated. This representative pig was in slow wave sleep (SW), as determined by a synchronized electroencephalogram (EEG), and then progressed into REM sleep, as determined by the desynchronized EEG and the eye-movement bursts seen in the electro-oculogram (EOG). The arrhythmias seen in the standard lead I electrocardiogram (ECG) were suppressed within 40 sec following the onset of REM sleep. Calibrations: amplitude = 500 μV; time = 10 sec. (From Skinner et al.[27] Reprinted by permission from *Circulation Research*.)

opposite effect, namely, a delay in the development of ventricular fibrillation. These investigators reached some unexpected conclusions: (a) slow wave sleep, but not REM sleep, has a deleterious influence on the ischemic heart; (b) REM sleep may be beneficial, because it delays the development of ventricular fibrillation during coronary artery occlusion; and (c) the heart rate changes during sleep do not correlate with the effects of slow wave or REM sleep on cardiac rhythm.

The explanation for the above changes remains unclear. It is curious that in the pigs with coronary artery occlusion, arrhythmia was reduced not only during REM sleep but also during wakefulness. These investigators[27] cited Baust and Bohnert,[25] who found in cats that reduction in sympathetic tone accounts for the slow tonic heart rates during REM sleep, whereas during slow wave sleep, bradycardia was due to increased parasympathetic tone. However, increased sympathetic tone is certainly an attribute of the awake state. Snyder, Hobson, and Goldfrank,[28] and others,[29,30] have demonstrated that heart rate and arterial blood pressure are higher during wakefulness than during sleep. Hemodynamic concomitants, as well as coronary artery flow changes, may indeed be linked to neural alterations during sleep stages and may influence the electrically unstable ischemic heart.

NEURAL FACTORS IN CARDIAC ARRHYTHMOGENESIS

What are the possible neurogenic mechanisms whereby sleep could induce fatal disturbances in heart rhythm? To address this question it is necessary to consider the influence of both limbs of the autonomic nervous system on cardiac electrophysiological properties.

Role of the Sympathetic Nervous System

There is a substantial body of information suggesting that peripheral sympathetic neural structures are primarily involved in mediating the autonomic nervous system influence on ventricular electrical stability. For example, it has been shown that the profibrillatory effects of central nervous system stimulation can be prevented by cardiac sympathectomy or by administration of sympatholytic drugs.[31–36] The direct effects of sympathetic neural influences can be demonstrated by electrical stimulation of the stellate ganglia. In normal animals, stimulation of cardiac sympathetic efferent fibers markedly lowers the threshold of the vulnerable period[37,38] and increases the incidence of spontaneous ventricular fibrillation during myocardial ischemia.[39] Conversely, stellate ganglionectomy increases the ventricular fibrillation threshold,[40] reduces susceptibility to cardiac arrhythmias during coronary artery occlusion,[41] and increases the capacity of the coronary arterial bed to dilate.[42]

The specific involvement of α-adrenergic receptors in neurally induced arrhythmias is not well understood. This uncertainty relates, in part, to the complexity of their influences, which include both direct actions on myocardial excitable properties[31] and indirect effects on insulin secretion,[42A] platelet aggregability,[43] and coronary hemodynamic function.[42,44] The latter consideration may be of particular importance in view of growing evidence implicating coronary vasospasm as a factor in the genesis of lethal arrhythmias. By contrast β_1-adrenergic receptors appear to be directly involved in mediating neurally induced vulnerability.[45–48] In particular, sympathetic agents have been shown to prevent stress-induced vulnerability to ventricular fibrillation during classical[49] and instrumental[50] conditioning, as well as during elicitation of an anger-like state.[51]

The possibility that surges in sympathetic activity may occur during sleep is suggested by our recent study of the effects of sleep on coronary hemodynamic function.[52] Dogs were chronically instrumented to allow for recording sleep stage and systemic and coronary hemodynamic function. The animals were studied during natural sleep, with the cycles divided into one minute epochs of either quiet wakefulness, or slow wave or REM sleep. The results are summarized in TABLE 1. The findings indicate that during slow wave sleep there are moderate but significant reductions in heart rate and coronary blood flow and an increase in coronary vascular resistance. In REM, the coronary blood-flow baseline is moderately elevated compared to slow wave sleep, and there are striking, episodic surges in flow. Coronary vascular resistance is reduced correspondingly. Heart rate and mean arterial pressure are also elevated during the flow surges, indicating that an increase in cardiac metabolic activity may be the basis for the coronary vasodilation. However, other factors, including imperceptible somatic activity, may be involved. Our preliminary data involving stellectomy suggest that coronary flow surges are abolished by this procedure, implicating direct involvement of the autonomic nervous system.

TABLE 1. Differential Effects of REM and Slow Wave Sleep (SWS) on Coronary Hemodynamic Function[52]

Function[a]	Awake[b]	SWS[b]	REM Baseline[b,c]	REM Surge[b,c]
MAP (mm Hg)	107 ± 4	106 ± 4	105 ± 7	111 ± 7
HR (beats/min)	85 ± 11	78 ± 10[d]	83 ± 10	102 ± 9[e]
CBF (ml/min)	33 ± 5	30 ± 4[d]	34 ± 4	52 ± 8[e]
CVR (mm Hg/ml/min)	3.6 ± 0.7	3.9 ± 0.7[d]	3.4 ± 0.7	2.5 ± 0.6[e]

[a]MAP, mean arterial pressure; HR, heart rate; CBF, coronary blood flow; CVR, coronary vascular resistance.
[b]Values are expressed as means ± SEM.
[c]Values at baseline and episodic surges of CBF, respectively; see text.
[d]$p < 0.02$ compared to awake and REM baseline.
[e]$p < 0.02$ compared to awake, SWS and REM baseline sleep.

The Parasympathetic Nervous System and Cardiac Arrhythmias

The prevailing view had been that vagal innervation did not extend to the ventricular myocardium. Clinical teaching had been in accord with this perception. If a tachycardia responded to cholinergic measures, the site of impulse formation was judged to be supraventricular. However, considerable data have now been amassed indicating that parasympathetic neural influences directly affect the inotropic, chronotropic, and electrophysiologic properties of the ventricles.[53–58] Kent et al.[53] demonstrated that vagus nerve stimulation increased the ventricular fibrillation threshold in both the normal and ischemic canine ventricle. They demonstrated, moreover, the cholinergic innervation of the specialized conducting system through which the antifibrillatory action of the vagus is thought to occur. Our understanding has been enhanced by the studies of Zipes and coworkers,[55,56,58] who utilized phenol to delineate the anatomical pathways mediating vagal influences on excitability of the normal and ischemic heart.

Results from our laboratory indicate that vagal influences are contingent upon the level of pre-existing cardiac sympathetic tone.[45,49] We observed that when sympathetic tone to the heart is augmented by thoracotomy,[59] sympathetic nerve stimulation,[46,59] or catecholamine infusion,[60] simultaneous vagal activation exerts a protective effect on ventricular vulnerability. Vagus nerve stimulation is without effect on vulnerability when adrenergic input to the heart is blocked by β-adrenergic antagonists.[59,61] The influence of vagus nerve activity on ventricular vulnerability appears to be due to activation of muscarinic receptors, since vagally mediated changes in vulnerability are prevented by atropine administration. Muscarinic agents have been shown both to inhibit the release of norepinephrine from sympathetic nerve endings[54,62] and to attenuate the response to norepinephrine at receptor sites by cyclic nucleotide interactions.[63] These mechanisms result in significant protection against ventricular fibrillation during acute myocardial ischemia (FIG. 4).

There is evidence indicating that sympathetic-parasympathetic interactions also modulate myocardial electrical stability in the conscious state.[51] This idea is supported by studies in which relatively small doses of atropine (0.05 mg/kg) were employed to block the effect of vagal efferent activity to the heart. When animals were exposed to an aversive environment where their catecholamine levels were elevated, vagal efferent blockade resulted in a substantial (50%) reduction in the threshold of the vulnerable

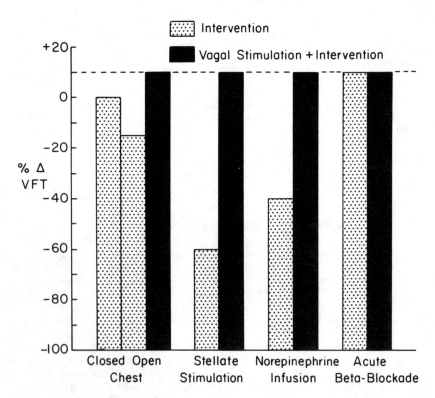

FIGURE 4. Influence of vagal stimulation in the presence of various levels of adrenergic tone. The effect on the ventricular fibrillation threshold (VFT) is demonstrable only when neural or humoral activity is increased. The particular intervention is specified below each stippled bar. (From Lown & Verrier.[49] Reprinted by permission from the *New England Journal of Medicine.*)

TABLE 2. Influence of Sleep Stage on Ventricular Refractoriness

	Heart Rate (beats/min)	Effective Refractory Period (msec)
Awake	170 ± 10	114 ± 4
REM	140 ± 7^b	124 ± 3^b
SWS[a]	140 ± 3^b	121 ± 2^b

Note: All determinations were made during fixed-rate pacing. Values are expressed as means ± SEM.
[a]SWS, slow wave sleep.
[b]$p < 0.05$.

period. In a nonstressful setting where their plasma catecholamine levels were low, vagal blockade in the animals was without effect on ventricular vulnerability.[64] Thus, tonic vagal activity can exert a significant influence on vulnerability to ventricular fibrillation in the conscious as well as the anesthetized state. The magnitude of the effect is related to the level of prevailing cardiac sympathetic tone.

Recently we have obtained evidence which suggests that alterations in vagal tone may modulate cardiac electrophysiologic properties during sleep.[65] Specifically, the effects of REM and slow wave sleep on ventricular refractoriness were studied in chronically instrumented cats. Electrodes were implanted to record electro-oculograms, electromyograms, and electroencephalograms for sleep-stage determination. A right ventricular catheter was employed for cardiac electrical testing using the single stimulus technique. Both REM and slow wave sleep significantly increased the effective refractory period (TABLE 2). This effect was independent of alterations in heart rate, as this variable was maintained constant by pacing. In addition, sleep shifted the timing of the vulnerable period later into diastole but did not alter the repetitive extrasystole threshold. These alterations were not prevented by bilateral stellectomy. However, when the muscarinic blocking agent atropine methyl nitrate was administered, the sleep-induced changes were completely abolished. These results suggest that the electrophysiologic changes associated with sleep are mediated through fluctuations in cardiac vagal tone.

NEUROCARDIAC MECHANISMS IN SIDS

Based on these considerations, how can sleep-induced changes in autonomic nervous system activity cause sudden death in infants? First, enhanced vagal discharge appears unlikely to be a factor in sudden death due to arrhythmias, since vagus nerve activity reduces rather than increases susceptibility to ventricular tachycardia and fibrillation. It is possible, however, that excess vagal tone, such as may occur during episodes of apnea, could lead to severe bradycardia and asystole.[66-69] Whether or not this influence would be sufficient to arrest the heart permanently remains to be determined.

Surges in sympathetic nervous system activity such as might occur during REM sleep also have the potential for precipitating sudden death in infants. However, based on the available data from experimental studies, it would appear that some underlying derangement in cardiac substrate would be necessary to result in life-threatening arrhythmias. To date, cogent evidence has not been obtained for a defect in the electrophysiologic function of the myocardium or its specialized conduction system in SIDS.[70-72] It is important to note, however, that ventricular premature beats and tachyarrhythmias have been observed in infants.[73,74]

Another possibility is that asymmetrical activation of the nervous system could lead to electrical inhomogeneities within the myocardium.[5] Highly relevant in this regard is the report of Kralios and Millar,[75] who have studied the functional development of cardiac sympathetic nerves in puppies between 1 and 6 weeks of age by measuring ventricular refractoriness at multiple sites. The developmental changes of the cardiac sympathetic nerves follow a distinct pattern. Namely, there is a regression of functional maturation in the third week of life in response to all the nerves tested except for the ventrolateral branch of the left stellate ganglion. These results suggest that there is regional sympathetic imbalance with left sympathetic predominance in the third week of development in the animals studied. These observations carry important implications. In particular, Schwartz and colleagues[76, 77] have suggested that the findings of Kralios and Millar,[75] of a time-limited dominance of left-sided cardiac nerves, may represent an explanation for the prolongation of QT interval that occurs, in normal babies, at the second and fourth months of life[76] (FIG. 5). These potential mechanisms are summarized in TABLE 3.

In summary, there are diverse mechanisms whereby the changes in autonomic tone which occur during sleep could result in the acute cardiac demise of infants. Whether the actual cause is singular or multiple remains to be determined.

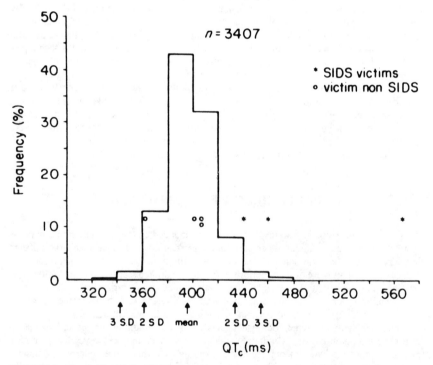

FIGURE 5. Distribution of the QT interval corrected for heart rate (QT$_c$) in newborns on the fourth day of life. The QT$_c$ of the 3 SIDS victims (*stars*) was 440, 460 and 563 msec, exceeding the mean by 2, 3 and 9 standard deviations, respectively. In contrast, the QT$_c$ of infants who died from causes other than SIDS (*open circles*) was within the normal range. (From Schwartz et al.[76] Reprinted by permission from *European Heart Journal*.)

TABLE 3. Summary of Potential Neurocardiac Mechanisms in SIDS

Autonomic Derangement	Cardiac Mechanism	Comments
Excess vagal activity due to sleep-induced apnea	Asystole	This could occur in association with hypoxia.[66-69] It is unclear whether the infant heart could be permanently arrested by sustained hypervagotonia.
	Asystole degenerating to ventricular fibrillation[16]	Cardiac arrest could lead to complete loss of blood pressure, leading to a massive reflex increase in sympathetic activity. This effect could in turn precipitate ventricular fibrillation.
Sleep-induced surges in sympathetic activity	Ventricular fibrillation	In the absence of functional derangement in the heart's susceptibility to fibrillation, it is unlikely that the increases in sympathetic activity observed during sleep are of a sufficient magnitude to trigger fibrillation. Arousal from sleep could be a factor.[15]
Developmental imbalance in sympathetic innervation to the heart[75]	Ventricular fibrillation	Experimental studies of cardiac electrophysiologic properties in puppies suggest that asymmetries in sympathetic innervation occur during development, a pattern of neural influence which has been shown to be highly arrhythmogenic. The prolongation of QT intervals which has been observed in infants is also suggestive of sympathetic nervous system imbalance.[77]

ACKNOWLEDGMENTS

The authors thank Sandra S. Verrier for her editorial assistance and Tina Bedard for typing the manuscript.

REFERENCES

1. BERGMAN, A. B., C. G. RAY, M. A. POMEROY, P. W. WAHL & J. B. BECKWITH. 1972. Studies of the sudden infant death syndrome in King County, Washington. III. Epidemiology. Pediatrics 49: 860–870.
2. FROGATT, P. & T. N. JAMES. 1973. Sudden unexpected death in infants. Evidence on a lethal cardiac arrhythmia. Ulster Med. J. 42: 136–152.
3. BURGESS, M. J. 1972. Miscellaneous effects upon the electrocardiogram. In Advances in Electrocardiography. R. C. Schlant & J. W. Hurst, Eds.: 367–375. Grune & Stratton. New York.
4. BURGESS, M. J., S. BLATT & J. A. ABILDSKOV. 1976. Observations pertinent to the prolonged QT syndromes (abstract). Am. J. Cardiol. 37: 125.
5. SCHWARTZ, P. J. 1987. The quest for the mechanisms of the sudden infant death syndrome: Doubts and progress. Circulation 75: 677–683.
6. BRODSKY, M., D. WU, P. DENES, C. KANAKIS & K. M. ROSEN. 1977. Arrhythmias

documented by 24-hour continuous electrocardiographic monitoring in 50 male medical students without apparent heart disease. Am. J. Cardiol. **39:** 390–395.

7. DeSILVA, R. A. 1982. Central nervous system risk factors for sudden cardiac death. Ann. N.Y. Acad. Sci. **382:** 143–161.

8. LOWN, B., M. TYKOCINSKI, A. GARFEIN & P. BROOKS. 1973. Sleep and ventricular premature beats. Circulation **48:** 691–701.

9. MONTI, J. M., L. E. FOLLE, C. PELUFFO, R. ARTUCIO, A. ORTIZ, O. SEVRINI & J. DIGHIERO. 1975. The incidence of premature contractions in coronary patients during the sleep-awake cycle. Cardiology **60:** 257–264.

10. PICKERING, T. G., L. GOULDING & B. A. COBERN. 1977. Diurnal variations in ventricular ectopic beats and heart rate. Cardiovasc. Med. **2:** 1013–1022.

11. PICKERING, T. G., J. JOHNSTON & A. J. HONOUR. 1978. Comparison of the effects of sleep, exercise and autonomic drugs on ventricular extrasystoles, using ambulatory monitoring of electrocardiogram and electroencephalogram. Am. J. Med. **65:** 575–583.

12. ROSENBLATT, G., E. HARTMAN & G. R. ZWILLING. 1973. Cardiac irritability during sleep and dreaming. J. Psychosom. **17:** 129–134.

13. SMITH, R., L. JOHNSON, D. ROTHFELD, L. ZIR & B. THARP. 1972. Sleep and cardiac arrhythmias. Arch. Intern. Med. **130:** 751–753.

14. WINKLE, R. A., M. G. LOPES, J. W. FITZGERALD, D. J. GOODMAN, J. S. SCHROEDER & D. C. HARRISON. 1975. Arrhythmias in patients with mitral valve prolapse. Circulation **52:** 73–81.

15. WELLENS, H. J. J., A. VERMEULEN & D. DURRER. 1972. Ventricular fibrillation occurring on arousal from sleep by auditory stimuli. Circulation **46:** 661–665.

16. SCHWARTZ, P. J. 1981. The sudden infant death syndrome. *In* Reviews in Perinatal Medicine. E. M. Scarpelli & E. V. Cosmi, Eds. Vol. 4: 475–524. Raven Press. New York.

17. KLEITMAN, N. 1963. Sleep and Wakefulness. University of Chicago Press. Chicago.

18. RUSHMER, R. F., O. A. SMITH, JR. & E. P. LASHER. 1960. Neural mechanisms of cardiac control during exertion. Physiol. Rev. **Suppl. 4:** 27–34.

19. SMITH, O. A., JR., S. J. JABBUR, R. F. RUSHMER & E. P. LASHER. 1960. Role of hypothalamic structures in cardiac control. Physiol. Rev. **Suppl. 4:** 136–141.

20. BOND, D. D. 1943. Sympathetic and vagal interaction in emotional responses of the heart rate. Am. J. Physiol. **138:** 468–478.

21. COHEN, D. H. & L. H. PITTS. 1968. Vagal and sympathetic components of conditioned cardioacceleration in the pigeon. Brain Res. **9:** 15–31.

22. JOUVET, M. 1969. Biogenic amines and the states of sleep. Science **163:** 32–41.

23. KOELLA, W. P., A. FELDSTEIN & J. S. CZICMAN. 1968. The effect of parachlorophenylalanine on the sleep of cats. Electroencephalogr. Clin. Neurophysiol. **25:** 481–490.

24. REITE, M., G. V. PEGRAM, L. M. STEPHENS, E. C. BIXLER & O. L. LEWIS. 1969. The effect of reserpine and monoamine oxidase inhibitors on paradoxical sleep in the monkey. Psychopharmacologia **14:** 12–17.

25. BAUST, W. & B. BOHNERT. 1969. The regulation of heart rate during sleep. Exp. Brain Res. **7:** 169–180.

26. BAUST, W., B. BOHNERT & O. RIEMANN. 1969. The regulation of the heart rate during sleep (abstract). Electroencephalogr. Clin. Neurophysiol. **27:** 626.

27. SKINNER, J. E., D. N. MOHR & P. KELLAWAY. 1975. Sleep-stage regulation of ventricular arrhythmias in the unanesthetized pig. Circ. Res. **37:** 342–349.

28. SNYDER, F., J. A. HOBSON & F. GOLDFRANK. 1963. Blood pressure changes during human sleep. Science **142:** 1313–1314.

29. BACCELLI, G., M. GUAZZI, G. MANCIA & A. ZANCHETTI. 1969. Neural and non-neural mechanisms influencing circulation during sleep. Nature **223:** 184–185.

30. COCCAGNA, G., M. MANTOVANI, F. BRIGNANI, A. MANZINI & E. LUGARESI. 1971. Arterial pressure changes during spontaneous sleep in man. Electroencephalogr. Clin. Neurophysiol. **31:** 277–281.

31. CORR, P. B. & A. D. SHARMA. 1982. Alpha- versus beta-adrenergic influences on dysrhythmias induced by myocardial ischaemia and reperfusion. *In* Advances in Beta-blocker Therapy II. A. Zanchetti, Ed.: 163–180. Excerpta Medica. Amsterdam.

32. ROSEN, M. R., R. B. ROBINSON & P. DANILO, JR. 1985. Developmental changes in

cardiac-autonomic interactions. *In* Cardiac Electrophysiology and Arrhythmias. D. P. Zipes & J. Jalife, Eds.: 159–164. Grune & Stratton. New York.

33. SCHWARTZ, P. J. & H. L. STONE. 1985. The analysis and modulation of autonomic reflexes in the prediction and prevention of sudden death. *In* Cardiac Electrophysiology and Arrhythmias. D. P. Zipes & J. Jalife, Eds.: 165–176. Grune & Stratton. New York.

34. ENGEL, B. T. & S. H. GOTTLIEB. 1970. Differential operant conditioning of heart rate in the restrained monkey. J. Comp. Physiol. Psychol. **73**: 217–225.

35. VERRIER, R. L. & E. L. HAGESTAD. 1985. Role of the autonomic nervous system in sudden death. *In* Sudden Cardiac Death. M. E. Josephson, Ed.: 41–63. F. A. Davis Company. Philadelphia.

36. VERRIER, R. L., A. CALVERT & B. LOWN. 1975. Effect of posterior hypothalamic stimulation on ventricular fibrillation threshold. Am. J. Physiol. **228**: 923–927.

37. GORMAN, R. R. 1979. Modulation of human platelet function by prostacyclin and thromboxane α_2. Fed. Proc., Fed. Am. Soc. Exp. Biol. **38**: 83–88.

38. VERRIER, R. L., P. THOMPSON & B. LOWN. 1974. Ventricular vulnerability during sympathetic stimulation: Role of heart rate and blood pressure. Cardiovasc. Res. **8**: 602–610.

39. HARRIS, A. S., H. OTERO & A. J. BOCAGE. 1971. The induction of arrhythmias by sympathetic activity before and after occlusion of a coronary artery in the canine heart. J. Electrocardiol. (San Diego) **4**: 34–43.

40. SCHWARTZ, P. J., N. G. SNEBOLD & A. M. BROWN. 1976. Effects of unilateral cardiac sympathetic denervation on the ventricular fibrillation threshold. Am. J. Cardiol. **37**: 1034–1040.

41. SCHWARTZ, P. J., H. L. STONE & A. M. BROWN. 1976. Effects of unilateral stellate ganglion blockade on the arrhythmias associated with coronary occlusion. Am. Heart J. **92**: 589–599.

42. SCHWARTZ, P. J. & H. L. STONE. 1977. Tonic influence of the sympathetic nervous system on myocardial reactive hyperemia and on coronary blood flow distribution in dogs. Circ. Res. **41**: 51–58.

42A. MAJID, P. A., C. SAXTON, J. R. W. DYKES, M. C. GALVIN & S. H. TAYLOR. 1970. Autonomic control of insulin secretion and the treatment of heart failure. Br. Med. J. **4**: 328–334.

43. PFISTER, B. & P. R. IMHOF. 1977. Inhibition of adrenaline-induced platelet aggregation by the orally administered alpha-adrenergic receptor blocker phentolamine (Regitine®). Eur. J. Clin. Pharmacol. **11**: 7–10.

44. MOHRMAN, D. E. & E. O. FEIGL. 1978. Competition between sympathetic vasoconstriction and metabolic vasodilation in the canine coronary circulation. Circ. Res. **42**: 79–86.

45. VERRIER, R. L. 1987. Mechanisms of behaviorally induced arrhythmias. Circulation. **76** (Suppl. I): I48–I56.

46. MATTA, R. J., R. L. VERRIER & B. LOWN. 1976. Repetitive extrasystole as an index of vulnerability to ventricular fibrillation. Am. J. Physiol. **230**: 1469–1473.

47. HOHNLOSER, S. H., R. L. VERRIER & B. LOWN. 1987. Influence of beta$_2$-adrenoceptor stimulation and blockade on cardiac electrophysiologic properties and serum potassium concentration in the anesthetized dog. Am. Heart. J. **113**: 1066–1070.

48. ROSENFELD, J., M. R. ROSEN & B. F. HOFFMAN. 1978. Pharmacologic and behavioral effects on arrhythmias that immediately follow abrupt coronary occlusion: A canine model of sudden coronary death. Am. J. Cardiol. **41**: 1075–1082.

49. LOWN, B. & R. L. VERRIER. 1976. Neural activity and ventricular fibrillation. N. Engl. J. Med. **294**: 1165–1170.

50. MATTA, R. J., J. E. LAWLER & B. LOWN. 1976. Ventricular electrical instability in the conscious dog. Effects of psychologic stress and beta adrenergic blockade. Am. J. Cardiol. **38**: 594–598.

51. VERRIER, R. L. & B. LOWN. 1984. Behavioral stress and cardiac arrhythmias. Annu. Rev. Physiol. **46**: 155–176.

52. KIRBY, D. A. & R. L. VERRIER. 1987. Differential effects of rapid eye movement and slow wave sleep on coronary hemodynamic function (abstract). Soc. Neurosci. Abstr. **13**: 740.

53. KENT, K. M., E. R. SMITH, D. R. REDWOOD & S. E. EPSTEIN. 1974. Beneficial

electrophysiologic effects of nitroglycerin during acute myocardial infarction. Am. J. Cardiol. **33:** 513–516.

54. LEVY, M. N. 1971. Sympathetic-parasympathetic interactions in the heart. Circ. Res. **29:** 437–445.

55. MARTINS, J. B. & D. P. ZIPES. 1980. Epicardial phenol interrupts refractory period responses to sympathetic but not vagal stimulation in canine left ventricular epicardium and endocardium. Circ. Res. **47:** 33–40.

56. ZIPES, D. P., M. J. BARBER, N. TAKAHASHI & R. F. GILMOUR, JR. 1985. Recent observations on autonomic innervation of the heart. *In* Cardiac Electrophysiology and Arrhythmias. D. P. Zipes & J. Jalife, Eds.: 181–189. Grune & Stratton. New York.

57. HOHNLOSER, S. H., R. L. VERRIER & B. LOWN. 1986. Effects of adrenergic and muscarinic receptor stimulation on serum potassium concentrations and myocardial electrical stability. Cardiovasc. Res. **20:** 891–896.

58. PRYSTOWSKY, E. N., W. M. JACKMAN, R. L. RINKENBERGER, J. J. HEGER & D. P. ZIPES. 1981. Effect of autonomic blockade on ventricular refractoriness and atrioventricular nodal conduction in humans. Evidence supporting a direct cholinergic action on ventricular muscle refractoriness. Circ. Res. **49:** 511–518.

59. KOLMAN, B. S., R. L. VERRIER & B. LOWN. 1975. The effect of vagus nerve stimulation upon vulnerability of the canine ventricle: Role of sympathetic-parasympathetic interactions. Circulation **52:** 578–585.

60. RABINOWITZ, S. H., R. L. VERRIER & B. LOWN. 1976. Muscarinic effects of vagosympathetic trunk stimulation on the repetitive extrasystole (RE) threshold. Circulation **53:** 622–627.

61. YOON, M. S., J. HAN, W. W. TSE & R. ROGERS. 1977. Effects of vagal stimulation, atropine, and propranolol on fibrillation threshold of normal and ischemic ventricles. Am. Heart J. **93:** 60–65.

62. LEVY, M. N. & B. BLATTBERG. 1976. Effect of vagal stimulation on the overflow of norepinephrine into the coronary sinus during cardiac sympathetic nerve stimulation in the dog. Circ. Res. **38:** 81–85.

63. WATANABE, A. M., J. P. LINDEMANN, L. R. JONES, H. R. BESCH, JR. & J. C. BAILEY. 1981. Biochemical mechanisms mediating neural control of the heart. *In* Disturbances in Neurogenic Control of the Circulation. F. M. Abboud, H. A. Fozzard, J. P. Gilmore & D. J. Reis, Eds.: 189–203. American Physiological Society. Bethesda, MD.

64. VERRIER, R. L. & B. LOWN. 1981. Autonomic nervous system and malignant cardiac arrhythmias. *In* Brain, Behavior, and Bodily Disease. H. Weiner, M. A. Hofer & A. J. Stunkard, Eds. Vol. 59: 273–291. Raven Press. New York.

65. FRANCIS, G. C., E. L. HAGESTAD & R. L. VERRIER. 1986. Influence of sleep stage on ventricular refractoriness (abstract). Physiologist **29:** 163.

66. GUILLEMINAULT, C., R. ARIAGNO, M. SOUQUET & W. C. DEMENT. 1976. Abnormal polygraphic findings in near-miss sudden infant death. Lancet **1:** 1326–1327.

67. GUILLEMINAULT, C., R. ARIAGNO, S. COONS, R. WINKLE, R. KOROBKIN, R. BALDWIN & M. SOUQUET. 1985. Near-miss sudden infant death syndrome in eight infants with sleep apnea-related cardiac arrhythmias. Pediatrics **76:** 236–242.

68. MOTTA, J. & GUILLEMINAULT, C. 1985. Cardiac dysfunction during sleep. Ann. Clin. Res. **17:** 190–198.

69. KELLY, D. H., H. GOLUB, D. CARLEY & D. C. SHANNON. 1986. Pneuomograms in infants who subsequently died of sudden infant death syndrome. J. Pediatr. **109:** 249–254.

70. MARON, B. J., C. E. CLARK, R. E. GOLDSTEIN & S. E. EPSTEIN. 1976. Potential role of QT interval prolongation in sudden infant death syndrome. Circulation **54:** 423–430.

71. KEETON, B. R., E. SOUTHALL, N. RUTTER, R. H. ANDERSON, E. A. SHINEBOURNE & D. P. SOUTHALL. 1977. Cardiac conduction disorders in six infants with "near-miss" sudden infant deaths. Br. Med. J. **2:** 600–601.

72. LIE, J. T., H. S. ROSENBERG & E. E. ERICKSON. 1976. Histopathology of the conduction system in the sudden infant death syndrome. Circulation **53:** 3–8.

73. SOUTHALL, D. P., D. G. VULLIAMY, M. J. DAVIES, R. H. ANDERSON, E. A. SHINEBOURNE & A. M. JOHNSON. 1976. A new look at the neonatal electrocardiogram. Br. Med. J. **2:** 615–618.

74. SOUTHALL, D. P., M. J. ORRELL, J. F. TALBOT, R. J. BRINTON, D. G. VULLIAMY, A. M. JOHNSON, B. R. KEETON, R. H. ANDERSON & E. A. SHINEBOURNE. 1977. Study of cardiac arrhythmias and other forms of conduction abnormality in newborn infants. Br. Med. J. 2: 597–599.

75. KRALIOS, F. A. & C. K. MILLAR. 1978. Functional development of cardiac sympathetic nerves in newborn dogs: Evidence for asymmetrical development. Cardiovasc. Res. 12: 547–554.

76. SCHWARTZ, P. J. & P. SALICE. 1984. Cardiac arrhythmias in infancy: Prevalence, significance and need for treatment. Eur. Heart J. (Suppl. B) 5: 43–50.

77. SCHWARTZ, P. J., M. MONTEMERLO, M. FACCHINI, P. SALICE, D. ROSTI, G. POGGIO & R. GIORGETTI. 1982. The QT interval throughout the first 6 months of life: A prospective study. Circulation 66: 496–501.

Upper Airway Reflex Control

J. G. WIDDICOMBE AND M. TATAR[a]

Department of Physiology
St. George's Hospital Medical School
London SW17 0RE
United Kingdom

INTRODUCTION

The upper airways are complex, both in terms of the muscles and effector tissues that control their patency and in terms of the afferent nervous inputs that can influence these structures. The patterns of reflex control differ for the various parts of the upper respiratory tract.

The larynx can dilate or constrict both during the normal pattern of breathing and in transient acts such as coughing and sneezing, where the changes in laryngeal caliber may be extreme.[1] Similarly, for the oropharynx, there are both physiological rhythmical changes during breathing and more extreme effects induced by activities such as swallowing.[2] Spontaneous changes in oropharyngeal caliber seem to be primarily dilative during inspiration, when the constrictor muscles of the pharynx do not seem to be involved. For the nose, the sketetal muscles of the palate and the nares play a major role in determining nasal airflow resistance in breathing, and the former are important in determining the balance of nasal and oral airflows.[3] Palatine muscle contraction is synchronized with that of the jaw muscles so that the mouth opens when nasal airflow is diverted in that direction. A further control system in the nose is the vascular bed,[4] congestion of which leads to nasal blockage and diversion of flow through the mouth in all but obligatory nose breathers. All the skeletal muscle systems for the larynx, oropharynx and nose, and also the vascular bed of the nose, are under reflex control, with respiratory modulation of activity and powerful reflex inputs that affect upper airway caliber.

REFLEXES FROM THE UPPER AIRWAY

Upper airway reflexes affecting breathing, with responses such as sneezing and also changes in spontaneous breathing patterns,[5-7] have been studied for a long time. The effect of such reflexes on upper airway patency has been less studied until recently. Negative pressure in the upper airways increases the respiratory contractions of the alae nasi, posterior cricoarytenoid, and genioglossus muscles, all of which dilate the upper airways[8-11] (FIG. 1). Muscles acting on the hyoid (geniohyoid and thyrohyoid) show a similar effect.[12] All these responses help to maintain upper airway patency during inspiration, since the muscles are inspiratory dilative in their action. The effect of positive pressure is more controversial, since it has been said to inhibit genioglossus[10,11] but also to increase hypoglossal (dilator) nerve activity.[13] In experimental animals these responses

[a]Usual address: Department of Pathophysiology, Comenius University, Faculty of Medicine, 037 53 Martin, CSSR.

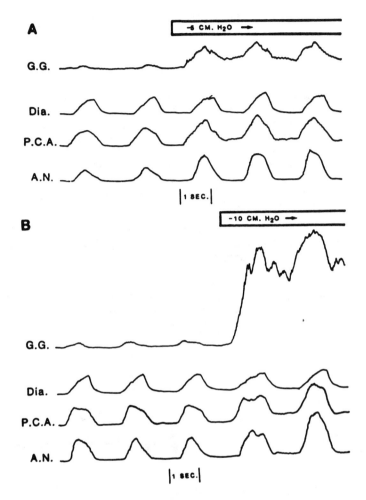

FIGURE 1. Responses in a dog of moving average of diaphragm (Dia.) and upper airway (G.G., P.C.A., and A.N.) muscles to upper airway negative pressure. **A:** electromyogram before and for the first 3 breaths during application of -5 cm H_2O to larynx in a representative animal. All upper airway muscles show increases in phasic activity; inspiratory time is minimally increased. **B:** -10 cm H_2O applied to nasopharynx of the same animal produced greater effects on inspiratory time and peak amplitude of upper airway muscles. G.G., genioglossus; P.C.A., posterior cricoarytenoid; A.N., alae nasi. (From Van Lunteren et al.[16] Reprinted with permission of the *Journal of Applied Physiology.*)

can be shown to be reflex by appropriate denervations. In man these denervations cannot be done, but indirect evidence suggests that the same reflexes are present. Expiratory resistive loading in man, which increases upper airway pressure, tends to close the glottis,[14,15] although continuous positive pressure in the upper airway does not have this effect. Nevertheless, the general pattern of experimental results both in animals and man indicates that reflexes from the upper respiratory tract have a powerful influence on upper respiratory tract patency, the stimulus certainly including airway pressure and possibly also airflow.

Reflexes from the Nose

In dogs and rabbits, negative pressure in the nose contracts the dilator muscles of the pharynx, larynx, and alae nasi (FIG. 2), and the effect is abolished by nasal mucosal anesthesia.[9,16] The upper respiratory tract responses are associated with a slowing of breathing.[17] The receptors for this reflex have not been identified, and it is difficult to visualize pressure receptors in the nose, which is a cavity surrounded by rigid bone.

Airflow in the nose is also a reflex stimulus,[5] and air puffed into the nose causes contraction of the alae nasi. Changes in contraction of the muscles of the pharynx and larynx do not seem to have been described. The recent description of receptors responsive to cold in the nose[19] has not yet been related to upper airway patency, but this is an important possibility.

The diving reflex, the apnea and multiple related reflex responses induced by water or cold applied to the face and nose,[5,20] includes laryngeal closure as an important component.[21] Changes in upper respiratory tract muscles other than those in the larynx do not seem to have been studied.

Chemical irritants in the nose may cause sneezing, associated with a powerful and transient change in laryngeal and upper airway caliber.[5,7] The same stimuli, when too weak to cause sneezing, also constrict the larynx in the expiratory phase[22] (FIG. 3).

We have recently studied the effect of mechanical stimulation of the nasal mucosa on

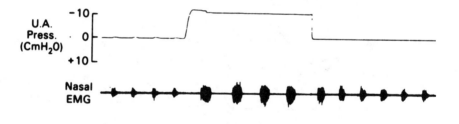

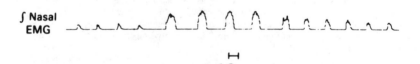

1 Sec.

FIGURE 2. Effect in a rabbit of negative upper airway pressure (U.A. Press.) on nasal electromyogram (EMG). U.A. pressure changes (**top trace**), direct nasal EMG (**middle trace**), and integrated nasal EMG (**bottom trace**) are shown. Phasic inspiratory activity present during control period increases markedly during negative pressure application, with an increase in inspiratory and expiratory times. (From Mathew.[9] Reprinted with permission from the *Journal of Applied Physiology*.)

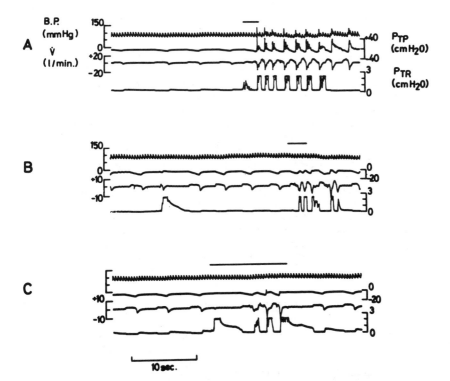

FIGURE 3. Effect of insufflation of ammonia vapor into nose of cat. Each trace shows, from top to bottom: signal (horizontal bar), blood pressure (B.P.), transpulmonary pressure (P_{TP}), lower tracheal flow ($\dot{V}$), and tracheal pressure (translaryngeal pressure P_{TR}, with saturation of pressure recorder corresponding to complete laryngeal closure). **A:** insufflation of 3 ml of 1:100 ammonia vapor into nose, with superior laryngeal nerves intact. Note sneezing, positive deflections of P_{TP}, and increase in laryngeal resistance in expiratory phase. **B:** insufflation of 3 ml of 1:1000 ammonia vapor into nose, with superior laryngeal nerves intact. Note the lack of sneezing and the increase in breathing frequency and laryngeal resistance. **C:** insufflation of 3 ml of 1:1000 ammonia vapor into nose, with superior laryngeal nerves cut. Note slowing of breathing and increase in laryngeal resistance. (From Szereda-Przestaszewska & Widdicombe.[22] Reprinted with permission from *Respiration Physiology*.)

upper airway resistance in dogs (M. Tatar and J. G. Widdicombe, unpublished results). When sneezing occurred, upper airway resistance during inspiration was greatly and significantly reduced. When there was not sneezing, upper airway resistance still decreased significantly, not only during stimulation but for some time (5–150 sec) after the stimulus. Thus, the upper airway dilator responses do not need to be secondary to the sneeze.

Reflexes from the Oropharynx

During swallowing, respiratory diaphragmatic activity is inhibited, as is that of the posterior cricoarytenoid muscle, the main laryngeal abductor.[2,5] Activity in the laryngeal adductors is enhanced. Inevitably, the pharyngeal constrictor muscles must be stimulated, although these have been little studied.

The aspiration reflex, induced by mechanical stimulation of the nasopharynx, consists of vigorous, repeated contractions of the diaphragm, and these are associated with laryngeal abductions in the inspiratory phase.[5,7,23] The afferent pathways for the aspiration reflex are probably the rapidly adapting receptors in the pharyngeal submucosa communicating with myelinated fibers in the glossopharyngeal nerves.[24]

A second group of pharyngeal receptors has been identified, those which respond to changes in pharyngeal pressure by maintained, slowly adapting discharge.[25] Their patterns of activity in various species (cat, dog, and rabbit) differ, but it seems likely that they are airway stretch-receptors with a considerable influence on breathing.[5] The action of pharyngeal stretch receptors on the upper respiratory tract probably constitutes a component of the reflex contractions of the dilator muscles in response to negative pressures and a component of the opposite response to positive pressures, since either change in pressure stimulates receptor activity in some species.[5,6] Denervation of the pharynx by cutting the glossopharyngeal nerves does not always reduce the upper airway muscle responses to changes in pressure, so the nose and larynx may also be reflexogenic zones. In general, the oropharyngeal reflexes have been rather neglected in relation to upper airway patency, although it seems probable that they are important.

Reflexes from the Larynx

The larynx is a site of some of the most powerful reflexes affecting both breathing and all parts of the respiratory tract. Its walls contain a large number, probably at least six types, of afferent end organs, which have not yet been categorized histologically or for their individual reflex actions.[5,26] They individually respond to pressure, flow, respiratory drive, osmolarity, temperature, and chemical irritants. In spite of this complexity of the afferent innervation of the larynx, there is general agreement that laryngeal stimuli cause reflex constriction of the larynx,[5,7,22,27] and this response seems to have a lower threshold than the reflexes inducing coughing or breathing changes[27] (FIG. 4). The responses are abolished by cutting the superior laryngeal nerves and may be absent in newborn animals, including humans.[28,29] The laryngeal reflex response may be related to the effect of inhalation of a histamine aerosol in healthy subjects and asthmatics, which causes expiratory constriction of the larynx.[30,31] A similar effect is seen spontaneously in patients with chronic bronchitis or asthma, and it seems likely that a laryngo-laryngeal reflex may be important in human airways disease.

The effects of pressure changes in the entire upper respiratory tract are very considerably reduced by cutting the superior laryngeal nerves,[9,17] indicating that a major component comes from the larynx. Distension or collapse of the larynx and oropharynx alone in dogs and rabbits causes reflex changes similar to those occurring with pressure changes in either the nose alone or the whole upper respiratory tract.[11,16] Local anesthesia to the larynx and oropharynx also prevents most of the reflex changes.[11] Thus, the larynx seems to be the major site of origin of reflexes induced by pressure changes in the upper respiratory tract. As indicated above, the actual nerve receptors have not been identified; but judging from patterns of activities of receptors, it seems plausible that the laryngeal pressure receptors are important in this respect. The upper respiratory tract responses to inhaled irritants reaching the larynx may be due to activation of the rapidly adapting irritant receptors found there.[5,26] The role on upper airway caliber of cold/flow receptors in the larynx does not seem to have been determined.[26]

REFLEXES FROM THE LOWER AIRWAYS

Reflexes from the lower airways and lungs affecting the upper airways have not been frequently studied, probably because experimental physiologists normally cannulate the trachea of the animals they study, thereby excluding the upper respiratory tract. Similarly in man, the use of a mouthpiece may greatly distort responses in the upper respiratory tract.

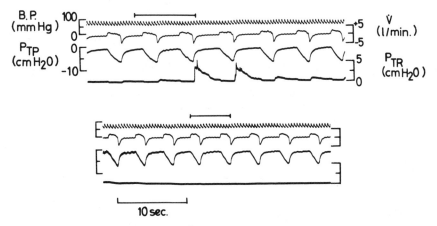

FIGURE 4. Effect of insufflation of $1:10^5$ ammonia vapor into larynx of cat before (**top**) and after (**bottom**) cutting superior laryngeal nerves. Note slight slowing of breathing, absence of expiratory efforts, and expiratory increase in laryngeal resistance before denervation. Each trace shows, from top to bottom: signal (horizontal bar), blood pressure (B.P.), transpulmonary pressure (P_{TP}), lower tracheal flow ($\dot{V}$), and translaryngeal pressure (P_{TR}). (From Szereda-Przestaszewska & Widdicombe.[22] Reprinted with permission from *Respiration Physiology*.)

Slowly Adapting Pulmonary Stretch Receptors

These nerve receptors, localized in a smooth muscle of the large airways, are responsible for the inhibition of breathing associated with the Hering-Breuer inflation reflex.[33-35] The reaction on the larynx is to arrest its intrinsic muscles and hold it partly open.[36] The action of the reflex on other muscles of the respiratory tract has been less studied. In preliminary experiments in the dog we have found that inflation of the lungs has little action on upper airway resistance above the larynx (M. Tatar and J. G. Widdicombe, unpublished results). The reflex seems to have little action on nasal vascular beds influencing nasal patency,[37] and its effect on airway dilator muscles in the nose and oropharynx consists of an inhibition that parallels phrenic activity.[5] Since breathing is arrested when the reflex is strongly stimulated, the degree of contraction of the upper airway muscles may be weak or absent during this phase.

Cough and Rapidly Adapting Lung Irritant Receptors

During coughing, whether induced from the larynx or the tracheobronchial tree, it is well established that constrictions of the larynx occur in the initial phase of expiratory muscle contraction.[7,38,39] What happens in the other muscles of the upper respiratory tract is less clear. We have recently measured oronasal resistance in anesthetised dogs, using a pharyngeal catheter for recording pressure. We found that, during coughing induced by stimulation of the trachea, oronasal resistance is significantly decreased in the inspiratory phase and that, after the coughing is complete, there remains a significant decrease in oronasal resistance during the expiratory phase of breathing. A similar stimulation of the trachea which was too weak to cause coughing also significantly reduced upper airways resistance in the expiratory phase (M. Tatar and J.G. Widdicombe, unpublished results). These results should be compared with the evidence that stimulation of rapidly adapting irritant receptors in the cat and dog, which does not cause coughing, causes a constriction of the larynx in the expiratory phase[33,40,41] (FIG. 5). Thus, there may be a difference between responses of the larynx and oronasal tract, or stimulation of tracheal receptors, if too weak to cause coughing, may have a different upper airway reflex response to that seen with stimulation of irritant receptors deeper in the lungs. It must also be borne in mind that the chemical means of stimulating lung irritant receptors in cats may also activate C-fiber endings.[33,34]

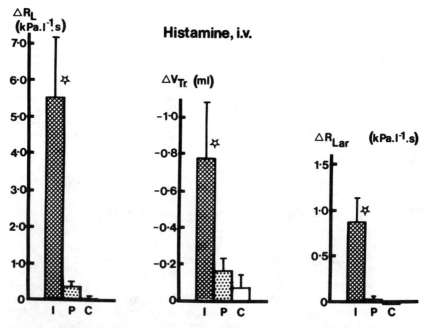

FIGURE 5. Effects of intravenous histamine stimulation of lung rapidly adapting irritant receptors on total lung resistance (R_L), tracheal volume (V_{Tr}) and laryngeal resistance (R_{Lar}) in dogs vagally intact (I), with partial vagal block (P), or with complete vagal blockade (C). Results are given as changes (Δ) from control. Star, $p < 0.05$. Note that the increases in all three variables due to histamine are abolished by vagal blockade. (From Jammes et al.[41] Reprinted with permission from *Clinical Respiratory Physiology*.)

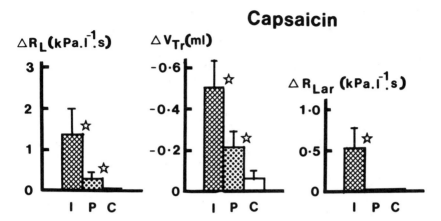

FIGURE 6. Effects of intravenous capsaicin stimulation of lung C-fiber receptors on total lung resistance (R_L), tracheal volume (V_{Tr}) and laryngeal resistance (R_{Lar}) in dogs vagally intact (I), with partial vagal block (P), or with complete vagal blockade (C). Results are given as changes ($\triangle$) from control. Star, $p < 0.05$. Note that the increases in all three variables due to capsaicin are abolished by vagal blockade. (From Jammes et al.[41] Reprinted with permission from *Clinical Respiratory Physiology*.)

C-Fiber Receptors

These are nerve endings with nonmyelinated fibers in the vagus nerves, which are stimulated by lung inflations and by pathological changes.[33,34] Their reflex actions on the upper respiratory tract include laryngeal constriction or closure during the apnea associated with the reflex[40,41] (FIG. 6). This response has been described for cats, rabbits, and pigs[42] and has recently been confirmed by us in dogs.[41] However, during the rapid shallow breathing that follows the apnea, there is a significant decrease in upper airway resistance associated with more powerful contractions of the genioglossus muscle (M. Tatar and J. G. Widdicombe, unpublished results). Thus, the C-fiber receptor reflex consists of two phases: a cessation of breathing associated with upper respiratory tract closure followed by rapid shallow breathing associated with more powerful contraction of the upper airway dilator muscles.

CONCLUSIONS

The upper respiratory tract is a complex anatomical structure with many skeletal muscle and vascular tissues which influence the caliber of its different components. Although these muscles normally exhibit respiratory variations in activity, with dilator responses generally corresponding to inspiration, a large number of reflexes from the respiratory system can influence their activity. These include the both powerful and transient changes in upper airway caliber seen in activities such as sneezing, swallowing and coughing. In addition, the phasic activity of the upper airway muscles is strongly affected by a variety of reflex inputs, including (1) physiological factors such as the pressures in the upper respiratory tract and the changes in pressure and volume of the lower airways and the lungs and (2) pathological factors such as the responses to upper and lower respiratory tract irritation and disease. In particular, lung conditions such as collapse, pneumonia, and edema may stimulate lung C-fiber and rapidly adapting irritant receptors, leading to laryngeal and upper airway constriction followed by dilatation; these responses may play a role in conditions such as respiratory distress syndrome and SIDS.

Although only the upper respiratory tract changes have been described in this report, they should be correlated with the changes in breathing and with the other physiological variables which the same afferent inputs may powerfully affect.

REFERENCES

1. BARTLETT, D., JR. 1986. Upper airway motor systems. *In* Handbook of Physiology. Section 3, The Respiratory System. Vol. II, Control of Breathing. N. S. Cherniack & J. G. Widdicombe, Eds.: 223–246. American Physiological Society. Bethesda, MD.
2. MILLER, A. J. 1982. Deglutition. Physiol. Rev. **62:** 129–184.
3. ECCLES, R. 1982. Neurological and pharmacological considerations. *In* The Nose: Upper Airway Physiology and the Atmospheric Environment. D. F. Proctor & I. B. Andersen, Eds.: 191–214. Elsevier. Amsterdam.
4. WIDDICOMBE, J. G. 1986. The physiology of the nose. *In* Clinics in Chest Medicine. J. H. Widdicombe, Ed.: 159–170. W. B. Saunders. Philadelphia, PA.
5. WIDDICOMBE, J. G. 1986. Reflexes from the upper respiratory tract. *In* Handbook of Physiology. Section 3, The Respiratory System. Vol. II, Control of Breathing. N. S. Cherniack & J. G. Widdicombe, Eds.: 363–394. American Physiological Society. Bethesda, MD.
6. WIDDICOMBE, J. G., G. SANT'AMBROGIO & O. P. MATHEW. 1988. Nervous receptors of the upper airway. *In* Respiratory Function of the Upper Airway. G. Sant'Ambrogio & O. P. Mathew, Eds. Marcel Dekker. New York. In press.
7. KORPAS, J. & Z. TOMORI. 1979. Cough and Other Respiratory Reflexes. S. Karger. Basel, Switzerland.
8. VAN LUNTEREN, E., K. P. STROHL, D. M. PARKER, E. N. BRUCE, W. B. VAN DE GRAAFF & N. S. CHERNIACK. 1984. Phasic volume-related feedback on upper airway muscle activity. J. Appl. Physiol. **56:** 730–736.
9. MATHEW, O. P. 1984. Upper airway negative-pressure effects on respiratory activity of upper airway muscles. J. Appl. Physiol. **56:** 500–505.
10. MATHEW, O. P., Y. K. ABU-OSBA & B. T. THACH. 1982. Influence of upper airway pressure changes on genioglossus muscle respiratory activity. J. Appl. Physiol. **52:** 438–444.
11. MATHEW, O. P., Y. K. ABU-OSBA & B. T. THACH. 1982. Genioglossus muscle responses to upper airway pressure changes: afferent pathways. J. Appl. Physiol. **52:** 445–450.
12. VAN DE GRAAFF, W. B., S. B. GOTTFRIED, J. MITRA, E. VAN LUNTEREN, N. S. CHERNIACK & K. P. STROHL. 1984. Respiratory function of hyoid muscles and hyoid arch. J. Appl. Physiol. **57:** 197–204.
13. HWANG, J. C., W. M. ST. JOHN & D. BARTLETT, JR. 1984. Afferent pathways for hypoglossal and phrenic responses to changes in upper airway pressure. Respir. Physiol. **55:** 342–354.
14. BRANCATISANO, T. P., D. S. DODD, P. W. COLLETT & L. A. ENGEL. 1985. Effect of expiratory loading on glottic dimensions in humans. J. Appl. Physiol. **58:** 605–611.
15. DAUBENSPECK, J. A. & D. BARTLETT, JR. 1983. Expiratory pattern and laryngeal responses to single-breath expiratory resistance loads. Respir. Physiol. **54:** 307–316.
16. VAN LUNTEREN, E., W. B. VAN DE GRAAFF, D. M. PARKER, J. MITRA, M. A. HAXHIU, K. P. STROHL & N. S. CHERNIACK. 1984. Nasal and laryngeal reflex responses to negative upper airway pressure. J. Appl. Physiol. **56:** 746–752.
17. MATHEW, O. P. & J. P. FARBER. 1983. Effect of upper airway negative pressure on respiratory timing. Respir. Physiol. **54:** 252–268.
18. DAVIES, A. & R. ECCLES. 1984. The effects of nasal airflow on the electromyographic activity of nasal muscles in the anaesthetised cat. J. Physiol. **358:** 102P.
19. GLEBOVSKY, V. D. & A. V. BEYEV. 1984. Stimulation of nasal cavity mucous trigeminal receptors with respiratory airflows. Sechenov Physiol. J. USSR **LLX:** 1534–1541.
20. ELSNER, R. & B. GOODEN. 1983. Diving and Asphyxia. Monographs of the Physiological Society, No.40. Cambridge University Press. Cambridge, UK.

21. BANTING, F. G., J. E. HALL, J. M. JANES, B. LEIBEL & D. W. LOUGHEED. 1938. Physiological studies in experimental drowning. Can. Med. Assoc. J. **39:** 226–228.
22. SZEREDA-PRZESTASZEWSKA, M. & J. G. WIDDICOMBE. 1973. Reflex effects of chemical irritation of the upper airways on the laryngeal lumen in cats. Respir. Physiol. **18:** 107–115.
23. TOMORI, Z. & J. G. WIDDICOMBE. 1969. Muscular, bronchomotor and cardiovascular reflexes elicited by mechanical stimulation of the respiratory tract. J. Physiol. (London) **200:** 25–50.
24. NAIL, B. S., G. M. STERLING & J. G. WIDDICOMBE. 1969. Epipharyngeal receptors responding to mechanical stimulation. J. Physiol. (London) **204:** 91–98.
25. HWANG, J. C., W. M. ST. JOHN & D. BARTLETT, JR. 1984. Receptors corresponding to changes in upper airway pressure. Respir. Physiol. **55:** 355–366.
26. MATHEW, O. P. & F. SANT'AMBROGIO. 1988. Laryngeal reflexes. *In* Respiratory Function of the Upper Airway. G. Sant'Ambrogio & O. P. Mathew, Eds. Marcel Dekker. New York. In press.
27. WYKE, D. B. & J. A. KIRCHNER. 1978. Neurology of the larynx. *In* Scientific Foundations of Otolaryngology. R. Hinchcliffe & D. Harrison, Eds.: 546–574. Heinemann. London.
28. HARDING, R. 1984. Function of the larynx in the fetus and newborn. Annu. Rev. Physiol. **46:** 645–659.
29. SASAKI, C. T. & M. SUZUKI. 1976. Laryngeal reflexes in cat, dog and man. Arch. Otolaryngol. **102:** 400–402.
30. COLLETT, P. W. T., T. P. BARNCATISANO & L. A. ENGEL. 1983. Changes in the glottic aperture during bronchial asthma. Am. Rev. Respir. Dis. **128:** 719–723.
31. HIGENBOTTAM, T. 1980. Narrowing of glottis opening in humans associated with experimentally induced bronchoconstriction. J. Appl. Physiol. **49:** 403–407.
32. HIGENBOTTAM, T. & J. PAYNE. 1982. Glottis narrowing in lung disease. Am. Rev. Respir. Dis. **125:** 746–750.
33. COLERIDGE, H. M. & J. C. G. COLERIDGE. 1986. Reflexes evoked from tracheobronchial tree and lungs. *In* Handbook of Physiology. Section 3, The Respiratory System. Vol. II, Control of Breathing. N. S. Cherniack & J. G. Widdicombe, Eds.: 395–430. American Physiological Society. Bethesda, MD.
34. SANT'AMBROGIO, G. 1982. Information arising from the tracheobronchial tree of mammals. Physiol. Rev. **62:** 531–569.
35. WIDDICOMBE, J. G. 1964. Respiratory reflexes. *In* Handbook of Physiology. Section 3, Respiration. Vol. I. W. O. Fenn & H. Rahn, Eds.: 585–630. American Physiological Society. Washington, DC.
36. PRESSMAN, J. J. & G. KELEMEN. 1955. Physiology of the larynx. Physiol. Rev. **35:** 506–554.
37. LUNG, M. A. & J. G. WIDDICOMBE. 1987. Lung reflexes and nasal vascular resistance in the anaesthetized dog. J. Physiol. (London) **386:** 465–474.
38. YOUNG, S. A., N. ABDUL-SATTAR & D. CARIC. 1987. Glottic closure and high flows are not essential for productive cough. Clin. Respir. Physiol. **23** (Suppl. 10): 115–185.
39. LEITH, D. E. 1977. Cough. *In* Respiratory Defense Mechanisms. J. D. Brain, D. F. Proctor & L. M. Reid, Eds. Part 2: 545–592. Marcel Dekker. New York.
40. STRANSKY, A. M., M. SZEREDA-PRZESTASZEWSKA & J. G. WIDDICOMBE. 1973. The effect of lung reflexes on laryngeal resistance and motoneurone discharge. J. Physiol. (London) **231:** 417–438.
41. JAMMES, Y., A. DAVIES & J. G. WIDDICOMBE. 1985. Tracheobronchial and laryngeal responses to hypercapnia, histamine and capsaicin in dogs. Clin. Respir. Physiol. **21:** 515–520.
42. AGGUGINI, G., M. G. CLEMENT & J. G. WIDDICOMBE. 1987. Lung reflexes affecting the larynx in the pig, and the effect of pulmonary microembolism. Q.J. Exp. Physiol. **72:** 95–104.

Airway Reflexes and the Control of Breathing in Postnatal Life[a]

P. JOHNSON

Nuffield Department of Obstetrics and Gynaecology
John Radcliffe Hospital
Headington, Oxford OX3 9DU
United Kingdom

Attempts to determine the cause of Sudden Infant Death Syndrome (SIDS) identified a hiatus in developmental physiology, both in man and animals. For example, the investigation of factors that could cause or underlie SIDS must take into account the observation that the incidence of all infant deaths, including most of those with explained causation (e.g., pneumonia, but excluding prematurity and some lethal congenital malformations), peaks between 2 and 4 months of age,[1,2] very close to the time of peak incidence claimed as unique for SIDS. It follows that a search for a cause for SIDS based on abnormality of respiratory control must also consider this postneonatal phase of development.

Until recently, concepts of cardiorespiratory control in the newborn were largely derived from studies either in the preterm human infant or in anesthetized newborn animals. These studies led to the superficially plausible but erroneous "apnea hypothesis,"[3] which in turn led to management (e.g., apnea monitors) and therapy (e.g., theophyline[4], usually applied to preterm infants with apnea. Neither the physiological concept nor the techniques applied to monitoring considered that cardiorespiratory failure was unlikely to be limited to, or indeed, was unlikely to be, central apnea. Obstructive apnea, hypoventilation or incoordination of cardiorespiratory function (e.g., temperature control) was not considered. Modulation or alteration of central thresholds such as arousal mechanisms was confused with changes in behavioral state, especially REM sleep—which was itself considered a vulnerable state because of "depressed" hypoxic and vagal reflexes.[5]

Physiological evidence for a multiphase postnatal development of cardiorespiratory function has been advanced previously.[6] The initial, and major, factor in this sequence is a large increase in both basal and actual metabolic rate which occurs soon after birth.[7] While this has been linked to thyroid function and has been shown to be essential for achievement of effective thermoregulation, thus ensuring immediate survival,[8] the longer-term effects on cardiorespiratory control have not been seriously considered. The inactivity of arterial chemoreceptors in early neonatal life[9] lends support to the view that nonchemoreceptor control of ventilation must sustain breathing during at least this period. An increasing dependance on mechanosensory (vagal) respiratory reflexes and chemical control of breathing with increasing postneonatal age has been suggested by earlier studies.[10] Yet the pursuit of mechanisms to explain the so-called biphasic ventilatory response to hypoxia, considered a characteristic of the newborn, still continues to focus on chemoreceptor function while disregarding major changes in metabolism. This paper summarizes recent work aimed at establishing the link between metabolic rate, thermoregulation, and effective breathing during postneonatal life. While emphasis is given to

[a]This work was funded in part by the Foundation for the Study of Infant Deaths.

262

airway reflexes during development, these observations are related to those studies which consider changes in homeostatic control close to the range of conditions operant during postneonatal development.

The winter prevalence for SIDS in temperate climates has led to the speculation that either cold or infection may play a role. The possibility that heat stress from overheating of infants in the cold weather could be a factor has been raised and was the subject of a study of infants observed at 27°C and 33°C.[11] It was hypothesized that apnea would occur at the higher temperature, as had been observed when preterm infants were "overheated" in early servoincubaters with unlimited upper temperatures, but the conditions used in this study failed to produce apnea. In addition, the investigators failed to appreciate that the higher ambient temperature used by them was actually within the thermoneutral range for newborn infants and that most newborns live below thermoneutrality. A notable response of tachypnea was, however, observed in the thermoneutral range.

So, before considering the role of respiratory reflexes, our recent studies in lambs[12,13] have followed the strategy of defining thermoneutrality and then testing close to the upper and lower temperature limits of comfort in order to determine what changes of the mechanisms directly involved in homeostasis occur with increasing age. Thus, the sequence of first-order adjustments, that is, making adaptive changes close to the zone of comfort, needs to be defined before any conclusions about a potential for developmental vulnerability can be made.

THERMONEUTRALITY

Thermoneutrality is usually defined as the ambient temperature at which metabolism is minimal while maintaining a normal body temperature. Although behavioral criteria are only sometimes considered, such factors as the stage of development at birth (e.g., whether altricial or precocial) and whether the species is polytocous or not are critical. In our studies, lambs reared in a comfortable environment (T_a, 16–20° C) on an *ad lib.* artificial milk supply were put at an ambient temperature (T_a) which was increased in 5° C steps of about 2 hr each from 0° C to 30° C. The requirement was that they should achieve sleep for a period of 30 min, so that we could measure at each temperature step the values during sleep for oxygen consumption, carbon dioxide production, heart rate, breathing frequency, amplitude and pattern—particularly the presence or absence of expiratory resistance to airflow (seen as prolonged chest or abdomen distension during the postinspiratory pause on the inductance plethysmograph signals)—and obtain arterial blood samples for Po_2, Pco_2, pH, T_3, T_4, cortisol, glucose, and NEFA (nonesterified fatty acids). This test was repeated for each animal at 4, 14, 30, 45, and, sometimes, 55 days of age.

The upper critical temperature (UCT), which was readily identified, was defined as the onset of sustained panting (breathing frequency above 150 per min with the mouth open), indicative of thermolysis. Most lambs still appeared to sleep at this point. Slow wave sleep (SWS), which is the predominant pattern of sleep, accounts for approximately 40% of total sleep time and occurs in 20 min episodes, whereas REM sleep is less than 10% of the total and occurs in episodes of 5 min or less (unpublished data). Thus, our studies were confined to SWS for this analysis. It was noticeable, however, that REM sleep episodes seemed to be longer and more plentiful close to the UCT.

The lower critical temperature (LCT) was defined as that T_a at which oxygen consumption rose above basal levels or shivering occurred. In this regard, the pattern of response during the progression from neonatal life was clearly from non-shivering (NST) to shivering thermogenesis (ST), with no loss in body temperature or obvious arousal.

Although both these responses were achieved during sleep, sleep onset was often longer in the cool environment and REM sleep was reduced, probably because it occurred for briefer intervals. Thus, although the protocol we used did not allow detailed analysis of sleep state effects of T_a close to the comfort range, there were neurobehavioral affects. The chamber used for these studies probably prevented the lambs from adopting any favorable thermoadaptive postural positions, in that they could not curl up.

The thermoneutral zone defined by these limits is shown in FIGURE 1. Although a postneonatal shift from NST to ST to meet thermogenic demand has been described for a number of species, it was notable in the studies described here that after 14 days of age (8/9 lambs at 14 days and 9/9 at 30 days), shivering occurred without any increase in V_{O_2} (oxygen consumption) above basal levels (FIGURE 1). Thus, a behavioral response (shivering) became the first response to temperature control outside thermoneutrality, with no other evidence of NST (i.e., no thyroid or metabolic response). However, it should be recalled that a decrease in the length of REM periods was also apparent as the LCT was approached. Thus, behavioral adaption, well described in the form of body posturing in the human infant, clustering in the litter or nesting species, and infant-maternal approximation in singleton species (the lamb lies against the rumen, 40° C, of the ewe in a cool environment), is closely linked to homeostatic control mechanisms.

In these studies, basal body temperature at thermoneutrality was observed to rise with postnatal age and may be a function of the increased basal metabolic rate and/or thyroid function, or the sequence in which the T_a was altered (i.e. starting from 5° C rather than 30° C would usually invoke thermogenesis in the younger lambs). However, the former explanation is favored because resting rectal temperatures in these lambs before study also increased with age. The rectal temperatures rose further when the lambs were either above or below thermoneutrality, except at 45 days of age, when thermal efficiency had developed so that the LCT exceeded our testing range, i.e., was below 5° C. Thus, despite having large effects on respiratory function, thermolysis, as well as thermogenesis, was relatively poorly developed and led to an increase in body temperature as part of the adaptive response. Thermovasomotor responses were not studied in these experiments.

Respiration and Thermoneutrality

Both breathing frequency and heart rate rose with postnatal age, although the effect on breathing frequency was most marked within the thermoneutral range in the young lamb.[13] Thus, although it is clear that cardiorespiratory performance is an integrated function in metabolic control, the respiratory system becomes involved in a greater variety of strategies to meet homeostatic needs as thermal efficiency matures.

We have previously demonstrated the mechanisms and importance of expiratory and "auxillary" inspiratory muscles in optimizing and regulating the respiratory cycle to meet ventilatory demands in health[14,15] and disease.[16] When this demand (i.e., the tonic sensory input) is high, usually breathing frequency or amplitude is such that there is little passive expiratory time for lung collapse (due to a soft chest wall) to occur. Either high-frequency, low-amplitude breathing (thermolysis) or low-frequency, high-amplitude breathing (thermogenesis) will meet this requirement. If, however, metabolic demand is minimal (i.e., outside the postnatal period where basal and actual metabolic rate is at its highest) and expiratory time is lengthened, the upper airway constrictor muscles are recruited, mainly by vagal afferents, to retard expiratory airflow. This not only maintains lung volume, but generates positive expiratory pressure during expiration. This generation of positive pressure is achieved either by elastic recoil of the chest or abdomen, which compresses the inspiratory lung volume against a closed or restricted outlet, or by the activation of expiratory forcing muscles, e.g., abdominal muscles, to empty the lung at

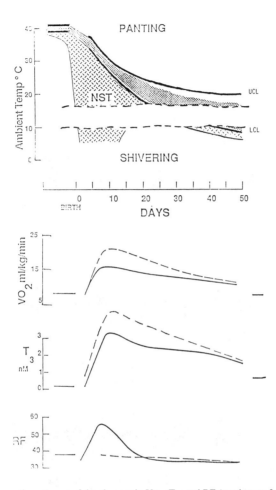

FIGURE 1. Schematic summary of the changes in V_{O_2}, T_3, and RF (respiratory frequency) related to the thermoneutral range (**upper panel**) in the lamb. Thermoneutrality (**dark hatched area**) is defined by the upper critical limit (UCL) of ambient temperature (T_a), where panting (thermolysis) is initiated, and the lower critical limit (LCL), where either an increase in V_{O_2} (non-shivering thermogenesis, NST: **light hatched area**) or shivering thermogenesis occurs (**upper panel**). The fall and widening in both these limits with increasing postnatal age is seen. The non-hatched area below the UCL starting at 14 days of age indicates the T_a in which dysrhythmic breathing occurs when the upper airway is bypassed. The **solid lines** (three **lower panels**) represent measurements at thermoneutrality; fetal (*far left*) and adult (*far right*) values are also shown. There is a large rise in all these variables, with a closely related time course. There was a similar rise in heart rate (not shown). Body temperature rose by 14 days of age to be significantly above that in fetal or adult life (not shown). The **broken lines** (three **lower panels**) represent the actual levels of these variables in a lamb living in a T_a of 15–20° C (comfortable) and clearly show that initially, at early postnatal ages, this T_a reflects a cool stimulus to metabolic rate, T_3, and respiratory frequency (which falls), while tidal volume and minute volume (not shown) increase to meet increased metabolism. Body temperature rose on cooling at all ages and also on warming above thermoneutrality (thermolysis), except at 45 days of age. This suggests that thermal efficiency is slow to develop, particularly for thermolysis.

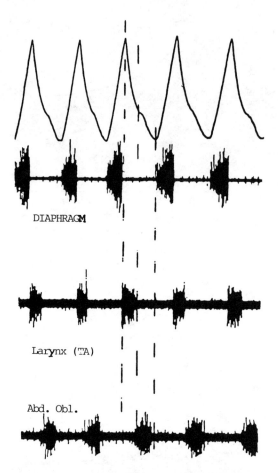

FIGURE 2. Respiratory muscle EMG activity during slow wave sleep in a healthy, 15-day-old lamb. The **upper trace** is the "sum" signal from inductance plethysmography (up is inspiration). The vertical black lines indicate the phases of expiration. As diaphragm activity (**second trace**) ceases (note there is no postinspiratory activity) the larynx (**third trace**) constricts during the first half of expiration, but ceases to do so as the abdominal oblique (Abd. Obl., **bottom trace**) becomes active and forces expiration during the latter half of expiration.

end-expiration (FIG. 2) or to force air through the glottis (when large distending pressures can be applied, perhaps to fluid-filled airways or non-uniformly expanded areas of lung).[16] In a previous series of experiments, hypoxia, which induces retarded expiratory airflow, increased the likelihood of overt respiratory failure if the upper airway was also bypassed, (i.e., functionally inactivated) between 2 and 5 weeks of postnatal age.[15] In our present studies, we have confirmed that the importance of these vagal mechanosensory mechanisms in ensuring rhythmic breathing is most obvious in the postneonatal period occurring *after* the basal metabolic rate has started to fall for T_a in the upper ranges of thermoneutrality. What was notable was that the respiratory dysrhythmia that occurred when the upper airway was bypassed, without significant change in arterial oxygen or carbon dioxide concentrations, was usually periodic with a frequency of 5–6 cycles per min. The metabolic rate was also lower in those animals that exhibited this periodic breathing. The possible relevance of these features will be discussed later.

Thyroid Function and Thermoneutrality

The basal levels of plasma triiodothyromine (T_3), as well as the short-term changes in response to cooling, decreased with postnatal age. These results taken together suggested that thyroid activity was directly involved in the regulation of basal metabolic rate as well as NST in early postnatal life.[12] There were no short-term changes in plasma cortisol, glucose or NEFA, although they decreased with age.

AIRWAY DEFENSE MECHANISMS

Most mammals tested[17] have powerful chemo- and mechanosensory receptor afferent pathways in the airways. The lamb, cat, monkey, and man have a concentration of taste-bud-like chemoreceptors greater than that seen on the tongue in the mucosa at the entrance to the larynx.[18] Although nasopharyngeal chemoreceptors also exist, stimulation of the laryngeal sensory pathways produces powerful arousal, swallowing, respiratory (apnea) and cardiovascular responses.[19] If the arousal responses and swallowing prove ineffective in clearing any offending material, apnea and bradycardia persist, often to profound hypoxia. However, hypertension and a redistribution of cardiac output, increasing the output to the central nervous system and heart and decreasing it to all other organs, (i.e., the diving response) occurs. In terms of defectiveness of function during sleep, as is claimed for some other responses during REM sleep,[5] it is important to realize that immediate arousal occurs in either sleep state if as little as 1 ml of water (but not warm saline) is applied to the aryepiglottic area. Under sedation or anesthesia, quite a different response is observed (FIG. 3). There is no initial arousal and swallowing is depressed. Apnea, bradycardia, hypertension, an increase in carotid blood flow, and a fall in abdominal aortic blood flow continue until the inhibitory fluid (water) is removed by saline. Recovery is almost instantaneous. In FIGURE 4, three sequences demonstrate the

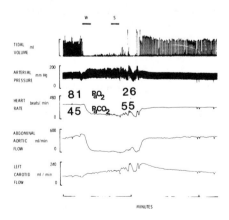

FIGURE 3. Effect of anesthesia on airway defense mechanisms. A record from a lamb under light urethane anesthesia, breathing spontaneously on air via a tracheostomy tube connected to a pneumotachograph (**top panel**). W indicates the point when water was applied to the mucosa of the laryngeal additus and immediate apnea occurred. Hypertension, bradycardia, a fall in aortic and an increase in carotid blood flow occurred (four **lower panels**). Pa_{O_2} fell from 81 to 26 mm Hg and Pa_{CO_2} rose from 44 to 55 mm Hg after 1 min of apnea (**center panel**). S (**top panel**) was the point at which saline was used to remove the water, and the onset of respiration followed with the rapid restoration of cardiorespiratory status.

effects of initiating apnea with the lamb initially hyperoxic, then normoxic, and, finally, hypoxic. The interaction between hypoxia and vagally mediated bradycardia can be distinguished in this way. Although hypoxia clearly contributes to the onset and degree of bradycardia, the major effect on heart rate is a vagally mediated, nonhypoxic bradycardia and hypertension. The changes in blood flow to specific organs during apnea (TABLE 1) confirm that the changes occurring in the ascending and descending aorta reflect these regional adaptive changes in blood supply. Absolute blood flow increased over twofold to the central nervous system and 60% to the myocardium, while cardiac output fell to 75% of control during hypoxic apnea. Undoubtedly, the sympathetically initiated vasoconstriction and hypertension contribute to this effect, partially as a result of baroreceptor stimulation. Combined and sympathetic blockade abolished nearly all these

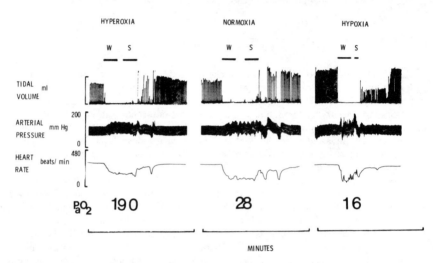

FIGURE 4. Effects of initiating apnea in a lamb initially hyperoxic (**left**), normoxic (**center**), or hypoxic (**right**). The cardiorespiratory sequence if a procedure similar to that in FIGURE 3 was performed when the lamb was initially hyperoxic (Pao$_2$, 190 mm Hg after 1 min of apnea), normoxic (Pao$_2$, 28 mm Hg after 1 min of apnea), or hypoxic (Pao$_2$, 16 mm Hg after 1 min of apnea). The magnitude and rapidity of the bradycardic response relates to the degree of hypoxia, although clearly the major effect was caused by stimulation of vagal afferents of the laryngeal mucosa. The inhibition overrides the hypoxic stimulus to respiration most obvious in the **right panel.**

adaptive responses (FIG. 5). These are classic, vagally mediated apneic responses, enhanced by hypoxia, in contrast to nonapneic responses, in which the hypoxic-induced hyperventilation stimulates heart rate, thus over-riding the hypoxic, carotid body-initiated bradycardia.[20] The intact diving response, with its ability to centralize the circulation, can mean a twofold conservation of oxygen stores.[21] Poor cardiac output or "fatigue" of the system by recurrent hypoxia can prevent this response and result in deterioration, although often with innocuous changes in heart rate.

Judging from experience with the preterm infant, bradycardia occurring without apnea is to be considered sinister. It may have at least two quite different causes. It may be due to obstructive apnea, where intrathoracic pressure or stretch receptors are triggered by large negative pressures. It may alternatively be due to airway vagal inhibitory reflexes

TABLE 1. Organ Blood Flow in Newborn Lambs Before and During Laryngeal Water-Induced Apnea When Hypoxia Occurred (Normoxia) and When Hypoxia was Prevented by the Prior Inhalation of Oxygen (Hyperoxia)

	Spontaneous Breathing[a]		Apnea[a]		
	Mean	SE	Mean	SE	Paired T Test
Normoxia[b]					
Head	24.5	4.1	41	7.6	$p < 0.005$
Brain	64	15.7	132	17.1	$p < 0.05$
Heart	200	44.8	325.5	54.6	$p < 0.005$
Small gut	160	24.7	46	7.8	$p < 0.005$
Kidneys	324	26.4	232	38.2	$p < 0.005$
Hyperoxia[c]					
Head	27	2.2	31	3.7	NS
Brain	60	8.3	80	12.7	NS
Heart	175	28.4	137	27.3	NS
Small gut	143	20.4	45	4.3	$p < 0.005$
Kidneys	353	47.3	307	60.4	NS

[a]ml/min/100g.
[b]$n = 8$.
[c]$n = 5$.

insufficient to inhibit breathing or to hypoxia which fails to stimulate vigorous breathing. In FIGURE 6 this former mechanism is tested by maintaining positive pressure ventilation at low tidal volume (FIG. 6a) or at increased tidal volume (FIG. 6b) during water-induced laryngeal apnea, and the latter mechanism is tested in FIGURE 6c. This demonstrates that airway afferent vagal input can be minimal, but still able to maintain ventilation, and fail to inhibit vagal and/or hypoxic-induced bradycardia. Vagal excitatory and inhibitory reflexes usually act, often in opposition, to produce the appropriate adaptive responses.

When these kind of studies were conducted in lambs of increasing age, it was found that prolonged central apnea, even when arousal and swallowing were abolished by anesthesia, only occurred in lambs less than 24 hr old. After that, breathing activity gradually broke through the central inhibition of breathing as asphyxia developed. It is

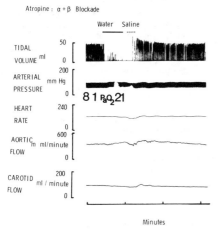

FIGURE 5. Recordings for a procedure similar to that described in FIGURE 3 performed on a lamb atropinized and under α- and β-sympathetic blockade. Hardly any adaptive changes took place during hypoxia, which occurred more rapidly (Pao$_2$, 21 mm Hg within 45 sec of apnea[21]).

worth noting that this form of apnea would be called central apnea, yet the airway is closed in response to a peripheral stimulus. Concomitant events such as hypoglycemia alter this ability to overcome inhibition of breathing and asphyxia could result. The potency and importance of arousal in response to upper airway stimulation cannot be overemphasized.

Although there is some evidence that irritant receptors can change from initiating apnea in the preterm infant to causing tachypnea in the full-term infant,[22] it is generally assumed that the role of inhibitory airway vagal reflexes decreases rapidly after birth.[23] This assumption is based on testing only one element of the Hering-Breuer tetrad of

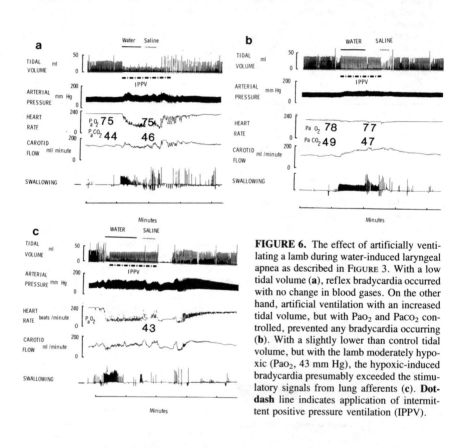

FIGURE 6. The effect of artificially ventilating a lamb during water-induced laryngeal apnea as described in FIGURE 3. With a low tidal volume (a), reflex bradycardia occurred with no change in blood gases. On the other hand, artificial ventilation with an increased tidal volume, but with Pao_2 and $Paco_2$ controlled, prevented any bradycardia occurring (b). With a slightly lower than control tidal volume, but with the lamb moderately hypoxic (Pao_2, 43 mm Hg), the hypoxic-induced bradycardia presumably exceeded the stimulatory signals from lung afferents (c). Dot-dash line indicates application of intermittent positive pressure ventilation (IPPV).

reflexes, namely, inflation apnea, and ignoring, in particular, the expiratory muscle activity invoked by applying or sustaining inflationary pressures.[24] Seemingly, expiration is regarded as passive, relying substantially on elastic recoil to restore the respiratory apparatus to its inspiratory starting position. Interest has focused on on-and-off-switch mechanisms governing inspiration, with little attention given to neural thresholds during expiration as possible determinants of inspiratory timing and, thus, rhythmogenesis. Our evidence in unanesthetized lambs and infants, using noninvasive measurements and intact upper airways, strongly refutes this view. Indeed, in the older lamb, where the basal metabolic rate is lower, the simple lack of an intact upper airway to enable the generation of expiratory pressure leads to prolonged expiration and, often, periodic apnea. Thus, the tonic drive from the high metabolic rate, mainly needed to meet thermogenesis, is progressively replaced by an expiratory positive pressure-induced tonic drive to breathing, before the chest wall becomes stabilized (ossification) with increasing age. Experimental studies in mature anesthetized animals such as those studies discussed in the paper by Widdicombe (this volume) have the limitation of investigating inspiratory control in isolation from expiratory muscle control, which is particularly susceptible to anesthetic effects.

Thus, our strategy has been to determine the developmental changes close to the operant range of conditions for the intact, unanesthetized animal before attempting to determine the role of reflex mechanisms that could be lethal.

HUMAN STUDIES

Studies on the full-term human infant, as a prelude to similar longitudinal studies on the development of thermoregulation and respiratory control in infants, have addressed the question of hypoxia at thermoneutrality[25] (before the peripheral arterial chemoreceptors could be expected to be fully active during air breathing[9]) and the relationship between metabolic rate and ambient temperature.[26]

Hypoxia at Thermoneutrality

In this study[25] it was found that 3-day-old infants placed in an incubator at 33° C (after residing in a ward at 27° C) responded to 15% hypoxia with an immediate fall in minute ventilation, which was sustained for the 10-min period with no increase in arterial carbon dioxide. There was therefore no biphasic ventilatory response but probably a decrease in basal metabolic rate. The majority of infants retarded expiratory airflow (REA) as they reduced breathing frequency in response to hypoxia (a so-called subclinical grunt). A minority, however, developed periodic breathing (PB), usually after a sigh. This latter group of infants were clearly different, even when breathing air, in that they had evidence of reduced ventilatory drive (lower Pao_2, lower minute ventilation (MV), and higher CO_2), which remained lower during hypoxia than in the former (REA) group. Despite having a lower Pao_2, they did not arouse; whereas the REA infants did, often more than once. The interesting feature was that the periodicity of periodic breathing during hypoxia was similar to the periodic oscillation in tidal volume observed in all the infants while air-breathing, regardless of sleep state. Attention to this similarity with the intrinsic variation in breathing pattern has been made before,[27] but convention has attributed it to feedback from an under- or over-damped chemoreceptor-induced oscillation. This oscillatory period coincides with thermovasomotor oscillations in skin perfusion which are often reflected in the heart rate pattern. Thus, a direct, higher central nervous system link between temperature control, metabolism, and cardiorespiratory control is indicated.

Although there were sleep state-related differences in both resting and hypoxic cardiorespiratory patterns, (e.g., MV and O_2 and CO_2 levels) the magnitude of the changes with hypoxia was not altered by sleep state.

Ambient Temperature, Metabolic Rate and Sleep State

In another group of full-term infants, the metabolic rate (Vo_2 and Vco_2) was measured at 27° C and 18° C. It was found that, in contrast to lambs[12] and cats[28], metabolic rate increased in REM sleep and that REM cycles tended to increase in length with decreasing T_a.[26] The former observation has been reported before[29] but the latter one is novel. Thus, the optimal sleep state for initiating a thermogenic response (primarily NST) was selected, presumably centrally, for the human infant, just as had occurred in the lamb, though with the opposite resulting preference in sleep state. It was also notable that increased body movements occurred in SWS; thus, behavioral activities to increase heat production (or loss) are also activated within the comfort zone.

There were no changes in body temperature in either of these studies, so the comfort zone was apparently not greatly exceeded by these tests.

These preliminary results, though testing short-term changes from a control state which was itself of relatively short duration, suggests that sleep state is another physiological behavior which is regulated in the process of temperature control.

DISCUSSION

Thus, although both long- and short-term studies of the changes at different postnatal ages are still needed, there is a basis for concluding that ambient temperature is closely linked to metabolic rate, especially in early postnatal life when the basal metabolic rate is high and provides an important tonic sensory input that directly influences the stability of breathing. A key to this tonic state, or threshold, is the degree of oscillation between .07 and 0.08 Hz. Changes in the amplitude and/or frequency of breathing can occur; either or both may be prominent. On the one hand, a barely perceptible oscillation under maximal drive can occur; on the other hand, periodic breathing, or apnea, can occur. This is the same oscillatory period that occurs in thermovasomotor oscillations and is normally seen as a peak in the power spectral analysis of the heart rate. The obvious coincidence in timing of these cardiac and respiratory patterns probably indicates the level (and thus potency) of thermal tonic sensory input. However, the maturation of vasomotor control of the peripheral circulation, and thus the ability of the circulatory system to lose or gain heat in the course of temperature regulation, is little known.[30]

Recently it has been shown that the ventilatory response to hypoxia in kittens, tested at or close to thermoneutrality, increases in parallel with increasing thermal efficiency over the first six weeks of life.[31] It was suggested that maturation of the carotid chemoreceptor pathway played a critical role in this sequence, because carotid body denervation in adult cats led to a fall in body temperature during hypoxia.[32] However, in the kittens, the addition of carbon dioxide during hypoxia substantially decreased the fall in body temperature, just as it had prevented respiratory failure during hypoxia in postneonatal lambs lacking upper airway control.[10] Although the Po_2 may not have fallen as low in this case as during hypoxia alone, it does seem that adding CO_2 would mimic an increase in metabolism, would be sensed as such, and would prevent heat-loosing responses from occurring.

The carotid body has been implicated in arousal during hypoxia,[33] though central mechanisms have been demonstrated.[34] Three-day-old infants who were breathing regularly aroused without a ventilatory response to hypoxia, but those with lower Po_2 who were breathing periodically did not.

The question of whether chemoreception or thermometabolism regulates breathing is important. Despite direct measurement of carotid sinus "chemoreceptor activity" in response to changes in O_2, and the change in threshold for O_2 tension described with increasing postnatal age,[9] the interaction with CO_2 appears to have been overlooked. For example, the ventilatory response to carbon dioxide is brisk and quantitatively similar to adult levels (indeed, some say greater) from birth. Yet basal levels of CO_2 are lower than in fetal life (the converse to O_2). Central and peripheral effects of CO_2, as also for O_2, are difficult to separate in the intact mammal.

Arousal of the central nervous system is a vital defense mechanism and is unlikely to be solely dependent on one pathway, namely, the carotid body. The threshold for arousal could also depend on the level of tonic input to the central nervous system, upon which respiratory rhythmogenesis during early postnatal life is also contended to depend. While we observed arousal to modest hypoxia and cooling when the tonic input was high, it was seldom observed during the onset of thermolysis. While this fits with a decreased tonic sensory input, it has to be set against the fact that the neonate, if given the option, chooses a high environmental temperature within the thermoneutral range.[35] Yet, one conclusion we came to is that thermoneutrality, though energetically optimal, may not be optimal for activating those mechanisms that maintain homeostasis, especially during sleep.

Although it has been known that cooling abolishes REM sleep, and although cooling is used for sleep deprivation studies in cats, it has been assumed that REM is a poikilothermic state.[28] Whether it is poikilothermic in some species, it is not in man, and the important issue seems to be that switching to the optimal sleep state, or behavior, is an integral part of temperature regulation *within* the comfort range.

In conclusion, it is impressive that neurobehavioral responses, including the organization of sleep state, appear closely linked to thermometabolic homeostatic mechanisms, even close to thermoneutrality. This relationship continues during major changes in the underlying regulatory processes (e.g., NST to ST) that occur with age. Thyroid function seems critical both in basal and short term adjustments to small changes in ambient temperature. Nonetheless, such factors as nutritional deprivation,[36] chronic hypoxia, and hostile environments before and after birth greater affect the time course of postnatal thermometabolic development.

Vagal reflexes tend to be considered inhibitory, and powerful upper airway inhibitory chemoreflexes have been described here which are a universal feature of mammalian defense mechanisms. They are inhibitory in order to be defensive; whether they can trigger damaging or fatal apnea normally in the intact animal is doubtful. Anesthesia, drugs, infection, or defective neural development, however, could conceivably convert a defensive response into a prolonged, unterminated one. On the other hand, airway mechanosensory reflexes acting in an important stimulatory or tonic role to ensure rhythmogenesis in the postneonatal period (as metabolic rate falls and, with it, respiratory frequency and heart rate), have not been actively considered before. The emphasis of this concept is on neural events in the expiratory phase of breathing and the recognition that mechanisms such as grunting are physiological, and not pathological, reflexes.[16] Infections or previous trauma (such as high-pressure artificial ventilation in the preterm infant) might damage or inactivate airway receptors and prevent their functioning in potentially pathological conditions. The implications for the development of respiratory control and abnormal airway reflex responses, and appropriate methods for testing them, are obvious.

REFERENCES

1. MINISTRY OF HEALTH. HMSO Publication No. 011321 0329. HMSO. London.
2. NORVENIUS, S. G. 1987. Sudden Infant Death Syndrome in Sweden. Acta Paediatr. Scand. **(Suppl):** 333.
3. STEINSCHNEIDER, A. 1972. Prolonged apnea and the sudden infant death syndrome: Clinical and laboratory observations. Pediatrics **50:** 646.
4. HUNT, C. E., R. T. BROUILLETTE & D. HANSON. 1983. Theophylline improves pneugram abnormalities in infants at risk for sudden infant death syndrome. J. Pediatr. **103:** 969–974.

5. HENDERSON-SMART, D. J. & D. J. C. READ. 1979. Reduced lung volume during behavioral active sleep in the newborn. J. Appl. Physiol. **46:** 1081–1085.
6. JOHNSON, P. 1985. The development of breathing. *In* The Physiological Development of the Fetus and Newborn. C. T. Jones, Ed.: 201–210. Academic Press. New York.
7. DAWES, G. S. & J. C. MOTT. 1959. The three-fold rise in metabolic rate in newborn lambs. J. Physiol. (London) **146:** 294–315.
8. BREALL, J. A., A. M. RUDOLPH & M. A. HEYMANN. 1983. Role of thyroid hormone in postnatal circulatory and metabolic adjustments. J. Clin. Invest. **73:** 1418–1424.
9. BLANCO, C. E., G. S. DAWES, M. A. HANSON & H. B. McCOOKE. 1984. The arterial chemoreceptors in fetal sheep and newborn lambs. J. Physiol. (London) **351:** 25–38.
10. FEWELL, J. E. & P. JOHNSON. 1981. The role of the larynx on the regulation of breathing during hypoxia in sleeping lambs. J. Physiol. (London) **320:** 57P.
11. STEINSCHNEIDER, A. & S. WEINSTEIN. 1983. Sleep respiratory instability in term neonates under hyperthermic conditions. Pediatr. Res. **17:** 35–41.
12. SYMONDS, M. E., D. C. ANDREWS, K. P. MAGEE & P. JOHNSON. The effect of ambient temperature on oxygen consumption and plasma triiodothyronine concentration in the developing lamb. *In* Fetal and Neonatal Development. C. T. Jones, Ed. Perinatology Press. In press.
13. ANDREWS, D. C., M. E. SYMONDS, K. P. MAGEE & P. JOHNSON. Respiratory rhythm and thermogenesis in the developing lamb. *In* Fetal and Neonatal Development. C. T. Jones, Ed. Perinatology Press. In press.
14. HARDING, R., P. JOHNSON & M. E. McCLELLAND. 1980. The expiratory role of the larynx during development and the influence of behavioural states. Respir. Physiol. **40:** 165–180.
15. HENDERSON-SMART, D. J., P. JOHNSON & M. E. McCLELLAND. 1982. Asynchronous respiratory activity of the diaphragm during spontaneous breathing in the lamb. J. Physiol. (London) **327:** 377–386.
16. JOHNSON, P. 1985. Prolonged expiratory apnoea and implications for control of breathing. Lancet **(Oct):** 877–879.
17. JOHNSON, P., D. M. SALISBURY & A. T. STOREY. 1975. Apnoea induced by stimulation of sensory receptors in the larynx. *In* Development of Upper Respiratory Anatomy and Function. J. F. Bosma & J. Showacre, Ed.: 160–178. United States Department of Health, Education and Welfare. Washington, D.C.
18. HARDING, R., P. JOHNSON & M. E. McCLELLAND. 1978. Liquid sensitive laryngeal receptors in the developing sheep, cat, and monkey. J. Physiol. (London) **277:** 409–422.
19. HARDING, R., P. JOHNSON, B. E. JOHNSTON, M. E. McCLELLAND & A. R. WILKINSON. 1976. Cardiovascular changes in newborn lambs during apnea induced by stimulation of laryngeal receptors with water. J. Physiol. (London) **256:** 35–36.
20. DE BURGH DALY, M. 1972. Interaction of cardiovascular reflexes. Sci. Basis Med. Annu. Rev. 307–332.
21. BUTLER, P. J. & D. R. JONES. 1971. The effect of variations in heart rate and regional distribution of blood flow on the normal pressor response to diving in ducks. J. Physiol. (London) **214:** 457–479.
22. FLEMING, P. J., A. C. BRYAN & H. E. BRYAN. 1978. Functional Immaturity of pulmonary irritant receptors and apnea in newborn preterm infants. Pediatrics **61:** 515–518.
23. CROSS, K. W., M. KLAUS, W. H. TOOLEY & K. WEISSER. 1960. The response of the newborn baby to inflation of the lungs. J. Physiol. (London) **151:** 551–565.
24. HERING, E. & J. BREUER. 1868. Die selbsteunung der athonung durch das nervus vagus. Sitz. Ungsber. Dtsch. Akad. Wiss. Wien **2(57):** 672–677.
25. ANDERSSON, D., A. SJOSTROM, G. GENNSER & P. JOHNSON. The effect of hypoxia and hyperoxia on breathing and ventilation in newborn infants during sleep. J. Develop. Physiol. In press.
26. FLEMING, P. J., M. R. LEVINE, Y. AZAZ & P. JOHNSON. The effect of sleep state on the metabolic response to cold stress in newborn infants. *In* Fetal and Neonatal Development. C. T. Jones, Ed. Perinatology Press. In press.
27. FINLEY, J. P. & S. T. NUGENT. 1983. Periodicities in respiration and heart rate in newborns. Can. J. Physiol. Pharmacol. **61:** 329–335.
28. PARMEGGIANI, P. L. 1979. Integrative aspects of hypothalmic influences on respiratory brain

stem mechanisms during wakefulness and sleep. *In* Central Nervous Control Mechanisms in Breathing. C. von Euler & H. Lagercrantz, Eds.: 53–60. Permagon Press. Oxford.

29. STOTHERS, J. K. & R. M. WARNER. 1978. Oxygen consumption and neonatal sleep state. J. Physiol. (London) **278:** 435–440.

30. OLUNSTEAD, C. H. E., J. R. VILLABLANCA, M. TARBINER & D. RHODES. 1979. Development of thermoregulation in the kitten. Physiol. Behav. **23:** 489–495.

31. BONORA, M. & H. GAUTIER. 1987. Maturational changes in body temperature and ventilation during hypoxia in kittens. Respir. Physiol. **68:** 359–370.

32. GAUTIER, H., M. BONORA, S. A. SCHULTZ & J. E. REMMERS. 1988. Hypoxic-induced changes in shivering and body temperature. J. Appl. Physiol. In press.

33. BOWES, G., E. R. TOWNSEND, L. F. KOZAR, S. M. BROMLEY & E. A. PHILLIPSON. 1981. Effect of carotid body temperature denervation on arousal response to hypoxia in sleeping dogs. J. Appl. Physiol. **51:** 70–75.

34. NEUBAUER, J. A., T. V. SANTIAGO & N. H. EDELMAN. 1981. Hypoxia arousal in intact and carotid chemodenervated cats. J. App. Physiol. **51(5):** 1294–1299.

35. HULL, J. & D. HULL. 1982. Behavioural thermoregulation in newborn rabbits. J. Comp. Physiol. Psychol. **96:** 143–147.

36. CONRADI, N. G., K. MUNTZING, P. SOURANDER & A. HAMBERGER. 1984. Effect of ambient temperature on rectal temperature in normal and malnourished rats during early postnatal development. Acta. Physiol. Scand. **121:** 147–153.

Chemical Control of Breathing in Early Life[a]

DAVID J. HENDERSON-SMART[b] AND GARY L. COHEN

Department of Perinatal Medicine
King George V Memorial Hospital
Sydney, Australia

INTRODUCTION

This review is mainly concerned with breathing responses to changing levels of oxygenation and acidosis (CO_2/pH). Emphasis is given to the major changes in chemical environment during the perinatal period and the effects that these and the concomitant central nervous system (CNS) development have on the integration of the chemical drives to breathe. Attention is drawn to the important interaction of breathing responses with other effects of chemostimulation on cardiac, CNS, and metabolic function. To facilitate understanding of the changes during development, current concepts of mature chemoreceptor physiology are briefly reviewed.

PHYSIOLOGY OF MATURE CHEMORECEPTOR RESPONSES

There is increasing evidence that chemoreceptors are essential for the maintenance of a normal breathing rhythm, particularly during sleep.[1] The traditional, general division of chemoreceptors into peripheral (arterial) oxygen sensors and central (medullary) CO_2 sensors is too simplistic and impedes the understanding of fetal and neonatal responses. Oxygen and CO_2 act both peripherally and centrally to alter breathing. A more useful concept is one in which peripheral receptors detect rapid changes in arterial blood gases (both O_2 and CO_2/pH) whereas central responses reflect slower (brain) tissue changes in O_2 supply and CO_2/pH. Although considerable advances in understanding have been made, there is still debate regarding the exact site of chemosensing within each tissue, the neurotransmitters involved, and the control of receptor sensitivity. For more detailed accounts, there are a number of excellent reviews[2-5] which should be consulted for additional references to the summary given below.

The Sensors

Arterial Chemoreceptors

The carotid bodies (CB), situated bilaterally at the bifurcations of the common carotid arteries, are the most important arterial chemoreceptors in humans. They have a dual role

[a]The authors' research program is supported by the National Health and Medical Research Council of Australia and the Australian Rotary Health Research Fund.
[b]To whom correspondence should be addressed at: Department of Perinatal Medicine, King George V Memorial Hospital, Missenden Road, Camperdown, NSW 2050 Australia.

in respiratory and cardiovascular control. The aortic bodies have chemoreceptor function in some animals, although their main role appears to be in cardiovascular regulation. In relation to their weight, the CB receive a large blood flow and have a very high rate of metabolism. The most abundant cell type in the CB is the glomus cell, which, together with the nerve endings of the glossopharyngeal afferents with which the glomus cells are in synaptic contact, probably makes up the chemotransducer for O_2 and CO_2. Glia-like sheath cells envelope the glomus cells. A small percentage of the endings on glomus cells are preganglionic nerves arising from the cervical sympathetic trunk. There is still argument as to whether there are glossopharyngeal efferents which might regulate receptor sensitivity. A more prevalent view is that receptor sensitivity is self-regulated by locally released neuromodulators and/or axon reflexes.[2]

Dopamine is the most abundant amine in the carotid body and is mainly synthesized and stored in the glomus cells. Smaller amounts of noradrenaline are present in both the glomus cells and sympathetic nerves. The turnover of these amines is rapid (1–2 hr), augmented by hypoxia, and probably dependent on afferent innervation. Smaller amounts of 5-hydroxytryptamine, met-enkephalin, substance P, neuropeptide Y, VIP (vasoactive intestinal polypeptide), and acetylcholine have also been found in the carotid body. The exact roles played in chemoreceptor function by these various substances, and neuro-modulators such as adenosine, are still debated.

Brainstem Chemoreceptors

For a long time it has been known that areas of the ventrolateral medulla are sensitive to changes in CO_2 and pH; this evidence has recently been reviewed.[2,5] However, there is still debate as to the precise site of chemoreception and whether the areas already defined are the only ones involved. Most workers agree that it is probably the hydrogen ion concentration, rather than CO_2 *per se,* that is the major stimulus,[2] although there is some evidence that CO_2 may have an effect independent of pH.[5]

Oxygen also acts centrally to influence breathing. This effect is seen in the normoxemic range and leads to a change in the intercept but not the slope of the CO_2 response, suggesting that direct hypoxic inhibition is not responsible.[6] The most likely explanation is that O_2 acts via an alteration of cerebral blood flow which then changes brain tissue CO_2. No specific site for the effects of central hypoxia has been found in adults, although this may not be so in the fetus (see below).

The Stimuli

Oxygen

In clinical medicine most emphasis is given to measuring Pao_2 as an indicator of adequate oxygenation of the organism overall. Yet oxygen supply to the tissues is much more dependent on the oxygen content of blood (Cao_2) and on blood flow. Chemoreceptor and other responses to changing oxygen levels, such as cerebral blood flow, show a hyperbolic relationship to Pao_2 but a more linear one to Cao_2. This suggests that it is the latter which is being measured. Arterial oxygen levels tend to change rapidly in response to variations in alveolar ventilation since body stores (mainly lungs and blood) are relatively small. This effect is even more pronounced in the newborn.[7]

Carbon Dioxide

There is increasing evidence that CO_2 effects are largely mediated via changes in pH.[2,5] Since the body stores of CO_2 are relatively large, tissue levels fluctuate more slowly. Arterial PCO_2 does change rapidly with variations in alveolar ventilation. With the slower breathing rates in adults, fluctuations with each breath have been estimated from pH measurements to be about 2–3 mm Hg.[4]

Oxygen/Carbon Dioxide Interaction

At the arterial chemoreceptors, a fall in O_2 and a rise in CO_2 act synergistically to augment breathing efforts. Centrally, these changes in O_2 and CO_2 tend to have opposing effects, possibly due to the cerebral vasodilator effect of hypoxia, which would lower brain tissue CO_2. Conversely, hyperoxia would have the opposite pattern of effects.

Physiological Effects of Chemoreceptor Stimulation

The effects of chemoreceptor stimulation due to a disturbance in blood or tissue gases depend on the magnitude of this stimulus in relation to other drives and priorities of the respiratory system. Much of the integration occurs in the brainstem, and this determines the level of drive to the various respiratory muscles. This activity is transmitted fully to the phrenic motor neurons, which have a predominantly respiratory input. Other motor neurons, such as the intercostals, have significant nonrespiratory excitatory and inhibitory inputs of central (e.g., reticular, vestibular and cerebellar) and spinal (e.g., proprioceptor) origin. Firing of these motor neurons depends on the magnitude of the respiratory drive as well as the balance of other inputs. Thus, a given output from the brainstem respiratory neurons will activate a variable set of muscles, depending on changing conditions such as behavioral state and posture, leading to variations in the way the respiratory pump achieves a desired ventilation. Some of these variations may be more efficient or stable than others. The situation is further complicated if there is an added load due to increased airways resistance or reduced compliance or if there are abnormalities in pulmonary perfusion. Consequently, in correcting an error in the levels of blood or tissue gases, there is a long and complicated route from chemoreceptor response to the modification of alveolar gas exchange. This has particular importance for the measurement of chemical responses, as discussed below.

Chemoreceptor stimulation also has nonrespiratory effects on the central nervous and cardiovascular systems. Arousal appears to be an important defense initiated by a decrease in oxygenation or an accumulation of CO_2. This CNS activation is reflected in excitation of many respiratory muscles, especially those with significant nonrespiratory inputs, such as upper airway, intercostal, and abdominal muscles. In adults, cortical arousal and voluntary activation of respiratory defenses may also be important. The arousal effects of chemostimulation appear to be largely dependent on the CB.[8]

Increased carotid body chemoreceptor afferent activity also enhances vasomotor output from the brainstem, including vagal slowing of heart rate and sympathetic peripheral vasoconstriction.[9] However, since this afferent activity also usually leads to activation of inspiratory neurons in the brainstem and more vigorous inflation of the lungs, both inhibitory to the cardiovascular effects mentioned above, the usual result is tachycardia. During apnea, when there is no inspiratory activity (central apnea) and/or when there is no lung inflation (obstructive apnea), vasomotor effects such as vagal bradycardia are revealed. Asphyxia during apnea thus activates an oxygen-conserving response which includes a reduction in cardiac output (work) via vagal bradycardia and redistribution of this reduced output to favor vital organs. Diving mammals have specialized in this chemoreceptor-augmented response,[10] and it may be particularly important in the fetus (see below). For further discussion of these cardiorespiratory interactions, see the paper by SPYER (this volume).

Measuring Responses

The technique for measuring responses depends on what one wants to measure. Determination of sensor function requires direct measurement of its output, for example, electrical recording of carotid sinus nerve afferents. This procedure requires general anesthesia, extensive dissection of the neck, division of the nerve, and teasing out of fine filaments which (it is hoped) will contain active chemoreceptor afferents. This difficult process is selective, and, while positive recordings are valid, they may not truly represent the overall response of the sensor. Direct recordings from brainstem respiratory neurons provide important information about the response of a given group of cells to a chemoreceptor stimulus and about their connections with other parts of the respiratory system. Careful control of conditions by anesthesia, paralysis, and mechanical ventilation, as well as the selective nature of the recordings, means that such information gives little indication of the overall integration of chemosensory information by the brainstem. Phrenic nerve recording does appear to give useful information relating to the output of the brainstem, at least to the major inspiratory muscle, the diaphragm. Again, general anesthesia is required, and information on the output to the other respiratory motor neurons, which may be important in determining respiratory pump function, is lacking. Electromyograms (EMG) can be recorded in multiple respiratory muscles during natural conditions to give a broader measure of the respiratory motor output in response to a chemoreceptor stimulus. Care must be taken when using these to infer timing of the respiratory cycle, since the pattern of activation can vary in different sites, even within a given muscle such as the diaphragm.[11]

Most studies in man and in intact animals have used minute ventilation to estimate the respiratory response to chemostimulation. This is easier than measuring alveolar ventilation, which is the factor that sets the levels of the blood gases and corrects the errors in them, as originally detected by the sensor. As long as minute ventilation and its components, tidal volume and frequency, are not used to infer details of sensor sensitivity, they are useful measures of the integrated response to a given stimulus. For further discussion of this topic, see Rebuck and Slutsky[12] and Sullivan[1].

With the recognition that it is an important response to chemoreceptor stimulation,[1] arousal has been determined more frequently. Most studies have used generalized movements, EMG activation, or electroencephalographic changes as measures of arousal. This is different from the sleep physiologists' view of arousal as a state of cortical activation which includes ability to cerebrate.

Oxygen

Inhalation of hyperoxic gas causes an immediate fall in minute ventilation, and this has been used to gauge the pre-existing hypoxic drive. Hypoxic tests usually employ either the steady-state response to inhalation of a hypoxic gas of fixed composition or the response to presentation of a gradient of increasingly hypoxic composition. In both of these tests it is preferable to maintain isocapnia since any ventilatory response will remove CO_2 and reduce the drive to breathe, but this is often not done. The steady-state method is easier to perform, but it may take 10 min to reach a true steady state in the adult. Due to the multiple effects of hypoxia in the newborn (see below), a steady state may never be reached in these cases. However, the immediate increase in ventilation which can be measured may be a useful indicator of peripheral chemoreceptor response.

Carbon Dioxide

In man, responses are usually expressed as the change in minute ventilation vs. the change in alveolar P_{CO_2} (P_{ACO_2}). In the steady state method, CO_2 is inhaled at a set level (e.g., 5% in air). This causes a rise in P_{ACO_2} and P_{aCO_2}, leading to narrowing of the gradient between this and brain tissue P_{CO_2}, which in turn rises and stimulates breathing. In adults, brain tissue CO_2 and ventilation continue to rise for about 4–6 min, until the blood/brain gradient is re-established and a steady state is reached.[12] This procedure is then repeated with different CO_2 levels to obtain a response line. Thus, this is a time-consuming test which is less suitable for rapid assessment in a defined behavioral state, particularly in the newborn. Furthermore, since it involves an 'open loop' system, there are difficulties assessing the stimulus: with a ventilatory response P_{aCO_2} falls.

An alternative method, published as a clinical test by Read,[13] utilizes rebreathing from a small bag containing O_2 and CO_2 at concentrations close to the mixed venous level. After a few breaths, an equilibrium is reached with approximately equal alveolar, arterial, brain tissue, and venous P_{CO_2}. Carbon dioxide builds up due to metabolic production and the absence of pulmonary excretion, leading to a progressive stimulus. Since an equilibrium has been achieved, P_{aCO_2} will closely reflect the stimulus in the medulla. The test is over in a few minutes and gives ventilation levels over a range of P_{aCO_2}. For further discussion of this method, see Read and Leigh[14] and others.[1,12]

Single-breath testing has also been employed as a rapid method. However, much higher concentrations of CO_2 (13%) are used, and the dose is dependent on the size of the single breath. It may be useful as a qualitative test, particularly to indicate an immediate CB response, but it is difficult to quantitate. There is also concern that such a large stimulus will excite airway receptors and modify breathing. Indeed, there is a possibility that lower levels of CO_2 in the airway, as in steady state or rebreathing, might modify the response.

CHEMICAL REGULATION DURING PERINATAL DEVELOPMENT

The Changing Chemical Milieu

The transition from fetal to adult life is associated with changes in the chemical environment. This is most marked at birth and in relation to oxygen. The fetus can be thought of as a highly specialized maternal tissue in equilibrium with placental mixed venous levels of oxygen (33 mm Hg) and carbon dioxide (46 mm Hg). Due to mixing in the heart, fetal carotid P_{aO_2} is 20–25 mm Hg. Oxygen supply to the fetus is ensured by the left shift in the curve for fetal hemoglobin/O_2 dissociation (i.e., higher O_2 saturation of the hemoglobin at low P_{aO_2}), the higher O_2-carrying capacity of this hemoglobin, and larger blood flows. The fetal circulation plays a major role in regulating the supply and distribution of O_2 and CO_2.

During the later phases of labor, P_{aO_2} levels fall further (to 15–20 mm Hg), P_{aCO_2} levels rise (50 mm Hg), and there is a combined respiratory and metabolic acidosis (pH

7.10–7.30). Following birth, the Pa_{O_2} rises rapidly to 60–90 mm Hg, while the Pa_{CO_2} falls to about 35 mm Hg, and there is a persisting metabolic acidosis during the first few days (pH 7.35, base deficit about 5 mmol/l).

Response to Hypoxia

Fetus

There are no data for the fetal response to hypoxia in humans. In the sheep, a reduction of Pa_{O_2} (to 12–15 mm Hg), achieved by giving the ewe 9% O_2 to breathe (plus 3% CO_2 to prevent hypocapnea), causes: (a) abolition of breathing movements, (b) an increase in slow wave sleep, (c) a reduction of metabolic rate, (d) inhibition of spinal motor neurons, and (e) cardiovascular responses. The physiological mechanisms underlying these responses have been reviewed by Dawes,[15] Hanson,[16] and Johnston and Walker.[17] Lesion experiments indicate that hypoxic inhibition of fetal breathing movements is mediated by the lateral part of the lower pons, in the region of the trigeminal nuclei. Similar hypoxic inhibition of breathing movements has been observed in the primate fetus.[18] The carotid chemoreceptors are active in the sheep fetus, although they respond at much lower Pa_{O_2} levels than those observed postnatally.[15] When freed from pontine inhibition, hypoxia augments fetal breathing.

Hypoxic facilitation of slow wave sleep is mediated at a suprapontine level. The reduction of metabolic rate is probably also under forebrain (hypothalamic) control, although sleep state changes, spinal inhibition, and cardiovascular effects of hypoxia also contribute by lowering oxygen consumption. Spinal inhibition is due to a direct effect of hypoxia on the brainstem, independent of the arterial chemoreceptors.

It is not clear whether the direct effects of hypoxia on the forebrain (behavior), pons (breathing inhibition), or brainstem (spinal motor inhibition) are mediated by the stimulation of specialized chemoreceptor cells or are nonspecific influences on neurons due to cerebral blood flow (CBF)/pH changes, and/or release of neuromodulators. Drugs that usually stimulate breathing, such as doxapram, caffeine, indomethacin and strychnine, do not prevent hypoxic inhibition. Neither do endogenous opiates appear to be involved, since naloxone infusion does not alter the response.[17]

Newborn

At the moment of birth, blood gas measurements in humans and other animals indicate that there should be powerful chemoreceptor drives to breathe. Carotid chemoreceptors do not appear to be essential for the initiation of air breathing[19], though, and are probably quickly silenced by the rise in Pa_{O_2} that occurs. Evidence for their relative inactivity during the first days after birth includes reduced ventilatory responses to hypoxia and hyperoxia in humans and an inability to detect chemoreceptor afferents in the lamb carotid sinus nerve. Presumably, other drives maintain breathing efforts at this time.

Resetting of the carotid chemoreceptors is probably triggered by the rise in blood oxygen levels. In the lamb, hyperoxia induced by mechanical ventilation of the fetus for a few days before birth causes premature resetting.[20] Conversely, maintaining rats in hypoxic environment during early postnatal life causes persistence of the immature inhibitory responses to hypoxia.[21]

In the adult, the immediate fall in ventilation caused by breathing a hyperoxic gas is attributable to withdrawal of peripheral chemoreceptor drive. During the first few days of postnatal life, the reduction in ventilation with 100% O_2 is less than in the adult,[22] consistent with inactivity of the carotid afferents during this resetting period. After a few minutes of hyperoxia, ventilation is elevated above control levels. In adults, a similar but less marked hyperventilation has been attributed to hyperoxic cerebral vasoconstriction, which leads to increased brain tissue CO_2.[23] Newborns appear to have more vigorous CBF responses to O_2 and these may be important during both hyperoxia and hypoxia.

During the first week of life for the full-term human infant, breathing hypoxic gas causes a transient increase in minute ventilation in the first min, followed by a decrease to, or below, the baseline level in the second and third min. Qualitatively similar "biphasic" ventilatory responses have been reported in the newborns of most species, although the magnitude of the late ventilatory decrease varies between species. Before proceeding to a discussion of the possible mechanisms underlying this allegedly unique biphasic response, it should be pointed out that even adult humans show a late decrease in ventilation during "isocapnic" hypoxia which, however, does not occur for about 10 min.[24] It may be more appropriate to take the broader view that the biphasic response is always present to some degree but is more dramatic in the immature, due to predominance of the CNS inhibitory effects of hypoxia, as observed in the fetus.

The initial increases in minute ventilation during breathing of hypoxic gas in full-term infants studied on the first day of life and in those that are born preterm is less than in full-term infants at later times. In a cool environment, the increase is absent. In animal studies, the initial stimulation of ventilation is due to activation of peripheral chemoreceptors, since it is abolished by CSN section.[25] These afferents continue to be activated throughout the hypoxic challenge and therefore cannot account for waning of the ventilatory response after the first min.[26,27] During the initial hyperventilation, P_{ACO_2} falls; this would be expected to reduce ventilatory drive. However, even when ventilation has fallen below control levels, the P_{ACO_2} remains low, suggesting that metabolic production is reduced. A reduction of metabolic rate during hypoxia has been observed in the fetus (see above), in newborns studied in a neutral thermal environment,[28] and in small adult animals in a cool one.[29] Reduction of CO_2 drive would be accentuated due to hypoxic cerebral vasodilatation and consequent reduction of brain tissue CO_2. If this latter mechanism accounted for the reduction of ventilation, then one would expect it to be transient, since there would be a gradual build-up of brain tissue CO_2 and re-establishment of the A-V (arterial-venous) difference. Yet in newborn kittens, ventilation is reduced for up to 40 min of hypoxia.[30] A further finding against a role of CO_2 is that adding it to the inspired air does not abolish the biphasic nature of the response.[31]

Changes in lung mechanics might also play a role in reducing the ventilatory response. Reduced compliance has been documented in infants[31] and monkeys,[32] and this could in part be related to the associated, raised functional residual capacity measured in primates.[32] Yet these compliance changes are present during the first min of hypoxia, when ventilation is increased.[32]

There has been interest in whether neuromodulators such as endorphins or adenosine might be involved in the biphasic response. It has been claimed that naloxone, an endorphin antagonist, reduces the decrease in ventilation induced by hypoxia.[33] This does not appear to be true for newborn monkeys,[34] anesthetized piglets,[35] or adult humans.[34] Adenosine increases in the brain during hypoxia, and analogues given intraperitoneally cause a reduction in ventilation, which is blocked by theophylline.[36]

Sleep State

In the past, little attention was given to controlling for the behavioral state, yet its influences are considerable. Since most newborns sleep during testing, it is now usual to distinguish between responses in quiet sleep (regular or slow wave sleep) and active sleep (rapid eye movement or paradoxical sleep). In preterm infants and animals that are more immature at birth, precise definition of sleep states can be difficult. Measurement of the immediate fall in ventilation with hyperoxia suggests that the resting hypoxic drive to breathe is similar during quiet and active sleep in the newborn infant.[37,38] In the preterm infant, Rigatto's group,[27] measuring the transient response to 15% O_2, showed that there was a sustained increase in ventilation during quiet sleep, a transient increase followed by a reduction during wakefulness, and predominantly a decrease during active sleep.

Animal studies employing an isocapneic gradient of hypoxia have shown that the responses during the active sleep state differ between species. Whereas calves,[39] lambs,[40] and puppies[40] each have a progressive ventilatory increment during quiet sleep, in active sleep, calves show no ventilatory response, lambs have a rate increment but little increase in ventilation, and puppies respond as in quiet sleep. Using steady-state hypoxia in a developmental study of puppies, Haddad et al.[41] found comparable increases in ventilation at older ages. However, the youngest animals showed a decrease in ventilation during quiet sleep. Further studies are needed to determine the reasons for these differing responses. Possibilities include differences in postnatal development of peripheral chemoreceptor drive, differences in brainstem integration of these drives during each sleep state, and variable stability of the respiratory pump during active sleep.

Response to Carbon Dioxide/Acidosis

Fetal responses to CO_2/acidosis have been reviewed recently.[15,17,42] Although it is difficult to compare fetal responses with those in the newborn, studies in sheep indicate that when breathing is present, it is augmented by elevating CO_2 or lowering pH. Responses have been obtained by delivering CO_2 via the ewe and acidifying the cerebral spinal fluid. When the fetus is in slow wave sleep, breathing is normally absent and cannot be induced by these methods.

The response of newborn infants to CO_2 gives a curve for minute ventilation vs. P_{ACO_2} with a slope similar to that seen for adults, although the curve is shifted to the left due to lower resting CO_2 levels. The tidal volume component of the ventilatory response assumes greater importance with postnatal development. In preterm infants, the slope of the ventilatory response is less and increases with postnatal growth.[27] Rigatto[27] suggests that this is due to immaturity of the central chemoreceptors rather than to mechanical differences in the respiratory pump, since diaphragm EMG responses are also reduced in the preterm infant. At a given low gestational age, infants with recurrent prolonged apnea have higher resting P_{ACO_2} levels and reduced CO_2 sensitivity. Further evidence of a link between CNS immaturity and apnea is the finding of less mature brainstem auditory-evoked responses in those with apnea.[43]

Sleep state also affects responses to CO_2. In full-term infants, the slope of the ventilatory response curve is less during active than quiet sleep.[44] This may be due to altered mechanical stability associated with rib-cage distortion in active sleep, since the diaphragmatic response is intact.[45] Other evidence suggests that rib-cage distortion does not account for the reduction of ventilatory responses in preterm infants.[27] As in adults,[1] it may be the random CNS activation, most marked in the "phasic" part of active sleep, that disrupts the ventilatory response.

CHEMOREFLEXES AND SUDDEN INFANT DEATH

Pathological Studies

A major difficulty in studying tissues of sudden infant death syndrome (SIDS) infants is finding adequate age-matched controls. Naeye et al.[46] claimed that carotid bodies (CB) were most commonly smaller but occasionally larger than controls. Others[47,48] have not been able to confirm this. Cole et al.[47] studied CB from 6 SIDS and 3 control infants and claimed that there were less dense-cored neurosecretory granules in the SIDS infants. Some doubt has been cast on the quality of the histological specimens examined,[2] though, and the finding has not been confirmed in a larger study by others.[48] Using a radio-enzyme assay method on homogenized CB, Perrin et al.[49] found a 10-fold increase in dopamine and a 3-fold increase in noradrenalin in SIDS-derived samples compared to controls. This is of particular interest, since dopamine is thought to inhibit carotid chemoreceptor function. Although dopamine levels rise in the CB with chronic hypoxia in the rat, the expected associated glomus cell hyperplasia is not present in SIDS.[49]

Studies of Infants at High Risk of SIDS

Differences in ventilatory and arousal responses to hypoxia and hypercapnea have been found in infants presenting with so-called near-miss SIDS (NMSIDS). Shannon et al.[50] found reduced steady-state ventilatory responses to inhalation of 5% CO_2 during quiet sleep in 11 infants with NMSIDS compared with 12 controls. Three of these NMSIDS infants subsequently died during sleep at home and no cause was found in the 2 for whom postmortems were performed. Hunt et al.,[51] using similar techniques, including nasal prongs, also found reduced ventilatory responses in NMSIDS. In contrast, Haddad et al.,[52] using only 2% CO_2 in a whole-body plethysmograph, found that mean minute ventilation was slightly higher in NMSIDS during both quiet and active sleep. However, overlap of the data for NMSIDS and controls was considerable.

Responses to hypoxia are also different in NMSIDS. When given 17% O_2, these infants switch to periodic breathing more commonly than do controls.[53] Caution is needed in interpreting these data, however, since Adamson et al.[54] have demonstrated a peak incidence of spontaneous periodic breathing at 1–2 months of age which is linked to postnatal rather than postmenstrual age. In the above study linking hypoxic induction of periodic breathing with NMSIDS,[53] the NMSIDS infants were studied at a mean postnatal age of 6 weeks compared with 10 weeks for the controls. In a study measuring minute ventilation in relation to end-expired Po_2 during stepwise reduction in inspired O_2, reduced responses were found in NMSIDS compared with controls, and the authors indicated that there was a concordance between hypoxic and hypercapnic responses, although no data were shown.[51] This observation would suggest a central defect in brainstem integration of these inputs.

A brainstem defect could also explain altered arousal thresholds in NMSIDS. Spontaneous,[55] as well as hypoxic and hypercapnic[56,57] arousals occur less frequently in NMSIDS. Furthermore, those infants who subsequently had episodes requiring resuscitation were the ones who had been least likely to arouse during hypoxia.[57] McGinty and Hoppenbrouwers[58] have previously suggested that a reticular formation defect could explain many of the behavioral and breathing disorders associated with SIDS. Histopathological evidence supports this view. Quattrochi et al.[59] found that reticular dendritic spines were excessive for the age of the infant in SIDS. This observation has been confirmed, and, together with the gliosis found,[60] suggests delayed development. The possibility of delayed development is consistent with many of the other findings in SIDS such as retention of brown fat, pulmonary smooth muscle and extramedullary erythropoiesis, as well as the delayed switching from fetal to adult hemoglobin.[61]

Since the altered function in NMSIDS infants has been observed after the life-threatening episode(s), it might be an effect rather than a cause of NMSIDS. Furthermore, although NMSIDS infants are at higher risk of dying in a manner similar to SIDS, it is not known if the anomalies found in their chemoresponses are applicable to SIDS in general.

These infants could instead represent a subgroup more closely related to infants with congenital central hypoventilation, who are thought to have an autonomic disorder.[62] Suggestions of a genetic link between altered chemoresponses and SIDS have come from studies of parents of SIDS victims showing reduced ventilatory responses to hypoxia, hypercapnia and flow resistive loading.[63]

CONCLUSION

A major problem in interpreting data on clinical problems such as NMSIDS is the paucity of normal physiological data on the development of chemical responses. Abundant data exist for the newborn period, when the infants are available for study. There is an urgent need to obtain good postneonatal measurements. In relation to SIDS, further attention could be focused on the integration of breathing responses to chemoreceptor stimulation and the other effects of asphyxia on the CNS, cardiovascular system, and metabolism. The role of sleep deprivation or other behavioral disturbances such as fear paralysis[64] need consideration. Persistence of immature systems in SIDS infants seems to be a hallmark of many studies; the hypoxic response is a prime candidate in this regard.

ACKNOWLEDGMENTS

The assistance of Deborah Edwards in editing this manuscript is gratefully acknowledged.

REFERENCES

1. SULLIVAN, C.E. 1980. Breathing in sleep. *In* Physiology in Sleep. J. Orem & C.D. Barnes, Eds.:213–272. Academic Press. New York.
2. BLEDSOE, S.W. & T.F. HORNBEIN. 1981. Central chemoreceptors and the regulation of their chemical environment. *In* Regulation of Breathing, Part I. T.F. Hornbein, Ed.:347–428. Marcel Dekker Inc. New York.
3. MCDONALD, D.M. 1981. Peripheral chemoreceptors. *In* Regulation of Breathing, Part I. T.F. Hornbein, Ed.:105–319. Marcel Dekker Inc. New York.
4. BISCOE, T.J. & P. WILLSHAW. 1981. Stimulus-response relationships of the peripheral arterial chemoreceptors. *In* Regulation of Breathing, Part I. T.F. Hornbein, Ed.:321–345. Marcel Dekker Inc. New York.
5. MILHORN, D.E. & F.L. ELDRIDGE. 1986. Role of ventrolateral medulla in regulation of respiratory and cardiovascular systems. J. Appl. Physiol. **61(4)**:1249–1263.
6. VAN BEEK, J.H., A. BERKENBOSCH, J. DEGOEDE & N. OLIEVIER. 1984. Effects of brain stem hypoxaemia on the regulation of breathing. Respir. Physiol. **57**:171–188.
7. HENDERSON-SMART, D.J. 1980. Vulnerability to hypoxemia in the newborn. Sleep **3**:331–342.
8. BOWES, G., E.R. TOWNSEND, S.M. BROMLEY, L.F. KOZAR & E.A. PHILLIPSON. 1981. Role of the carotid body and afferent vagal stimuli in the arousal response to airway occlusion in sleeping dogs. Am. Rev. Respir. Dis. **123**:644–647.
9. ANGELL-JAMES, J.E. & M. DE BURGH DALY. 1969. Cardiovascular responses in apnoeic asphyxia: Role of arterial chemoreceptors and the modification of their effects by a pulmonary vagal inflation reflex. J. Physiol. (London) **201**:87–104.
10. DE BURGH DALY, M. & J. E. ANGELL-JAMES. 1979. The "diving response" and its possible clinical implications. Int. Med. **1(2)**:12–19.
11. HENDERSON-SMART, D.J., P. JOHNSON & M.E. MCCLELLAND. 1982. Asynchronous respi-

ratory activity of the diaphragm during spontaneous breathing in lambs. J. Physiol. (London) **327:**377–391.

12. REBUCK, A.S. & A.S. SLUTSKY. 1981. Measurement of ventilatory responses to hypercapnia and hypoxia. *In* Regulation of Breathing, Part II. T.F. Hornbein, Ed.:745–772. Marcel Dekker Inc. New York.

13. READ, D.J.C. 1967. A clinical method for assessing the ventilatory response to carbon dioxide. Australas Ann. Med. **16:**20–32.

14. READ, D.J.C. & J. LEIGH. 1967. Blood-brain tissue Pco_2 relationships and ventilation during breathing. J. Appl. Physiol. **23:**53–70.

15. DAWES, G.S. 1984. The central control of fetal breathing and skeletal muscle movements. J. Physiol (London) **346:**1–18.

16. HANSON, M.A. 1986. Peripheral chemoreceptor function before and after birth. *In* Reproductive and Perinatal Medicine. III, Respiratory Control and Lung Development in the Fetus and Newborn. B.M. Johnston & P.D. Gluckman, Eds.:311–330. Perinatology Press. Ithaca, New York.

17. JOHNSTON, B.M. & D.W. WALKER. 1986. Respiratory responses to changes in oxygen and carbon dioxide in the perinatal period. *In* Reproductive and Perinatal Medicine. III, Respiratory Control and Lung Development in the Fetus and Newborn. B.M. Johnston & P.D. Gluckman, Eds.:279–310. Perinatology Press. Ithaca, New York.

18. MARTIN, C.B., Y. MURATA, R.H. PETRIE & J.T. PARER. 1974. Respiratory movements in fetal rhesus monkeys. Am. J. Obstet. Gynecol. **119:**939–948.

19. HERRINGTON, R.T., H.S. HARNED, J.I. FERREIRO & C.A. GRIFFIN, III. 1971. The role of the central nervous system in perinatal respiration: Studies of chemoregulatory mechanisms in the term lamb. Pediatrics **47(5):**857–864.

20. BLANCO, C.E., M.A. HANSON, H.B. McCOOKE & B.A. WILLIAMS. 1987. Studies of chemoreceptor resetting after hyperoxic ventilation of the fetus in utero. *In* Chemoreceptors in Respiratory Control. J.A. Ribero & D.J. Pallot, Eds.:221–227. Croom Helm. Kent.

21. EDEN, G.J. & M.A. HANSON. 1987. Effects of chronic hypoxia on chemoreceptor function in the newborn. *In* Chemoreceptors in Respiratory Control. J.A. Ribero & D.J. Pallot, Eds.: 369–376. Croom Helm. Kent.

22. GIRARD, F., A. LaCAISSE & P. DeJOURS. 1960. Le stimulus O_2 ventilatoire à la periode neonatale chez l'homme. J. Physiol. (Paris) **52:**108–109.

23. ELLINGSON, R.J. 1972. Development of wakefulness-sleep cycles and associated EEG patterns in mammals. *In* Sleep and the Maturing Nervous System. C.D. Clemente, D.P. Purpura & F.E. Meyer, Eds.: 166–174. Plenum Academic Press, New York.

24. KAGAWA, S., M.J. STAFFORD, T.B. WAGGENER & J.W. SEVERINGHAUS. 1982. No effect of naloxone on hypoxia-induced ventilatory depression in adults. J. Appl. Physiol. Respir. Environ. Exercise Physiol. **52(4):**1030–1034.

25. BUREAU, M.A., J. LaMARCHE, P. FOULON & D. DALLE. 1985. Postnatal maturation of respiration in intact and carotid body-denervated lambs. J. Appl. Physiol. **59(3):**869–874.

26. SCHWIELER, G. 1968. Respiratory regulation during postnatal development in cats and rabbits and some of its morphological substrate. Acta Physiol. Scand. Suppl. **304:**10–85.

27. RIGATTO, H. 1984. Control of ventilation in the newborn. Annu. Rev. Physiol. **46:**661–674.

28. TAYLOR, P.M. 1960. Oxygen consumption in new-born rats. J. Physiol. (London) **154:** 153–168.

29. HILL, J.R. 1959. The oxygen consumption of new-born and adult mammals. Its dependence on the oxygen tension in the inspired air and on the environmental temperature. J. Physiol. (London) **149:**346–373.

30. BONORA, M., D. MARLOT, H. GAUTIER & B. DURON. 1984. Effects of hypoxia on ventilation during postnatal development in conscious kittens. J. Appl. Physiol. Respir. Environ. Exercise Physiol. **56(6):**1464–1471.

31. BRADY, J.P. & E. CERTI. 1966. Chemoreceptor reflexes in the newborn infant: Effects of varying degrees of hypoxia on heart rate and ventilation in warm environment. J. Physiol. (London) **184:**631–645.

32. LaFRAMBOISE, W.A., R.D. GUTHRIE, T.A. STANDAERT & D.E. WOODRUM. 1983. Pulmonary mechanics during the ventilatory response to hypoxia in the newborn monkey. J. Appl. Physiol. Respir. Environ. Exercise Physiol. **55(3):**1008–1014.

33. DE BOECK, C., P. VAN REEMPTS, H. RIGATTO & V. CHERNICK. 1984. Naloxone reduces decrease in ventilation induced by hypoxia in newborn infants. J. Appl. Physiol. Respir. Environ. Exercise Physiol. 56(6):1507–1511.
34. MAYOCK, D.E., W.A. LAFRAMBOISE, R.D. GUTHRIE, T.A. STANDAERT & D.E. WOODRUM. 1986. Role of endogenous opiates in hypoxic ventilatory response in the newborn primate. J. Appl. Physiol. 60(6):2015–2019.
35. LONG, W.A. & E.E. LAWSON. 1984. Neurotransmitters and biphasic respiratory response to hypoxia. J. Appl. Physiol. Respir. Environ. Exercise Physiol. 55:483–488.
36. RUNOLD, M., H. LAGERCRANTZ & B.B. FREDHOLM. 1986. Ventilatory effect of an adenosine analogue in unanesthetized rabbits during development. J. Appl. Physiol. 62(1):255–259.
37. BOULTON, D.P.G. & S. HERMAN. 1974. Ventilation and sleep state in the newborn. J. Physiol. (London) 240:66–77.
38. FAGENHOLTZ, S.A., K. O'CONNELL & D.C. SHANNON. 1976. Chemoreceptor function and sleep state in apnea. Pediatrics 58:31–36.
39. JEFFREY, H.E. & D.J.C. READ. 1980. Ventilatory responses of newborn calves to progressive hypoxia in quiet and active sleep. J. Appl. Physiol. 48:892–895.
40. HENDERSON-SMART, D.J. & D.J.C. READ. 1979. Ventilatory responses to hypoxia during active sleep in the newborn. J. Dev. Physiol. 1:195–208.
41. HADDAD, G.G., M.R. GANDHI & R.B. MELLINS. 1982. Maturation of ventilatory response to hypoxia in puppies during sleep. J. Appl. Physiol. Respir. Environ. Exercise Physiol. 52(2):309–314.
42. BISSONNETTE, J.M. & A.R. HOHIMER. 1986. Central neurogenesis of respiration in the fetus. In Reproductive and Perinatal Medicine. III, Respiratory Control and Lung Development in the Fetus and Newborn. B.M. Johnston & P.D. Gluckman, Eds.:237–248. Perinatology Press. Ithaca, New York.
43. HENDERSON-SMART, D.J., A.G. PETTIGREW & D.J. CAMPBELL. 1983. Clinical apnea and brain stem neural function in preterm infants. N. Engl. J. Med. 308:353–357.
44. HONMA, Y., D. WILKES, M.H. BRYAN & A.C. BRYAN. 1984. Rib cage and abdominal contributions to ventilatory response to CO_2 in infants. J. Appl. Physiol. Respir. Environ. Exercise Physiol. 56(5):1211–1216.
45. HAGAN, R. & A.G. GULSTON. 1981. The newborn: Respiratory electromyograms and breathing. Aust. Paediatr. J. 17:230–231.
46. NAEYE, R.L., R. FISHER, M. RYSER & P. WHELAN. 1976. Carotid body in sudden infant death syndrome. Science 191:567–569.
47. COLE, S., L.B. LINDENBERG, F.M. GALIOTO, P.E. HOWE, A.C. DEGRAFF, J.M. DAVIS, R. LUBKA & E.M. GROSS. 1979. Ultrasound abnormalities of the carotid body in sudden infant death syndrome. Pediatrics 63:13–16.
48. PERRIN, D.G., E. CUTZ, L.E. BECKER & A.C. BRYAN. 1984. Ultrastructure of carotid bodies in sudden infant death syndrome. Pediatrics 73:646–651.
49. PERRIN, D.G., E. CUTZ, L.E. BECKER, C.E. BRYAN, A. MADAPALLIMATUM & M. SOLE. 1984. Sudden infant death syndrome: Increased carotid-body dopamine and noradrenaline content. Lancet 8402:535–537.
50. SHANNON, D.C., D.H. KELLY & K. O'CONNELL. 1977. Abnormal regulation of ventilation in infants at risk for sudden infant death syndrome. N. Engl. J. Med. 297:747–750.
51. HUNT, C.E., K. MCCULLOCH & R.T. BROUILLETTE. 1981. Diminished hypoxic ventilatory responses in near-miss sudden infant death syndrome. J. Appl. Physiol. Respir. Environ. Exercise Physiol. 50(6):1313–1317.
52. HADDAD, G.G., H.L. LEISTNER, T.L. LAI & R.B. MELLINS. 1981. Ventilation and ventilatory pattern during sleep in aborted sudden infant death syndrome. Pediatr. Res. 15:879–883.
53. BRADY, J.P., R.L. ARIAGNO, J.L. WATTS, S.L. GOLDMAN & B.S. DUMPIT. 1978. Apnea, hypoxemia, and aborted sudden infant death syndrome. Pediatrics 62:686–691.
54. ADAMSON, T.M., S.M. CRANAGE, J.E. MALONEY, M. WILKINSON & F.E. WILSON. 1984. Periodic breathing: Its occurrence and relation to birth in preterm and term infants. Aust. Paediatr. J. 20:340.
55. COONS, S. & C. GUILLEMINAULT. 1985. Motility and arousal in near miss sudden infant death syndrome. J. Pediatr. 107:728–732.
56. MCCULLOCH, K., R.T. BROUILLETTE, A.J. GUZZETTA & C.E. HUNT. 1982. Arousal

responses in near-miss sudden death syndrome and in normal infants. J. Pediatr. **101(6):**911–917.

57. VAN DER HAL, A.J., A.M. RODRIGUEZ, C.W. SARGENT, A.G. PLATZKER & T.G. KEENS. 1985. Hypoxic and hypercapneic arousal responses and prediction of subsequent apnea of infancy. Pediatrics **75:**848–854.

58. MCGINTY, D.J. & T. HOPPENBROUWERS. 1983. The reticular formation, breathing disorders during sleep, and SIDS. *In* Sudden Infant Death Syndrome. J.T. Tildon, L.M. Roeder & A. Steinschneider, Eds.:375–400. Academic Press. New York.

59. QUATTROCHI, J.J., P.T. MCBRIDE & A.J. YATES. 1984. Brainstem immaturity in sudden infant death syndrome: A quantitative rapid Golgi study of dendritic spines in 95 infants. Brain Res. **325:**39–48.

60. BECKER, L.E. 1983. Neuropathological basis for respiratory dysfunction in sudden infant death syndrome. *In* Sudden Infant Death Syndrome. J.T. Tildon, L.M. Roeder & A. Steinschneider, Eds.:99–114. Academic Press. New York.

61. GIULIAN, G.G., E.F. GILBERT & R.L. MOSS. 1987. Elevated fetal haemoglobin levels and sudden infant death syndrome. N. Engl. J. Med. **316:**1122–1126.

62. GUILLEMINAULT, C., J. MCQUITTY, R.L. ARIAGNO, M.J. CHALLAMEL, R. KOROBKIN & R.E. MCCLEAD, JR. 1982. Congenital central hypoventilation syndrome in six infants. Pediatrics **70:**684–694.

63. SCHIFFMAN, P.L., B. FRIEDMAN, T.V. SANTIAGO & N.H. EDELMAN. 1984. Effect of naloxone on ventilatory control in parents of victims of sudden infant death syndrome. Am. Rev. Respir. Dis. **130:**964–968.

64. KAADA, B. 1986. Sudden Infant Death Syndrome. The Possible Role of "the Fear Paralysis Reflex." Norwegian University Press. London.

Lung Surfactant and Sudden Infant Death Syndrome[a]

COLIN MORLEY[b], CHARLES HILL, AND BETTY BROWN

Department of Paediatrics
University of Cambridge
Addenbrooke's Hospital
Cambridge, England

INTRODUCTION

In 1982 we first reported that babies who died from Sudden Infant Death Syndrome (SIDS) appeared to have abnormal surfactant in their lungs.[1] In this paper we will update those results now that we have analyzed surfactant from 111 babies who died from SIDS. These samples will be compared with a total of 144 different surfactant specimens from living babies or babies who have died from other conditions. For simplicity these 144 specimens will be referred to as "controls."

MATERIALS AND METHODS

In this study, SIDS was diagnosed by the pathologists if the baby died suddenly and unexpectedly and no other cause of death could be found. Surfactant was obtained at autopsy by saline lavage of the lungs from 111 babies who had died from SIDS (mean age, 114 days; range, 22 to 365). Of these, 39% showed histological evidence of lung inflammation which was presumed to be related to infection but was not considered to be serious enough to have been the cause of death. The mean age of the babies dying from SIDS who had lung inflammation was 122 days, range, 42 to 280 days.

Control cases are always a problem in SIDS research because babies who die are seldom normal. However, to determine whether the surfactant from SIDS cases was abnormal it will be compared with that from several "control" groups. The first control group ("mature") consisted of 17 babies who died between 14 days and 1 yr of age from diseases other than SIDS and who had minimal lung pathology (mean age at death, 134 days; range, 32 to 308). They died from asphyxia (1 baby), heart disease (8), pericarditis (1), malrotation (1), encephalopathy (2), hydrocephalus (1), Reye's syndrome (1), road accident (1), and drowning (1). In the second control group, tracheal aspirates were collected, in collaboration with Dr. David Southall, from 14 living infants up to 2 yr of age (mean age, 173 days; range, 112 to 644) who had tracheostomies performed for upper airway problems. These aspirates were intended to represent surfactant samples from normal living infants. However, it must be remembered that these children would have had more respiratory infections than normal children, and this may have altered the

[a]This project was funded by the University of Cambridge Baby Research Fund, Action Research for the Crippled Child, and the Foundation for the Study of Infant Deaths.
[b]To whom correspondence should be addressed at: Department of Paediatrics, Level E8, Addenbrooke's Hospital, Cambridge, CB2 2QQ. UK.

composition of their surfactant. To overcome this problem, we initially tried to collect tracheal aspirates from healthy babies undergoing anesthesia, but they did not have sufficient secretions to collect and analyze. The third control group was 15 full-term babies who died within 2 weeks of birth but who had normal lungs (mean age, 4 days, range 0.5 to 14). Seven died from asphyxia and 8 from congenital heart disease. The surfactant composition from all these babies is compared with 35 pharyngeal aspirates obtained from full-term, healthy newborn babies. To determine whether surfactant was altered by infection, specimens were obtained from babies who died within 8 months of birth, 11 from septicemia (mean age, 84 days; range, 1 to 196) and 15 from pneumonia (mean age, 84 days; range, 1 to 224). The final comparison group was 37 very premature babies who died in the acute phase of hyaline membrane disease (HMD; mean gestational age, 29 weeks; range, 21 to 38).

The postmortem specimens were all obtained by lavaging the lungs at the autopsy; in consequence, any possible postmortem change in composition would affect them all (for details see Hill et al.[2]).

The specimens were centrifuged at 300 × g for 5 min to remove the debris, and the larger samples were freeze-dried. The phospholipids were extracted by a modified Folch technique and separated by two-dimensional thin-layer chromatography using the technique of Hill.[3] The phospholipid spots on the plates were identified by comparison with standards and then quantified by phosphorus estimation; quantities were expressed as a percentage of the total phospholipid present.

The major surfactant phospholipids are phosphatidylcholine, lysophosphatidylcholine, phosphatidylglycerol, phosphatidylethanolamine, phosphatidylserine, phosphatidylinositol, and sphingomyelin. Although all the phospholipids were examined as part of this study, for simplicity only the values for phosphatidylcholine and sphingomyelin will be shown in this paper, because they exhibited the most interesting differences between SIDS and control specimens. The data for the other phospholipid analyses have been published.[2]

RESULTS

The main phospholipid present in lung surfactant is phosphatidylcholine; its level (mean % ± SE) in specimens from SIDS babies and each group of control cases is shown in FIGURE 1. Since the SIDS group with evidence of possible infection has a phosphatidylcholine level (63.8 ± 1.1%) similar to the other SIDS infants (62.2 ± 1.1%), these values are combined (FIG. 1). Although the mature infants have a higher level (66.2 ± 2.1%), it is not significantly different from the SIDS babies. Whereas the tracheal aspirate samples (T/A) have a value (70.8 ± 2.0%) which is significantly higher ($p < 0.01$) than the SIDS samples, it is similar to the value from the mature infants. The group with the highest level of phosphatidylcholine is the full-term newborn babies (76.1 ± 1.5%). This value is not significantly different from the level obtained for pharyngeal aspirates (P/A) taken at birth from mature babies (73.6 ± 1.3%). The value for both these groups is significantly higher than the SIDS babies ($p < 0.001$). The fact that the specimens taken at comparable ages from living and dead babies are similar shows that surfactant does not deteriorate significantly after death (for further details on this point, see Hill et al.[2]). Those babies who died from pneumonia have low levels (60.2 ± 2.9%), which are similar to those from the SIDS babies. However, the babies who died from septicemia have levels (69.6 ± 3.9%) which are comparable to the values seen in samples from mature infants and in the specimens obtained by tracheostomy (70.8 ± 2.0%). The similarity in levels of phosphatidylcholine in SIDS and pneumonia may suggest that SIDS is related to lung infection. The last comparison is with babies who died from hyaline membrane disease (HMD) in the first 2 days after birth. The value for these babies (57.7 ± 1.7%) is lower than for the SIDS babies ($p < 0.05$) and very much lower than the values for the other groups, except for the babies who died of pneumonia.

In summary, the data in FIGURE 1 show that the phosphatidylcholine level in surfactant from SIDS babies is lower than in specimens from babies of similar age and/or full-term babies and is surprisingly similar to the level in specimens from both very premature babies who have died from severe HMD and babies who have died from pneumonia.

Sphingomyelin levels are shown in FIGURE 2. These are relatively low in the

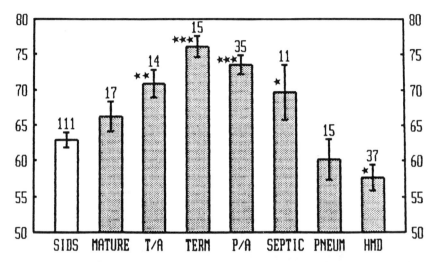

FIGURE 1. The level of phosphatidylcholine as a percentage of the total phospholipid in the lung wash for each of the groups. The results are expressed as the mean (± SE) with differences analyzed using Student's *t* test. The significant differences compare SIDS with other groups: *, $p < 0.05$; **, $p < 0.01$; ***, $p < 0.001$. Numbers above brackets indicate number of infants in each group. SIDS, babies who died of SIDS; MATURE, babies who died from diseases other than SIDS at age 14 days to 1 yr (minimal lung pathology); T/A, tracheal aspirates from living infants who had tracheostomies for upper airway problems; TERM, full-term babies with normal lungs who died within 14 days of birth; P/A, pharyngeal aspirates from full-term, healthy newborns; SEPTIC, babies who died from septicemia; PNEUM, babies who died from pneumonia; HMD, very premature babies who died in the acute phase of hyaline membrane disease. See MATERIALS AND METHODS for further details.

specimens which should have normal surfactant i.e., tracheostomy specimens (3.4 ± 1.0%), samples from full-term babies (3.3 ± 0.5%), and pharyngeal aspirates (3.8 ± 0.6%). By contrast, the percentage is high in the SIDS group (11.5 ± 0.6%), the pneumonia group (11.4 ± 1.0%) and the babies who died from HMD (12.4 ± 1.0%); it is intermediate in the mature infants (7.2 ± 0.9%) and the septicemia group (8.9 ± 2.1%).

As "mature" infants have intermediate levels of phosphatidylcholine and sphingo-myelin which are similar to those found in the septicemic babies, the data may indicate that the lungs of the "mature" infants were not absolutely normal.

Since surfactant appears to be abnormal in SIDS, it is possible that it might be a useful marker for the condition. The ratio of phosphatidylcholine to sphingomyelin, which is the best discriminator, may be a useful index. A ratio of 10:1 was chosen as the discriminant level, because 90% of SIDS cases have a ratio lower than this value. TABLE 1 shows the incidence of values below the cut-off level of 10:1 for the ratio of phosphatidylcholine to sphingomyelin in surfactant samples from each group. From these results, it can be calculated that if this ratio is used to classify surfactant obtained from the lungs of a dead infant, it would have a sensitivity of 87% and a specificity of 59%.

Surfactant is important for the maintenance of normal lung function. A change in surfactant composition is only important if it causes an alteration in its physical properties. FIGURE 3 shows the surface tension versus area of normal surfactant compared with specimens from 5 SIDS babies. When mature surfactant is placed on a surface tension trough and compressed by 50% of its surface area, it produces a surface tension of almost

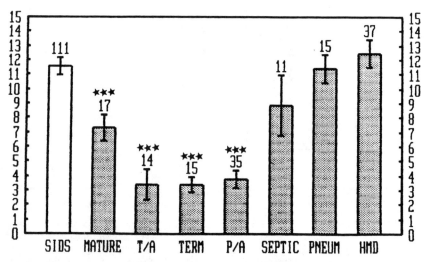

FIGURE 2. The level of sphingomyelin as a percentage of the total phospholipid in the lung wash for each of the groups. The results are expressed as the mean ($\pm$ SE) with differences analyzed using Student's t test. The significant differences compare SIDS with other groups: *, $p < 0.05$; **, $p < 0.01$; ***, $p < 0.001$. For definitions of groups, see FIGURE 1 and MATERIALS AND METHODS.

zero, as shown by the solid loop line in FIGURE 3. The most important physical property of surfactant is to sustain a low surface tension, which maintains alveolar patency. It can be seen (FIG. 3) that when the surfactant obtained from SIDS babies is compressed, the surface tension does not fall below 20 mN/m.

The inability of the surfactant from SIDS cases to produce low surface tensions under pressure means that this surfactant would be likely to compromise normal lung function, predisposing these babies to smaller alveolar size and a lower lung volume. In this situation, alveolar collapse during expiration might occur, particularly if the other mechanisms which maintain the functional residual capacity, such as intercostal and diaphragmatic muscle tone and laryngeal activity, were inadequate. Without adequate surfactant, alveolar edema would also occur.

TABLE 1. The Incidence in Surfactant Samples from Each Group of a Phosphatidylcholine: Sphingomyelin Ratio Less than 10:1

Group[a]	Incidence	(%)
Pneumonia	14/15	(93)
SIDS	97/111	(89)
HMD	31/37	(84)
Septicemia	6/11	(55)
Mature infants	7/17	(41)
Pharyngeal aspirate	4/35	(11)
Tracheal aspirate	2/14	(14)
Full-term infants	3/15	(20)

[a]For definition of groups, see FIGURE 1 and MATERIALS AND METHODS.

DISCUSSION

The data presented in this paper show that the surfactant obtained from the lungs of babies who have died from SIDS is very abnormal compared with the composition of surfactant from babies who have died from other conditions or are alive but had tracheostomies. The problem with all postmortem studies of SIDS is that satisfactory control cases are rare, because very few healthy babies in the same age range die suddenly and most of those who do were not particularly healthy. For this reason we have compared

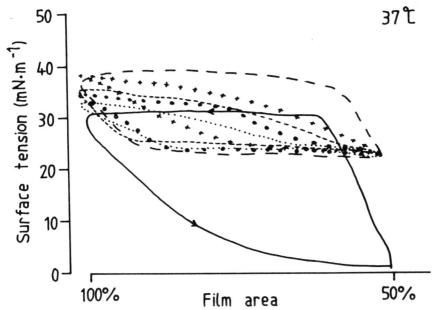

FIGURE 3. Surface tension versus film area of mature normal surfactant (**solid line**) and of 5 specimens of surfactant obtained from the lungs of babies who died from SIDS (**lines of crosses, dots, or dashes,** respectively). Each sample was spread from a surface particle to an equilibrium monolayer at 37°C on a subphase of 0.9% saline; each monolayer was then compressed by 50% of its area.

the surfactant composition from the SIDS babies with the surfactant composition from premature babies who are known to have died with abnormal surfactant, i.e., babies with HMD. Surprisingly, the surfactant composition from the SIDS babies is much nearer to that from HMD babies than to that from "normal" babies of a similar age. It also resembles the surfactant from babies who died from pneumonia and is very different from the surfactant obtained from the newborn full-term babies.

The biological significance of this difference in composition in SIDS rests in the surface-active properties of the phospholipids. A reduction in the amount of saturated phosphatidylcholine in the surfactant raises the minimum surface tension formed during compression and predisposes to a smaller alveolar size and potential atelectasis during expiration, particularly if the other mechanisms which maintain the functional residual capacity of the lung are temporarily inadequate. Evidence for such a problem may only be manifest in the live infant, however, because the pressure/volume loops of postmortem lungs from SIDS infants are reported by Fagan and Milner to be normal.[4] Although these lungs show small areas of atelectasis and considerable edema, the histology does not reveal large areas of collapse.

The reason for the high levels of sphingomyelin in the SIDS cases cannot easily be explained. It may have come from cell membranes and be a marker of cell damage.

The cause of the surfactant defect in SIDS is not clear. In this study we divided the SIDS cases into those with no signs of lung pathology and those with some evidence of infection. One of the intriguing features of the results is the almost complete homogeneity between the composition of surfactant obtained from these two groups of babies. Viral infections may cause little tissue damage, and it is also possible that some of the apparently uninfected SIDS babies had an infection which was not apparent. It is impossible from this data to determine whether the surfactant abnormality predisposed to the infection or whether infection caused the abnormal surfactant. There is evidence that viral pneumonitis can cause surfactant abnormalities.[5,6] It is therefore possible that the surfactant abnormality in the SIDS babies may be secondary to undetected viral infections.[7] This possibility may have bearing on the fact that the age for the peak incidence of deaths from SIDS is also the age for the peak incidence of infant respiratory virus infections, which is at the nadir of infant immunity. However, no single virus has been implicated, and even when viruses are found, it is not possible to know whether they are the cause of the problem or passive pathogens. Particularly in this age group, when viral infections are so common, it is not surprising that some children will actually be infected or show incidence of a recent infection at the time of death.

It is a well-known fact that SIDS rarely occurs in the first 2 weeks of life. This may be because normal babies secrete a large amount of surfactant after birth to facilitate and maintain normal lung expansion and the remnants of this surfactant persist for many days. During this time, the ability of the surfactant to support normal lung patency and function would be much greater than in the subsequent weeks when the surfactant supply and composition might have been changed by infections.

It is interesting to consider which mechanisms may be involved in the alteration in surfactant composition with a viral infection. During viral infections children breathe faster, which would cause more surfactant to be lost from the lungs. This would stimulate the type II cells to increase their synthesis and release of surfactant. During the final stages of surfactant synthesis, the phosphatidylcholine is remodeled from having one saturated and one unsaturated fatty acid chain to having two saturated fatty acids. It may be possible that either the virus infection interferes with this final enzymatic process or the increased release of surfactant causes it to be released prematurely, in a more unsaturated form.

In conclusion, we are not in a position to say whether the abnormal surfactant we have found in the babies who died from SIDS is the main factor predisposing to their deaths, a contributory cause, or even a coincidental finding. However, because the change in surfactant composition, whether pathological or developmental, is such a constant feature of SIDS, it is likely in a high proportion of cases to be a fundamental component of the pathogenesis of the sudden death.

Finally, we would like to suggest that abnormal lung surfactant be considered part of the etiology of sudden unexpected infant death. We would like to speculate that this abnormality may be secondary to damage of the type II cells by viral infection. How this causes death is unclear. It may be a primary factor, but it is more likely that it exaggerates the effects of a hypoxic episode so that the infant is suddenly overwhelmed. It is possible that the infant has an episode of expiratory apnea, very similar to the breath-holding attacks of older infants. During this apnea, the lung volume is considerably reduced. Babies who have abnormal surfactant would be liable to develop very low lung volumes and a high level of right-to-left shunting of blood. Under these circumstances, they could become very hypoxic within seconds. If for some reason they could not gasp their way out of this apnea, they would soon die.

ACKNOWLEDGMENTS

We would like to thank Dr. A. Barson and Professor A. Gresham for their help collecting the specimens.

REFERENCES

1. MORLEY, C. J., C. M. HILL, B. D. BROWN, A. J. BARSON & J. A. DAVIS. 1982. Surfactant abnormalities in babies dying from sudden infant death syndrome. Lancet **i:** 1320–1332.
2. HILL, C. M., B. D. BROWN, C. J. MORLEY, J. A. DAVIS & A. BARSON. 1988. Pulmonary surfactant: 2. In sudden infant death syndrome. Early Hum. Dev. **16:** 153–162.
3. HILL, C. M., B. D. BROWN, C. J. MORLEY, J. A. DAVIS & A. BARSON. 1988. Pulmonary surfactant 1. In immature and mature babies. Early Hum. Dev. **16:** 143–151.
4. FAGAN, D. G. & A. D. MILNER. 1985. Pressure volume characteristics of the lungs of sudden infant death syndrome. Arch. Dis. Child. **60:** 471–485.
5. TYRRELL, D. A., M. MIKA-JOHNSON, G. PHILLIPS, W. H. J. DOUGLAS & P. J. CHAPPLE. 1979. Infection of cultured human type 2 pneumocytes with certain respiratory viruses. Infect. Immun. **26:**621–629.
6. LOOSLI, C. G., S. F. STINSON, D. P. RYAN, M. S. HERTWECK, J. D. HARDY & R. SEREBRIN. 1975. The destruction of type 2 pneumocytes by airborne influenza PR8-A virus: Its effect on surfactant and lecithin content of the pneumonic lesions of mice. Chest **67:**7S–14S.
7. WILLIAMS, A. L., E. C. UREN & L. BRETHERTON. 1984. Respiratory viruses and sudden infant death. Br. Med. J. **288:**1491–1493.

The Role of Pulmonary Surfactant in SIDS

R. A. GIBSON

Department of Pediatrics
Flinders Medical Centre
Bedford Park
South Australia 5042

E. J. McMURCHIE

C. S. I. R. O. Division of Human Nutrition
Majors Road
O'Halloran Hill
South Australia 5158

In order to discuss the role of pulmonary surfactant in SIDS I would like to first of all review the role of pulmonary surfactant in the lung. The model generally accepted by a number of workers is that for all practical purposes we can consider the unit of the lung, the alveolus, as a spherical structure made up of alveolar type I cells.[1] At numerous locations around the sphere, type II pneumocytes are located (FIGURE 1). The internal surface of the alveolar sphere is considered to be covered by a thin aqueous layer, and, like all aqueous layers, the surface is subject to surface tension. Using this model, it is possible to recognize that this surface tension results in a force that either will tend to cause fluid (from interstitial space) to fill the alveolar cavity or will collapse the alveolus, or both. For any given sphere (or alveolus) this force (P) is given by the Laplace equation, which is written as $P = 2T/R$. Even with the most rudimentary knowledge of mathematics, it is possible to tell a number of things from this equation. The first is that the force tending to collapse the alveolus (or, more properly, the force required to support it) is dependent on the surface tension (T); the higher the surface tension, the higher the pressure required to support the sphere. The second important thing to be seen from the equation is that the pressure is also dependent on the radius (R) of the sphere in such a way that the smaller the size of the sphere (and thus its radius), the higher the pressure required to support it. This means that very small alveoli are harder to keep open (i.e., require more pressure) than larger alveoli. Now, while it is not possible for the body to regulate in any immediate way the size of alveoli in the lung, it can regulate the surface tension of the air/aqueous interface. This of course is performed by pulmonary surfactant which is secreted from the lamellar bodies in the type II pneumocytes and forms a layer over the internal aqueous lining of the alveolus.

Pulmonary surfactant actually performs two separate roles.[2] Firstly, surfactant lowers the surface tension of the air-water interface to acceptable levels, probably about 20 mN/m. Secondly, it provides a rigid structural support to the inside of the alveolus. Surfactant is composed chiefly of disaturated phosphatidylcholine (DSPC) which, because of its two constituent saturated fatty acids (generally palmitic acid), is able to form a layer of closely packed molecules on the surface of the aqueous lining. When on exhalation the radius of the alveolus is decreased and the layer of surfactant is compressed, it forms a rigid layer which provides mechanical support that further compensates for and perhaps even obliterates any residual effects of surface tension. Thus, because of its combined effect of reducing the surface tension of the internal aqueous layer lining the lung and providing mechanical support, the presence of the surfactant DSPC means that little or no pressure is required to keep all the alveoli of the lung open in the normal child.

We wondered several years ago whether there was any relationship between SIDS and the chemical composition of pulmonary surfactant, since an undoubted result of SIDS was that the infant at some point stopped breathing. In addition, some workers have reported areas of atelectasis in the lungs of infants succumbing to SIDS, and death from SIDS was often preceded by a minor respiratory-tract infection.[3] The model in our minds at that time was that the infants who subsequently succumbed to SIDS could be analogous to premature infants who develop hyaline membrane disease or respiratory distress syndrome (HMD/RDS), a condition known to be partially due to surfactant insufficiency and immaturity.[4] Generally surfactant from HMD/RDS infants is much lower in DSPC content than is that from normal full-term infants, and lung collapse is a constant threat.

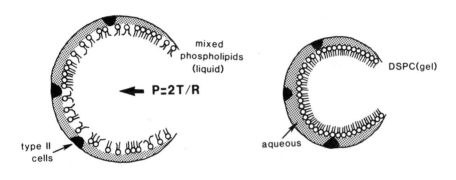

EXPANDED   CONTRACTED

FIGURE 1.   Schematic model of the alveolus as a spherical structure lined by a thin aqueous layer (**shading**) onto which is spread a layer of pulmonary surfactant (mixed phospholipids) secreted from lamellar bodies in type II pneumocytes (**dark patches**). The force (**P**) required to support the alveolus and prevent its collapse is dependent on the surface tension (**T**) and inversely dependent on the radius (**R**) of the alveolus (sphere). Upon exhalation, the expanded alveolus (*left*) becomes contracted (*right*) and the layer of surfactant (**liquid**) is compressed, forming a rigid structure (**gel**) which provides mechanical support. DSPC, disaturated phosphatidylcholine. See text for further discussion of surfactant function.

MATERIALS AND METHODS

In our first study[5,6] we examined the surfactant obtained by lung lavage at autopsy of 40 infants who died of SIDS and 12 infants who died from other causes. The classification of SIDS was made according to standard practice at the Adelaide Children's Hospital; it was made only if the death was unexpected from a detailed history and if autopsy examination failed to find a cause of death. For the control group, death was caused by liver disease (1 infant), drowning (1), motor vehicle accidents (6), heart failure (2), neck trauma (1) and renal failure (1). The number of males and females in the control group was equal while in the SIDS group 24 (60%) were males. The age range of the subjects and the postmortem interval of control and SIDS infants is shown in TABLE 1 (Study I). Subsequent to this, in 1986, we examined a further 25 SIDS and 4 control infants (TABLE 1, Study II) and currently, in 1987, we have so far examined the lung lavage and lamellar

TABLE 1. Comparison between SIDS and Control Infants Studied: Age at Death and Time to Postmortem Examination

	Study I		Study II	
	Control	SIDS	Control	SIDS
No. of infants	12	40	4	25
Age (wk)				
Mean	77 ± 17	23 ± 3	32 ± 20	16 ± 10
Range	1–168	4–89	1–85	3–39
Time to postmortem (hr)				
Mean	21 ± 3	26 ± 4	14 ± 11	27 ± 19
Range	14–36	2–77	5–29	3–54

body surfactant from 13 SIDS and 3 control infants. All of the control subjects in these latter studies died in motor vehicle accidents.

The details of our lung-washing procedure have been described in detail elsewhere, as has the method for the separation of DSPC from surfactant lipids.[5,6] Briefly, the procedure, which is based on the method of Mason et al.,[7] involves complexing all unsaturated phospholipids with osmium tetroxide and subsequently separating the DSPC by thin-layer chromatography. Currently we are also separating the lamellar bodies from excised lung tissue obtained at autopsy from SIDS and control infants. The lamellar bodies are isolated from lung homogenates by differential and sucrose density gradient centrifugation[8] and the lipids analyzed by the methods referred to above.

RESULTS AND DISCUSSION

We have not attempted in any of our studies to quantitate the amount of surfactant or surfactant lipids present in the lavage material, as the yield of lavage fluid varies enormously from subject to subject. However, we have examined the surfactant lipids in detail. The phospholipid class distribution of the total lipids from the lung-lavage samples examined in two studies is shown in TABLE 2. Phosphatidylcholine (PC), at 58–64% of the total, was the predominant phospholipid class present, but no difference was seen in

TABLE 2. Phospholipid Class Distribution in the Surfactant of Lung Lavage Samples from SIDS and Control Infants

	Study I		Study II	
Phospholipid[a]	Control[b] (n = 12)	SIDS[b] (n = 40)	Control[b] (n = 4)	SIDS[b] (n = 25)
PC	57.9 ± 2.9	60.7 ± 0.9	63.9 ± 8.1	64.1 ± 5.2
PG	10.8 ± 0.7	10.3 ± 0.5	8.2 ± 0.5	6.8 ± 2.1
Sph.	12.0 ± 1.3	11.4 ± 0.5	6.6 ± 2.6	10.0 ± 3.7
PE	9.3 ± 1.0	9.2 ± 0.4	10.5 ± 4.0	10.5 ± 2.7
PS & PI	10.2 ± 0.6	8.2 ± 0.5	8.9 ± 0.6	8.6 ± 1.4
% DSPC	77 ± 4[c]	66 ± 2[c]	64 ± 8[c]	56 ± 8[c]

[a]PC, phosphatidylcholine; PG, phosphatidylglycerol; Sph., sphingomyelin; PE, phosphatidylethanolamine; PS, phosphatidylserine; PI, phosphatidylinositol; DSPC, disaturated phosphatidylcholine.
[b]Percentage of total phospholipid.
[c]Percentage of total PC.

the level of PC when the source of the lipids was SIDS rather than control infants. This result contrasts markedly with that published by Morley and coworkers,[9] who reported a reduced proportion of PC and some other phospholipids in lavage surfactant lipids obtained from infants who died of SIDS. It should be stressed, however, that there are important methodological differences between the study of Morley's group and ours; it may well be that the extremely low values they report for the percentage of DSPC present in surfactant from SIDS infants are to some extent due to their method of separating disaturated phospholipids.

Our further investigations of the PC fraction did, however, reveal differences between the SIDS and control groups (TABLE 2). In Studies I and II, the percentage of DSPC in the PC fraction of lavage surfactant lipids was higher in the samples from control infants than from SIDS infants, and in study I, at least, this difference was significant ($p < 0.01$). A similar result was reported by Morley and colleagues.[9]

Because lavage surfactant almost certainly represents surfactant that was secreted from the alveoli some considerable time before death, there exists the possibility that some of the changes reported here may be due to extracellular breakdown of surfactant lipids. Although we have evidence that this is probably minimal in degree (and would tend to reduce differences between SIDS and control samples rather than account for them), it was obviously necessary to obtain a source of surfactant which was more stable. Lamellar

TABLE 3. Disaturated Phosphatidylcholine (DSPC) Content of Total Phosphatidylcholine from Surfactant Lipids in Lung Lavage Samples or Lamellar Bodies: Comparison of Control and SIDS Infants

Infants	n	DSPC[a]	
		Lavage	Lamellar Body
Control	3	77 ± 4	60 ± 5
SIDS	13	66 ± 2	47 ± 7

[a]Percentage of total phosphatidylcholine.

bodies, which are known to contain stored surfactant, are an ideal source of material. In an analysis of isolated lamellar bodies as well as lung lavage specimens, our results to date for a limited experimental series (13 SIDS, 3 control samples) are similar to those we obtained in previous studies, that is, no significant difference in percentage PC between SIDS (85%) and control (79%) infants and a reduced proportion of DSPC in the PC fraction in SIDS infants as compared with control infants (TABLE 3).

These observed changes in the DSPC content of lung surfactant in SIDS would be expected to induce changes in its biophysical properties, particularly at its site of action, the air-aqueous interface of the alveolus.[10,11] In a separate study reported earlier[12] and in a study reported in this volume, MORLEY has consistently found that surfactant from SIDS infants and infants who died from pulmonary infection reduces the surface tension to a value no lower than about 20 mN/m, while control surfactant apparently ablates all surface tension (i.e., apparently reduces it to zero). However, it is probable that this apparently zero value for the surface tension came about as an artifact of the surface tension measurement[2] and that what is actually being measured is the ability of control surfactant to provide mechanical support to the internal surface of the alveolar air-aqueous interface in a sort of "igloo" effect. Thus, the surfactant from SIDS, which is less saturated (i.e., contains less DSPC), is not able to be compressed and provides less structural support against the force (surface tension) tending to collapse the alveoli.

Talbert and Southall[1,13] have argued quite elegantly that an abnormal surfactant of the type described in this paper could give rise to a lowered alveolar volume and could, under certain conditions, lead to alveolar collapse. It may well be that the results reported by ourselves and by Morley's group indicate that, whether as a result of a congenital abnormality and/or as a result of infection, the lungs of SIDS infants are predisposed to irreversible collapse. We therefore believe the decreased proportion of saturated PC in pulmonary surfactant to be a factor in SIDS.

REFERENCES

1. TALBERT, D.G. & D.P. SOUTHALL. 1985. Spherical alveoli and sudden infant lung collapse syndrome. Lancet ii: 217–218.
2. BANGHAM, A.D. 1987. Lung surfactant: How it does and does not work. Lung 165: 17–25.
3. BEAL, S.M. 1983. Some epidemiological factors about sudden infant death syndrome (SIDS) in South Australia. In Sudden Infant Death Syndrome. J.T. Tilton, L.M. Roeder and A. Steinschneider, Eds.: 15–28. Academic Press. New York.
4. IKEGAMI, M., H. JACOBS & A. JOBE. 1983. Surfactant function in respiratory distress syndrome. J. Pediatr. 102: 443–447.
5. GIBSON, R.A. & E. J. McMURCHIE. 1986. Changes in lung surfactant lipids associated with the sudden infant death syndrome. Aust. Paediatr. J. 22: 77–80.
6. GIBSON, R.A. & E.J. McMURCHIE. 1987. Decreased lung surfactant disaturated phosphatidyl-choline in sudden infant death (SIDS). Early Hum. Dev. In press.
7. MASON, R.J., J. NELLENBOGEN & J.A. CLEMENTS. 1976. Isolation of disaturated phosphatidylcholine with osmium tetroxide. J. Lipid Res. 17: 281–284.
8. POWER, J.H.T., M.E. JONES, H.A. BARR & T.E. NICHOLAS. 1986. Analysis of pulmonary phospholipid compartments in the unanethetized rat during prolonged periods of hyperpnea. Exp. Lung Res. 11: 105–128.
9. MORLEY, C.L., C.M. HILL, B.D. BROWN, A.J. BARSON & J.A. DAVIS. 1982. Surfactant abnormalities in babies dying from sudden infant death syndrome. Lancet i: 1320–1323.
10. BANGHAM, A.D., C. MORLEY & M. PHILLIPS. 1979. The physical properties of an effective lung surfactant. Biochim. Biophys. Acta 573: 552–556.
11. BANGHAM, A.D. 1980. Breathing made easy. New Sci. 85: 408–410.
12. MORLEY, C.J., R.J. DAVIES, C.M. HILL & M.E. HEATH. 1985. Alveoli and abnormal surfactant. Lancet i: 1329–1330.
13. TALBERT, D.G. & D.P. SOUTHALL. 1985. A bimodal form of alveolar behaviour induced by a defect in lung surfactant—possible mechanism for sudden infant death syndrome. Lancet i: 727–728.

Periodic Breathing

DOROTHY H. KELLY,[a]

DAVID W. CARLEY, AND DANIEL C. SHANNON

Children's Service
Massachusetts General Hospital
Boston, Massachusetts

Periodic breathing (PB) has been described in normal adults[1] and newborns[2] who are living at high altitude. It has also been noted in adults with central nervous system (CNS) disturbances,[3,4] in cardiac failure,[5–9] and during hypoxemia.[10,11] It has been found in excessive amounts in the preterm infant[12] and in some full-term infants,[13] as well as in some infants who have apnea of infancy (AOI),[14,15] in some who are victims of the sudden infant death syndrome (SIDS) and have a history of AOI or a family history of SIDS,[16] and in some who are siblings of SIDS victims (SS).[17] In addition, studies by Southall *et al.*[18] have suggested a relationship between PB and SIDS in some apparently normal infants who had no family history of SIDS.

Because PB with a very similar pattern is found in multiple clinical settings, including apnea and sudden death, and because the origins of PB in an individual subject are unexplained, a computer model of respiratory control was developed.[19] By using this model, one can determine the specific type and magnitude of changes in the respiratory control system which are necessary to generate an unstable breathing pattern. The maximum instability is demonstrated in this model by a pattern of periodic respirations alternating with periodic apnea.[20]

Respiratory control has been studied by many physiologists, using multiple variables[21–25] to describe the three basic components of the control system: (1) the controller, which represents the CNS input for directing ventilation, (2) the controlled system or total body gas storage, and (3) the feed-back delay or time necessary for blood to travel from the controlled system to the controller. In general, these models describe an equilibrium among the key components. This equilibrium encourages restabilization following a disturbance (e.g., a sigh) if the loop gain is substantially less than 1.0. However, if the gain exceeds 1.0, instability is perpetuated, as demonstrated by oscillatory breathing which grows to a maximum and is sustained. These models have not been experimentally validated, primarily because they included 15 or more physiological variables which, basically, are impossible to measure on any one subject at any one time.

Carley and Shannon[19] have developed a minimal model that includes 5 physiological variables, all of which are measured in about 20 min in adults. Loop gain depends on the interaction of these 5 variables and determines the relative stability of the chemoreceptor control system. These variables are (1) central chemosensitivity to carbon dioxide, (2) mixed venous P_{CO_2}, (3) cardiac output, (4) circulation delay, and (5) mean lung volume for CO_2 (functional residual capacity of the lungs plus half of the mean tidal volume). This model has now been validated in awake ($n = 15$) and asleep ($n = 22$) young healthy adults. In addition, a simulation model has been developed[26] that allows manipulation of variables singly or in combinations.

[a]Mailing address: Pediatric Pulmonary Laboratory, Massachusetts General Hospital, Boston, MA 02114.

METHODS

The computer simulation model[26] was used to alter the 5 variables individually and in combinations in order to change loop gain. Respiratory patterns generated by this model before, during, and following these changes were recorded.

In order to validate the model, the 5 variables were measured on each subject and the individual loop gain was calculated. The breathing pattern was measured at rest, using a calibrated inductance plethysmograph, before and after a two-breath challenge with CO_2 ($\triangle P_{CO_2}$ averaged 4 mm Hg) against a background of air, 15% O_2, and 12% O_2; hypoxia was used in order to amplify chemoreceptor sensitivity, increase loop gain and, therefore, promote instability. An index of relative stability was developed by comparing the power spectral density of the respiratory signal centering at 0.05 Hz following the CO_2 pulse to the preceding baseline normalized for the change in P_{ACO_2}. The value of the relative stability measured from the recorded responses at the loop gain calculated from the measured variables was then compared to that predicted by the model.

RESULTS

Periodic breathing was repeatedly generated by the computer simulation model using small changes in values of the variables, in the range typical for an infant. These changes included (1) increasing the time delay 1.75 times, (2) decreasing functional residual capacity by 25%, and (3) increasing chemosensitivity to CO_2 by a factor of 2. Analysis of the relationship between loop gain and PB demonstrated that sustained PB was generated when the loop gain was ≥ 1.0.

In the adult subjects, PB was uniformly provoked ($n = 13$) by a CO_2 pulse if the calculated loop gain for the subject was increased to a value ≥ 1.0 by the breathing of an hypoxic gas mixture. Even before a CO_2 pulse was given, PB was also seen in some subjects breathing 12% O_2 at loop gains ≥ 1.0. On three occasions, PB occurred when the loop gain was 0.8–1.0, but never when it was less than 0.72 ($n = 69$).

DISCUSSION

Periodic breathing is seen in a variety of clinical settings. From the computer model tested in this study, it is predicted that PB will occur when the interactions among the five variables of the model, that together characterize the controller, controlled system and time delay, result in a loop gain ≥ 1.0. In addition, when this computer model was applied to the healthy adult male subjects, both awake and asleep, it accurately predicted the breathing pattern generated by amplifying the controller gain. Thus, by measuring the 5 physiological variables in the adult subject and calculating the loop gain, one can anticipate the relative stability of the breathing pattern at a frequency of about 0.05 Hz. We plan to test the model on adults in whom various variables are altered to further validate its ability to predict instability. We also plan to validate the model in infants in whom computer simulations predict that reduced FRC will be one of the factors most likely to provoke instability. If, by using this computer model, we can accurately predict the breathing pattern of specific infants, we may also be able to determine the physiological variable(s) producing PB in a particular infant. By understanding the physiological cause of this breathing pattern, a more rational approach to therapy should be possible.

In summary, PB is naturally inherent in the ventilatory control system. It becomes apparent when abnormalities, affecting one or more of the components of the system, enhance the loop gain above a critical level. Although it has been seen in infants in association with several pathophysiolocial conditions, including AOI and SIDS, we do not understand either its origin or its value as a predictor of morbidity or mortality. It is hoped that with further development of this computer model in infants, the significance of PB in AOI, SS, and SIDS will be better understood.

REFERENCES

1. DOUGLAS, C.G. & J.B.S. HALDANE. 1909. The causes of periodic or Cheyne-Stokes respiration. J. Physiol. (London) **38**: 401–419.
2. DEMING, J. & A.H. WASHBURN. 1935. Respiration in infancy. Am. J. Dis. Child. **49**: 108–124.
3. JACKSON, J.H. 1895. Neurological abstracts: XV. Superior and subordinate centers of the lowest level. Lancet **1**: 476–478.
4. ROSENBACH, O. 1880. Real-encyclopedie der gasammten Haikunde. Dr. Albert Culenberg **3**: 5150.
5. CHEYNE, J.A. 1818. A case of apoplexy in which the fleshy part of the heart was converted into fat. Dublin Hosp. Rep. **2**: 216–223.
6. STOKES, W. 1854. The diseases of the heart and the aorta. Dublin, Hodges & Smith **326**: 323–324.
7. PEMBREY, M.S. 1908. Observations on Cheyne-Stokes respiration. J. Pathol. Bacteriol. **12**: 258–266.
8. KLEIN, O. 1930. Untersuchungen uber das Cheyne-Stokesche arthmungsphanomen. Vehr. Dtsch. Ges. Inn. Med. **42**: 217–222.
9. PRYOR, W.W. 1956. Cheyne-Stokes respiration in patients with cardiac enlargement and prolonged circulation time. Circulation **4**: 223–228.
10. WAGGENER, T.B., P.J. BRUSIL, R.E. KRONAUER & R. GABEL. 1977. Strength and period of oscillations in unacclimatized humans at high altitude. Physiologist **20**: 9.
11. WEST, J.B., R.M. PETERS, G.K.H. AKSNES, J.S. MILLEDGE & R.B. SCHOENE. 1986. Nocturnal periodic breathing at 6300 and 8050 m. J. Appl. Physiol. **61**: 280–287.
12. CHERNICK, V. 1981. The fetus and newborn. *In* Regulation of Breathing. T.B. Hornbein, Ed.: 1164. Marcel Dekker Inc. New York.
13. KELLY, D.H., L.M. STELLWAGEN, E. KATZ & D.C. SHANNON. 1985. Apnea and periodic breathing in normal full term infants during the first 12 months. Pediatr. Pulmonol. **1**: 215–219.
14. KELLY, D.H. & D.C. SHANNON. 1979. Periodic breathing in infants with near-miss sudden infant death syndrome. Pediatrics **63**: 355–360.
15. KEENS, T.G., S.M.E.P. BOOKOUT & A.C.G. PLATZKER. 1982. Pneumograms do not predict subsequent apnea in near-miss sudden infant death syndrome infants (abstract). Clin. Res. **30**: 150A.
16. KELLY, D.H., H. GOLUB, D.W. CARLEY & D.C. SHANNON. 1986. Pneumograms in infants who subsequently died of SIDS. J. Pediatr. **109**: 249–254.
17. KELLY, D.H., A.M. WALKER, L. CAHEN & D.C. SHANNON. 1980. Periodic breathing in siblings of sudden infant death syndrome victims. Pediatrics **66**: 515–520.
18. SOUTHALL, D.P., J.M. RICHARD, E.A. SHINEBOURNE, C.I. FRANKS, A.J. WILSON & J.R. ALEXANDER. 1983. Prospective population-based studies into heart rate and breathing patterns in newborn infants: Prediction of infants at risk of SIDS. *In* Sudden Infant Death Syndrome. J.T. Tildon, L.M. Roeder & A. Steinschneider, Eds.: 621. Academic Press. New York.
19. CARLEY, D.W. & D.C. SHANNON. 1985. A minimal control system model of periodic breathing. *In* Proceedings of the 11th Northeast Bioengineering Conference: 361–364. IEEE Publication No. 85CH2203-8. IEEE. Worchester, MA.
20. CARLEY, D.W. 1985. The Stability of Respiratory Control in Man: Mathematical and

Experimental Analyses. Ph.D. Thesis. Massachusetts Institute of Technology. Cambridge, MA.

21. GRODINS, F.S., J.S. GRAY, K. SCHROEDER, A.I. NORINS & R.W. JONES. 1954. Respiratory responses to CO_2 inhalation; a theoretical study of a nonlinear biological regulator. J. Appl. Physiol. **7:** 283–306.

22. MILHORN, H. & A.C. GUYTON. 1965. An analog computer analysis of Cheyne-Stokes breathing. J. Appl. Physiol. **20:** 328–333.

23. LONGOBARDO, G.S., N.S. CHERNIACK & A.P. FISHMAN. 1966. Cheyne-Stokes breathing produced by a model of the human respiratory system. J. Appl. Physiol. **21:** 1839–1846.

24. GRODINS, F.S., J. BUELL & A. BART. 1967. A mathematical analysis and digital simulation of the respiratory control system. J. Appl. Physiol. **22:** 160–276.

25. KHOO, M.C., R.E. KRONAUER, K.P. STROHL & A.S. SLUTSKY. 1982. Factors inducing periodic breathing in humans: A general model. J. Appl. Physiol. Respir. Environ. Exercise Physiol. **53:** 644–659.

26. CARLEY, D.W. & D.C. SHANNON. A minimal mathematical model of human periodic breathing. J. Appl. Physiol. In press.

Postneonatal Development of Respiratory Oscillations[a]

PETER J. FLEMING,[b] MICHAEL R. LEVINE,
ANDREW M. LONG, AND JOHN P. CLEAVE

University of Bristol
Departments of Child Health, Physiology, and Mathematics
Bristol Maternity Hospital
Bristol BS2 8EG
United Kingdom

INTRODUCTION

There is some evidence that in many, if not all, infants who die of SIDS the final sequence of events is cessation of breathing followed, after a variable delay, by cardiac arrest. The lack of any detectable major physical abnormality in the lungs or respiratory musculature leads to the conclusion that this cessation of breathing is due to the failure of the respiratory control system normally responsible for the maintenance of regular respiration. The search for ways in which the respiratory control system might fail has led to many investigations of breathing pattern in infants and many attempts to recognize differences in the patterns of breathing between normal infants and those deemed, by epidemiological risk scoring, to be at increased risk of SIDS.

Such attempts to identify altered patterns of breathing presuppose that for a control system to fail, it must behave in some abnormal or faulty way. The study of other control systems (e.g., in engineering) shows that such failure does not necessarily signify a detectable pre-existing fault or abnormality. It is equally possible that a particular combination of circumstances or events may expose a vulnerability within a *normally* functioning control system and thus lead to failure. Changes with age in a developing control system may mean that apparently identical stimuli at different ages will give rise to widely differing responses. In an attempt to understand the ways in which catastrophic failure might arise, we have therefore sought to investigate and characterize the development of the control of respiration in normal infants.

The dynamic performance of a control system such as that of respiration, which consists of several interdependant and interacting feedback loops, can be investigated—

1. by characterizing the spontaneously occurring oscillations in the system;
2. by investigating the pattern of recovery after a brief, naturally occurring disturbance.

Hathorn[1] and Waggener[2] have used different techniques to characterize the continuous oscillations in respiration in newborn infants. Hathorn[1] used the technique of cross-covariance analysis of the relationship between tidal volume (VT) and respiratory

[a]These studies were supported by a grant (No. 45) from the Foundation for the Study of Infant Deaths.

[b]To whom correspondence should be addressed at: Department of Child Health, Bristol Maternity Hospital, Southwell Street, Bristol BS2 8EG, U.K.

frequency (f) in normal full-term and preterm infants. He showed that there are continuous oscillations in both VT and f. In quiet sleep (QS) these oscillations are usually out of phase with each other, whilst in rapid eye movement (REM) sleep their phase relationship is highly variable. Waggener[2] showed that the variability of respiratory pattern in infants in REM sleep could be closely approximated by the effects of numerous, superimposed oscillations of different periods (6–87 sec). The occurrence of apnea in REM, an apparently random event, was shown to correspond closely with the trough of one or more of these oscillations. Neither of these investigators attempted to define the changes with age.

We have used the pattern of breathing after a sigh in QS as a means of characterizing the response of the respiratory control system to spontaneous disturbances.[3] The pattern of change in breath-by-breath minute ventilation (Ve; i.e., VT × f) can be described mathematically in terms of the behavior of a linear second-order differential equation. (see FIGS. 1 and 2). The oscillation in Ve which follows a sigh occurring in the first few days

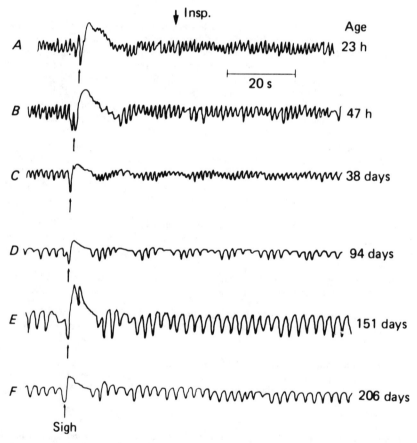

FIGURE 1. A series of 6 respiratory traces from one infant in QS at the ages shown. A spontaneous sigh (**small arrow**) is shown near the *left* of each trace. Inspirations are shown by downward deflections, as at the **large arrow** (Insp.). s, sec; h, hr. (Reproduced from Fleming *et al.*[3] with permission from the Physiological Society.)

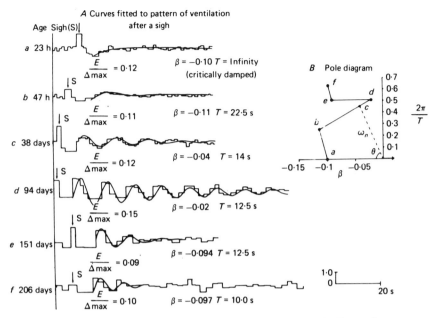

FIGURE 2. (A) Curves fitted to the patterns of ventilation after a sigh. The respiratory traces shown in FIGURE 1, processed and displayed as fractional deviation from the mean of Ve. Inset (*bottom, right*) is the scale for ordinate and abscissa. Superimposed on each response curve is the fitted cosine curve from which are derived the values for the damping factor, β, and the period of oscillation, T, given with each curve, together with the error of fitting, $E/\triangle$max. (B) An S-plane pole diagram in which the values for β and T from curves a–f (in A) have been plotted on the axes β and $2\pi/T$. (Reproduced from Fleming *et al.*[3] with permission from the Physiological Society.)

after birth of the full-term infant is highly damped, with a period (T) greater than 20 sec. With increasing age of the infant, the period of oscillation gradually shortens, to approximately 10 sec by 5–7 months of age. This increasing rapidity of response is accompanied by a progressive decrease in damping, so that between 1 and 3 months of age most infants show a prolonged oscillation in Ve after a sigh. Beyond 3 months of age, the damping again increases, so that by 5–7 months the response is highly damped. Thus, a similar, naturally-occurring disturbance can have very different effects at different ages.

In preterm infants a similar pattern was observed, but was much more variable, and the changes were more closely related to postnatal age than to postconceptional age.[4]

This technique of analysis of the responses to spontaneous disturbances can only be applied to sections of fairly regular respiration, as occur in QS. In REM sleep the extremely variable respiratory pattern makes the application of this technique inappropriate.

We have therefore developed a technique of digital filtering which allows the identification and quantification of oscillations in both QS and REM sleep.

METHODS AND SUBJECTS

The results to be presented were obtained by reanalysis of some of the recordings from the longitudinal study of normal infants previously reported.[3] The infants were all born normally, at full term, to healthy mothers. There were no significant perinatal problems, and no infants needed resuscitation at birth. Informed consent was obtained and the infants' mothers were present for most of the recordings.

For the purposes of the present report, recordings from 6 infants have been examined. Five or 6 recordings were made on each infant, at ages from 14 hr to 210 days. Each recording was for the duration of a daytime sleep period (40–180 min).

Respiration was recorded by means of the Bristol four-lead transthoracic impedance pneumograph[5] and the barometric plethysmograph.[6] Expired CO_2 was recorded by means of a catheter sampling from close to the face at a flow rate of 100 ml/min through an infrared analyzer (Beckman LB2). This use of 3 parallel systems to record respiration allowed recognition of movement artifacts and airway obstruction.[3] Sleep state was determined from bilateral recordings of EEG and electrooculogram (EOG);[7] respiratory pattern was not used as a criterion of sleep state. All signals were recorded onto a chart recorder (Devices M19), and the respiratory signals were recorded onto FM tape (Racal Store 4). Respiratory signals were later sampled at 50 Hz, using the analog-to-digital converter of a laboratory minicomputer (DEC PDP 11/34), and stored on disks.

We have previously described the program to identify breaths on the respiratory recordings.[3,8] This program produces sequential plots of breath-by-breath VT and f, and their product, Ve. For the purpose of this paper, only the plots of Ve will be considered. In order to allow comparisons between babies, and between recordings at different ages, Ve was plotted as the fractional deviation from the mean Ve (V̄e) for each study, i.e., as (Ve − V̄e)/ V̄e.

Using a program developed in our laboratory, the plots of breath-by-breath Ve were smoothed by sampling at 0.5-sec intervals and then averaged over an 8-sec moving window centered on the point being considered. The output of this moving time-averaging program was plotted on a compressed scale (see FIG. 3). Sections of these compressed plots were then subjected to Fourier analysis to determine their frequency components in both QS and REM sleep.

RESULTS

In all 6 infants the filtered plots of Ve showed characteristic patterns of oscillation, which changed with age and with sleep state. FIGURE 3 shows a 15-min section of respiratory recording from one infant (No. 29) at age 112 days, together with the filtered plot of Ve produced for this section of recording. The time of transition from REM sleep to QS is shown on both the raw, recorded signal and the filtered Ve plot (bidirectional arrow). There is a continuous oscillation with a period of 15 sec during REM sleep, whilst in QS these oscillations are less marked and are interrupted by the highly damped oscillations which follow the sighs.

FIGURE 4 shows a sequence of 5 plots of Ve for sections of respiration, each lasting 30 min, at ages from 23 hr to 206 days, for the baby (No. 26) whose respiratory traces are depicted in FIGURES 1 and 2. The duration of periods of QS and REM sleep are shown. In the first two recordings (FIGS. 4A and 4B), within 48 hr of birth, there are continuous irregular oscillations with a period of 20–25 sec during both QS and REM sleep, though the amplitude of oscillation is greather during REM sleep. By 38 days (FIG. 4C), the period of the continuous oscillation during REM sleep has shortened to 15 sec. The period of oscillations during QS has also shortened to 15 sec, but these oscillations have now become discontinuous. In QS, the oscillations are predominantly those which follow sighs, and, as previously demonstrated,[3] at this age these oscillations are damped out after 4 or 5 cycles (see FIG. 2). At 94 days (FIG. 4D) a similar pattern occurs. The relatively underdamped oscillations after sighs in QS (see FIG. 2) are clearly shown, whilst in REM sleep the oscillations are undamped and continuous. In the final line (F) of FIGURE 4, at 206 days of age, the continuous oscillations during REM sleep are still clearly seen, whilst in QS the oscillations are of very much smaller amplitude. The pattern of respiration after a sigh in QS is highly damped with no continued oscillation.

FIGURE 5 shows a similar sequence of recordings from another infant (No. 22), at ages from 15 hr to 107 days. As in the first study discussed (infant No. 29, FIG. 3), there is again a pattern of irregular, continuous oscillation during both REM sleep and QS, though in this infant, by 41 hr of age (FIG. 5B) the oscillations during QS have decreased in

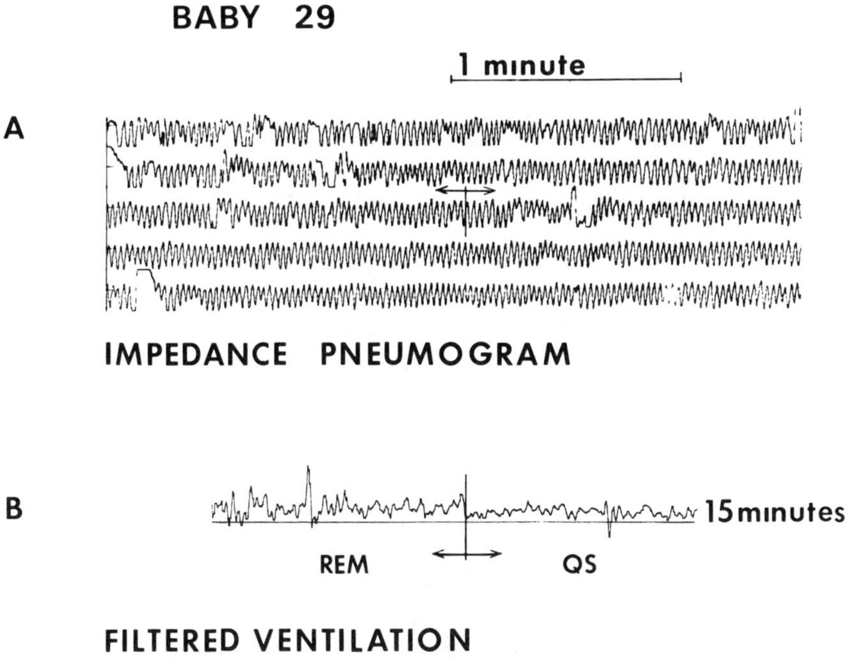

BABY 29

FIGURE 3. (A) 15-min section of respiratory trace from an infant (No. 29) aged 112 days and (B) a filtered, compressed plot of Ve for the same section of recording. The transition from REM sleep to QS is shown (*vertical line with horizontal, bidirectional arrow*). There is a continuous oscillation with a period of 15 sec in REM sleep. In QS this oscillation is of much smaller amplitude and is interrupted by the damped oscillations which follow the sighs.

amplitude except for the first minute or so after a sigh. With increasing age, the period of the dominant oscillation shortens, and the distinction between REM sleep and QS becomes more clear. The oscillations during REM sleep remain continuous, whilst those during QS occur mainly after sighs and then die away after a variable period. In the recordings at 32 and 78 days of age (FIGS. 5C and 5D), the sighs in QS are followed by relatively underdamped oscillations which continue for 4–9 cycles. By 107 days (FIG. 5E), there is little continuous oscillation during QS and no detectable oscillation after a sigh, whilst in REM sleep there are continuous oscillations of high amplitude.

A similar pattern of development was seen in all 6 infants. Oscillations were

BABY 26

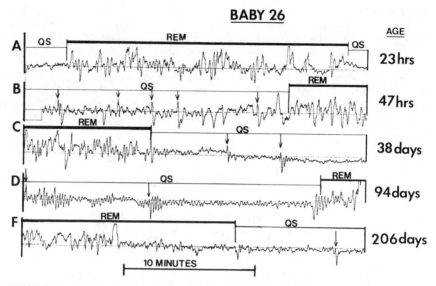

FIGURE 4. Compressed, filtered plots of Ve from 5 recordings (**A–D, F**) at different ages of infant No. 26, the infant whose respiratory traces at various ages are shown in FIGURES 1 and 2. The *arrows* show the times of occurrence of sighs in QS. See text for discussion of recordings **A–D, F**; plot for recording at 151 days of age, **E**, is not shown.

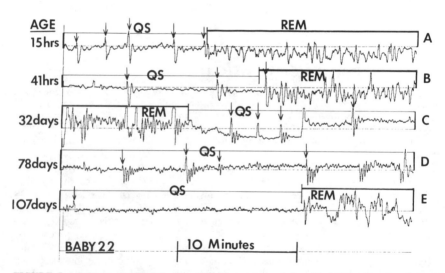

FIGURE 5. Compressed, filtered plots of Ve from another infant (No. 22) at the ages shown (**A–E**). The *arrows* show the times of occurrence of sighs in QS. See text for discussion.

continuous in REM sleep at all ages. In QS the oscillations were continuous in the first day or two after birth but with increasing age became discontinuous, occurring mainly after sighs. In the first few days after birth the occurrence of a sigh did not necessarily lead to any interruption of the underlying oscillation. Beyond the first few days, spontaneous sighs seemed to entrain a damped oscillation of similar period to the continuous oscillations during REM sleep at the same age.

FIGURE 6 shows the results of the Fourier analysis of the recordings in QS and in REM sleep for the studies of infant No. 26, at 23 hr, 38 days, and 206 days of age, which are shown in FIGURE 4. These patterns confirm the complex nature of the oscillations but clearly show that in REM sleep and in QS, at each age, there are striking similarities in the frequency composition of the oscillations. FIGURE 7 shows the results of the Fourier

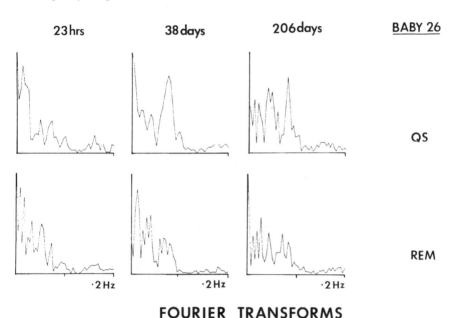

FOURIER TRANSFORMS

FIGURE 6. Fourier transforms of sections of the compressed plots of Ve, in QS (**upper panels**) and in REM sleep (**lower panels**), shown in FIGURES 4A, C, and F, respectively, for infant No. 26 at ages 23 hr, 38 days, and 206 days. The scale for the abscissa is 0–0.2 Hz. See text for discussion of patterns.

analysis for 3 of the sections of recording shown in FIGURE 5, at ages 15 hr, 32 days, and 107 days. These patterns confirm the presence of similarities in frequency composition of the oscillations during QS and REM sleep at each age. Both FIGURES 6 and 7 show an increasing contribution from higher frequency components with increasing age. This change is most marked between the studies on the first day and those at 38 (FIG. 6) or 32 days (FIG. 7), respectively.

DISCUSSION

The results of this study confirm our previous observations[3] that the major oscillations which can be detected in Ve during QS are those which follow spontaneous deep breaths.

The features of these oscillations change with age in a characteristic way: the period shortens progressively, whilst the damping initially decreases to a minimum between 1 and 3 months and subsequently increases, so that by 5–7 months the pattern of response is rapid and highly damped. The present series of studies shows that in the first few days after birth the irregularity of the respiratory pattern after sighs in QS is due to underlying continuous and irregular slow oscillations of relatively low amplitude. There is commonly no interruption of these underlying oscillations after a sigh.

The presence of continuous oscillations in Ve during REM sleep has been described before,[2] but the pattern of change with age has not been documented. The striking continuity of the oscillations during REM sleep at all ages and the fact that these

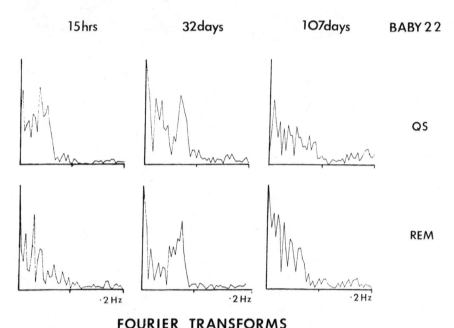

FOURIER TRANSFORMS

FIGURE 7. Fourier transforms of sections of the compressed plots of Ve, in QS (**upper panels**) and in REM sleep (**lower panels**), from infant No. 22, shown in FIGURES 5A, C, and E, at ages 15 hr, 32 days, and 107 days. The scale for the abscissa is 0–0.2 Hz. See text for discussion of patterns.

oscillations, although irregular, are relatively unaffected by body movements suggest the operation of a feedback control system operating at a high gain.

The continuity between the irregular oscillations occurring in periods of QS and of REM sleep in the first few days of life and the striking similarities of the Fourier transforms for each suggest that a common control system may be operating in both states.

Despite the clear differences between oscillations occurring during periods of QS and of REM sleep in older infants, there were similarities in the changes with age of the Fourier transforms for the two states, with a progressive increase in the higher frequency components. This suggests that the same underlying control system may also be operating to give rise to the oscillations in the older infants.

We have previously demonstrated theoretically[9,10] and experimentally[8] that the oscillations which follow sighs in QS are compatible with the operation of the peripheral chemoreceptor-mediated response to Pco_2. In this model, the changes with age in damping of the oscillations could be accounted for by a number of possible changes in the parameters of the model, e.g., an increase in cardiac output as a proportion of lung volume, an increase in signal transit time, or a combination of these changes.

Recent studies in adults[11] and in infants[12-14] have shown that in humans, unlike most other species which have been studied, the metabolic response to thermal stress is more marked in REM sleep than in QS. The continuous oscillations which we have shown would also be compatible with the known characteristics of the vasomotor response to thermal stress.[15] These vasomotor responses can affect blood gases by changing blood flow.

Thus, it is interesting to speculate on the possibility that the continuous oscillations of Ve in REM sleep may be related ultimately to thermoregulatory activity rather than to the requirements of respiratory control alone.

Whatever the underlying mechanisms responsible for these oscillations, the striking changes with age and the differences between patterns during QS and REM sleep lead to great difficulties in the definition of "normal" and "abnormal" patterns. The wide differences in rates of development between infants, with similar patterns appearing at widely differing ages, further limits the value of any attempt to define a single recording as "normal" or "abnormal" on the basis of an analysis of the pattern of oscillation. Further investigation of the nature of the oscillations in respiration may allow a better understanding of the interactions of the various feedback loops involved and the ways in which the developing control system might fail.

REFERENCES

1. HATHORN, M.K.S. 1978. J. Physiol. (London) **285:** 85–99.
2. WAGGENER, T.B., A.R. STARK, B.A. COHLAN & I.D. FRANTZ. 1984. J. Appl. Physiol. **57:** 536–544.
3. FLEMING, P.J., A.L. GONCALVES, M.R. LEVINE & S. WOOLLARD. 1984. J. Physiol. (London) **347:** 1–16.
4. LONG, A.M., P.J. FLEMING, M.R. LEVINE & J.P. CLEAVE. 1986. Early Hum. Dev. **14:** 135.
5. FLEMING, P.J., M.R. LEVINE & A. GONCALVES. 1982. Pediatr. Res. **16:** 1031–1034.
6. FLEMING, P.J., M.R. LEVINE, A. GONCALVES & S. WOOLLARD. 1983. J. Appl. Physiol. **55:** 1924–1931.
7. ANDERS. T., R. EMDE & A. PARMELEE. 1971. A Manual of Terminology, Techniques and Criteria for Scoring of States of Sleep and Wakefulness in Newborn Infants. UCLA, Brain Information Service, BRI Publications Office. California.
8. FLEMING, P.J., M.R. LEVINE, A.M. LONG & J. CLEAVE. 1986. *In* Physiology of the Fetal and Neonatal Lung. D.V. Walters, L.B. Strang, & F. Geubelle, Eds.: 107–124. MTP Press. Lancaster, UK.
9. CLEAVE, J.P., M.R. LEVINE & P.J. FLEMING. 1984. J. Theor. Biol. **108:** 261–183.
10. CLEAVE, J.P., M.R. LEVINE, P.J. FLEMING & A.M. LONG. 1986. J. Theor. Biol. **119:** 299–318.
11. PALCA, J.W., J.M. WALKER & R.J. BERGER. 1986. J. APPL. PHYSIOL. **613:** 940–947.
12. STOTHERS, J.K. & R.M. WARNER. 1978. J. Physiol. (London) **278:** 435–440.
13. DARNALL, R.A. & R.L. ARIAGNO. 1982. Pediatr. Res. **16:** 512–514.
14. FLEMING, P.J., M.R. LEVINE, Y. AZAZ & P. JOHNSON. 1987. *In* Fetal and Neonatal Development. C.T. Jones, Ed. Academic Press. London. In Press.
15. KITNEY, R.I. 1984. Automedica **5:** 289–310.

Pathophysiology of Sudden Upper Airway Obstruction in Sleeping Infants and Its Relevance for SIDS[a]

B. T. THACH, A. M. DAVIES, AND J. S. KOENIG

Mallinckrodt Department of Pediatrics
Washington University School of Medicine, and
St. Louis Children's Hospital
St. Louis, Missouri 63110

INTRODUCTION

The focus of this conference concerns cardiac and respiratory mechanisms that could be causes of the Sudden Infant Death Syndrome. This paper concerns perhaps the oldest theory for SIDS, the upper airway obstruction theory. At the outset it is appropriate to ask, what kind of causal mechanism should we be looking for? What characteristics should be required for a potential SIDS mechanism? We feel that 4 characteristics are required. First, the mechanism should be known to cause death in man—or at least it should be theoretically capable of causing death. Second, it should be capable of producing *sudden* death—that is, death occurring within minutes, or several hours at the longest. Third, the mechanism should be without antecedent alarming symptoms—thus, capable of causing *unexpected* death. Finally, when death occurs, it should be *unexplained* by the case history, postmortem, and death-scene investigation. That is to say, such investigations should not reveal conclusive evidence of the lethal mechanism. Other desirable features might include an explanation for the SIDS age distribution or the association of SIDS with sleep or respiratory infection. However, the way in which SIDS is currently defined makes the 4 primary characteristics listed above paramount.

Over the past several years, our research group has focused on mechanisms of upper airway obstruction which might be capable of producing sudden asphyxia and death in infants. Obviously, complete upper airway obstruction, if sufficiently prolonged, produces rapid, silent death. Furthermore, it is generally accepted that the postmortem findings in such deaths are indistinguishable from those of SIDS.[1] The challenge, then, is to determine what kinds of airway obstruction could occur suddenly in an ostensibly healthy child and leave no compelling evidence, either on the body or at the scene of the death, as to cause of the obstruction. We can think of 4 mechanisms which meet these criteria: (1) occlusion of the mouth and nose by compression or by foreign objects, (2) pharyngeal airway obstruction due to failure of airway-maintaining mechanisms, (3) airway obstruction associated with the laryngeal chemoreflex, and (4) similar obstruction during infantile "breathholding."

ORAL-NASAL OCCLUSION (SUFFOCATION)

Occlusion of the external airway, causing death by accidental suffocation, was until recent times the generally accepted mechanism for SIDS. Over the past 20 to 30 years this

[a]This work was supported by funding from the NIH, Grant HD-10993.

theory has lost general acceptance for 2 reasons. First, it was realized that the assignment of suffocation as the cause of an infant's death usually depends on circumstantial evidence only—this mechanism can rarely be conclusively proved. Therefore, with the actual cause of death in doubt, it was deemed cruel to add to the mental anguish of the parents of a SIDS victim by rendering a diagnosis that suggests parental negligence.[2] Second, those who viewed SIDS as having a single cause rejected the suffocation theory, since for many infants who died suddenly and unexpectedly, suffocation was clearly not the cause of death.

There are 3 situations involving unexpected infant deaths in which suffocation has been implicated: (1) sharing a bed with an adult or sibling, (2) entrapment or wedging of the infant's head against a mattress, and (3) sleeping in the face-down posture. A recent report has provided indirect but reasonably convincing evidence of the accidental death of an infant from overlying by a parent sharing a bed with the infant.[3] Older, but fairly well documented, SIDS studies also found overlying to be a cause of infant deaths.[4] More recent reports indicate that as many as 48% of SIDS deaths occur in a bed-sharing situation.[5] Additionally, it is worth noting that death of the newborn due to overlying is common in some domestic species.[6] Where human deaths are concerned, however, it is practically impossible to prove conclusively that the infant's airway was completely occluded (or the chest compressed) and, therefore, that suffocation was the cause of death in a bed-sharing situation. Hence, it is nearly always justifiable to make the diagnosis of SIDS in cases in which overlying is suspected.[1] For this reason, overlying should be viewed as a causal mechanism for SIDS, since it clearly meets the fourth as well as the other three of our required criteria for SIDS mechanisms. Moreover, if we accept the possibility that SIDS may have multiple causal mechanisms, there is no need to discard overlying as a cause of SIDS on the grounds that it is not implicated in all SIDS cases.

One situation where there appears to be a general consensus about asphyxiation as a proven cause of unexpected infant deaths is in cases involving occlusion of the mouth and nose by plastic bags or sheeting.[7] It is interesting to note that most of these deaths have occurred in infants under 6 months of age and also that death occurred in the infant's crib. Similarly, there is apparent agreement among forensic pathologists that a substantial number of deaths of infants under 6 months of age have occurred when the infant's heads became wedged between cribbars or between the crib and mattress.[7,8] The infants' pattern of motor activity, combined with his limited ability to defend his airway, may render infants in this 2-to-6-month age range particularly vulnerable to such accidents when unattended by an adult. Furthermore, if an infant can be asphyxiated by plastic sheeting or by head entrapment, it seems reasonable to assume that an infant would be vulnerable to the same outcome if trapped beneath a sleeping parent sharing the same bed. The infant's survival in this situation would depend on the parent's awakening; however, arousal from sleep can be depressed for many reasons.

Up to 25% of SIDS infants are found with the face positioned directly down, against the bedding.[9] It is entirely plausible that the weight of the infant's head might be sufficient to compress the nose and mouth in this position. It has been stated that a child cannot be suffocated by "ordinary" bed clothing and that if the nose is compressed by a pillow or mattress, the child will adjust his posture sufficiently to obtain an airway.[1] However, it has not been appreciated that the two studies on which these beliefs are based[2,10] would, by modern standards, be termed "anecdotal" since they contain minimal actual data regarding living infants and since they fail to provide an adequate description of the research protocol, methods or subjects. The authors of these widely quoted studies were actually trying to prove that *most* sudden deaths in infants are not due to accidental suffocation; they never maintained that accidental suffocation *cannot* happen.

In summary, there seems to be a consensus among forensic pathologists that reasonably well documented accidental suffocation does occur in young infants and is by no means rare. Moreover, from the standpoint of airway defensive capability, the young infant appears to be particularly vulnerable to this form of death. However, current diagnostic and investigative techniques are inadequate to indicate how much of what is currently diagnosed as SIDS is accounted for by these mechanisms.

PHARYNGEAL OCCLUSION (OBSTRUCTIVE SLEEP APNEA)

A number of laboratory and clinical observations have contributed to an increased understanding of the neuromuscular mechanisms that maintain pharyngeal patency.[11] These observations indicate that upper airway patency is contingent on a balance between airway-dilating and airway-constricting forces. Achieving such a balance is important, as the pharynx is essentially a floppy tube with little intrinsic rigidity. Commonly encountered airway-constricting forces include airway suction during inspiration and airway compression caused by neck flexion. These forces are opposed by the airway-dilating effect produced by contraction of upper airway muscles (e.g., geniohyoid, genioglossus, and sternohyoid).

Clinical observations have provided indirect evidence that muscle activity is important for upper airway patency.[12] Additional evidence for the role of upper airway muscles comes from studies of upper airway elastance. Such studies have used the transmural airway pressure that coincides with pharyngeal closure, (the "airway closing pressure," AWCP) as a reflection of upper airway elastance.[13,15] Upper airway elastance has two components: an "intrinsic" elastance component provided by the elastance of soft tissues and relaxed muscles and an "added" elastance component provided by the contraction of upper airway dilating muscles (see FIGS. 1A and 1B). Upper airway intrinsic elastance (i.e. AWCP) has been assessed in animals and in human infants who died of natural causes. These studies suggest that the intrinsic elastance of the human infant airway is insufficient to withstand the upper airway collapsing force of the inspiratory suction of average breaths—hence, we suspect that the added elastance supplied by upper airway muscles is more or less constantly required for upper airway patency. Studies of AWCP and tongue-muscle activity during respiratory occlusion maneuvers in human infants reveal that AWCP varies in proportion to muscle electrical activity (see FIG. 1), which is added evidence that these muscles contribute to increasing upper airway elastance.[15]

The tone of upper airway muscles is regulated by several reflex mechanisms. These reflex pathways and their effects on airway patency are illustrated in FIGURE 2. Such reflexes are probably quite important, because the inspiratory activity of the diaphragm and upper airway-dilating muscles must be balanced in order to prevent airway closure. From studies in infants and adults with obstructive sleep apnea (OSA), we know that airway closure can rapidly occur during the middle of an inspiratory effort. Thus, the delicate balance between airway-dilating and airway-constricting forces is tenuous and can rapidly be upset. On the basis of numerous studies in animals and in humans, it appears that several reflex mechanisms regulating airway muscle tone act to maintain this balance. For example, chemoreceptor stimuli (either increased arterial CO_2 or decreased O_2) stimulate the airway dilating muscles.[16] Therefore, increasing asphyxia would favor airway patency. Similarly, in animal studies, stimuli resulting from suction pressures in the nose, pharynx, or larynx rapidly stimulate activity of the upper airway dilating muscles.[17] Hence, the suction pressure in the airway during obstructive apnea should stimulate reflexes that would tend to restore airway patency (see FIG. 3). Also, in recent studies of sleeping infants, we have found that maneuvers which suddenly increase upper airway suction pressure cause a rapid inhibition of thoracic inspiratory muscles.[18] Such a reflex could contribute to preserving upper airway patency by preventing the upper airway closing pressure from being reached during the course of an inspiratory effort.

Failure of these complex pharyngeal airway-stiffening mechanisms appears to be the basis for obstructive sleep apnea in patients with a variety of disorders, many of which are associated with anatomical narrowing of the upper airway (e.g., micrognathia, choanal stenosis, obesity, enlarged adenoids or tonsils). When the lumen of the nasopharyngeal airway is reduced in diameter by enlarged adenoids, for example, resistance to airflow is increased and inspiratory suction increases downstream from the constriction. Periodically, this suction overcomes the force exerted by the airway-maintaining muscles and the

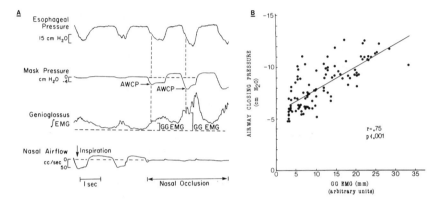

FIGURE 1. (A) The effect of nasal occlusion on tongue muscle activity and pharyngeal patency. Polygraphic tracings of respiratory activity during sleep in a 14-day-old, full-term infant with micrognathia. The infant is breathing through a nasal mask with an attached flow meter. A catheter records pressure in the mask. Genioglossus muscle (GG) electrical activity (EMG) was measured with intramuscular fine-wire electrodes. When the nasal mask airway is occluded, the GG EMG of the first occluded breath increases, indicating a mechanoreceptor-mediated reflex which increases muscle activity. The additional increase in GG EMG activity in the second occluded breath probably reflects combined chemoreceptor- and mechanoreceptor-mediated reflexes. Following occlusion of the nasal airway, the pharyngeal airway closes midway during the inspiratory efforts (at *vertical dashed lines*), as indicated by a plateau in the mask pressure. The airway pressure at which pharyngeal closure occurs is the airway closing pressure (AWCP). Note the decrease in the AWCP in the second occluded breath, which correlates with an increased level of GG EMG activity at the moment of closure. (B) A plot of airway closing pressure vs. the amount of GG EMG activity at the time of closure for multiple nasal occlusion trials like those shown in **A**. There is a correlation between the amount of GG EMG activity and the amount of negative pressure needed to cause airway closure. The linear regression equation is: AWCP $= -0.21$(GG EMG) $- 5.75$. In this equation, AWCP reflects total pharyngeal airway elastance, which has two components: (i) the "intrinsic" elastance of the pharyngeal tissues and relaxed pharyngeal muscles, as reflected by the y-intercept value (-5.75) and (ii) an "added" elastance component provided by the contractile force of pharyngeal airway dilating muscles ($-k \times$ GG EMG; here, k is -0.21). (Reprinted from Roberts *et al.*[15] with permission from the *Journal of Applied Physiology*.)

walls of the oropharynx collapse inward (see FIG. 4). Such obstructive episodes characteristically occur during sleep, probably because the airway-maintaining muscles have reduced activity during sleep. Of potential relevance to SIDS is the fact that patients with OSA have more severe episodes of apnea during upper respiratory tract infections. In some infants, no obvious source of airway narrowing can be found.[19,20] Therefore, motor control of tongue muscles or airway-maintaining reflexes may be abnormal in these infants.

As regards SIDS, it is relevant to note that young infants with Pierre-Robin syndrome have a high mortality (20–30%).[21] Often deaths in such infants occur suddenly and unexpectedly, when the infants have been discharged from the hospital.[22,24] Such cases reportedly have only minimal findings, associated with intrathoracic petechiae and pulmonary edema, similar to that seen in SIDS cases.[24] Acute airway obstruction is the presumed cause of deaths from Pierre-Robin syndrome, although the precise events leading to death are unclear, as deaths generally occur when the infant is unattended.

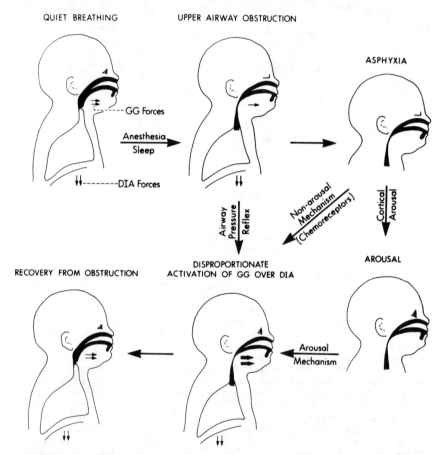

FIGURE 2. Schematic illustration of an obstructive sleep apnea (OSA) episode, illustrating reflex pathways potentially involved in recovery from obstruction. Both sleep and general anesthesia have the effect of depressing upper airway dilating muscles (GG Forces) more than chest wall inspiratory muscles (DIA Forces). In certain individuals, particularly those with increased nasal resistance, the balance of forces required for pharyngeal airway patency may be upset so that inspiratory suction pressure causes pharyngeal closure. Such OSA episodes typically terminate with spontaneous recovery of airway patency. Three reflex pathways that cause disproportionate activation of upper airway muscles over chest muscles are potentially involved in this recovery. These reflex pathways are (1) airway mechanoreceptor pressure reflexes originating in the upper airway and, possibly, also from lung stretch reflexes, (2) respiratory chemoreceptor reflexes responsive to asphyxia, and (3) a cortical arousal pathway probably mediated by respiratory chemoreceptors.

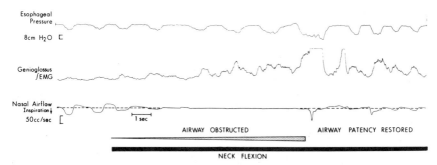

FIGURE 3. Tracings showing occurrence and resolution of upper airway obstruction associated with experimental neck flexion in a 2-month-old micrognathic infant. The sleeping infant's neck was gently flexed by the investigator during the period indicated by **black bar.** During the period of airway obstruction, note increase in inspiratory drive (Esophageal Pressure) and progressive increase in baseline and peak inspiratory genioglossus electromyographic (EMG) activity. After about 10 sec, behavioral arousal, increased neck extensor tone, and swallowing was noted; these activities coincided with further increases in EMG activity and recovery of airway patency, although the infant's neck remained flexed. (Reprinted from Roberts *et al.*[15] with permission of the *Journal of Applied Physiology.*)

AIRWAY OBSTRUCTION WITH THE LARYNGEAL CHEMOREFLEX

A third mechanism leading to upper airway obstructive episodes has been termed the "laryngeal chemoreflex." Receptors at the entrance to the larynx have been identified which, when stimulated by various fluids, give rise to a spectrum of responses: apnea, airway closure, swallowing, coughing, and arousal from sleep. These various responses are viewed as airway protective, since, collectively or individually, they would have the effect of preventing pulmonary aspiration of fluid pooled in the upper airway. Recent studies by ourselves and others suggest that this reflex likely plays a significant role in prolonged apneic spells in certain infants[25,26,27] (see Fig. 5).

In lambs, Johnson and co-workers[28] and others have shown that chemical stimulation of the larynx provokes not only swallowing but also very prolonged apnea. In our own recent studies, we have found that a very small bolus of warmed physiological saline (0.04 ml) delivered to the pharynx of a normal sleeping infant will elicit various airway protective responses including swallowing, brief central apnea, and obstructed inspiratory efforts.[29] We feel that this may be an important normal physiological mechanism for removal of upper airway secretions during sleep. In contrast, in preterm infants with a history of apnea of prematurity, the episodes of swallowing, central apnea, and obstructed inspiratory efforts included in the spectrum of responses to pharyngeal saline were more prolonged.[26,27] Of particular significance is the observation that spontaneous prolonged apneic spells in such infants are nearly identical to saline-induced episodes.[26] These observations suggest that an abnormality of normal airway-protective mechanisms plays an important role in the etiology of apnea of prematurity. We have speculated that accumulation of upper airway secretions acts as a trigger for spontaneous apneic spells. In further recent studies, we have found that the pattern of airway obstruction during apnea associated with respiratory syncytial viral (RSV) infection in young infants is similar to that elicited with pharyngeal fluid boluses.[30] This observation suggests that the apnea typically associated with RSV infection is similar to apnea of prematurity and may also involve the laryngeal chemoreflex.

In subsequent studies in infants, we have found that water is a much more potent stimulus than saline in eliciting these responses, including the prolonged apnea, thus indicating that the reflex pathway involves chemoreceptors capable of differentiating water from saline.[27] Such a chemoreceptor reflex has been implicated in prolonged apnea associated with gastroesophageal reflux and regurgitation in infants. Herbst et al.[32] and also Spitzer et al.[33] found a temporal relationship between occult reflux of gastric contents into the esophagus and episodes of prolonged obstructive or mixed apnea in young infants. Additionally, Menon and co-workers[34] found an increased incidence of prolonged mixed and obstructive apnea associated with swallows immediately following overt regurgitation episodes in young infants (see FIG. 5). Collectively, these observations suggest that in certain infants symptomatic upper airway obstruction and apnea can be triggered by reflux or regurgitation of gastric contents into the pharynx. The distinctive pattern of such spells, and also spells occurring during feedings,[36] suggests involvement of the laryngeal chemoreflex.

In summary, it seems that the upper airway receptors regulating aspiration-preventive reflexes can serve as a trigger for prolonged airway obstruction and apnea. In infants,

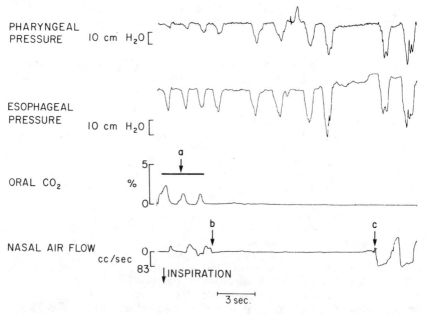

FIGURE 4.   Tracings demonstrating how a sudden increase in upper airway resistance can trigger an episode of spontaneous obstructive apnea. The subject was a 2-week-old micrognathic infant born at term. Prior to the episode, airflow is occurring through nose and mouth (**arrow a**). At **arrow b,** the infant spontaneously closes his mouth, the only remaining route for airflow being the nose. This results in increased pharyngeal suction pressure; note the more negative pharyngeal inspiratory pressures just prior to complete airway closure. With the next inspiratory effort, nasal airflow begins but soon returns to zero, signifying complete airway closure. The next 4 breaths remain completely obstructed. Since pharyngeal pressure mimics esophageal pressure, we know that closure occurs above the pharyngeal catheter tip, i.e., in the upper pharynx. At **arrow c,** airflow is spontaneously re-established during inspiration, probably as a result of the reflex mechanisms regulating upper airway muscle tone which are illustrated in FIGURES 1–3. (Reprinted from Roberts et al.[51] with the permission of the Journal of Applied Physiology.)

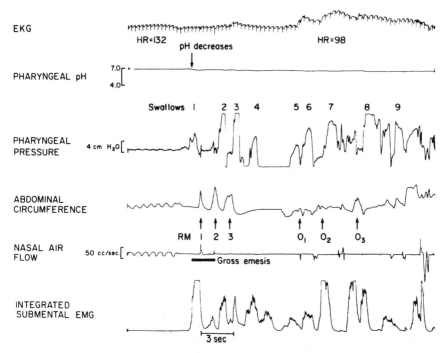

FIGURE 5.   Tracings showing episode of regurgitation in a preterm infant, followed by prolonged apnea with bradycardia. During period of absent nasal airflow, oral CO_2 tracing (not shown) indicated absent oral airflow. **Arrows O_1 to O_3** indicate obstructed breaths during apnea. A brief period of central apnea occurs between swallows **4** and **5**. Expulsive abdominal movements (RM **arrows 1–3**) are typically associated with regurgitation in infants. A similar pattern of swallows, obstructed breaths, central apnea and bradycardia is often observed during spontaneous prolonged apnea that is not associated with regurgitation in preterm infants. This pattern can also be experimentally produced by stimulating the upper airway with minute boluses of saline or water. HR, heart rate. (Reprinted from Menon *et al.*[34] with permission from the *Journal of Pediatrics.*)

significant asphyxia during these episodes has been documented[36] and, in animal studies, death has resulted.[35]

INFANTILE BREATHHOLDING RESPONSE (INFANTILE SYNCOPE)

The Valsalva maneuver is a common physiological response, typically associated with vigorous motor activity in young infants, as well as a variety of other normal infant behaviors, including coughing, crying, and abdominal expulsive maneuvers. Moreover, in infants, a Valsalva response is usually seen in conjunction with painful, frightening or annoying stimuli[37,38] (see FIG. 6). Apneic spells associated with "squirming" motor activity in preterm infants and asphyxial episodes termed "breathholding spells" in older infants appear to consist of a single, prolonged Valsalva maneuver or a series of briefer maneuvers[38] (see FIG. 7). Thus, the normal breathholding response to pain or emotional stimuli usually results in a brief but marked reduction in ventilation; in certain infants,

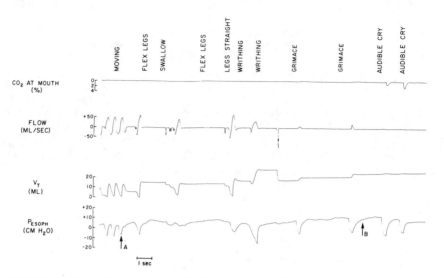

FIGURE 6. Polygraphic tracings and behavioral observations illustrating the pattern of breathing during "squirming" in a preterm infant showing the smooth transition from a silent breathing pattern to crying. Onset of "squirming" activity at **arrow A.** Note appearance of Valsalva maneuvers indicated by positive esophageal pressure and airway closure (Flow) at end inspiration. Note that the pattern of breathing in "squirming" and crying are very similar. Onset of crying at **arrow B.** Note appearance of CO_2 in expired oral air occurring with cry, signaling transition to oral breathing. Flow, nasal air flow; V_T, integrated flow (tidal volume); P_{ESOPH}, esophageal pressure. (Reprinted from abu-Osba et al.[38] with permission from the *American Review of Respiratory Disease.*)

though, this activity can progress to severe asphyxia with loss of consciousness. In a "simple" breathholding spell an infant who is crying suddenly holds its breath until cyanosis appears. In contrast, during "severe" breathholding spells, this cyanotic phase is rapidly followed by a syncopal episode and, often, a brief seizure. Recovery then occurs promptly with a sudden gasp.

Such breathholding spells are quite common; up to 5% of normal children experience one or more severe spells during the first six years of life. Simple spells are still more common. The pathophysiology of respiratory and circulatory events during spells is complex.[39] Loss of consciousness and the seizure are the result of cerebral hypoxia. The hypoxia is believed to result from either reduced arterial oxygen tension, reduced cerebral perfusion, or a combination of these two factors. During these spells, arterial oxygen tension has been observed to decrease extremely rapidly, reaching 30% saturation within 40 sec of the onset of breathholding. Several observations can potentially explain this rapid fall in PaO_2. These observations include prolonged breathholding at end expiration, obstructed inspiratory efforts, and low lung volume during spells.[40,41]

Cardiovascular changes are also prominent during breathholding spells. In many cases, a period of asystole has been documented just prior to loss of consciousness, supporting the argument that decreased cerebral blood flow produces cerebral hypoxia. It has been observed that the infant performs a Valsalva maneuver during spells. This maneuver might produce intra-atrial shunting of venous blood and also might impede venous return to the heart. Maulsby and Kellaway[37] suggested that the respiratory and cardiovascular events are both the end result of an accentuated response to pain or emotional disturbance. They observed that experimental ocular compression produced not only cardiac asystole but also a Valsalva maneuver and breathholding in children with a history of breathholding spells. Therefore, some infants may have a predominance of the respiratory response and others a predominance of the cardiovascular response. In either case, acute cerebral hypoxia is the end result.

Recently, Kaada[42] has advanced the interesting theory that these infantile respiratory and cardiovascular responses to pain or emotion may actually represent a very old phylogenetic behavioral pattern present in many mammalian species. This behavior, termed "death feigning," is often accentuated in newborn and juvenile animals and is widely viewed as an adaptive behavior promoting survival in the wild. In Kaada's view, through an as yet ill-defined physiological malfunction, recovery of circulation and breathing during "death feigning" might fail to occur, with the end result that sudden death would occur as a consequence of a frightening experience. Recently, Southall[43] has

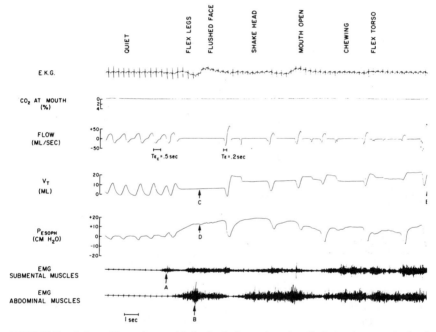

FIGURE 7. Polygraphic tracings and behavioral observations (*top line*) showing an episode of "squirming" motor activity and associated respiratory changes in a preterm infant. Tracings are: electrocardiogram (E.K.G.), CO_2 sampled at the mouth, nasal air flow (Flow), integrated flow (V_T), esophageal pressure (P_{ESOPH}) and submental and abdominal muscle electromyograms (EMG). Onset of "squirming" episode first appears as submental muscle electromyographic activity (**arrow A**), soon followed by abdominal muscle electromyographic activity (**arrow B**), movement artifacts in the electrocardiographic baseline (E.K.G.), and observations of leg flexion and "flushed face." Note changes in the respiratory pattern that appear simultaneously with the motor activity. These respiratory changes include Valsalva maneuvers characterized by a plateau configuration of the tidal volume (V_T) trace (**arrow C**), increased esophageal pressure (**arrow D**), and the abdominal muscle electromyographic activity (**arrow B**) already mentioned. The flat CO_2 trace indicates an absence of oral air exchange. Note greatly reduced minute volume during motor activity compared to control period. Arterial oxygen usually falls during such episodes. Obstructed inspiratory efforts and bradycardia may occur in some infants. This breathing pattern, when associated with marked hypoxemia and bradycardia, is closely similar to that of the typical breathholding spells that have been studied most extensively in older children. (Reprinted from abu-Osba *et al.*[38] with permission from the *American Review of Respiratory Disease.*)

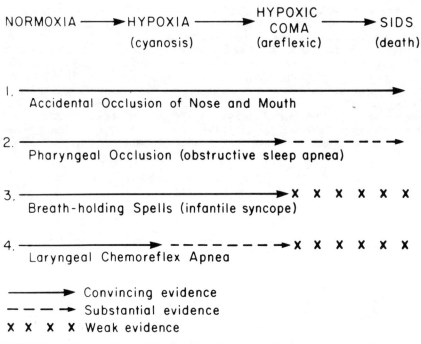

FIGURE 8. Schematic diagram of the hypothetical sequence of events immediately prior to death in SIDS caused by respiratory failure. Also depicted is the strength of the documentation that various SIDS mechanisms can actually cause sudden death. Thus, there is strong evidence (**solid line**) that occlusion of the nose and mouth (e.g. by plastic sheeting) has caused infant deaths, whereas the evidence that the laryngeal chemoreflex can cause deaths is weak (**xxxxxx**). However, there is strong evidence that this laryngeal reflex can produce significant hypoxia in infants[25,26] and, probably, occasionally (**dashed line**) causes hypoxic coma when infants experience prolonged apnea during feedings.[36]

made a similar suggestion on the basis of studies in infants with spells identical to, or, at least, very similar to, severe breathholding spells. Although its relation to SIDS is obscure, infantile breathholding likely plays a prominent role in many ''near-miss SIDS'' cases (e.g., ''apparent life-threatening episodes'').

EVALUATION OF POTENTIAL SIDS MECHANISMS

The 4 potentially fatal mechanisms outlined above meet most of our 4 criteria for SIDS mechanisms reasonably well. One outstanding problem with several of these mechanisms, however, is that although they can produce severe asphyxia, they apparently are rarely if ever lethal. This criticism applies to breathholding spells in particular. Historically, such spells have been viewed as medically benign by most pediatricians. In FIGURE 8 we have outlined the probable sequence of events that occur when SIDS results from ventilatory failure. Although acute asphyxia can very rapidly render an infant comatose, it is clear from clinical experience and experimental evidence that potent physiological mechanisms for promoting spontaneous recovery from severe asphyxia, termed ''auto-resuscitation'' mechanisms, will be operative.[44-46] For example, it is very well known that in the typical severe breathholding spell the infant loses consciousness (i.e., "hypoxic coma") but then spontaneously recovers without evidence of ill effects. On the other hand, one can certainly argue that an infant would be much more vulnerable to death during hypoxic coma than during normoxia and, furthermore, there is substantial evidence that all 4 SIDS mechanisms discussed here can and do cause hypoxic coma in young infants. For death to occur in an unattended infant who has reached the stage of hypoxic coma, auto-resuscitation (via the gasping mechanism) must fail. This mechanism, although quite robust in most situations, can fail in certain circumstances. Topical anesthesia of the upper airway prevents auto-resuscitation in the rabbit model;[47] subtle compromise of the cardiovascular or respiratory systems might conceivably have a similar effect. Following this line of thought, one wonders if certain common postmortem findings in SIDS which have been termed "agonal" and assumed to be non-contributory to death might actually have played a key role in the sequence of events leading to death by impairing auto-resuscitation. Examples of such findings which might be relevant to the sequence of events leading to death include the observation of the face-directly-down posture, aspiration of gastric contents, and pulmonary edema.[1,19]

Also, it should be stressed that there is a need for improved techniques to identify the specific mechanisms of death in SIDS victims. The pathological studies of Beckwith[48] and Krous[49,50] on petechiae have been valuable with respect to supporting the hypothesis of airway obstruction as a cause of death. Improved techniques of death-scene investigation might also be sought. Using eyewitness accounts to reconstruct the position of the infant in the crib, after removal of the body, is a very crude means of assessing the status of the infant's airway at the time of death. It is clear that support for the theory of accidental asphyxiation as a mechanism of death in SIDS will require better techniques to document the precise position of the infant at the time of death.

Finally, it is well to bear in mind the implications of accepting the possibility that SIDS may have multiple causal mechanisms. In the past, many SIDS theories have been rejected because they could not adequately explain circumstances surrounding the "typical" SIDS case. For example, much thought has been devoted to explaining the peak incidence of SIDS at 3 months of age. In this context, apnea of prematurity has been viewed as an unlikely cause of SIDS by some, because such apnea decreases postnatally and, hence, does not explain the peak of SIDS at 3 months. On the other hand, if one accepts a multiple-cause hypothesis for SIDS, then the pattern of incidence for SIDS would reflect the summed incidences of the various causes, which could have peaks of incidence at different ages (FIG. 9). In our view, any potential mechanism for SIDS that

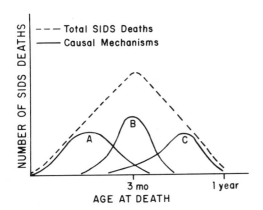

FIGURE 9. Schematic graph illustrating the age-related incidence of 3 (A,B,C) hypothetical causes of SIDS and their contribution to total SIDS deaths. Thus, 3 mechanisms with peak incidences occurring at different ages might produce a summed peak incidence at 3 months of age, like that currently reported for SIDS.

meets the 4 criteria stated above should be carefully considered, even if it fails to explain all the circumstances in the "typical" SIDS death. From this perspective, all of the 4 mechanisms discussed here could play a role in SIDS.

REFERENCES

1. VALDES-DAPENA, M. A. 1967. Sudden and unexpected death in infancy: A review of the world literature 1954–1966. Pediatrics **39**: 123–138.
2. WOOLEY, P. V. 1945. Mechanical suffocation during infancy: A comment on its relation to the total problem of sudden death. J. Pediatr. **26**: 572–575.
3. BASS, M., R. E. KRAVATH & L. GLASS. 1986. Sudden Infant Death: Death scene investigation. N. Engl. J. Med. **315**: 100–105.
4. GEERTINGER, P. 1968. Sudden Death in Infancy. Charles C. Thomas. Springfield, MA.
5. LUKE, J. L. 1978. Sleeping arrangements of sudden infant death syndrome victims in the District of Columbia—A preliminary report. J. Forensic Sci. **23**: 379–83.
6. GLASTONBURY, J. R. W. 1977. Preweaning mortality in the pig. Pediatr. Vet. J. **53**: 310–314.
7. KRAUS, J. F. 1985. Effectiveness of measures to prevent unintentional deaths of infants and children from suffocation and strangulation. Public Health Rep. **100**: 231–239.
8. BASS, M. 1979. Asphyxial crib death. N. Engl. J. Med. **296**: 555–556.
9. VALDES-DAPENA, M. 1977. Sudden unexplained infant death, 1970 through 1975. *In* Pathology journal. S. G. Sommers & P. P. Rosen, Eds. Vol. 12: 117–145. Appleton Century Crofts. New York.
10. BOWDEN, K. 1950. Sudden death or alleged accidental suffocation in babies. Med. J. Aust. **37**: 65–72.
11. BLOCK, A. J., J. FAULKNER, R. L. HUGHES, J. REMMERS & B. T. THACH. 1984. Factors influencing upper airway closure. Chest **86**: 114–122.
12. REMMERS, J. E., W. J. DEGROOT, E. K. SAUERLAND & A. M. ANCH. 1978. Pathogenesis of upper airway occlusion during sleep. J. Appl. Physiol. Respir. Environ. Exercise Physiol. **44**: 931–938.
13. WILSON, S. L., B. T. THACH, R. T. BROUILLETTE & Y. K. ABU-OSBA. 1980. Upper airway patency in the human infant: Influence of airway pressure and posture. J. Appl. Physiol. **48**: 500–504.
14. BROUILLETTE, R. T. & B. T. THACH. 1979. A neuromuscular mechanism maintaining extrathoracic airway patency. J. Appl. Physiol. **46**: 772–779.
15. ROBERTS, J. L., W. R. REED, O. P. MATHEW & B. T. THACH. 1986. Control of the respiratory activity of the genioglossus muscle in micrognathic infants. J. Appl. Physiol. **61**: 1523–1533.
16. BROUILLETTE, R. T. & B. T. THACH. 1980. Control of genioglossus muscle as an accessory muscle of inspiration. J. Appl. Physiol. **49**: 801–808.
17. MATHEW, O. P., Y. K. ABU-OSBA & B. T. THACH. 1982. Influence of upper airway pressure changes on genioglossus muscle respiratory activity. J. Appl. Physiol. **51**:2.
18. MATHEW, O. P., B. T. THACH, Y. K. ABU-OSBA, R. T. BROUILLETTE & J. L. ROBERTS. 1982. Regulation of upper airway maintaining muscles during progressive asphyxia. Pediatr. Res. **18**: 819–822.
19. BROUILLETTE, R. T., S. K. FERNBACH & C. E. HUNT. 1982. Obstructive sleep apnea in infants and children. J. Pediatr. **100**: 31–40.
20. YITZCHAK, F., R. E. KRAVATH, C. P. POLLAK & E. D. WEITZMAN. 1983. Obstructive sleep apnea and its therapy: Clinical and polysomnographic manifestations. Pediatrics **71**: 737–742.
21. MONROE, C. W. & K. OGO. 1972. Treatment of micrognathia in the neonatal period. Plast. Reconstr. Surg. **50**: 317–325.
22. WILLIAMS, A. J., M. A. WILLIAMS, C. A. WALKER & P. G. BUSH. 1981. The Robin anomalad (Pierre Robin syndrome)—A follow up study. Arch. Dis. Child. **56**: 663–668.
23. DENNISON, W. M. 1965. The Pierre-Robin syndrome. Pediatrics **36**: 336.
24. FOREST, H. & A. G. GRAHAM. 1963. The Pierre-Robin syndrome. Scott. Med. J. **8**: 16–24.

25. PERKETT, E. A. & R. L. VAUGHN. 1982. Evidence for a laryngeal chemoreflex in some human preterm infants. Acta Paediatr. Scand. **71**: 969–972.
26. PICKENS, D. L., G. L. SCHEFFT & B. T. THACH. 1988. Prolonged apnea associated with upper airway protective reflexes in apnea of prematurity. Am. Rev. Resp. Dis. **137**:113–118.
27. DAVIES, A. M., J. S. KOENIG & B. T. THACH. 1987. Potency of saline and water in eliciting prolonged apnea, a laryngeal chemoreflex response, in human infants. Pediatr. Res. **21**: 447A.
28. JOHNSON, P., D. M. SALISBURY & A. T. STOREY. 1975. Apnea induced by stimulation of sensory receptors in the larynx. *In* Symposium on Development of Upper Respiratory Anatomy and Function. J. F. Bosma & J. Showacre, Eds.: 160–183. U.S. Government Printing Office. Washington, D.C.
29. PICKENS, D. L., G. L. SCHEFFT & B. T. THACH. 1986. Ventilatory and airway protective responses to pharyngeal stimulation in sleeping infants. Fed. Proc. Fed. Am. Soc. Exp. Biol. **45**: 318.
30. PICKENS, D. L., G. L. SCHEFFT, B. T. THACH. 1987. Prolonged apnea in infants with respiratory syncytial virus (RSV) infection is similar to apnea of prematurity and laryngeal chemoreflex (LC) apnea. Pediatr. Res. **21**: 504A.
31. DAVIES, A. M., J. S. KOENIG & B. T. THACH. 1988. Upper airway responses to saline and water in preterm infants. J. Appl. Physiol. In press.
32. HERBST, J. J., L. S. BOOK & S. D. MINTON. 1979. Gastroesophageal reflux causing respiratory distress and apnea in newborn infants. J. Pediatr. **95**: 763–768.
33. SPITZER, A. R., J. T. BOYLE, N. M. TUCHMAN & W. W. FOX. 1984. Awake apnea associated with gastroesophageal reflux: A specific clinical syndrome. J. Pediatr. **104**: 200–205.
34. MENON, A., G. SCHEFFT & B. T. THACH. 1985. Apnea associated with regurgitation in infants. J. Pediatr. **106**: 625–629.
35. DOWNING, S. E. & S. C. LEE. 1975. Laryngeal chemosensitivity: A possible mechanism for sudden infant death. Pediatrics **55**: 640–649.
36. ROSEN, C. L., D. G. GLAZE & J. D. FROST. 1984. Hypoxemia associated with feeding in the preterm infant and full-term neonate. Am. J. Dis. Child. **138**: 623–628.
37. MAULSBY, R. & P. KELLAWAY. 1964. Transient hypoxic crises in children. *In* Neurological and Electroencephalographic Correlative Studies in Infancy. P. Kellaway & I. Petersen, Eds.: 349–360. Grune and Stratton, Inc. New York.
38. ABU-OSBA, Y. K., R. T. BROUILLETTE, S. L. WILSON & B. T. THACH. 1982. Breathing pattern and transcutaneous oxygen tension during motor activity in preterm infants. Am. Rev. Respir. Dis. **125**: 382–387.
39. THACH, B. T. 1985. Sleep apnea in infancy and childhood. *In* Symposium on Sleep Apnea Disorders. S. T. Thawley, Ed. Medical Clinics of North America.
40. PEIPER, A. 1963. Cerebral Function in Infancy and Childhood. Consultants Bureau. New York.
41. GAUK, E. W., L. KIDD & J. S. PRICHARD. 1963. Mechanisms of seizures associated with breathholding spells. N. Engl. J. Med. **268**: 1436–1441.
42. KAADA, B. 1986. Sudden Infant Death Syndrome: The Possible Role of the Fear Paralysis Reflex! Norwegian University Press and Oxford University Press. Oslo and New York.
43. SOUTHALL, O. P., D. G. TALBERT & P. JOHNSON. 1985. Prolonged expiratory apnea: A disorder resulting in episodes of severe arterial hypoxemia in infants and young children. Lancet **2**: 571–577.
44. GUNTHEROTH, W. G. 1982. Crib Death: The Sudden Infant Death Syndrome: 2–3. Future Publishing Company. Mount Kisko, N.Y.
45. LAWSON, E. E. & B. T. THACH. 1977. Respiratory patterns during progressive asphyxia in newborn rabbits. J. Appl. Physiol. **43**: 468–474.
46. MATHEW, O. P., B. T. THACH, Y. K. ABU-OSBA, R. T. BROUILLETTE & J. L. ROBERTS. 1984. Regulation of upper airway maintaining muscles during progressive asphyxia. Pediatr. Res. **18**: 819–822.
47. ABU-OSBA, Y. K., O. P. MATHEW & B. T. THACH. 1981. An animal model for airway sensory deprivation producing obstructive apnea with postmortem findings of sudden infant death syndrome. Pediatrics **68**: 796–800.
48. BECKWITH, J. B. 1970. Observations on the pathological anatomy of the sudden infant death

syndrome. *In* Sudden Infant Death Syndrome. A. B. Bergman, J. B. Beckwith & C. G. Ray, Eds. Univ. Washington Press. Seattle and London.

49. KROUS, H. F. 1984. The microscopic distribution of intrathoracic petechiae in sudden infant death syndrome. Arch. Pathol. Lab. Med. **108:** 77–79.

50. KROUS, H. F. & J. JORDAN. 1984. A necropsy study of distribution of petechiae in non-sudden infant death syndrome. Arch. Pathol. Lab. Med. **108:** 75–76.

51. ROBERTS, J. L., W. R. REED, O. P. MATHEW, A. MENON & B. T. THACH. 1985. Assessment of pharyngeal airway stability in normal and micrognathic infants. J. Appl. Physiol. **58:** 290–300.

Mechanisms for Abnormal Apnea of Possible Relevance to the Sudden Infant Death Syndrome[a]

DAVID P. SOUTHALL[b,c]

Cardiothoracic Institute
Brompton Hospital
London, United Kingdom

DAVID G. TALBERT

Institute of Obstetrics
Queen Charlotte's Hospital
London, United Kingdom

Two strategies based on an ability to record in combination vital physiological parameters from non-invasive sensors over long time periods have been applied to researching the mechanisms responsible for SIDS. The first has involved the prospective collection of clinical and physiological data on large numbers of infants, some of whom have subsequently suffered SIDS. The second has been an in-depth study of cyanotic episodes in infants and young children.

STRATEGY 1: PROSPECTIVE PHYSIOLOGICAL STUDIES OF INFANTS WHO SUFFERED SIDS

In the first of 3 such non-intervention studies, 24-hr tape recordings of ECG and breathing movements on 9,856 infants yielded 29 infants who subsequently suffered SIDS.[1,2] Analysis of these data showed that cardiac arrhythmias, pre-excitation, prolonged heart-rate-corrected QT intervals, and prolonged apneic pauses were *not* a feature of the SIDS cases. When compared with surviving controls matched by age, gestation, and birthweight, the SIDS cases did *not* show significantly increased numbers of short apneic pauses or quantities of periodic breathing.[3] Nevertheless, recordings taken in the first week of life showed a tendency for the SIDS cases to have higher values for these latter parameters. When the 12 preterm SIDS cases were blindly compared with surviving controls matched by gestation, birthweight, and postnatal age (in collaboration with Dr. Yount at the University of Oregon), there was in the SIDS group a significantly larger quantity ($p < 0.05$) of a specific pattern of heart-rate variability and breathing

[a]These studies were funded by the British Heart Foundation, the Foundation for the Study of Infant Death, Nellcor, Healthdyne, the Nuffield Foundation, the Hayward Foundation, the New Moorgate Trust, Smiths Charity, the National SIDS Foundation, the National Heart and Chest Hospitals, and the Joseph Levy Foundation.
[b]Funded by Nellcor and the National SIDS Foundation.
[c]To whom correspondence should be addressed at: The Cardiothoracic Institute, Fulham Road, London SW3 6HP, U.K.

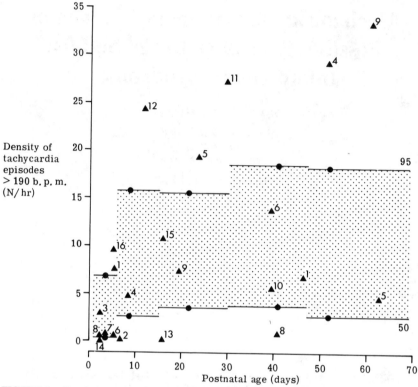

FIGURE 1. Density of tachycardic episodes (number/hr) plotted against postnatal age at time of recording. The control data consist of 321 recordings on 230 randomly selected infants. The 50th and 95th percentiles for each age subgroup (separated by a **stippled area**) are shown for the controls as **solid circles** plotted at the median age of each age subgroup with the age range for the subgroup indicated by a **horizontal line** through the circle. Each SIDS recording is plotted as a **triangle.** b.p.m., beats per min. From Southall *et al.*[6] Reprinted with permission from the *European Journal of Pediatrics.*

movements. This pattern consisted of episodes of bradycardia accompanied by altered patterns of breathing movements, including the termination of the bradycardia by a large-amplitude inspiratory movement.[4]

Analyses of heart-rate variability in full-term ($\geq$ 37 weeks gestation) SIDS cases and controls matched by age, birthweight, and gestation (in collaboration with Dr. A. Wilson at the University of Sheffield) showed in the SIDS cases significantly higher overall mean heart rates ($p < 0.05$)[5] and significantly increased quantities of sinus tachycardia ($p < 0.01$).[6] In the latter observations, 7 of the 16 SIDS cases showed values for sinus tachycardia which exceeded the 95th percentile for the controls (FIG. 1) These findings were not due to an increased amount of the awake state (as shown by an integrated analysis of heart rate and respiratory rate variabilities, done in collaboration with Dr. R. Harper at the University of California, Los Angeles).[7] Episodes of sinus tachycardia predominantly occurred in association with crying but appeared to reach higher levels and to last for longer in the SIDS cases compared with controls. Computerized analysis of-beat-to-beat heart-rate variability, including time-series spectral analysis, (in collaboration with Dr. I. Valimaki and Dr. K. Antila at the University of Turku) showed that, although there appeared during the state of regular breathing to be a reduced heart-rate variability in the SIDS cases compared with controls matched for age, gestation, and birthweight, this did not reach significance.

Follow-up into early childhood of the 9,856 infants from this study has been achieved with the help of the birth and death central registration center at the Office of Population, Censuses and Surveys.[8] All have now passed their 5th birthdays, and analysis of all deaths occurring between 1 and 5 yr of age has shown that out of a total of 15 deaths, 5 were sudden, unexpected, and without adequate cause of death identified at postmortem. Two of these 5 deaths, one at 16 months and 1 at 42 months of age, were similar to SIDS in their presentation in that apparently healthy children were placed in bed and found dead some hours later; one of these children had a sibling with cyanotic breathholding episodes. The remaining 3 children died during cyanotic episodes. In 2 there had been a history of many previous such episodes, and a diagnosis of prolonged expiratory apnea[9-11] (cyanotic breathholding) had been previously established. In the third child there had been no previous cyanotic episodes, although a sibling had suffered cyanotic breathholding spells.

The clinical features of the fatal episode were most explicable by prolonged expiratory apnea[9-11] (partial or complete absence of ventilation with evidence of ventilatory perfusion mismatch). Cyanotic breathholding occurs in 2.8% of all children,[12] and, therefore, in the 9,856 children recruited one might have anticipated 276 cases. Since 2, perhaps 3, of the children studied died from this condition, the risk of sudden death between the ages of 1 and 5 yr in patients having prolonged expiratory apnea can be computed to be around 1%. Although a fatal outcome affects a relatively small proportion of such patients, this form of prolonged apnea appears to be a major contributor to sudden deaths in this age group.

In the second prospective study, standard ECG recordings were performed on 7,254 infants born in 2 hospital centers (Doncaster and West Dorset).[13] Fifteen of these infants subsequently suffered SIDS. Examination of their heart-rate-corrected QT intervals showed no significant differences between the SIDS cases and the survivors. Although these data show that measurement of the QT interval in the neonatal period is not predictive of SIDS, we know anecdotally that a long QT interval may be associated with sudden death in infancy that is registered as SIDS[14] and that this disorder of ventricular excitability may not always be associated with a prolongation of QT interval on the ECG.[15] A proportion of SIDS cases, probably (in our opinion) a very small proportion, may therefore result from this disease. One of the main problems with this disorder of enhanced ventricular excitability is the inherent lack of precision with which it is possible to measure the end of the QT interval on ECG recordings. There is a need to be able to document with more objectivity the presence of this disorder.

A third prospective study, which has recently commenced (July 1986), involves 12-hr, overnight tape recordings of beat-to-beat arterial O_2 saturation (from a modified pulse oximeter), breathing movements (from an abdominal pressure capsule), airflow (from a thermistor sampling from one nostril) and ECG. These recordings are being performed on all infants discharged from the neonatal intensive care units of 3 hospitals in South Yorkshire. Recordings are being made at the time of discharge from the units, at home around 4–6 weeks later, and during an intercurrent respiratory tract infections suffered by these infants during their first 6 months of life. The tape recordings will not be analyzed until the infants have reached 1 yr of age; as with the previous prospective studies, they are being checked for quality and then stored away. However, in the event of any infant suffering SIDS, his or her tape recording(s) will immediately be compared with matched controls and a sequential analysis pursued. If a significantly predictive pattern is found on the recordings from SIDS victims, the study design will be changed to include analysis of all tapes as they are recorded and the treatment of any respiratory patterns found to be predictive of sudden death.

STRATEGY 2: INVESTIGATION OF INFANTS AND YOUNG CHILDREN SUFFERING CYANOTIC/APNEIC EPISODES

Between 1983 and 1986, we investigated 131 infants with unexplained cyanotic or apneic episodes. No cause was identified in 81 of these cases; usually these were infants who had isolated episodes without recurrence. Of the remaining 50 cases, 44 had prolonged expiratory apnea (apnea with evidence of ventilatory perfusion mismatch),[9-11] 1 had seizure-induced apnea (see FIG. 2 and the published report[16]), 2 had sleep-related upper airway obstruction[17] and 2 had maternally imposed apnea (smothering see Fig. 3 and the published report[18]). In one case, abnormal apnea was identified but its precise mechanism remained a mystery.

The severity of the hypoxemia in apnea with ventilatory perfusion mismatch (VPM), in imposed apnea, and in seizure-induced apnea suggest that all 3 may contribute to SIDS. The hypoxemia associated with sleep-related upper airway obstruction, although in some cases severe and frequent, was rarely prolonged. In all of the episodes documented by our overnight recordings during sleep-related obstruction, the hypoxemia was terminated within 20 sec, either by arousal from sleep or by a series of larger amplitude breaths.

Since apnea with VPM represented in our experience the most frequent cause of cyanotic episodes during infancy and early childhood, this condition will now be described in detail.

In 14 of the 44 cases of apnea with VPM, the infants had cyanotic episodes which began when they were awake and which were usually precipitated by an attempt to cry or with crying following a noxious stimulus. This type of presentation, which was most prevalent in the older infant (> 4 months of age) and young child, has previously been described as cyanotic breathholding.[12,19] Although a sudden attempt to cry was the most frequent stimulus to begin a cyanotic episode, the duration of this cry was variable. Sometimes the cry would be 5–10 sec in duration before its character altered, expiratory sound ceased, and cyanosis rapidly followed, usually within 5–6 sec. At other times the expiratory sound of the cry would not occur, but, rather, the mouth would remain open and cyanosis would begin 5–6 sec after the beginning of the response to the noxious stimulus.

All of the remaining 30 patients with apnea and VPM were infants under 4–6 months of age when the cyanotic episodes occurred. These episodes could begin following crying or an attempt to cry when the infant was awake, as described above, or when the infant was asleep or feeding. Cyanotic episodes occurred in 9 of these 30 cases during respiratory tract infections (pertussis in 6 patients,[20] respiratory syncytial virus in 2 and herpes simplex pneumonitis in 1). In the remaining 21 cases, 11 presented as apparent life-threatening events (''near-miss'' SIDS), 7 occurred in preterm infants who had reached full term but had cyanotic episodes which were delaying their discharge from the neonatal intensive care unit, and 3 occurred in the surviving twins of SIDS victims.

The hallmark of this form of abnormal apnea is the rapidity of onset and the severity of the arterial hypoxemia (documented by indwelling arterial lines and by pulse oximetry). This feature gives rise to the concept of ventilatory perfusion mismatch (VPM). There is considerable evidence to support the hypothesis that alveolar atelectasis, with its consequent disturbances of lung receptor function, is the underlying mechanism for the VPM and for the ensuing disturbances of respiratory control.[11,21] Some of the findings constituting this evidence will now be presented.

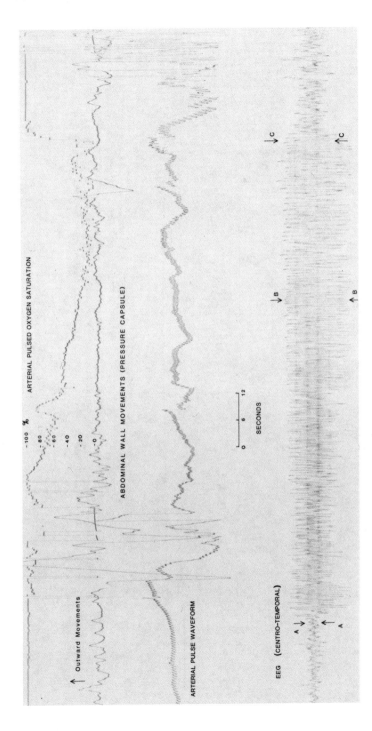

FIGURE 2. Multichannel recording showing seizure activity in the EEG (**arrows A–C**) preceding an episode of severe hypoxemia (duration around 72 sec) associated with a prolonged pause in breathing movements. At the end of the episode of hypoxemia, there is a bradycardia (as shown by the timing of pulse waveforms). A recovery in oxygenation takes place following a large breath (gasp) occurring before the end of the seizure. The total response time of the oximeter (physiological plus electronic) has a mean value of 6 sec. (From Southall *et al.*[16] Reprinted with permission from *Developmental Medicine and Child Neurology*.)

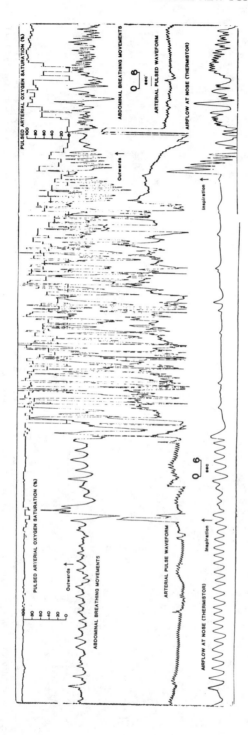

FIGURE 3.   Recording taken at the time of an episode of cyanosis due to imposed asphyxia in a 21-month-old child. There is the sudden onset, during relatively regular breathing, of a period of large breathing movements which persists for 94 sec. This apneic event ends abruptly with a large inspiratory flow coinciding with a relatively small abdominal breathing movement (as measured by a pressure capsule transducer). Towards the end of the large breathing movements, there appears to be a short episode in which expiratory pauses followed each breath. During the large body movements, the oxygen and arterial pulse waveform signals are uninterpretable. (From Southall *et al.*[18] Reprinted with permission from the *British Medical Journal*.)

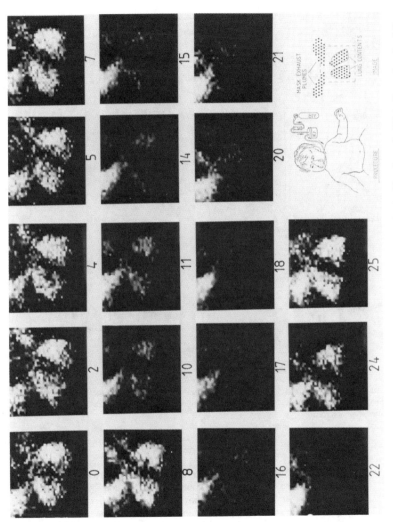

FIGURE 4. Sequential scintograms on a child, 29 months of age, during a cyanotic episode. **Numbers** (0–25) indicate time (sec) from an arbitrary starting point (0). From 0 to 8 sec, there is a stable volume of gas within both lungs. Comparing **frame 10** (sec) with **frame 8** (sec), there is a loss of krypton from both lungs. From 10 sec to 15 sec, there is a period of instability before a complete loss of gas for a period of 9 sec.

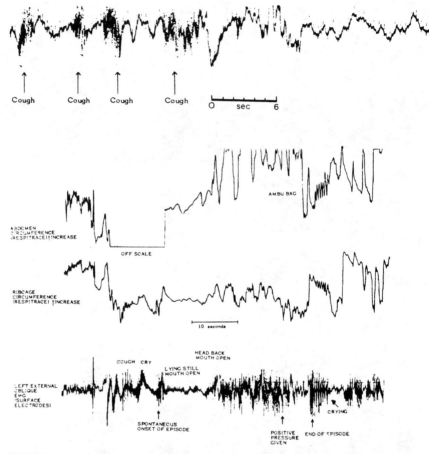

FIGURE 5. Recording during an episode of cyanosis in a 9-month-old boy. **Upper panel** shows the ability of the expiratory muscle EMG signal to detect coughing. For the first 10 sec of the cyanotic episode, no expiratory muscle EMG is detected. Subsequently, bursts of activity occur up until the time of resuscitation.

The rapidity and severity of the arterial hypoxemia (for instance, a PaO$_2$ of 16 mm Hg at 20 sec following the onset of the apnea) cannot be explained by an intracardiac right-to-left (R-L) shunt. Contrast echocardiography during cyanotic episodes showed no evidence of R-L transfer of blood at the atrial or ventricular level. Since ventilation scans (see below) have shown an extremely rapid fall in gas content of both lungs (with 4 sec of the onset of the attack; see FIG. 4), the R-L shunt is likely to be occurring within the lungs. This could arise from active expiration continuing to a state of low lung volume, from widespread alveolar atelectasis, or from a combination of the two. Recordings of expiratory muscle EMG during those cyanotic episodes which began without crying have shown that for the first 10 sec or so of the apnea there is no evidence of active expiration (FIG. 5). Thereafter, there are bursts of active expiratory muscle EMG but no evidence of

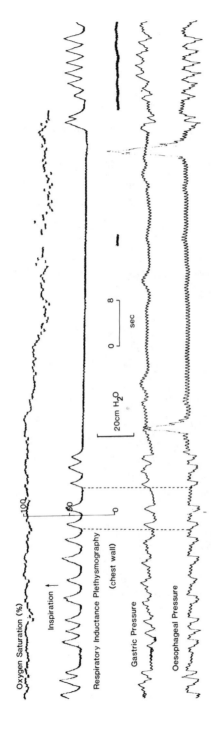

FIGURE 6. An episode of prolonged apnea, 55 sec in duration, during sleep in a 30-month-old child with cyanotic episodes due to apnea with ventilatory perfusion mismatch. From the gastric and esophageal pressure signals, there is no evidence of expiratory activity to explain the onset or maintenance of the prolonged apnea. The large, transient excursions of the esophageal pressure signal might reflect swallowing but, since they do not appear on the gastric pressure trace, cannot be due to expiratory activity.

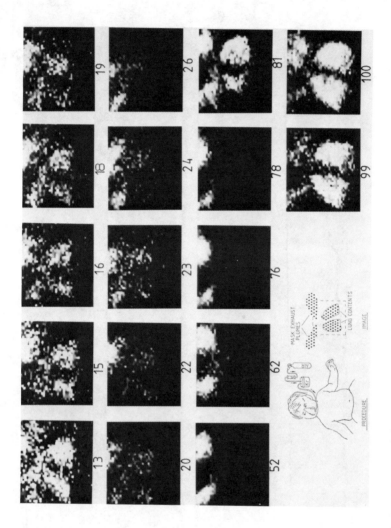

FIGURE 7a. Scintogram sequence during a cyanotic episode. **Numbers** indicate time (sec) from an arbitrary starting point. From a relatively stable period preceding **frame 13** (sec), an unstable sequence follows up to **frame 24** (sec), after which the lungs appear empty of krypton for a period of 52 sec. At around **frame 81** (sec), there is a sudden inflow of gas into both lungs, which eventually become stable at **frames 99** and **100** (sec). For scintograms between 81 and 99 sec, see FIGURE 7b.

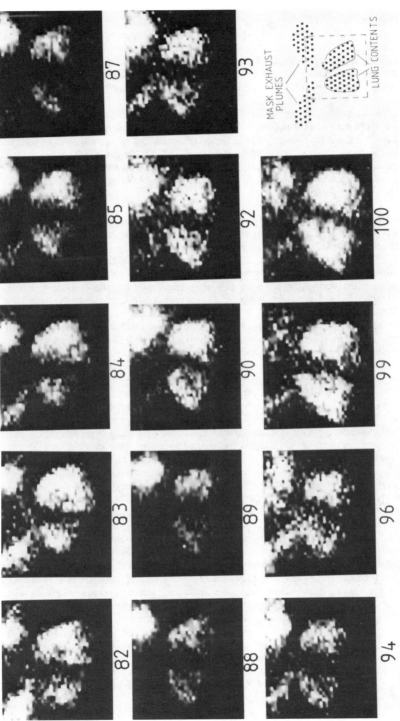

FIGURE 7b. Recovery sequence between **frames 81** and **99** (sec) of FIGURE 7a. There are rapid changes in the distribution of gas between lungs and throughout each lung; for example, compare **frames 89** and **90** (sec).

sustained expiratory efforts. During an episode of prolonged apnea occurring in a sleeping, 30-month-old child who had frequent, awake-onset cyanotic attacks, there was no evidence that expiratory activity initiated or maintained the apnea (FIG. 6). Therefore, although the apneic episode may be brought on by crying, and there may be bursts of expiratory activity during the apneic episode, these data suggest that active expiration continuing to the state of low lung volume is not the primary cause of the absent ventilation and R-L shunt at low lung volume.

Studies of 2 patients, aged 6 and 21 months, in whom prolonged apnea was imposed by total upper airway obstruction,[18] showed that, despite major physical activity and, therefore, increased O_2 consumption, a period of around 72 sec elapsed before falls in PaO_2 sufficient to produce the loss of consciousness and the changes in EEG characteristic of cerebral hypoxia occurred. In contrast, episodes of apnea with VPM are associated with the loss of consciousness and changes in EEG due to cerebral hypoxia within 25–30 sec from the onset of the apnea.

Krypton ventilation scans during 2 cyanotic episodes in a child with apnea accompanied by VPM showed a rapid (FIG. 4) and sometimes prolonged (FIG. 7a) loss of gas from within both lung fields. During forced expiration and breathholding in 6 adults with normal lung function, breathholding at end-expiration was only possible for short time periods (< 15 sec) and there was retention of krypton within the lungs, representing residual volume. In the child with apnea, there was a fall in krypton and, moreover, lung scans during the periods immediately following recovery from the cyanotic episodes showed rapid changes in the distribution of the gas within different areas of the lungs (see FIG. 7b).

Microlaryngoscopy during cyanotic episodes in children with this disorder has shown adduction of the vocal cords. However, this laryngeal closure is not the primary problem, since cyanotic episodes continue in the presence of nasotracheal intubation and tracheostomy. Moreover, the inspiratory waveform pattern typical of airway obstruction (FIG. 8) is not seen during cyanotic episodes in these patients.

The presence of an abnormal expiratory breathing-movement waveform typical of expiratory braking (grunting) was, however, seen in 7 of the 14 patients in the group who had awake-onset cyanotic attacks (FIG. 9). In most of these patients, this pattern was most prevalent immediately following a cyanotic attack and may have been associated with attempts to restore functional residual capacity and to reopen areas of atelectasis. In one child it was present throughout the awake state. This kind of expiratory braking is typical of that in patients with reduced lung compliance due to the alveolar atelectasis resulting from a deficiency of lung surfactant.

The presence of prolonged apneic pauses during sleep in a small proportion (4 out of 14) of those patients with an awake-onset presentation (FIG. 10) could be explained by the hypothesis that areas of atelectasis suck open large airways, thereby inappropriately stimulating stretch receptors and initiating an absence of inspiratory drive.[11,21]

Between their clinically obvious cyanotic attacks, the younger infants (at < 4–6 months of age) with apnea and VPM show episodes of abnormal hypoxemia awake, during sleep and feeding. These dips in O_2 saturation (SaO_2) are related to 4 patterns of breathing and occur in varying quantities in different infants. They are most prevalent in those who are or have been preterm. We suspect, but as yet have not proven, that they reflect the dynamic occurrence of small areas of atelectasis resulting from a defect in lung surfactant and are aided by the compliant nature of the young infant's chest wall. For a given degree of defect in surfactant, the number of such dips in SaO_2 per sleep period may correlate with the degree of compliance of the chest wall; a factor which may explain why dips in SaO_2 during sleep are much less frequent in the older infant and young child with this problem.

The 4 types of breathing pattern seen in young infants during sleep-related dips in SaO_2 are as follows:

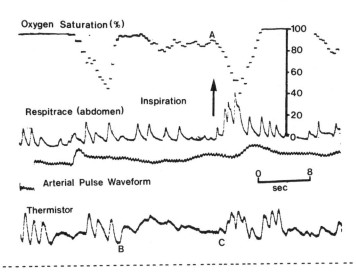

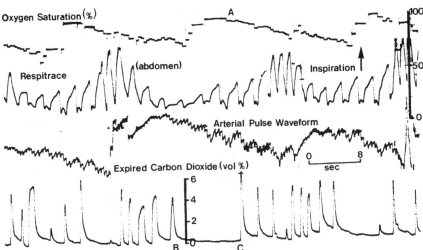

FIGURE 8. Upper panel: recording from an infant with apnea and VPM shows an episode of hypoxemia, beginning at **A** (*top tracing*), associated with continued breathing movements and absent airflow at the nose, as shown by the thermistor signal (**B** to **C**, *bottom tracing*). **Lower panel:** recording from a young child with sleep-related upper airway obstruction shows an episode of hypoxemia, beginning at **A** (*top tracing*), associated with continued breathing movements but absent airflow at the nose, as shown by the end-tidal CO_2 signal (**B** to **C**, *bottom tracing*). Unlike those in the upper panel, the inspiratory waveforms of the respitrace signal are abnormal. Inspiration is biphasic, showing an initially rapid and subsequently slower movement; the latter reflects an increase in airway resistance. (From Southall.[22] Reprinted with permission from *Pediatrics*.)

1. Prolonged (> 15 sec) pauses in inspiratory efforts (FIG. 11a).
2. Inspiratory efforts present but inspiratory airflow absent (FIG. 11b). This pattern may also occur in sleep-related upper airway obstruction, but in this latter condition there is evidence of increased inspiratory airway resistance on the inspiratory breathing-movement waveform,[17,22] a feature which is not seen in apnea with VPM (FIG. 8).
3. An initial pause in inspiratory efforts, followed by inspiratory efforts without inspiratory airflow (previously termed "mixed apnea").
4. Continued inspiratory efforts and continued inspiratory airflow (FIG. 11c). Again, this also is a pattern which may be seen in sleep-related upper airway obstruction, but the abnormal inspiratory breathing-movement waveform of this latter condition is not seen in apnea with VPM (FIG. 8). This fourth type of breathing pattern is further evidence in support of the atelectasis hypothesis, since it is otherwise difficult to explain the presence of severe hypoxemia during continued breathing.

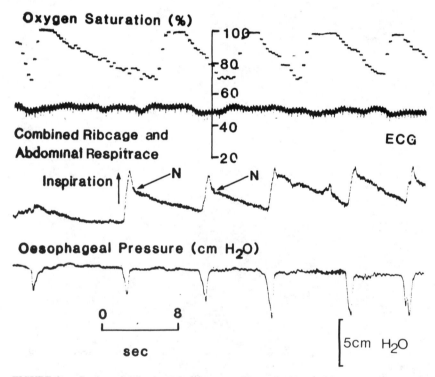

FIGURE 9. Section of a daytime recording on a 27-month-old girl, immediately following a cyanotic episode accompanied by a loss of consciousness. Inspiration and the early part of expiration are rapid, but at N expiration becomes retarded (expiratory braking). Associated with this pattern of breathing, there are short episodes of hypoxemia. The magnitudes of the increases in chest wall area with each breath (obtained from the respiratory inductance signal) are not correlated with the amplitudes of the esophageal pressure excursions, suggesting a breath-to-breath variability in compliance. (From Southall and Talbert.[11] Reprinted with permission from Elsevier and the editor, M. A. Hollinger.)

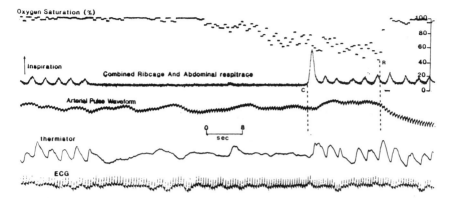

FIGURE 10. Section of an overnight recording on a 27-month-old girl. During sleep there is a cessation of breathing movements for 48 sec without bradycardia and with hypoxemia. The total response time of the pulse oximeter in this child is C − R (16 sec). (From Southall and Talbert.[11] Reprinted with permission from Elsevier and the editor, M. A. Hollinger.)

FIGURE 12 provides further evidence for alveolar atelectasis. It shows an episode of hypoxemia in a 9-week-old, previously preterm infant with cyanotic episodes. This hypoxemia is associated with continued inspiratory movements but the absence of airflow. The inspiratory movements do not show evidence of increased inspiratory resistance, and the thermistor signal shows the presence of cardiac artifact, implying that the airway is fully open. Moreover, the inspiratory airflow at the time of recovery from this apneic episode is delayed with respect to an inspiratory effort, suggesting the gradual expansion of an area of atelectasis.

Since our studies have shown that apnea with VPM is the most frequent cause of prolonged apnea in infancy and we are suggesting that prolonged apnea may be a major cause of SIDS, we must determine how well the characteristics of this disorder conform to the known epidemiology and pathology of SIDS.[22]

The following features of the epidemiology of SIDS support the apnea with VPM hypothesis. Firstly, the characteristic age distribution of SIDS, that is, a sparing of the neonatal period and an increased incidence between 6 weeks and 4 months of age, could follow the development of alveoli within the lungs. From around 6 weeks of age, alveoli multiply in number,[23] producing many structures of small radius which provide, in the presence of a defective surfactant, the ideal substrate for atelectasis.

Secondly, the increased incidence of SIDS in low birthweight infants and in the infants of drug-dependent and smoking mothers might be related to the disturbances in fetal breathing reported as prenatal complications in these circumstances.[24-26] Disturbances in fetal breathing could influence the normal development of the lungs, possibly predisposing to a postnatal surfactant defect.

Thirdly, the known association between respiratory tract infections and SIDS may be related to their production of a disturbance in the functioning of the type 2 cell or of an abnormality in the substrate of the surfactant. The association between clusters of SIDS cases and epidemics of pertussis[27] and respiratory syncytial virus infection[28] may also be relevant to our findings that these infections may produce apnea with VPM.[20]

Finally, the relationships between poor socioeconomic conditions and sudden infant death may relate to this disorder by effects mediated both prenatally and postnatally. Before birth, poverty is associated with retardation of intrauterine growth, smoking and drug dependency, conditions which have been shown to disturb fetal breathing (see

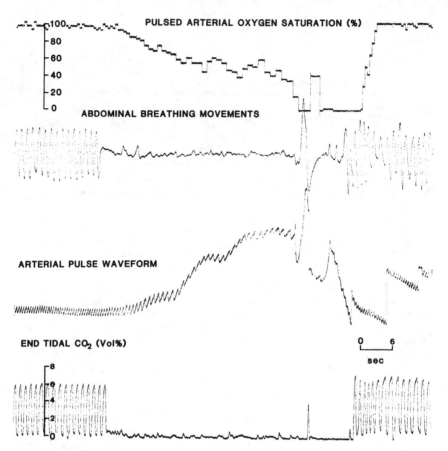

FIGURE 11a. Section of an overnight recording in a previously preterm infant aged 24 weeks (postconceptional age, 49 weeks) with cyanotic episodes due to apnea with VPM and an associated pertussis infection. A prolonged absence of inspiratory efforts ("central apnea") for 37 sec is associated with hypoxemia and bradycardia (as demonstrated by the arterial pulses).

above). Postnatally, it is associated with an increased incidence of respiratory tract infections, which, again, might produce apnea with VPM or trigger a fatal episode in an infant predisposed to this condition. Poverty may also produce preterm birth, which is also a factor associated with an increased incidence of SIDS, both alone and through its association with bronchopulmonary dysplasia. It is possible that the long-term ventilatory therapy given to some of these latter infants may be responsible for a subsequent defect in lung surfactant or its substrate. Unfortunately, at this stage we must recall that prolonged apneic episodes may also, in a very small proportion of cases, result from imposed asphyxia, a condition that is more likely to occur under circumstances of socioeconomic deprivation.

Overheating has recently been implicated in some examples of SIDS.[29] This disturbance could predispose to apnea with VPM by its possible adverse effects on the functioning of lung surfactant[30] and predispose to seizure-induced apnea through its propensity to lower the threshold for convulsions.[31]

The following features of the pathology of SIDS support the apnea with VPM hypothesis. Pulmonary edema is found at postmortem in over 90% of SIDS victims.[32] Since there is no cardiac lesion to explain this edema, we suspect that it results from a defect within the lungs. Abnormalities of the control of surface tension are known to be accompanied by a suction of fluid from the pulmonary capillaries to within the alveoli; such changes could occur during a terminal episode of widespread alveolar atelectasis.

Petechial hemorrhages are found in approximately 75% of SIDS victims and have a characteristic distribution[33] which suggests the generation of large negative intrathoracic pressures at end-expiration.[34] This would typify the situation in apnea with VPM arising at the time of a gasp or series of gasps attempting to re-open the lung and ventilate areas of widespread atelectasis.

The possibility that chronic intermittent hypoxemia occurred prior to death in a major proportion of SIDS victims was first suggested by Naeye.[35] Subsequently, the presence of some of the tissue markers suggestive of this hypothesis has been substantiated.[36] Recently, new support for this hypothesis has been provided by Guilian et al.,[37] who identified increased levels of fetal hemoglobin in SIDS victims compared to age-matched controls. The frequent hypoxemic episodes documented in some infants with apnea and VPM would be supported by these postmortem findings.

Finally, the evidence of respiratory tract infections demonstrated at postmortem in over 75% of SIDS cases could be relevant to apnea with VPM through mechanisms described above.

One important postmortem study which is contrary to the defective-surfactant hypothesis is that produced by Fagan et al.,[38] who reported no difference in the pressure/volume characteristics of the lungs in SIDS victims compared with controls. This study has, however, been criticized in 3 respects. Firstly, the studies were not carried out at the low lung-volumes necessary to demonstrate a surfactant defect;[39] secondly, the temperature at which the studies were performed was not controlled;[39] and, finally—and perhaps of most importance—postmortem changes in the surfactant subphase may have tended to nullify any difference between SIDS cases and controls.[40] Further studies are clearly needed in this area.

In summary, it would appear that if, as supported by the observations of clinical physiology, apnea with evidence VPM is indeed due to a defect in lung surfactant, then the epidemiology and pathology of SIDS would support defective lung surfactant as a

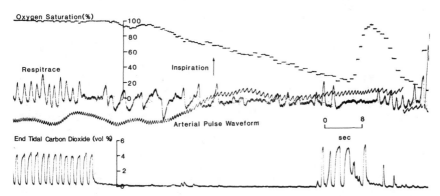

FIGURE 11b. Section of a recording taken at 4 weeks of age in a full-term infant with cyanotic episodes. An absence of airflow (measured by an expired CO_2 signal) for 50 sec is associated with continued breathing movements and hypoxemia.

major mechanism for SIDS. Imposed asphyxia and seizure-induced apnea could also be contributory causes, but, on the basis of our own studies, these mechanisms would be relatively rare causes of sudden infant death.

In conclusion, infants destined to suffer SIDS do not have cardiac arrhythmias, prolonged apneic pauses, pre-excitation, or prolongation of the QT interval. Infants at risk do, however, have higher heart rates and larger quantities of sinus tachycardia than survivors. Four main mechanisms can produce cyanotic episodes in early infancy. These are apnea with ventilatory perfusion mismatch, seizure-induced apnea, imposed asphyxia, and sleep-related upper airway obstruction. Apnea with VPM is the most prevalent and has many characteristics which suggest that it could be a major cause of SIDS. Some infants may have this disorder from birth; others may acquire it as the direct result of certain respiratory tract infections, in particular, those resulting from pertussis and respiratory syncytial virus. On the basis of our findings, attempts to prevent SIDS should

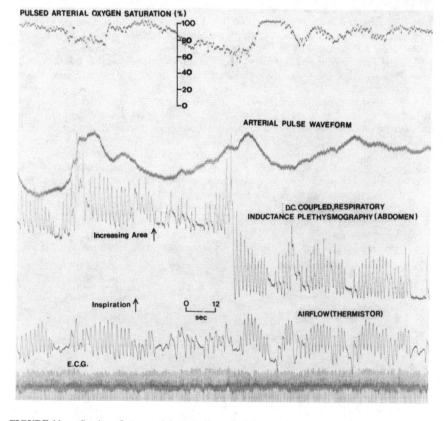

FIGURE 11c.   Section of an overnight recording on a full-term infant, 11 days of age, with a type 1 herpes simplex respiratory tract infection and cyanotic episodes. There is a dip in Sao_2 accompanied by a change in the pattern of—but not an interruption of—breathing movements, continued inspiratory airflow, and a slight slowing of heart rate. The breathing-movement and airflow signals show evidence of expiratory braking. The sudden change in DC position of the inductance plethysmography signal is due to an electronic reset mechanism. (From Southall and Talbert.[11] Reprinted with permission from Elsevier and the editor, M. A. Hollinger.)

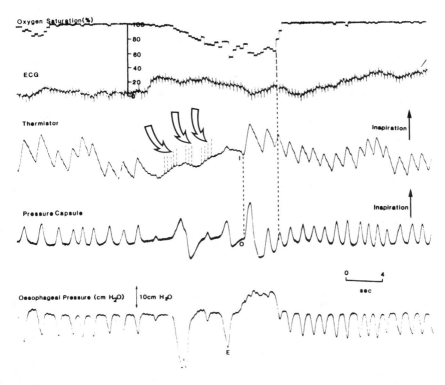

FIGURE 12.   An episode of hypoxemia from an overnight recording on a previously preterm infant who had suffered a series of apparent life-threatening (cyanotic) episodes at home at the age of 62 days (postconceptional age, 40 weeks). There are continued inspiratory efforts and movements but no inspiratory airflow. During the absence of airflow, small amplitude signals on the thermistor tracing (marked with **dotted lines** at **curved arrows**) are present and align with each ECG complex. Probably representing oscillations in airflow associated with each heart beat, they confirm that the airway is open and that the absent airflow is *not* due to inspiratory efforts which are ineffective because of airway obstruction. At **I** on the thermistor signal, inspiratory airflow resumes, coinciding with an outward movement of the pressure capsule signal (**O**) but against a positive esophageal pressure. The sharp rise in Sao_2 indicates the arrival of a bolus of oxygenated blood at the pulse oximeter probe following the time interval required for circulatory transport to the toe. It is possible that the inspiratory airflow at **I** is produced by the delayed effect of the inspiratory effort at **E** and is then responsible for the increase in Sao_2. (From Southall and Talbert.[11] Reprinted with permission from Elsevier and the editor, M. A. Hollinger.)

concentrate on improving prenatal and early postnatal care and reducing the incidence of respiratory tract infections during the first 6 months of life.

ACKNOWLEDGMENTS

We thank Jane Lang for her invaluable help in preparing this report.

REFERENCES

1.   SOUTHALL, D.P. *et al.* 1983. Identification of infants destined to die unexpectedly during infancy: Evaluation of predictive importance of prolonged apnoea and disorders of cardiac

rhythm or conduction. First report of a multicentred prospective study into the sudden infant death syndrome. Br. Med. J. **286:** 1092–1096.

2. SOUTHALL, D.P. *et al.* 1982. Prolonged apnea and cardiac arrhythmias in infants discharged from neonatal intensive care units: Failure to predict an increased risk for SIDS. Pediatrics **70:** 844–851.

3. SOUTHALL, D.P., J.M. RICHARDS, V.A. STEBBENS, A.J. WILSON, V. TAYLOR & J.R. ALEXANDER. 1986. Pauses, periodicity, and regularity of breathing movements, heart and respiratory rates in 16 full-term infants who suffered SIDS. Pediatrics **78:** 787–796.

4. YOUNT, J.E., J.R. ALEXANDER, V.A. STEBBENS & D.P. SOUTHALL. 1987. Cardiorespiratory patterns in preterm infants suffering SIDS: Positive results from a controlled, blinded analysis (abstract). Poster presented at the New York Academy of Science Meeting, The Sudden Infant Death Syndrome: Cardiorespiratory Mechanisms and Interventions. May 24–27. Como, Italy.

5. WILSON, A.J., V. STEVENS, C.I. FRANKS, J. ALEXANDER & D.P. SOUTHALL. 1985. Respiratory and heart rate patterns in infants destined to be victims of sudden infant death syndrome: Average rates and their variability measured over 24 hours. Br. Med. J. **290:** 497–501.

6. SOUTHALL, D.P., V. STEVENS, C.I. FRANKS, R.G. NEWCOMBE & A.J. WILSON. 1988. Sinus tachycardia in term infants preceding sudden infant death. Eur. J. Pediatr. **147:** 74–78.

7. SCHECHTMAN, V.L., R.M. HARPER, K.A. KLUGE, A.J. WILSON & D.P. SOUTHALL. 1987. Cardiac patterns in normal infants and victims of SIDS (abstract). Sleep Research Neuroscience Meeting, Copenhagen, 1987. In press.

8. SOUTHALL, D.P., V.A. STEBBENS & E.A. SHINEBOURNE. 1987. Sudden and unexpected death between one and five years. Arch. Dis. Child. **62:** 700–705.

9. SOUTHALL, D.P., D.G. TALBERT, P. JOHNSON *et al.* 1985. Prolonged expiratory apnoea: A disorder resulting in episodes of severe arterial hypoxaemia in infants and young children. Lancet **2:** 571–577.

10. SOUTHALL, D.P., D.G. TALBERT, P. JOHNSON *et al.* 1985. Prolonged expiratory apnoea and hypoxaemia. Lancet **2:** 1125–1126.

11. SOUTHALL, D.P. & D.G. TALBERT. 1987. Sudden atelectasis apnoea braking syndrome (SAABS). *In* Current Topics in Pulmonary Pharmacology. M.A. Hollinger, Ed.: 210–281. Elsevier. New York.

12. LOMBROSO, C.T. & P. LERMAN. 1967. Breath holding spells (cyanotic and pallid infantile syncope). Pediatrics **39:** 563–581.

13. SOUTHALL, D.P., W.A. ARROWSMITH, V. STEBBENS & J.R. ALEXANDER. 1986. QT interval measurements before sudden infant death syndrome. Arch. Dis. Child. **61:** 327–333.

14. SOUTHALL, D.P., W.A. ARROWSMITH, J.R. OAKLEY, G. McENERY, R.H. ANDERSON & E.A. SHINEBOURNE. 1979. Prolonged QT interval and cardiac arrhythmias in two neonates; Sudden infant death syndrome in one case. Arch. Dis. Child. **54:** 776–779.

15. RUTTER, N. & D.P. SOUTHALL. 1985. A family with life-threatening cardiac arrhythmias mistakenly diagnosed as epilepsy. Arch. Dis. Child. **60:** 54–56.

16. SOUTHALL, D.P., V. STEBBENS, N. ABRAHAM & L. ABRAHAM. 1987. Prolonged apnoea with severe hypoxaemia resulting from complex partial seizures. Dev. Med. Child Neurol. **29:** 784–789.

17. SOUTHALL, D.P., C.B. CROFT, H. IBRAHIM, A. GURNEY, R. BUCHDAHL & J.O. WARNER. 1988. Sleep associated upper airway obstruction in infants and young children. Submitted, Eur. J. Pediatr.

18. SOUTHALL, D.P., V.A. STEBBENS, S.V. REES, M.H. LANG, J.O. WARNER & E.A. SHINEBOURNE. 1987. Apnoeic episodes induced by smothering: Two cases identified by covert video surveillance. Br. Med. J. **294:** 1637–1641.

19. GAUK, E.W., L. KIDD & J.S. PRICHARD. 1963. Mechanism of seizures associated with breath-holding spells. N. Engl. J. Med. **268:** 1436–1441.

20. SOUTHALL, D.P., M.G. THOMAS & H.P. LAMBERT. 1988. Severe hypoxaemia in infants with pertussis. Arch. Dis. Child. In press.

21. TALBERT, D.G. & D.P. SOUTHALL. 1985. A bimodal form of alveolar behaviour induced by a defect in lung surfactant: A possible mechanism for sudden infant death syndrome. Lancet **1:** 727–728.

22. SOUTHALL, D.P. 1988. Role of apnea in the sudden infant death syndrome: A personal view. Pediatrics **80:** 73–84.
23. BOYDEN, E.A. & D.H. TOMPSETT. 1965. The changing patterns in the developing lungs of infants. Acta Anat. **61:** 164–192.
24. ROBERTS, A.B., D. LITTLE & S. CAMPBELL. 1978. 24 hour studies of fetal respiratory movements and fetal body movements in five growth-retarded fetuses. *In* Recent Advances in Ultrasound Diagnosis. A. Kurjak, Ed.: 192–193. Excerpta Medica. Amsterdam.
25. GOODMAN, J.D.S., F.G.A. VISSER & G.S. DAWES. 1984. Effects of maternal cigarette smoking on fetal trunk movements, fetal breathing movements and fetal heart rate. Br. J. Obstet. Gynaecol. **91:** 657–661.
26. RICHARDSON, B.S., J.P. O'GRADY & G.D. OLSEN. 1984. Foetal breathing movements and the response to CO_2 in patients on methadone maintenance. Am. J. Obstet. Gynecol. **150:** 400–405.
27. NICOLL, A. & A. GARDNER. 1988. Whooping cough and unrecognised postperinatal mortality. Arch. Dis. Child. **63:** 41–47.
28. WILLIAMS, A.L., E.C. UREN & L. BRETHERTON. 1984. Respiratory viruses and sudden infant death. Br. Med. J. **288:** 1491–1493.
29. STANTON, A.N. 1984. Overheating and cot death. Lancet **2:** 1199–1201.
30. GOERKE, J. & J. GONZALES. 1981. Temperature dependence of dipalmitoyl phosphatidyl choline monolayer stability. J. Appl. Physiol. **51:** 1108–1114.
31. NEGMAN, M.E. 1939. The relation of convulsions and hyperthermia. J. Pediatr. **14:** 190–202.
32. KROUS, H.F. 1984. Sudden infant death syndrome: Pathology and pathophysiology. Pathol. Ann. **19:** 1–14.
33. KROUS, H.F. 1984. The microscopic distribution of intrathoracic petechiae in sudden infant death syndrome. Arch. Pathol. Lab. Med. **108:** 77–79.
34. BECKWITH, J.B. 1970. Observations on the pathological anatomy of the sudden infant death syndrome. *In* Proceedings of the Second International Conference on Causes of Sudden Death in Infants. A.B. Bergman, J.B. Beckwith & C.G. Ray, Eds.: 83–102. Univ. Washington Press. Seattle.
35. NAEYE, R.L. 1980. Sudden Infant Death. Sci. Am. **242:** 56–62.
36. MERRITT, T.A. & M.A. VALDES-DAPENA. 1984. SIDS research update. Pediatr. Ann. **13:** 193–207.
37. GIULIAN, G.G., E.F. GILBERT & R.L. MOSS. 1987. Elevated fetal hemoglobin levels in sudden infant death syndrome. N. Engl. J. Med. **3l6:** 1122–1126.
38. FAGAN, D.G. & A.D. MILNER. 1985. Pressure volume characteristics of the lungs in sudden infant death syndrome. Arch. Dis. Child. **60:** 471–473.
39. SOUTHALL, D.P. & D.G. TALBERT. 1985. Pressure volume characteristics of the lungs in sudden infant death syndrome (letter). Arch. Dis. Child. **60:** 1104–1105.
40. GIBSON, R.A. & E.J. McMURCHIE. 1986. Changes in lung surfactant lipids associated with the sudden infant death syndrome. Aust. Paediatr. J. Suppl.: 77–80.

Cardiorespiratory Interactions in Heart-Rate Control[a]

K. M. SPYER AND M. P. GILBEY

Department of Physiology
Royal Free Hospital School of Medicine
Rowland Hill Street
London NW3 2PF
United Kingdom

INTRODUCTION

The growing interest in the etiology of the sudden infant death syndrome (SIDS) has led to a reawakening of interest in the subject of the physiological control and organization of cardiorespiratory interactions. The most notable physiological manifestation of such an interaction is sinus arrhythmia, and the basis for much of current thinking about its origin lies in the work of Anrep.[1,2] He showed convincingly that the respiratory-related fluctuations in heart rate resulted from 2 mechanisms: first, a regulation of the vagal outflow to the heart by those neural processes that generate respiratory rhythm and reside in the brainstem; second, reflex inputs that are activated on inflation of the lungs. These act together to produce tachycardia during inspiration and a slowing of the heart in expiration.

The major output pathway for heart-rate control appears to be the vagus. Recent studies have shown that the sensitivities of the baroreceptor and chemoreceptor controls of vagal outflow are markedly affected by respiratory state. A brief stimulus to either, if timed to occur during expiration, is effective; but one timed to occur during inspiration is ineffective in activating cardiac vagal efferent fibers or slowing the heart.[3] Indeed, potent influences of respiration on the efficacy of a wide range of cardiovascular and respiratory reflexes are well illustrated, and many of the non-linearities in the control of the heart during reflexes involving numerous different receptors can be accounted for by the influences that these elicit concomitantly on respiration.[4] It must also be stressed that equivalent changes are produced in the sympathetic outflow to the heart and blood vessels, and respiration strongly influences the effectiveness of reflex inputs to sympathetic neurones.[5]

These observations have led my laboratory to seek to determine the central mechanisms mediating these interactions. We have used a wide range of neurophysiological approaches in an attempt to unravel the synaptic processes that lead to the respiratory patterning of vagal[6] and sympathetic discharge.[7] Our first hypothesis was that important interactions that would account for the influences of lung inflation on both heart rate and reflex inputs to cardiac vagal efferents occurred at the level of the nucleus of the tractus solitarius (NTS). This hypothesis was based on the fact that the major cardiovascular and respiratory afferents terminate in the NTS,[8] and the input from slowly adapting vagal stretch-afferents might modulate reflex transmission at this level. However, a series of

[a]The work of the laboratory is supported by grants from the British Heart Foundation and the Medical Research Council.

studies has failed to reveal any effective action of this input on either baroreceptor, sinus (SN), or aortic (AN) nerve inputs.[9-11] Equally, central respiratory inputs were ineffective in influencing either the afferent terminals of the baroreceptors, SN, and AN, or the NTS neurones affected by these inputs.[10] In consequence, our major investigations have been directed to the preganglionic vagal and sympathetic neurones and have taken the form of analyzing their basic firing patterns and the mechanisms that elicit their respiratory-related periodicities. This review will concentrate on this subject and will seek to place our observations in the context of the link between respiratory apnea and bradycardia, which may be the basis of SIDS.

METHODS

In the studies to be reported, attempts have been made to record the activity of CVMs (cardiac vagal motor neurons) in the cat and SPNs (sympathetic preganglionic neurons) in both cat and rat, in situations where the two components of respiration—the central drive and lung inflation—could be desynchronized to assess their independent actions. Accordingly, in both species anesthetized animals were artificially ventilated, pneumothoracotomized and paralyzed. Full experimental details are given in two recently published papers.[6,7] Microelectrodes have been used to record in the cat, both extracellularly and intracellularly, from CVMs identified by their antidromic responses to stimulation of the intrathoracic cardiac vagal branches.[6,12,13,14] In some experiments, multibarreled micropipettes were used to allow the ionophoresis of the excitant amino acid, DL-homocysteate, acetylcholine and atropine. In a few cats, SPNs at T2–3 level have been studied. These were identified by their antidromic response to stimulation of the white rami. In the rat, SPNs were identified in the gray matter of T2 upon stimulation of the ipsilateral cervical sympathetic nerve. Both single and multibarreled microelectrodes were used to record extracellularly from SPNs. In both species, a record of phrenic nerve activity was taken as an indicator of central respiratory activity. Tracheal pressure was recorded also to monitor lung inflation.

RESULTS

Cardiac Vagal Motor Neurons

From the results of our neurophysiological investigations, it is established that CVMs in the cat are located within the nucleus ambiguus.[12,13] Under the conditions of our experiments, these neurons only rarely displayed ongoing activity although they were readily activated antidromically. Indeed, the anesthetized cat is known to have a "low" vagal tone. However, in those neurons that were active (see FIG. 1A), and also in those which were induced to fire by the microionophoresis of the excitant amino acid, DL-homocysteate, onto them, the discharge was correlated with the central respiratory cycle. Invariably they fired during expiration, with a period of silence during inspiration (FIG. 1A). The most notable period of activity was in phase-1 expiration, or postinspiration,[15] with a variable discharge during stage-II expiration (see FIG. 1A). Notably, their discharge followed central respiratory activity and not lung inflation. In this context, it is necessary to stress that inflation volumes of less than 30 ml were used; but, whilst a clear and reproducible influence of central respiratory activity was noted, no discharge in phase with lung inflation has been apparent in any of our studies.[6,12,13,14] Whilst the data from extracellular studies provide an indication of the pattern of

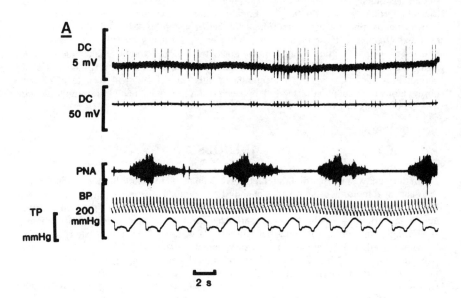

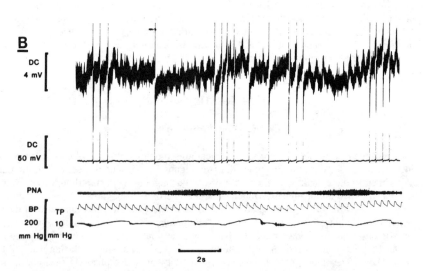

FIGURE 1. **A:** extracellular recording from a CVM. **B:** intracellular recording from a CVM. Traces, from *top* to *bottom,* in each panel: high and low gain recordings of CVM activity (DC), phrenic nerve activity (PNA), femoral arterial blood pressure (BP) and tracheal pressure (TP). (Reproduced from Gilbey *et al.*[6] with permission from the *Journal of Physiology.*)

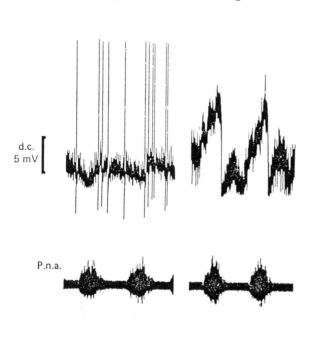

FIGURE 2. A: intracellular recording from a CVM showing changes in membrane potential in relation to phrenic nerve activity. Passage of negative hyperpolarizing current (1 nA for 3 min) resulted in reversal of the hyperpolarizing waves. B: recording taken after current injection ended. In each panel, *upper trace* is high gain DC recording of membrane potential (d.c.) and *lower trace* is phrenic nerve activity (P. n. a.). (Reproduced from Gilbey *et al.*[6] with permission from the *Journal of Physiology.*)

modulation, the synaptic events underlying the modulation can only be revealed using intracellular recordings. As shown in FIGURE 1B, impaled CVMs reveal a pattern of membrane potential during the respiratory cycle that accounts for the discharge seen in extracellular recordings. Most striking is the period of membrane hyperpolarization during inspiration, followed by a rapid repolarization at the cessation of inspiration and then subsequent depolarization during postinspiration, with a further and variable depolarization occurring later in expiration. The hyperpolarization during inspiration is a consequence of a wave of Cl^--dependent i. p. s. p. s., since the induced hyperpolarization can be reversed in polarity by injection of either DC hyperpolarizing currents (1–2 nA) or Cl^- (FIG. 2) and appears to be mediated by a muscarinic cholinergic mechanism. The membrane potential changes were accompanied by falls in membrane input-resistance of up to 45% during inspiration. Together, the hyperpolarization and lowered membrane resistance dramatically alter the sensitivity of CVMs to excitatory inputs; the e. p. s. p. s. generated by the baroreceptors, which are the major excitatory input to CVMs,[6,14] are diminished during inspiration, to the extent of almost total attenuation during the latter part of inspiration (FIG. 3).

This pattern of central respiratory influence, culminating in a direct inhibition of CVMs in phase with inspiration, provides a clear explanation for the respiratory modifications of the baroreceptor-vagal reflex. During inspiration, the influence of the baroreceptors and other excitatory inputs are maintained at subthreshold levels, and it is only during expiration that CVMs are brought to discharge by baroreceptor stimulation.

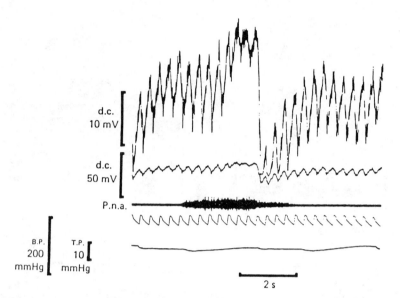

FIGURE 3. Respiratory modulation of pulse-rhythmic e. p. s. p. s. Recording in a cell in which i. p. s. p. s. had been reversed previously by Cl⁻ injection (3 nA for 5 min). Further details in text. Traces, from *top* to *bottom:* high and low gain DC recordings of membrane potential (d.c.), phrenic nerve activity (P. n. a.), femoral arterial blood pressure (B. P.) and tracheal pressure (T. P.). (Reproduced from Gilbey *et al.*[6] with permission from the *Journal of Physiology.*)

The period of postinspiration is particularly important, since at this time CVMs are particularly excitable. Postinspiration is a functionally critical period in the patterning of respiratory activity.[15,16] Changes in the activity of medullary postinspiratory neurons, which are no doubt strongly influenced in their action by the strength of peripheral reflex inputs, can, through inhibitory and excitatory actions on other medullary respiratory neurons, either produce a postinspiratory apnea or turn the system to rapid shallow breathing. A wide range of inputs may be effective in modifying postinspiratory state; chemoreceptor and superior laryngeal inputs, amongst others, intensify postinspiratory activity and will excite CVM discharge. Accordingly, at this time of transition in the patterning of respiration, circumstances may involve respiratory suppression and brady-cardia concomitantly to provoke a potentially life-threatening situation.

Sympathetic Preganglionic Activity

Whilst vagal preganglionic neurons can be functionally classified on the basis of their patterns of response and innervation,[13] the classification of SPNs is not as yet well defined. Indeed, whilst there are numerous reports of respiratory-related discharges in sympathetic outflows, it is only with single-unit recordings that the mechanisms generating the various patterns can be established. To this end, we have studied the activity of SPNs relaying in the cervical sympathetic nerve by recording from their cell bodies in the intermediolateral cell column at T2.[7] Three distinct patterns of nerve discharge were observed in both SPNs with ongoing activity and those induced to fire by the ionophoresis of glutamate (FIG. 4). These comprised a group with maximal discharge in phase with inspiration (see FIG. 4), one with maximal discharge in expiration, and, finally, one with activity unaffected by central respiratory activity. Many of these neurons were studied in animals in which bilateral vagotomy had been effected to remove reflex inputs resulting from inflation of the lungs. The activity of all 3 groups appears to be susceptible to baroreceptor inhibition.[17] Interestingly, the "inspiratory" sympathetic group of neurons appeared refractory to the effects of ionophoretically applied glutamate in postinspiration, and it was notable that with increasing levels of glutamate, an inspiratory-ramp discharge became more prevalent in their discharge (FIG. 1). This implies that the neurons are receiving a pattern of input not dissimilar to that driving inspiratory intercostal motor neurons. In contrast, the expiratory-firing group showed a tendency to tonic discharge in the absence of central respiratory activity (induced by hyperventilation), implying that their expiratory-firing pattern was imposed by inhibition during inspiration, as in the case of CVMs (see above), or by disfacilitation. In a few cases, SPNs in the cat have been impaled and show respiratory-related changes in membrane potential. These observations indicate that sympathetic neurons are in many cases receiving central respiratory-drive potentials similar to those received by respiratory motor neurons.

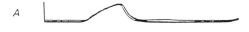

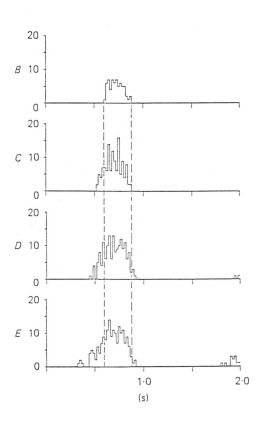

FIGURE 4. Periphrenic histograms. B, C, D and E: the effect of the ionophoretic application of glutamate, using currents of 10, 30, 50, and 100 nA, respectively, on the type "A" discharge of a glutamate-activated, and, otherwise, silent neuron (twenty sweeps, 20 msec bins). A: the average superimposed phrenic activity during the periods when B, C, D, and E were accumulated. Observe that the timing of the off-switching changes little compared with the advance of onset of the inspiratory synchronous discharge. (Reproduced from Gilbey et al.[7] with permission from the Journal of Physiology.)

DISCUSSION

The data presented in this review have indicated that in the anesthetized cat (and rat), the neural networks generating respiratory activity act not only to drive respiratory motor neurons but also to impose patterns of activity in the vagal and sympathetic outflows. Functionally, this may provide a mechanism for the integration of cardiovascular and respiratory control, although in many circumstances it may act at a barely liminal level. An alteration in either a peripheral afferent input(s) or a central drive may, however, lead to a more clearly established correlation. The tendency in postinspiration is for cardiac vagal activity to be enhanced, and any substantial chemoreceptor or laryngeal input can intensify this. Similarly, in many sympathetic neurons, postinspiration is a phase of minimal excitability, although whether this is the case in fibers innervating the stellate ganglion—and hence affecting the heart—remains to be determined.

The influence of respiration is not limited to autonomic outflows. Many neurons in the reticular formation exhibit patterns of discharge with marked respiratory-related periodicities.[18] One motor output with a striking respiratory rhythm is that of hypoglossal motor neurons. Hypoglossal neurons innervating the genioglossus muscle of the tongue have a marked respiratory rhythm and, in a recent study, have been shown to be particularly active in inspiration and postinspiration.[19] The importance of the activity of the tongue to prevent relapse and airway obstruction has been noted, and, clearly, sleep apnea is complicated by the relaxation of the tongue. Interestingly, we have demonstrated that, in a situation in the anesthetized cat when hypoglossal activity was minimal, a stimulus to the hypothalamic defense area provoked a marked postinspiratory discharge in the hypoglossal nerve (Richter, Gilbey, and Spyer, unpublished observation) at a time when postinspiratory activity in the phrenic neurogram was absent. Such hypothalamic stimulation also evoked an inhibition of CVM discharge.[20] In effect, arousal stimuli largely overcame the deleterious effects of apnea. It is possible that a laryngeal stimulus might also serve as a safety mechanism provoking postinspiratory activity and hence relieving airway obstruction.

So far, we have concentrated on the central respiratory component of sinus arrhythmia. Our studies have failed to reveal a potent influence of slowly adapting vagal pulmonary stretch on the activity of CVMs. Others have demonstrated effects on the performance of the baroreceptor-vagal reflex,[9] but the baroreceptor control of vascular resistance has been shown to be uneffected.[21] Whatever the case, as lung stretch-inputs reflexly modify central respiratory activity, under normal patterns of respiration, with lung inflation and central rhythm synchronized, an influence is certain to be manifest. In other studies we have sought to determine whether respiratory effects on the baroreceptor reflex occur during the initial processing of the reflex at the level of the NTS. Our results are unequivocal; NTS neurons receiving excitatory inputs from SN and the arterial baroreceptors are not influenced by either lung inflation or central respiratory activity. This would indicate that the effects noted in our report must be mediated at other stages in the reflex pathway, but, evidently and most importantly, through synaptic actions at the level of the autonomic motor neurons.

ACKNOWLEDGMENTS

Several colleagues have made valuable contributions to the studies reviewed.

REFERENCES

1. ANREP, G. V., W. PASCUAL & R. ROSSLER. 1936. Respiratory variations of heart rate. I. The reflex mechanism of the respiratory arrhythmia. Proc. R. Soc. London Ser. B. **119:** 191–217.

2. ANREP, G. V., W. PASCUAL & R. ROSSLER. 1936. Respiratory variations of heart rate. II. The central mechanism of respiratory arrhythmia and the inter-relationships between central and reflex mechanisms. Proc. R. Soc. London Ser. B **119:** 218–230.

3. POTTER, E. K. 1981. Inspiratory inhibition of vagal responses to baroreceptor and chemoreceptor stimuli in the dog. J. Physiol. (London) **316:** 177–190.

4. DALY, M. DE BURGH. 1985. Interactions between respiration and circulation. *In* Handbook of Physiology. The Respiratory System. Vol. II, Chapter 16: 529–594. American Physiological Society. Bethesda, MD.

5. DAVIS, A. L., D. I. MCCLOSKEY & E. K. POTTER. 1977. Respiratory modulation of baroreceptor and chemoreceptor reflexes affecting heart rate through the sympathetic nervous system. J. Physiol. (London) **272:** 691–703.

6. GILBEY, M. P., D. JORDAN, D. W. RICHTER, & K. M. SPYER. 1984. Synaptic mechanisms involved in the inspiratory modulation of vagal cardio-inhibitory neurones in the cat. J. Physiol. (London) **356:** 65–78.

7. GILBEY, M. P., Y. NUMAO & K. M. SPYER. 1986. Discharge patterns of cervical sympathetic preganglionic neurones related to central respiratory drive in the rat. J. Physiol. (London) **378:** 253–265.

8. JORDAN, D. & K. M. SPYER. 1986. Brainstem integration of cardiovascular and pulmonary afferent activity. Prog. Brain Res. **67:** 295–314.

9. JORDAN, D. & K. M. SPYER. 1979. Studies on the excitability of sinus nerve afferent terminals. J. Physiol. (London) **297:** 123–134.

10. MIFFLIN, S. W., K. M. SPYER & D. J. WITHINGTON-WRAY. 1986. Lack of respiratory modulation of baroreceptor inputs in the nucleus of the tractus solitarius of the cat. J. Physiol. (London) **376:** 33P.

11. RICHTER, D. W., D. JORDAN, D. BALLANTYNE, M. MEESMAN & K. M. SPYER. 1986. Presynaptic depolarization in myelinated vagal afferent fibres terminating in the nucleus of the tractus solitarius in the cat. Pfluegers Arch. **406:** 12–19.

12. MCALLEN, R. M. & K. M. SPYER. 1976. The location of cardiac vagal preganglionic motooneurones in the medulla of the cat. J. Physiol. (London) **258:** 187–204.

13. MCALLEN, R. M. & K. M. SPYER. 1978. Two types of vagal preganglionic motoneurones projecting to the heart and lungs. J. Physiol. (London) **282:** 353–364.

14. MCALLEN, R. M. & K. M. SPYER. 1978. The baroreceptor input to cardiac vagal motoneurones. J. Physiol. (London) **282:** 365–374.

15. RICHTER, D. W. 1982. Generation and maintenance of the respiratory rhythm. J. Exp. Biol. **100:** 93–107.

16. RICHTER, D. W., D. BALLANTYNE & J. E. REMMERS. 1987. The differential organization of medullary post-inspiratory activities. In press.

17. NUMAO, Y. & M. P. GILBEY. 1987. Effects of aortic nerve stimulation on cervical sympathetic preganglionic neurones in the rat. Brain Res. **401:** 190–194.

18. LANGHORST, P., M. LAMBERTZ & G. SCHULZ. 1981. Central control and interactions affecting sympathetic and parasympathetic activity. J. Autonomic Nerv. Syst. **4:** 149–163.

19. MIFFLIN, S. W., K. M. SPYER & D. J. WITHINGTON-WRAY. 1986. Respiratory modulation of hypoglossal motoneurones in the cat. J. Physiol. (London) **382:** 61P.

20. SPYER, K. M. 1984. Central control of the cardiovascular system. *In* Recent Advances in Physiology. Chap. 6. P. F. Baker, Ed.: 163–200. Churchill Livingstone. Edinburgh.

21. DALY, M. DE BURGH, J. WARD & L. M. WOOD. 1986. Modification by lung inflation of the vascular responses from the carotid body chemoreceptors and other receptors in dogs. J. Physiol. **378:** 13–30.

SIDS, Near-Miss SIDS and Cardiac Arrhythmia

CHRISTIAN GUILLEMINAULT

Sleep Research Center
Stanford University School of Medicine
Stanford, California 94305

INTRODUCTION

The imprecise phrase "sudden infant death syndrome" (SIDS) is used to describe the abrupt and puzzling death of infants. The vagueness of the term mirrors our ignorance of the underlying problems, and the use of "syndrome" is probably unfortunate, as it implies that we have at least some clinical clues. We have, in fact, no clues; and this so-called syndrome is defined by negative findings and from information gained through epidemiological surveys. But without clinical clues, there is no certainty that the variables found in surveys are at all relevant to the problem under investigation. Moreover, some clues important to a subgroup of infants may be masked by the statistical analyses required in epidemiological surveys. This may lead to the very debatable belief that there is only one etiology of the unexplained death of infants. If we study the end-result—the dead infant—retrospectively, we may once again miss the subtle precipitating event responsible for the tragic outcome. The quest for understanding of SIDS is confounded by many paradoxes, some as simple as equating the findings from premature infants with those from the full-term. We acknowledge the many state-of-the-art difficulties plaguing any research protocol, as well as the limitations of our own presentation. But despite histological evaluations of infant victims compared with appropriate controls, sophisticated epidemiological surveys, and prospective population investigations, with the methods of data collection and the technology currently available, SIDS research is still mainly focused on 2 populations that, from the evidence of retrospective studies, are supposedly more at risk (although only to a very limited extent) of unexplained, abrupt death: siblings of SIDS victims, and infants who have suffered the so-called near-miss SIDS (a vaguely defined population).

The 2 theories most frequently favored over the past 20 years in searching for a common pathway to this tragic occurrence are a *cardiac theory* that proposes the sudden appearance of a lethal arrhythmia[1] and a *respiratory theory* that suggests an abrupt interruption of air exchange.[2] Undoubtedly, these two basic mechanisms have little chance to be denied as causes of abrupt, unexplained death in infants! But even the postmortem examinations have not clarified these issues significantly.[3] Our contribution to the SIDS issue has the stamp of our time: it involves a patient population that has rarely died of SIDS, despite the overall slightly elevated SIDS occurrence compared with the two populations mentioned above. It is also limited by the technology used and the variables investigated.

One hypothesis that has been considered is that the states-of-alertness-dependent controls of vital functions may be impaired or incompletely functioning in early infancy. Sudden, unexpected death could be precipitated, in infancy, secondary to a dysfunction involving the different sleep/wake regulatory activities of the autonomic nervous system (ANS): the controls exercised by the ANS on vital functions vary, depending on the states of alertness.[4] The sympathetic-parasympathetic balance not only depends on the 3 major states, wakefulness, non-rapid eye movement (NREM) and rapid eye movement (REM) sleep, but also is influenced by tonic or phasic events during REM sleep. In infancy, sympathetic and parasympathetic tones will mature at different speeds and there will be reorganization of the state-dependent controls as a function of age. Prematurity will add a new difficulty; we have some knowledge about the changes in state-related sympathetic-parasympathetic balances in full-term animal (mammal) models and infants, but our understanding of the speed of change of these two state-related influences is still very nebulous. It is possible that the combination of an abnormal ANS setting and sleep contributes to abrupt death, particularly if dysfunction of a vital variable is added to these two factors. This hypothesis would allow for different types of abrupt organ failures, i.e., cardiac or ventilatory. The state-dependent ANS dysfunction may only be a risk factor for sudden significant health problems. If, secondary to an external challenge, the ANS is significantly stimulated, the existence of the state-dependent ANS dysfunction may be responsible for abrupt death.

Experimental Investigations

We did 24-hr polygraphic monitoring of near-miss SIDS infants during sleep and wakefulness. We evaluated the frequency at which we observed significant cardiac arrhythmias and examined their relationship to the sleep/wake cycle, respiratory events, and behavior known to induce vagal tone, particularly phasic events of REM sleep, such as, defecation, urination, loud screaming, etc.

METHOD OF INVESTIGATION

Recruitment of Subjects

Near-Miss SIDS

The term "near-miss SIDS" is now often replaced by "infant with life-threatening event."[5] Independently of the terminology employed, we can distinguish these infants as a group who were considered to be "healthy" but presented an abrupt event very frightening for their caretakers. The infants may have appeared blue, pale, limp, or stiff. Vigorous stimulation, mouth-to-mouth breathing, or cardiopulmonary resuscitation may have been used to revive them. These infants, after hospitalization and pediatric work-up, had no specific diagnosis and were sent to our unit for a 24-hr polygraphic monitoring during wake and sleep. All infants reviewed here were full-term, and their unexplained event occurred between 3 weeks and 6.5 months of age. Most, but not all, were placed on a home monitor. One percent of the infants we examined subsequently died abruptly, and, after autopsy, the term "SIDS" appeared on their death certificates. Five of these 6 infants died before, and one after, near-systematic use of the home monitor. In the latter case it is unclear whether the monitor was in use at the time of death. One death occurred in a child who had had repetitive "life threatening events." During a rehospitalization, a respiratory arrest, which occurred despite care by highly trained medical personnel, had left this child severely brain-damaged due to anoxic lesions. Within six weeks, the child suffered another respiratory arrest, which was fatal.

Siblings of SIDS Victims

Fifty-one full-term siblings of SIDS victims were examined; nearly all were between 15 days and 4 weeks of age. These examinations were on an elective basis; the siblings were in no distress and had no reported health problems. A small subset of 5 highly selected siblings of SIDS victims, who snored at night between the ages of 6 and 18 months and developed symptoms of obstructive sleep apnea syndrome (OSAS),[6] were subjects of a special research protocol. None of the siblings reported here died during the first 2 years of life, the duration of our follow-up.

Recording Techniques

During the 24-hr study, mothers were allowed to sleep in the research area and to remain for the entire procedure. They participated in the infants' routine care. Monitoring lasted for 24 hr, except for some 4.5 and 6-month-old infants who were monitored for only 12 nocturnal hours. Variables monitored during the 24 hr included recordings of electroencephalogram (C_3/A_2-C_4/A_1), electro-oculogram, digastric electromyogram, and electrocardiogram from one lead (V2). Respiration was measured using several devices: abdominal and thoracic strain gauges initially and non-calibrated respiratory inductive plethysmography in later years. Nasal and oral thermistors, measurements of the percentage of CO_2 in the expired gases, monitored through a nasal or oral catheter (Beckman LB2 CO_2 analyzer), and oxygen saturation measured using an ear oximeter (Waters Instrument Co.) were also used initially. When they became available, transcutaneous oxygen and carbon dioxide electrodes (Kentron Co.) were added to the protocol. Finally, a 24-hr Holter electrocardiogram concurrent with the polygraphic study was recorded in 62 near-miss-SIDS infants and 26 age-matched controls. Behavioral observations were also made during the recordings.

Data Analysis

States of alertness, i.e., wake, REM sleep, and NREM sleep, were scored in 30-sec epochs. For infants at 3 and 6 weeks of age, we used criteria outlined in *A Manual of Standardized Terminology, Techniques and Criteria for the Scoring of States of Sleep and Wakefulness in Newborn Infants*.[7] For infants of 3 months of age or over, sleep was scored using criteria previously outlined and derived from the adult scoring criteria.[8] Over the past 2 years, we have also used a technique based on activity level that can indicate sleep states.[9]

Respiratory events were classified by types: central, mixed, and obstructive or periodic breathing, as previously defined.[10] Respiratory events were also tabulated by duration, i.e., 3 to 6 sec, 6 to 10 sec, 10 to 15 sec, and longer than 15 sec. The amount of oxygen desaturation, expressed as the percentage of oxygen saturation (ear oximetry) or in mm Hg (for the transcutaneous electrodes), was noted. The amount and type of significant cardiac arrhythmias were tabulated. When a 24-hr Holter ECG was obtained, we correlated the polygraphic recording based on the machine clock and the continuous ECG recording with the Holter ECG. Data were entered into a DEC PDP-11 computer for analysis after sleep states had been hand-scored. The 24-hr Holter ECG was also analyzed using a computer program developed by the Stanford Division of Cardiology, which provides standard arrhythmia evaluation and determines the R–R interval. The R–R intervals are graphically displayed in msec as a function of time, with an increase in heart rate shown as a decrease in R–R interval and a decrease in heart rate as an increase in R–R interval.[11,12]

RESULTS

Cardiorespiratory Findings During Sleep

SIDS Victims

None of the polygraphic recordings of the near-miss-SIDS infants who later died of what was designated as SIDS presented (a) cardiac abnormalities, including long Q–T syndrome, or (b) respiratory "pathology," either as defined by the American Academy of Pediatrics[13] (i.e., none had an apnea longer than 20 sec) or as defined by our own polygraphic study of control infants during sleep (i.e., none had a central apnea longer than 15 sec during sleep). However, the recordings of these infants who later died were not "normal" compared with those from our study of normal controls.[10] Based upon the 24-hr polygraphy done in our laboratory—a similar setting to that used in the study described in this paper—using similar equipment, we calculated "normative data" extracted from our control infant population, with limits of ±2 standard deviations (SD) from mean results.[10] The variables considered were "respiratory pauses" lasting > 3 sec, which were classed as central, mixed, or obstructive, according to established definition. We also considered drops in oxygen tension, the importance of bradycardia, or the presence/absence of marked sinus arrhythmia. When the infants who subsequently became SIDS victims were monitored after their first "near-miss event," we found the following abnormalities:

1. An increase of greater than 2 SD over control values in the number of mixed and obstructive respiratory events lasting between 3 and 10 sec during sleep (observed in 4 infants)
2. The following combination: an increase of greater than 2 SD over control values in the number of total respiratory events which lasted between 3 and 10 sec during sleep and which occurred in association with a respiratory obstructive pause with a duration of 10 sec, a 20-torr decrease in oxygen tension (transcutaneous Po_2), and a progressive bradycardia with at least one R–R interval at the end of apnea indicating a heart rate of 39 per minute (observed in 1 infant)
3. The combination of an increase of greater than 2 SD over control values in the number of total respiratory events lasting between 3 and 10 sec during sleep together with an esophageal pH which was below 4 during a total of 6% of the 24-hr monitoring (observed in 1 infant). (We have not collected a sufficient amount of normative data on esophageal pH to use our own criteria; we have used those in the literature, considering esophageal reflux "normal" if it occurred for up to 5% of the 24-hr recording time.[14])

Near-Miss-SIDS Infants

All the findings presented below were obtained on "near-miss" infants who are presently alive. Infants have had regular follow-ups for from 4 (in the case of those most recently observed) to 16 months.

Investigation of the Long Q–T Syndrome. A systematic study of Q–T interval from polygraphic recordings was done for 100 near-miss-SIDS infants. Some of these infants were examined independently by Dr. Maron (National Institutes of Health) as part of a larger investigation of the role of elongated Q–T in SIDS. None was identified as having abnormally long Q–T interval.

Identified Cardiac Arrhythmias. Following the analyses, we subdivided the significant identifiable arrhythmias seen in the 24-hr polygraphic monitoring into 5 groups, each based on one of the following characteristics:

1. Bradycardia below 45 beats per min sustained for 5 sec (noted in full-term infants 3 to 12 weeks old)
2. Bradycardia below 40 beats per min sustained for 5 sec (noted in full-term infants 14 to 18 weeks old)
3. Isolated episodes of second-degree atrioventricular conduction block:
    a. Mobitz type I
    b. Mobitz type II
4. Sinus arrest longer than 2 sec
5. Other arrhythmias.

Out of 594 near-miss-SIDS infants—

a. 22 (3 to 17 weeks old) had at least one bradycardic episode below 45 beats per min;
b. 3 (14 to 18 weeks old) had bradycardias below 40 beats per min;
c. 1 (9 weeks old) had a second-degree atrioventricular induction block identified as Mobitz type I;
d. 11 (3 to 8 weeks old) had at least one sinus arrest of a duration between 2 and 5 sec;
e. 1 (5.5 months old) had several sinus arrests of a duration between 7 and 30 sec (mostly during wake);
f. 3 (4, 6, and 9 weeks old) had bradycardia with a shift from a sinusal to a nodal rhythm, a progressive broadening of the QRS complex, and the appearance of negative T waves for 4, 5 and 6 beats, respectively.

None of the control infants had any of the above arrhythmias during their 24-hr monitoring.

Relationship between Observed Arrhythmias in Near-Miss SIDS and Respiratory Variables

With one notable exception, nearly all the reported variables occurred in conjunction with abnormal breathing events during NREM sleep. Significant bradycardia, second-degree atrioventricular conduction block, and a switch to nodal rhythm with development of negative T wave were all seen during mixed and obstructive respiratory events leading to oxygen desaturation. Significant bradycardia was never seen at the beginning of the apnea but always occurred several seconds into the event and while the infant was struggling against a closed airway (Muller maneuver).

Sinus Arrest

The most common cardiac arrhythmia seen in our population was sinus arrest, and the reported population could clearly be subdivided into 2 groups. In the 11 infants of subgroup A, the sinus arrest was clearly secondary to a respiratory event, while in infant B it was not.

Subgroup A

One infant had a 2-sec sinus arrest and a central apnea concurrently. All other infants had clearly identified, mixed and obstructive apneas before the sinus arrest, which occurred before any of the infants had a bradycardia below 45 beats per min for 5 sec. However, 9 of the 11 infants had repetitive apneic events associated with bradycardia within 5 min of the sinus arrest. Six of the 11 infants had several sinus arrests associated with apnea during the 24-hr polygraphic recording. When several sinus arrests occurred, they were clustered within a period of 30 min, always during NREM sleep.

oxygen tension

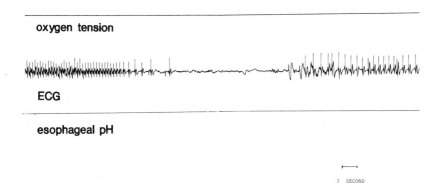

ECG

esophageal pH

1 SECOND

FIGURE 1. Polygraphic monitoring during quiet sleep (**center trace**). Presence of an isolated 7-sec sinus arrest unassociated with apnea in a 5.5-month-old, full-term male infant presenting unexplained color changes and occasional limpness. Note that oxygen tension (**top trace**) and esophageal pH (**bottom trace**) remain constant at normal values.

Infant B

For several weeks, this infant had been noted to become blue and limp while in his mother's arms. An occasional jerking, or an upward gaze with associated limpness, suggested a seizure disorder. Several clinical EEGs, a 12-lead ECG, and a pediatric work-up had revealed no abnormality. The possibility of an "apnea of infancy" problem was raised. An initial 24-hr polygraphic monitoring was done at 5.5 months of age. During placement of the esophageal pH probe, after the infant was attached to the cardiac monitor but before hard-copy recording was begun, a cardiac arrest of several seconds was noted on the scope of the monitor. During the following polygraphic recording, a 7-sec sinus arrest was recorded during quiet sleep, despite normal oxygen tension, normal breathing and normal esophageal pH (see FIGURE 1). Successive polygraphic monitoring and a 24-hr Holter ECG were obtained. Forty-eight hours after the initial recording, while the screaming and voiding infant was again being readied for cardiorespiratory monitoring, the cardiac monitor signaled an arrest for a period of 15 sec, as evaluated on the scope, which resulted in the infant's becoming blue and limp. There was no hard copy recorded for this event. The subsequent polygraphic monitoring revealed only a 3-sec sinus arrest during sleep, once again not secondary to any abnormal respiratory event. Follow-up monitorings with continuous Holter ECGs demonstrated the presence of several sinus arrests of duration between 20 and 30 sec (see FIGURE 2). All long arrests were associated with screaming at full voice; one was clearly associated with voiding (and perhaps bowel movement).

Negative Findings

As often emphasized, ventricular arrhythmia is, most commonly, considered the number-one candidate for "lethal arrhythmia" (despite the fact that a 30-sec sinus arrest could most probably be considered a significant risk factor in an infant). Despite drops in oxygen tension to a level of 25–30 torr in certain infants, with a combination of hypoventilation due to closely clustered repetitive apneas and a mixed or obstructive apnea occurring in an infant with an oxygen share already significantly depleted, ventricular arrhythmia was never observed in our population.

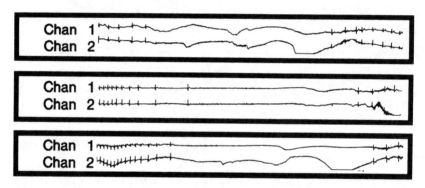

FIGURE 2. Long asystoles in a 5.5-month-old infant. Holter ECG recordings in the same infant as in FIGURE 1. The 30-sec segments from the 24-hr ambulatory ECG recordings were obtained when the infant was awake, crying and voiding (**top segment**), or when crying (**middle** and **lower segments**). The sinus arrest without rhythm escape can be noted. (Holter ECG tracings courtesy of Paul Pitlick, M.D., Pediatric Cardiology, Stanford University Medical Center.)

Comparative Study of Heart Rate and Body Movements during Sleep

In 1984 we reported[15] a comparative study of 6 near-miss-SIDS infants and 6 age-matched controls. Each infant had polygraphic monitoring as well as Holter ECG that was analyzed by computer. Systematic R–R evaluation indicated that during quiet sleep, without respiratory irregularities, near-miss-SIDS infants had (a) a faster heart rate than controls, (b) a decreased variability in heart rate compared with age-matched controls, and (c) a decrease in "movement time" compared with the controls during the same period of analysis.

COMMENTS

Heart-Rate Variability and Near-Miss SIDS

Leistner and colleagues[16] have already reported on an increase in heart rate in near-miss SIDS. Harper and colleagues[17] also noted this phenomenon in near-miss SIDS and in siblings of SIDS victims, particularly during quiet (NREM) sleep. Why heart rate increases in not clear. Harper *et al.*[17] attribute it to a decrease in vagal activity. Leistner and colleagues [16] disagree and support the hypothesis that an increase in sympathetic activity is responsible for the changes. Our data, obtained on only 6 near-miss-SIDS infants and 6 controls, confirm the phenomenon but do not shed much new light on the mechanisms involved. However, it must be emphasized that we observed in our population a decrease not only in heart-rate variability but also in body movements during NREM sleep. Of course, these observations constitute an "association," and the two elements may not be related. But heart-rate variability during sleep is linked to several factors. Mazza and colleagues[18] have shown that there is a direct relationship between heart rate and beat-to-beat variability in sleeping infants. Variability decreases with faster heart rates. Harper and colleagues[17] indicated that, during NREM sleep, there is very little heart-rate variability not related to respiration. Several groups also emphasized that a decrease in cardiac-rate variation is present in infants with respiratory distress syndrome (RDS)[19,20] and in infants with prenatal anoxia.[21] It is interesting to note that in these infants, as in near-miss SIDS, hypotonia of shoulders and trunk occurs.[22] There is no doubt that small body-movements will increase heart-rate variability. It has been hypothesized[23,24] that the decrease in small body-movements noted in near-miss-SIDS populations larger than the one reported here reflects a decrease in arousal response during sleep that seems to occur in near-miss-SIDS infants.[25,26] We hypothesize that the decrease in heart-rate variability (noted in infants who also present a decrease in small body-movements) is also related to this decrease in arousal response through a decrease in small body-movements during sleep and perhaps through other mechanisms that impinge on the ANS.

Cardiac Arrhythmias and Sleep in Our Infant and Young Adult Population

As indicated, most of the significant cardiac arrhythmias seen during sleep were secondary to apneas and hypoventilation. Of the respiratory-related cardiac arrhythmias, only one was secondary to central apnea; all the others were secondary to mixed and obstructive events and were seen during the Muller maneuver done during obstructive sleep apnea (OSA). The cardiac rhythm changes seen in our study were very similar to those reported in children and adults with OSA.[27] In a review of the literature on cardiac arrhythmia associated with OSA, Shepard[28] concluded that, with the exception of premature ventricular complexes (PVCs), sinus arrest and marked sinus bradycardia (<30 beats per min) were the predominant significant cardiac arrhythmia reported in adults, while ventricular tachycardia was seen in only 3% of the populations studied. The ventricular ectopies were shown to increase significantly in adults when drops in oxygen saturation associated with OSA were below 65 to 60%. Hemodynamic study has not been done on infants or children presenting with OSA, but it has been widely performed in adults; significant changes in systemic-, pulmonary arterial-, and pulmonary wedge-pressures can be monitored. The changes are due to multifactorial elements: hypoxia, the secondary effect of the Muller maneuver with increasing left ventricle transmural pressure, changes in cardiac output and stroke volume, and changes in venous return. Similar changes probably occur during OSA in infants.

We have also reported that young adults may present during REM sleep significant sinus arrest not associated with respiratory events.[29] Since publication of our article, we have had an additional 2 adults and 2 children referred to us with similar findings. Infant B, previously mentioned, is moderately different, inasmuch as his long sinus arrests were prominent during wake in association with very specific behaviors. In our children and adults, we hypothesized that a parasympathetic tone dysfunction existed, leading to the periods of profound asystole unassociated with any form of escape rhythm. Undoubtedly such asystole can lead to syncope and could probably be responsible for abrupt, unexplained death. In our young adults, extensive invasive electrophysiological studies and right heart catheterizations (not performed on infant B) indicated an anatomically and physiologically normal cardiovascular system.

In summary, we have described infants who presented significant sinus arrest during wake and sleep. These sinus arrests, in our view, could have led to abrupt, unexplained death. Their causes were different and, in all cases, were ignored during the early weeks of life. In most cases, the infants who presented these events outgrew their problem by the end of their first year.

REFERENCES

1. JAMES, T. N. 1985. Crib death: Editorial comment. J. Am. Coll. Cardiol. **5:** 1185–1187.
2. KELLY, D. H. & D. C. SHANNON. 1982. Sudden infant death syndrome and near miss sudden infant death syndrome: A review of the literature 1964 to 1982. Pediatr. Clin. North Am. **29:** 1241–1261.
3. BECKWITH, J. B. 1983. Chronic hypoxemia in the sudden infant death syndrome: A critical review of the data base. *In* Sudden Infant Death Syndrome. J. T. Tildon, L. M. Roeder & A. Steinschneider, Eds.: 145–160. Academic Press. New York.
4. OREM, J. & J. BARNES, Eds. 1981. Physiology in Sleep. Academic Press. New York.
5. FISHER, B. 1985. Crib death: The unsolved mystery of SIDS. Pul. Med. Technol. **2:** 36.
6. GUILLEMINAULT, C., G. HELDT, N. POWELL & R. RILEY. 1986. Small upper airway in near miss SIDS infants and their families. Lancet **i:** 402–407.
7. ANDERS, T., R. EMDE & A. PARMELEE, Eds. 1971. A Manual of Standardized Terminology, Techniques and Criteria for the Scoring of States of Sleep and Wakefulness in Newborn Infants. Brain Research Institute, Univ. of California, Los Angeles. Los Angeles, CA.
8. GUILLEMINAULT, C. & M. BOUQUET. 1979. Sleep states and related pathology. *In* Advances in Perinatal Neurology. R. Korobkin & C. Guilleminault, Eds.: 225–247. Spectrum Publications. New York.
9. KAYED, K., P. E. HESLA & D. ROSJO. 1979. The acticulographic monitor of sleep. Sleep **2:** 253–260.
10. GUILLEMINAULT, C., R. ARIAGNO, R. KOROBKIN, L. NAGEL, R. BALDWIN, S. COONS & M. OWEN. 1979. Mixed and obstructive sleep apnea and near miss for SIDS: 2. "Near miss" and normal control infants: comparison over age. Pediatrics **64:** 882–891.
11. FITZGERALD, J. W., R. R. CLAPPIER & D. C. HARRISON. 1974. Small computer processing of ambulatory electrocardiogram computers in cardiology. *In* IEEE Biomedical Proceedings, Vol. 3. Institute of Electrical and Electronic Engineers, Inc. Bethesda, MD.
12. LOPES, M. G., J. W. FITZGERALD, D. C. HARRISON & J. S. SCHROEDER. 1975. Diagnosis and quantification of arrhythmias using an improved R–R plotting system. Am. J. Cardiol. **35:** 816–823.
13. AMERICAN ACADEMY OF PEDIATRICS. TASK FORCE ON PROLONGED APNEA. 1978. Prolonged apnea. Pediatrics **61:** 651–652.
14. BOIX-OCHOA, J., J. M. LAFUENTE & J. M. GIL-VERNET. 1980. Twenty-four hour esophageal pH monitoring in gastro-esophageal reflux. J. Pediatr. Surg. **15:** 74–78.
15. GUILLEMINAULT, C., S. COONS & R. WINKLE. Cardiac abnormalities during sleep and near miss SIDS infants. *In* Sudden Infant Death Syndrome: Risk Factors and Basic Mechanisms. R. M. Harper & H. J. Hoffman, Eds. Pergamon. New York. In press.
16. LEISTNER, H. L., G. G. HADDAD, R. A. EPSTEIN, T. L. LAI, M. A. F. EPSTEIN & R. B. MELLINS. 1980. Heart rate and heart rate variability during sleep in aborted sudden infant death syndrome. J. Pediatr. **97:** 51–55.
17. HARPER, R. M., B. LEAKE, T. HOPPENBROUWERS, M. B. STERMAN, D. J. McGINTY & J. HODGMAN. 1978. Polygraphic studies of normal infants and infants at risk for the sudden infant death syndrome: Heart rate and variability as a function of state. Pediatr. Res. **12:** 778–785.

18. MAZZA, N. M., M. A. F. EPSTEIN, G. G. HADDAD, H. S. LAW, R. B. MELLINS & R. A. EPSTEIN. 1980. Relation of beat-to-beat variability to heart rate in normal sleeping infants. Pediatr. Res. **14:** 232–235.

19. KERO, P. 1974. Heart rate variation in infants with the respiratory distress syndrome. Acta Paediatr. Scand. Suppl. **250:** 1–70.

20. RUDOLPH, A. J., C. VALLBONA & M. M. DESMOND. 1965. Cardiodynamic studies in the newborn. III. Heart rate patterns in infants with idiopathic respiratory distress syndrome. Pediatrics **35:** 551–559.

21. MIYAZAKI, S., K. WATANABE & K. HARA. Heart rate variability in full-term normal and abnormal newborn infants during sleep. Brain Dev. **1:** 57–60.

22. KOROBKIN, R. & C. GUILLEMINAULT. 1979. Neurologic abnormalities in near miss for sudden infant death syndrome infants. Pediatrics **64:** 369–384.

23. COONS, S. & C. GUILLEMINAULT. 1982. Ontogeny of sleep in near miss sudden infant death syndrome (abstract). Sleep Res. **11:** 82.

24. HOPPENBROUWERS, T., D. JENSEN, J. HODGMAN, R. M. HARPER & M. STERMAN. 1982. Body movements during quiet sleep in subsequent siblings of SIDS. Clin. Res. **30:** 136a.

25. GUILLEMINAULT, C., R. ARIAGNO, R. KOROBKIN, S. COONS, M. OWEN-BOEDDIKER & R. BALDWIN. 1981. Sleep parameters and respiratory variables in "near miss SIDS" infants. Pediatrics **68:** 354–360.

26. MCCULLOCH, K., R. T. BROUILLETTE, A. J. GUZZETTA & C. E. HUNT. 1982. Arousal responses in near miss SIDS and normal infants. J. Pediatr. **101:** 911–917.

27. GUILLEMINAULT, C. 1984. Diagnosis, pathogenesis and treatment of the sleep apnea syndromes. Ergeb. Inn. Med. Kinderheilkd. [Rev. Intern. Med. Pediatr.] **52:** 1–57.

28. SHEPARD, J. W. 1985. Gas exchange and hemodynamics during sleep. Med. Clin. North Am. **69:** 1243–1264.

29. GUILLEMINAULT, C., P. POOL, J. MOTTA & A. GILLIS. 1984. Sinus arrest during REM sleep in young adults. N. Engl. J. Med. **311:** 1006–1010.

Cardiorespiratory Control during Sleep[a]

R. M. HARPER,[b] R. C. FRYSINGER, J. D. MARKS,
J. X. ZHANG, AND R. B. TRELEASE

Department of Anatomy and the Brain Research Institute
University of California, Los Angeles
Los Angeles, California 90024-1763

Any attempt to determine the mechanisms of failure in the sudden infant death syndrome (SIDS) should consider the role of functional circumstances that appear to accompany fatal episodes. An association of SIDS events with sleep states appears to be one such major circumstance, although that association may be only an approximate, temporal one, with the fatal event occurring during waking following a sleep episode. Knowledge of the association of sleep states with SIDS should direct our attention to those brain mechanisms that are modified by sleep state and might affect respiratory and cardiac control mechanisms. Moreover, even the name of the syndrome indicates that SIDS occurs suddenly; the circumstances of death normally do not include prolonged respiratory failure or signs indicative of life-threatening, prolonged cardiac failure. Thus, one would expect that a cataclysmic event, or a very unique combination of events, perhaps compounded by long-standing conditions, would be associated with death. The combination of circumstances of sleep state and sudden failure would suggest disturbance of central integration mechanisms.

Structures within the brain are affected differently by sleep and waking states, and some of these areas of the brain have profound effects on cardiac and respiratory patterning. The pontine brainstem, for example, gives rise to large phasic EEG spikes during rapid eye movement (REM) sleep that are coincident in time with large changes in motor membrane potentials, phasic movements of the extremity involved, and alterations in tone of the diaphragm.[1,2,3,4] These pontine structures appear to alter reflex and motor patterning during REM sleep in such a fashion as to dissociate influences from more rostral brain areas and to exert, compared to the standards of control patterns during waking, unusual, all-encompassing modulation of motor reflex activity. The dissociative effects are great enough to abolish or greatly reduce large blood pressure rises elicited by electrical stimulation of the central nucleus of the amygdala[5] or respiratory-cycle timing elicited by electrical stimulation of the orbital frontal cortex.[6]

Forebrain structures underlie a synchronization of brain electrical activity during quiet sleep that provides the potential for interaction between brain structures but elicits a burst-pause mode of neuronal discharge in motor areas which accompanies considerable regularity in respiratory and cardiac motor control. Quiet sleep can greatly diminish both the excitatory properties of single-pulse stimulation to forebrain areas[7] and the phasic discharge relationships of neurons to the respiratory cycle.[8] However, the very large dissociative effects observed during REM sleep are not apparent in this state. Thus, in

[a]This work was supported by Grant HL-22418 from the National Heart, Lung, and Blood Institute and Grant HD-22695 from the National Institute of Child Health and Human Development, National Institutes of Health.
[b]Author to whom correspondence should be sent.

considering the potential roles that various brain structures might play in disturbance of breathing or cardiac patterning, we must examine the effects of sleep state on these brain structures.

A number of systems that exert descending influences, both voluntary and involuntary, project from suprapontine sites and interact with brainstem regions regulating cardiac and respiratory patterning. These systems may be susceptible to dysfunction, and the susceptibility to dysfunction may itself be a function of sleep state.

A portion of the involuntary descending influence is that of diencephalic temperature-regulating structures. Perturbation of temperature-regulating areas in the anterior hypothalamus will elicit appropriate respiratory responses to such manipulations; however, that pattern of response is lost during REM sleep.[9] REM sleep thus abolishes a major protective mechanism, the ability to dissipate core temperature appropriately. This dissociation of temperature control during REM sleep may have major implications for infant survival if core temperature is elevated by some mechanism such as infection, swaddling, or sustained peripheral constriction from abnormal sympathetic discharge, such as might occur during seizure discharge. SIDS victims often show elevated core temperature after death,[10] and an inability to dissipate heat might be suspected.

The activity of particular brain structures may be subject to disturbances in function. One such disturbance is the occurrence of focal seizures of temporal lobe origin. These dysfunctions are of particular interest because the signs of seizure discharge may not be apparent from scalp EEG recordings, and motor signs suggestive of cortical and voluntary motor involvement might be minimal. However, structures in the temporal lobe region have exceptional potential to modify cardiac and respiratory patterning (FIG. 1).

It is the objective of this manuscript to demonstrate that suprapontine structures, particularly structures mediating affective aspects of behavior, exert profound influences on cardiac and respiratory patterning and that disturbances in these forebrain structures may elicit patterns of activity that are disruptive to normal function. Further, it is an objective to demonstrate that the close integration of cardiac and respiratory patterning results in aberrant control of one system if the other is disturbed and that sleep states can accentuate this aberrant control.

Suprapontine influences that normally affect cardiorespiratory interactions include voluntary motor control mechanisms. Interruption of voluntary motor pathways by stroke or other forms of lesion results in a failure to breath on command. This syndrome should be distinguished, of course, from the "Ondine's Curse" syndrome described by Severinghaus and Mitchell,[11] which is a loss of automatic respiratory patterning, particularly during sleep. The effects of voluntary motor pathway lesions would be immediately apparent by loss of other voluntary motor activity; whereas seizure discharge in voluntary motor pathways would be accompanied by severe motor involvement. Except for occasional reports of hypotonia and overall diminished movement in SIDS siblings,[12] there is little evidence that infants at risk for SIDS exhibit disturbed motor patterns. There is also little evidence of generalized motor seizure discharge, although the presence of seizure activity in infants can lead to prolonged apnea,[13] and the presence of seizures in infants manifesting apnea leads to a poorer prognosis.[14,15] Thus, although infants at risk might show signs of seizure discharge, it is unlikely that SIDS victims have, as a primary disorder, a disturbance in the descending *voluntary* motor system.

Patients with loss of voluntary control of breathing, however, can respond with appropriate diaphragmatic movements to affective stimuli, e.g., they can make appropriate diaphragmatic movements in laughter (Younes, personal communication). The maintenance of respiratory function to such affective input in the presence of voluntary motor lesions suggests that alternative descending "drives" to respiration exist and that these "drives" can incorporate higher, i.e., cortical, input (e.g., the sense of emotional appreciation). The mechanisms for controlling respiratory musculature during such

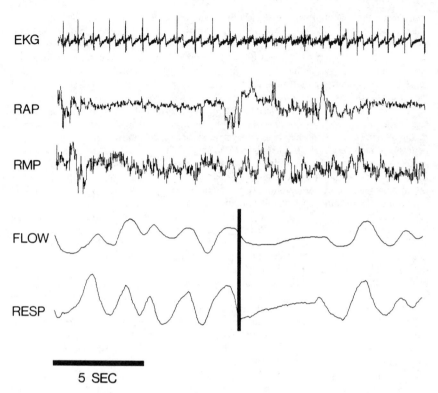

FIGURE 1. The powerful influence of excitation of a limbic forebrain area on respiratory patterning. A single paired-pulse electrical stimulation (**vertical bar**), delivered to the right anterior pes (RAP) of a patient undergoing depth electrode monitoring for localization of temporal lobe seizure discharge, results in a central apnea. Tracings (*top* to *bottom*): EKG, electrocardiogram; RAP, right anterior pes EEG; RMP, right mid-pes EEG; FLOW, nasal airflow; RESP, thoracic movements.

affective behavior involve suprapontine and probably cortical areas for integration of the response, and the descending influence must be exerted by projections other than those of the voluntary pathways. It now appears that particular "affective" regions of the temporal lobe can incorporate cortical responses and project massively to brainstem cardiorespiratory areas.

One limbic forebrain area that projects heavily to the parabrachial pons and to the nucleus of the solitary tract is the central nucleus of the amygdala (ACE, FIG. 2). This structure, which receives afferent activity from a wide range of cortical and subcortical areas, appears to mediate autonomic and respiratory components of aversive conditioning. The ACE projects to the parabrachial area of the pons (which includes the nucleus parabrachialis medialis and Kolliker-Fuse nuclei) and to the periaqueductal gray area, as well as to the nucleus of the solitary tract.[16,17] The parabrachial pons may be involved in mediating sleep state-related respiratory timing differences, since evidence from studies employing stimulation, recording, or lesions[18-21] suggests involvement of this pontine area in the central nervous system's control of respiratory phase switching. The periaqueductal gray area, which apparently mediates a portion of the cardiovascular response to a defense reaction,[22] has projections to laryngeal motor neurons in the cat and rabbit[23] and to the ventrolateral portion of the nucleus of the solitary tract, which is a prominent medullary respiratory area. Thus, both the parabrachial pons and the periaqueductal gray area, which receive heavy projections from the ACE, appear to be strategically located to mediate aspects of cardiovascular control, as well as aspects of respiratory musculature functioning. At least part of this respiratory muscle functioning is related to upper airway activity. The ACE receives cortical inputs by way of cortical projections to neighboring amygdaloid nuclei, i.e., lateral, basal, and basal accessory nuclei,[17] and, in the rabbit, receives direct projections from the insular cortex.[24] Thus, anatomical evidence suggests that the ACE has the potential for integrating aspects of cortical input to brainstem areas mediating respiratory and autonomic control patterning.

The evidence that the ACE can affect both cardiovascular and respiratory patterning is considerable. Single-pulse electrical stimulation of the ACE at a rate slightly higher than the respiratory rate will result in entrainment of the respiratory cycle, an effect that is abolished when the subject enters quiet sleep.[7] Train electrical stimulation of the ACE results in apneusis and a dramatic rise in blood pressure;[5] the blood pressure response is

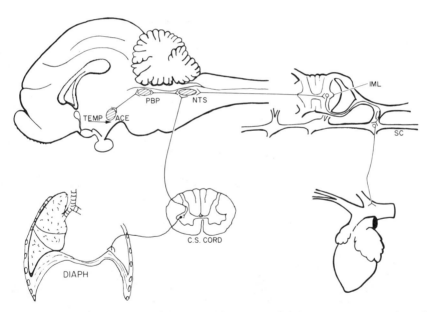

FIGURE 2. Schematic diagram of some brain structures involved in integrating cardiovascular and respiratory control. The central nucleus of the amygdala (ACE), which receives cortical input as well as input from subcortical regions, projects heavily to the parabrachial pontine nucleus (PBP) and to the nucleus of the solitary tract (NTS). The NTS in turn projects to sympathetic preganglionic neurons of the intermediolateral column (IML) of the spinal cord, which then modulates postganglionic fibers in the sympathetic chain (SC). These neurons can directly affect the heart and constrict the vasculature. The NTS can also alter diaphragmatic activity (DIAPH) through cervical spinal cord (C.S. CORD) projections. For clarity, projections from the ACE to the periaqueductal gray area are not shown; the periaqueductal gray area projects to upper airway motor neurons in addition to a number of cardiovascular-related structures. Diencephalic structures also integrate descending temperature control influences (TEMP).

nearly abolished during REM sleep. Pharmacological,[25] electrolytic,[26] and cold blockade[27] studies of the ACE suggest that this structure mediates major, but specific, components of aversive aspects of affective conditioning. Cold blockade, for example, results in abolition of a conditioned blood-pressure and respiratory-rate response, but not an aversively conditioned heart-rate response.[27] The projections of the ACE to the periaqueductal gray area are also of interest, since the excitatory pharmacological stimulation of the periaqueductal gray area results in an extreme defense reaction.[22]

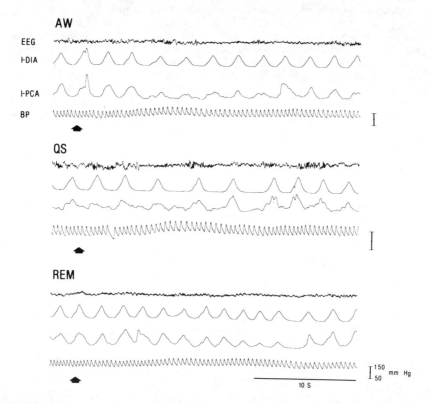

FIGURE 3. Integrated diaphragmatic (I-DIA) and posterior cricoarytenoid (I-PCA) EMG (electromyographic) responses to transient hypertension elicited by phenylephrine infusion (**arrows**) in one cat during sleep and waking states. Note the initial respiratory slowing in waking (AW **upper panel**) and quiet sleep (QS **middle panel**), the delayed slowing in REM sleep (**lower panel**), and the relatively greater diminished amplitude of laryngeal motor activity in response to transient hypertension. BP, blood pressure (mm Hg). Tracings in each panel, from *top* to *bottom*, respectively: EEG, I-DIA, I-PCA, and BP. (Reprinted from Marks and Harper[32] with permission from *Experimental Neurology*.)

A prominent aspect of a number of amygdaloid structures is an extraordinary sensitivity to seizure discharge. Seizures can be "kindled" (i.e., repetitive exposure to short bursts of train electrical stimulation results in a lowered threshold for convulsive seizures[28]) very much more easily in amygdaloid (and hippocampal) structures than in other brain areas. There is the potential for focal seizure discharge to elicit pronounced cardiovascular or respiratory consequences.[29,30] Seizure discharge in deep temporal lobe structures, such as in the structures of the ACE, may not be observable on surface EEG recordings; focal discharge often is observable only with indwelling electrodes or strategically placed sphenoidal electrodes.

Extreme activation of either the respiratory motor system or the parasympathetic or sympathetic motor system, such as might be attained during seizure discharge, results in a marked effect on one system by the other. A rapid elevation of arterial pressure, for example, results in an inhibition of diaphragmatic activity, an effect that is enhanced during sleep.[31] Although this effect is marked in the diaphragm, the blood-pressure effect is even more pronounced on a laryngeal dilator, the posterior cricoarytenoid[32] (FIG. 3), and leads to a phase dissociation of diaphragmatic and laryngeal activity as well. A very rapid rise in arterial pressure following, for example, an obstructive apnea or seizure discharge in limbic structures might result in an induction of apnea or a prolongation of an obstructive apnea. Respiratory patterning in turn can gate vagal efferent flow to the heart and can gate the occurrence of pressor-induced arrhythmias.[33]

If SIDS results from seizure discharge in brain areas that mediate affective responses, several predictions might be made. One would expect that seizures, and thus respiratory- or cardiac-related failures, would occur during sleep, since sleep enhances epileptic discharge. The instances of failure would be sudden, and they might be silent. Signs of sustained apneusis in SIDS victims, resulting from hyperactivation of this limbic arousal site, might also occur. Upper airway petechiae might be present as a result of extended inspiration against an excessive seizure-induced laryngeal muscle activation, and edema might be present. Conditions exacerbating the potential for seizure discharge, such as sleep deprivation, might precede a fatal event. One might also find relatively elevated core temperatures after death. Many of these characteristics, of course, are descriptive of the signs associated with circumstances surrounding SIDS.[10,34,35]

One might expect to find gradations in response to excitation of these affective areas and instances in which nonfatal episodes occur after the peak incidence of risk. Indeed, infantile breathholding episodes, elicited by extreme emotional responses, are a well-known entity, although the mechanism of action or treatment is not known (Thach, personal communication).

An unexplained aspect of this suggested effect of seizure discharge is the relationship of temporal lobe seizure activity to the "window of risk" for SIDS. It may be that the age period of 2–4 months is a time of particular risk for the development of complex partial epilepsy or that suprapontine mechanisms essential for the suppression of temporal lobe seizures have not yet matured in the infants.

This suggestion of seizure-elicited dysfunction of affective brain areas is highly speculative and may bear no relationship to the question of mechanisms underlying SIDS. However, one objective of this proposal is to demonstrate that, in addition to conventional "voluntary" motor control over respiratory patterning, these limbic forebrain structures have powerful descending influences on cardiovascular and respiratory brainstem areas. Moreover, areas within these suprapontine areas are relatively seizure-prone and have activities that are heavily mediated by sleep state. These structures undoubtedly play a major role in normal regulation of cardiac and respiratory control and may also make a substantial contribution to disturbances in such control.

REFERENCES

1. CHASE, M. H. 1983. Synaptic mechanisms and circuitry involved in motoneuron control during sleep. Int. Rev. Neurobiol. **24:** 213–258.
2. CHASE, M. H., S. ENOMOTO, T. MURAKAMI, Y. NAKAMURA & M. TAIRA. 1981. Intracellular

potential of medullary reticular neurons during sleep and wakefulness. Exp. Neurol. **71:** 226–233.

3. OREM, J. 1980. Neuronal mechanisms of respiration in REM sleep. Sleep **3:** 251–267.

4. SIECK, G. C., R. B. TRELEASE & R. M. HARPER. 1984. Sleep influences on diaphragmatic motor unit discharge. Exp. Neurol. **85:** 316–335.

5. FRYSINGER, R. C., J. D. MARKS, R. B. TRELEASE, V. L. SCHECHTMAN & R. M. HARPER. 1984. Sleep states attenuate the pressor response to central amygdala stimulation. Exp. Neurol. **83:** 604–617.

6. MARKS, J. D., R. C. FRYSINGER & R. M. HARPER. 1987. State-dependent respiratory depression elicited by stimulation of the orbital frontal cortex. Exp. Neurol. **95:** 714–729.

7. HARPER, R. M., R. C. FRYSINGER, R. B. TRELEASE & J. D. MARKS. 1984. State-dependent alteration of respiratory cycle timing by stimulation of the central nucleus of the amygdala. Brain Res. **306:** 1–8.

8. ZHANG, J. X., R. M. HARPER & R. C. FRYSINGER. 1986. Respiratory modulation of neuronal discharge in the central nucleus of the amygdala during sleep and waking states. Exp. Neurol. **91:** 193–207.

9. PARMEGGIANI, P. L. 1980. Temperature regulation during sleep: a study in homeostasis. *In* Physiology in Sleep. J. Orem & C. D. Barnes, Eds.: 98–143. Academic Press. New York.

10. STANTON, A. N. 1984. Overheating and cot death. Lancet **24:** 1199–1201.

11. SEVERINGHAUS, J. W. & R. A. MITCHELL. 1962. Ondine's curse—failure of respiratory center automaticity while awake. Clin. Res. **10:** 122.

12. HOPPENBROUWERS, T., D. JENSEN, J. HODGMAN, R. HARPER & M. STERMAN. 1982. Body movements during quiet sleep (QS) in subsequent siblings of SIDS. Clin. Res. **30:** 136A.

13. WILLIS, J. & J. B. GOULD. 1980. Periodic alpha seizures with apnea in a newborn. Dev. Med. Child Neurol. **22:** 214–222.

14. MONOD, N., N. PAJOT & S. GUIDASCI. 1972. The neonatal EEG: statistical studies and prognostic value in full-term and pre-term babies. Electroencephalogr. Clin. Neurophysiol. **32:** 529–544.

15. OREN, J., D. KELLY & D. C. SHANNON. Identification of a high-risk group for sudden infant death syndrome among infants who were resuscitated for sleep apnea. Pediatrics **77:** 495–499, 1986.

16. HOPKINS, D. A. & G. HOLSTEGE. 1978. Amygdaloid projections to the mesencephalon, pons and medulla oblongata in the cat. Exp. Brain Res. **32:** 529–547.

17. PRICE, J. L. & D. G. AMARAL. 1981. An autoradiographic study of the projections of the central nucleus of the monkey amygdala. J. Neurosci. **1:** 1242–1259.

18. BERTRAND, F. & A. HUGELIN. 1971. Respiratory synchronizing function of nucleus parabrachialis medialis: pneumotaxic mechanisms. J. Neurophysiol. **34:** 189–207.

19. COHEN, M. I. 1971. Switching of the respiratory phases and evoked phrenic responses produced by rostral pontine electrical stimulation. J. Physiol. (London) **217:** 133–158.

20. EULER, C. VON, I. MARTTILA, J. E. REMMERS & T. TRIPPENBACH. 1976. Effects of lesions in the parabrachial nucleus on the mechanisms for central and reflex termination of inspiration in the cat. Acta Physiol. Scand. **96:** 324–337.

21. ST. JOHN, W. M., R. L. GLASSER & R. A. KING. 1971. Apneustic breathing after vagotomy in cats with chronic pneumotaxic center lesions. Respir. Physiol. **12:** 239–250.

22. BANDLER, R. Brain mechanisms of aggression as revealed by electrical and chemical stimulation: Suggestion of a central role for the midbrain periaqueductal grey region. *In* Progress in Psychobiology and Physiological Psychology. A. Epstein & A. Morrison, Eds. Vol. 13. Academic Press. New York. In press.

23. DAVIS, P. J. & B. S. NAIL. 1984. On the location and size of laryngeal motoneurons in the rat and rabbit. J. Comp. Neurol. **230:** 13–32.

24. KAPP, B. S., J. S. SCHWABER & P. A. DRISCOLL. 1985. The organization of insular cortex projections to the amygdaloid central nucleus and autonomic regulatory nuclei of the dorsal medulla. Brain Res. **360:** 355–360.

25. GALLAGHER, M., B. S. KAPP & J. P. PASCOE. 1982. Enkephalin analogue effects in the amygdala central nucleus on conditioned heart rate. Pharmacol. Biochem. Behav. **17:** 217–222.

26. KAPP, B. S., R. C. FRYSINGER, M. GALLAGHER & J. HASELTON. 1979. Amygdala central nucleus lesions: Effects on heart rate conditioning in rabbit. Physiol. Behav. **23:** 1109–1117.
27. ZHANG, J. X., R. M. HARPER & H. NI. 1986. Cryogenic blockade of the central nucleus of the amygdala attenuates aversively conditioned blood pressure and respiratory responses. Brain Res. **386:** 136–145.
28. GODDARD, G. V. 1967. Development of epileptic seizures through brain stimulation at low intensity. Nature **214:** 1020–1021.
29. HARPER, R. M. 1986. State-related physiological changes and risk for the sudden infant death syndrome. Aust. Paediatr. J. **22** (Suppl. 1): 55–58.
30. HARPER, R. M. & R. C. FRYSINGER. Suprapontine mechanisms underlying cardiorespiratory regulation: Implications for the sudden infant death syndrome. *In* Sudden Infant Death Syndrome: Risk Factors and Basic Mechanisms. R. M. Harper & H. J. Hoffman, Eds. PMA Publishing. New York. In press.
31. TRELEASE, R. B., G. C. SIECK, J. D. MARKS & R. M. HARPER. 1985. Respiratory inhibition induced by transient hypertension during sleep in unrestrained cats. Exp. Neurol. **90:** 173–186.
32. MARKS, J. D. & R. M. HARPER. 1987. Differential inhibition of the diaphragm and posterior cricoarytenoid muscles induced by transient hypertension across sleep states in intact cats. Exp. Neurol. **95:** 730–742.
33. TRELEASE, R. B., G. C. SIECK & R. M. HARPER. 1983. Cardiac arrhythmias induced by transient hypertension during sleep-waking states. J. Auton. Nerv. Syst. **8:** 179–191.
34. STERMAN, L. T. 1975. Sudden infant death syndrome infants and subsequent siblings: Relationship of sleep-waking and feeding behaviors. Unpublished Thesis. Univ. of California, Los Angeles. Los Angeles.
35. BECKWITH, J. B. 1973. The sudden infant death syndrome. Curr. Probl. Pediatr. **3:** 1–36.

Physiological Approaches to Respiratory Control Mechanisms in Infants

Assessing the Risk for SIDS[a]

R. HAIDMAYER[b] AND T. KENNER[b]

Institute of Physiology
University of Graz
Austria

INTRODUCTION

Sudden infant death syndrome (SIDS) remains the single leading cause of infant death, accounting for nearly one half of all deaths in infants between 28 days and 1 year of age. Results of pathological studies in autopsies of victims of SIDS have indicated that a number of infants may have had chronic hypoxemia prior to death.[1,2] Physiological studies have demonstrated abnormal patterns of breathing, including apnea, in infants who subsequently died of SIDS, and in "near-miss" SIDS infants.[3,4] Group mean differences in cardiorespiratory patterns during hypoxia and hypercapnia stress-tests have been discussed for high-risk groups.[5-7]

The purpose of this report is to attempt to describe the regulatory behavior of respiration during sleep by means of statistical parameters and to identify infants with deviating respiratory patterns probably implying a risk for SIDS. We also tested the hypothesis that siblings of SIDS infants exhibit a different respiratory behavior compared with controls. In addition, we tested the usefulness of hypoxia-challenge tests for identifying infants at increased risk for SIDS. Since sleep apnea syndrome in infants has been related to an immaturity of respiratory control mechanisms,[8,9] we studied the coordination of sucking and swallowing during feeding. The control centers for these functions are closely linked to respiration control in the medulla oblongata.[10,11]

SUBJECTS AND METHODS

The study was performed on 646 normal infants (gestational age 38–40 weeks, $n = 323$; gestational age < 38 weeks, $n = 323$) and 201 infants with clinical signs of sleep apnea syndrome (SAS; gestational age 38–40 weeks, $n = 81$; gestational age < 38 weeks, $n = 120$) up to 1 year of age. All of the SAS infants were supposed to be at increased risk for SIDS. The control group consisted of 458 males and 188 females, versus 110 males and 91 females in the risk group. None of the infants investigated had demonstrable symptoms of pulmonary, cardiac or cerebral diseases; they were admitted to

[a]This study was supported by the Austrian Research Fund.
[b]Address for correspondence: Physiologisches Institut, Karl-Franzens-Universität Graz, Harrachgasse 21/V, A-8010 Graz, Austria.

the department of pediatrics or pediatric surgery for treatment or diagnosis of diseases not related to the respiratory tract.

The group at risk for SIDS consisted of infants who had been observed to suffer from frequent sleep apneas of more than 15 sec in duration and/or periodic breathing episodes exceeding 5% of total sleep time during non-REM sleep. Furthermore, infants with bradycardia (heart rate < 80 beats/min from 0 to 1 month of age, < 70 beats/min from 1 to 3 months of age, < 60 beats/min at > 3 months of age) or pronounced drops of pO_2-values were also assigned to the group of infants at risk for SIDS. Twenty-five infants of this group had experienced a near-miss SIDS event. In addition, we investigated 28 siblings of SIDS victims, 2 siblings of near-miss infants, and 20 siblings of infants with SAS. Another study was performed on 16 pairs of twins in whom at least one of each pair showed clinical symptoms of SAS.

Respiratory waveform recordings were performed either by means of impedance pneumography or strain-gauge plethysmography. By using the second method, actual variations of tidal volume can be estimated from recordings of chest wall and abdominal excursions. All measurements were recorded on an 8-channel strip chart recorder and on analogue tapes for automatic analysis by a digital computer.[12] In addition to respiration, we continuously recorded heart rate and transcutaneous pO_2- and pCO_2-values (Radiometer).

In order to describe the ventilatory behavior, frequency distributions of sleep apneas, breathing intervals, and variations of tidal volume were computed. From the frequency distribution of sleep apneas (all respiratory pauses of > 3 sec were noted), we calculated the probabilities for the occurrence of apneas of a certain duration according to age,[13] and we computed a characteristic weighted apnea factor.

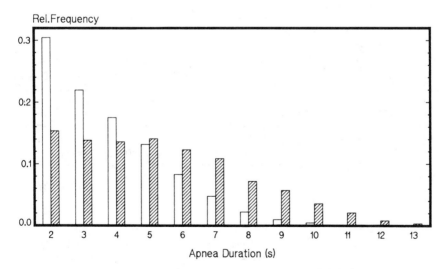

FIGURE 1. Frequency distribution of sleep apneas of control infants (**open bars**, $n = 646$) and infants of the at-risk group with clinical signs of sleep apnea syndrome (**hatched bars**, $n = 201$). The apnea durations (sec) were rounded to integer numbers; each class corresponds to a duration of the indicated number of seconds (s).

In earlier papers,[14] we used the mean apnea value (MA-value), expressed as the integral of all respiratory spells in sec per min of recording:

$$MA = 1/T \sum_{t=3}^{t_{max}} h(t)t$$

The definition of a weighted apnea factor (GA-value) is described below:

$$GA = 1/T \left(-\sum_{t=3}^{t_{max}} h(t)\ln p(t)t \right)$$

The summation is performed over all apnea durations (t to t_{max}) found in a particular baby during observation period T, and the individual frequency distribution $h(t)$ of apneic periods t of an infant is plotted. The term $p(t)$ is the age-specific probability distribution of the occurrence of an apnea. Thus, the GA-value considers the content of diagnostic information in apneas of different durations[15] by giving added weight to the longer apneas.

Sleep states (non-REM and REM) were defined according to criteria based on electro-oculogram (EOG) recordings, observations of sleep behavior, and regularity of respiratory and heart activities. All periods with properties showing a discrepancy among these criteria were classified as undefined sleep.

In order to examine the properties of respiratory control, we performed tests with hypoxic gas mixtures in a limited number of infants. The infants breathed room air or 15% oxygen in nitrogen through a respiratory face mask. The gas was delivered at a flow-rate of 10 l/min through a T-tube, which was connected with the face mask by a pneumotachograph. Alterations of respiration during hypoxia were evaluated as the percentage deviation from a mean basic value observed when the infants were breathing air.

Investigations on coordination of sucking, swallowing, and breathing were performed by measurements of intra-oral pressure, using a specially adapted rubber nipple attached via a pressure transducer. Laryngeal movements during swallowing were recorded by using a strain-gauge device.

Therapy with aminophylline was performed in most of the SAS infants after the first sets of measurements. Aminophylline was administered orally (first day: 6 mg/kg body weight, twice a day; second to fourth day: 4 mg/kg, three times a day; fifth day to sixth week: 3 mg/kg, three times a day). Serum concentrations were monitored continuously.

In order to investigate the influence of chronic hypoxemia on the characteristics of red blood cells, we performed measurements of the density of red cell concentrates (prepared by centrifugation at 5000 rpm for 20 min) by means of a density measuring device (DMA602: Paar KG, Graz) based on the so-called mechanical oscillator principle.[16] The temperature within the measuring cell was adjusted to 20°C by means of an ultrathermostat.

RESULTS

In the group of infants regarded to be at increased risk for SIDS, we could demonstrate that respiratory behavior during sleep deviates statistically significantly from the standard (control) pattern. The at-risk group reveals a differently shaped pattern for the frequency distribution of apneas during sleep compared to the distribution for normal control infants (FIG. 1), which can be approximated by an exponential function.[15]

To evaluate the respiratory pattern of the infants, a characteristic value (GA-value) was computed from the distribution of apneas. By means of this weighted apnea factor, the biological importance of prolonged apneas can be more adequately taken into account. In TABLE 1, we have compared the GA-values of at-risk infants with age-matched control infants and found significant differences between the 2 groups. In addition, the positive effect of aminophylline on the respiratory pattern can be characterized by the significant lowering of the GA-values during and after therapy, independent of gestational age (TABLE 1). In FIG. 2, we have plotted the course of the GA-values with increasing age of the control and at-risk infants. It is evident that the characterization of the respiratory pattern during sleep by the GA-value is more-or-less unaffected by the age of the infant. Thus, it can be excluded that the positive effective of aminophylline on respiration in infants at risk could simply reflect diminishing GA-values due to the aging process during the 6-week therapy.

Besides the apneic behavior, there are also differences between the 2 groups with respect to respiratory rate during non-REM sleep. As can be seen in FIG. 3, the frequency distribution of mean respiration periods is shifted towards longer periods in the at-risk group, indicating that there is also general hypoventilation in this group during non-apneic cycles.

In this connection, we also found significantly lower mean pO_2-values during sleep in at-risk infants with clinical signs of sleep apnea syndrome (SAS) when compared with age-matched controls (TABLE 2). The influence of the chronic hypoxemia due to SAS on erythrocytes is evident by the increasing 2,3-diphosphoglycerate (2,3-DPG) and potas-

TABLE 1. Comparison of Respiratory Behavior (Mean GA-Values) during Sleep in Control Infants and in Infants with SAS (Sleep Apnea Syndrome), before, during, and after Therapy with Aminophylline.

| | Control | | SAS | | | | | |
| | | | Before Therapy | | During Therapy | | After Therapy | |
	GA[a]	n	GA[a]	n	GA[a]	n	GA[a]	n
Age group 1 : 0–30 days old								
Total	6.0 ± 4.2	101	39.4 ± 27.4	62	17.5 ± 13.6	24	20.7 ± 17.0	2
Mature	5.6 ± 4.2	83	33.2 ± 19.4	26	14.3 ± 11.2	11	20.7 ± 17.0	2
Premature	7.6 ± 4.4	18	43.8 ± 31.4	36	20.3 ± 15.2	13		
Age group 2 : 31–60 days old								
Total	5.2 ± 6.8	214	28.5 ± 25.3	94	9.7 ± 9.5	95	13.1 ± 13.6	17
Mature	4.9 ± 8.8	110	24.4 ± 18.0	40	8.2 ± 7.7	44	14.2 ± 16.1	12
Premature	5.5 ± 3.8	104	31.2 ± 29.2	54	10.9 ± 10.7	51	10.7 ± 4.6	5
Age group 3 : 61–90 days old								
Total	4.6 ± 3.5	173	32.3 ± 25.2	27	8.6 ± 9.0	74	6.5 ± 6.3	55
Mature	4.4 ± 3.5	65	34.4 ± 31.7	11	8.9 ± 11.0	28	7.5 ± 6.8	22
Premature	4.7 ± 3.5	108	30.9 ± 20.6	16	8.4 ± 7.6	46	5.8 ± 6.0	33
Age group 4 : 91–120 days old								
Total	4.2 ± 3.2	83	23.8 ± 21.5	13	9.1 ± 10.6	38	5.3 ± 4.3	42
Mature	3.8 ± 3.2	30	29.4 ± 28.7	4	11.0 ± 11.6	16	4.7 ± 3.9	18
Premature	4.4 ± 3.1	53	21.3 ± 19.1	9	7.8 ± 9.8	22	5.7 ± 4.6	24
Age group 5 : > 120 days old								
Total	3.6 ± 3.2	75	23.6 ± 15.0	5	12.1 ± 15.9	26	6.8 ± 10.5	65
Mature	3.1 ± 3.1	35			17.8 ± 25.8	8	6.5 ± 11.1	30
Premature	4.0 ± 3.3	40	23.6 ± 15.0	5	9.6 ± 8.6	18	7.1 ± 10.0	35

Note: Duration of aminophylline therapy is 6 weeks; therefore the composition of the different age groups is not constant.
[a]Mean ± SD.

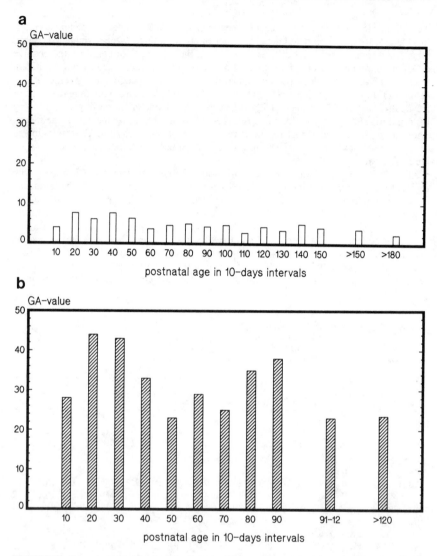

FIGURE 2. GA-values (weighted apnea factor) with increasing postnatal age in (*a*) control infants (**open bars**, $n = 644$) and (*b*) infants at risk for SIDS (**hatched bars**, $n = 198$).

sium concentrations in red blood cells (TABLE 2). There seems to be a close relationship between these changes and the decreases in mean densities of erythrocytes.

To evaluate possible hereditary components in conjunction with respiratory disorders and SIDS, we studied siblings of SIDS victims, of near-miss SIDS infants, and of SAS infants. As demonstrated in TABLE 3, only 2 out of 28 siblings of SIDS victims had severe symptoms of sleep apnea syndrome. Twenty-three of these siblings were completely without conspicuous respiratory symptoms. On the other hand, siblings of SAS infants and of near-miss infants showed clinical signs of SAS with a much higher frequency. A

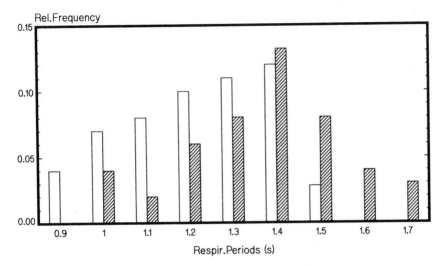

FIGURE 3. Frequency distribution of mean respiration periods (s, sec) in control infants (**open bars**, $n = 74$) and infants at risk for SIDS (**hatched bars**, $n = 29$) during non-REM sleep; only non-apneic periods have been considered for evaluation.

TABLE 2. Hypoxemia and Blood Chemistry: Infants with SAS (Sleep Apnea Syndrome) Compared to Normal Control Infants

	Control Infants	n	SAS Infants	n	p
Density of erythrocytes (g/ml)	1.0938 ± 0.002	16	1.0909 ± 0.002	11	<0.01
Potassium (eryth.)[a] (mmol/l)	97.02 ± 6.15	19	106.83 ± 6.33	10	<0.01
Potassium (serum)[b] (mmol/l)	5.1 ± 0.7	19	4.6 ± 0.3	10	NS
ATP (eryth.)[a] (mmol/l)	51.37 ± 9.29	28	49.95 ± 7.29	10	NS
2,3-DPG (eryth.)[a] (mmol/l)	5.29 ± 0.37	15	6.49 ± 0.75	11	<0.01
Mean tc-pO_2[c] during sleep (mm Hg)	80.8 ± 9.7	22	65.9 ± 10.1	11	<0.01

[a]Concentration in erythrocytes.
[b]Concentration in serum.
[c]Transcutaneous pO_2.

TABLE 3. Comparison of Respiratory Behavior (Mean GA-Values) during Sleep in Siblings of SIDS Victims, Near-Miss SIDS Infants, and SAS Infants.

Sibling	n	Mean GA (±SD)	Mean Age (weeks)	Mean Gestational Age (weeks)	SAS[a] (n)	?SAS[b] (n)
SIDS	28	8.3 ± 9.0	8.1 ± 5.4	39.6 ± 2.2	2	3
Near-Miss SIDS	2	24.1 ± 7.6	6.5 ± 0.7	39.5 ± 0.7	2	0
SAS[a]	20	31.6 ± 33.8	9.6 ± 5.6	34.2 ± 1.9	10	4

[a]SAS, sleep apnea syndrome.
[b]?SAS, questionable-borderline SAS.

TABLE 4. Respiratory Behavior (Mean GA-Values) during Sleep and Respiratory Symptoms in 16 Pairs of Twins

		First Twin			Second Twin		
Pair	Gestational Age	Mean GA	Age[a] (weeks)	Symptoms[b]	Mean GA	Age[a] (weeks)	Symptoms[b]
1	32	78.0	3	SAS	62.0	20	SAS
2	35	44.1	28	SAS	4.1	24	None
3	34	154.8	8	SAS	42.3	8	SAS
4	35	21.3	18	SAS	15.0	6	?SAS
5	35	25.9	5	SAS	22.4	3	?SAS
6	35	69.3	8	SAS	14.8	12	None
7	36	31.4	3	SAS	60.5	5	SAS
8	34	103.2	4	SAS	15.8	6	?SAS
9	35	29.5	6	SAS/N-M	18.7	7	SAS/N-M
10	31	55.9	12	SAS	7.2	14	None
11	36	25.5	3	SAS	5.5	8	None
12	34	34.5	6	SAS	30.9	6	SAS
13	35	43.3	12	SAS	42.3	16	SAS
14	31	35.8	10	SAS/SIDS	5.5	12	None
15	35	27.4	6	SAS	34.1	6	SAS
16	34	33.0	7	SAS	3.9	8	None

[a]Age at time of examination.
[b]SAS, sleep apnea syndrome; N-M, near-miss for SIDS; None, no conspicuous respiratory symptoms; ?SAS, questionable-borderline SAS.

comparison of respiratory behavior in twins with SAS is shown in TABLE 4. Only 6 out of 16 SAS twins were without conspicuous symptoms with respect to respiratory behavior, and a twin brother of a near-miss infant had a near-miss event himself. It is noteworthy that the twin of the SIDS victim shown in TABLE 4 (first twin of pair no. 14) did not reveal any signs of respiratory disorders.

One of the most critical functions of the respiratory control system is the reaction to hypoxia. Therefore, we tested the respiratory response of some at-risk infants and control infants to moderate hypoxia (FIG. 4). When breathing 15% oxygen in nitrogen, all infants responded in a similar way, which can be described as a "biphasic response." After a transient increase of ventilation, a marked ventilatory depression can be observed. There were no pronounced differences between younger (6–60 days of age, FIG. 4a) and older (62–153 days of age, FIG. 4b) control infants. In contrast, the ventilatory depression in the at-risk group was more distinct in comparison with the control group, especially in the younger infants. Furthermore, the time-course of the transcutaneous pO_2-values (FIG. 5) indicates that normal control infants are able to reach a steady state during hypoxia and to maintain their pO_2-values at a constant lower level. At-risk infants, firstly, have lower pO_2-values than control infants during sleep, and, secondly, show a more pronounced and continuing fall of pO_2 to a critical range (FIG. 5).

On the assumption that SAS is the consequence of an immaturity of respiratory control mechanisms or of certain functions of the autonomic nervous system, we also investigated the coordination of breathing, sucking, and swallowing during bottle feeding. The control mechanisms for these activities are located in the medulla oblongata, closely linked to the respiratory center. In a study of 40 control infants (mean age: 66.8 ± 31.9 days, mean birthweight: 2841 ± 887 g), a good coordination of sucking and swallowing became evident, as demonstrated in a typical example shown in FIGURE 6. Sucking was always

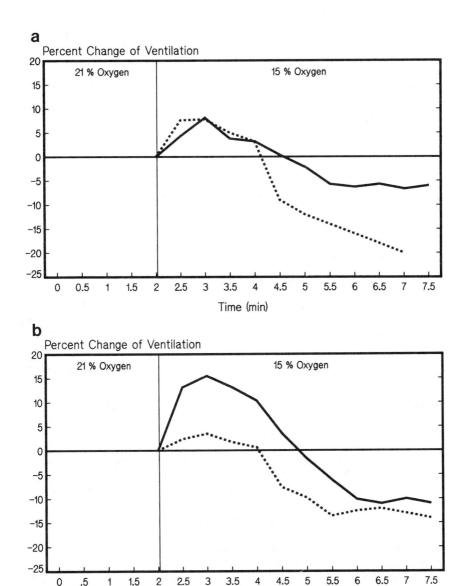

FIGURE 4. Ventilatory response to hypoxia (% deviation of ventilation from a mean basic value measured during normoxia) of control infants (**solid lines**) and infants at risk for SIDS (**dotted lines**) for (*a*) infants of postnatal age 6–60 days and (*b*) infants of 62–153 days of age. In *a*, *n* = 18 for control, 13 for at-risk, infants. In *b*, *n* = 25 for control, 19 for at-risk, infants.

immediately followed by swallowing, and respiration was almost regular in this group after a short apnea (2 to 8 sec) when bottle feeding was started. In contrast to control infants, most of the infants with SAS (n = 15, mean age: 66.4 ± 41.1 days, mean birthweight: 2541 ± 634 g) had an irregular coordination of sucking and breathing. In 11 infants, sucking activities interrupted breathing. Periods of sucking alternated with periods of breathing. Repeated apneas up to 15 sec were observed in these infants, and pO_2-values, which decreased during feeding, were significantly lower after feeding (76.4 ± 8.9 mm Hg before feeding, 68.6 ± 9.4 mm Hg after feeding; $p < 0.01$). A typical example of this behavior is shown in FIGURE 7 for a near-miss infant with severe symptoms of SAS.

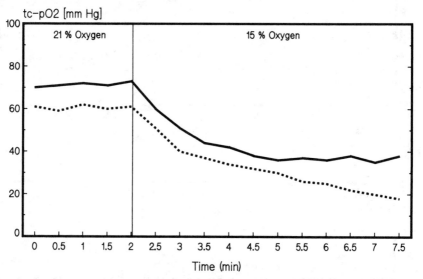

FIGURE 5. Time-course of transcutaneous pO_2-values (tc-pO_2) during hypoxia in control infants (**solid line**, n = 43) and infants at risk for SIDS (**dotted line**, n = 32).

DISCUSSION

We have described the incidence in the first 12 months of life of apneas during sleep in a sample of normal infants and of infants assumed to be at increased risk for SIDS. We were able to demonstrate that the frequency distribution of apnea duration differs in the 2 groups. In agreement with the findings of Kelly *et al.*,[17] control infants predominantly had apneas shorter than 10 sec, while apneas of more than 15 sec were not recorded in this group. On the other hand, numerous prolonged sleep apneas were demonstrated in infants at risk and especially in near-miss infants, as has also been reported by other investigators.[18,19]

We are aware of the fact that the term "at risk for SIDS" may be problematical. Since we do not yet know the underlying cause for SIDS, the prediction of risk for SIDS is still more uncertain than for other diseases. Our current knowledge about the possible

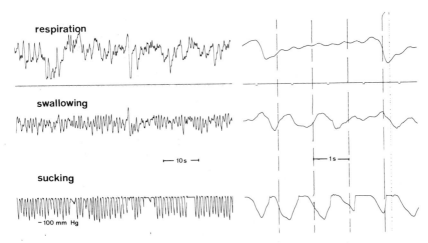

FIGURE 6. Recording showing the coordination of sucking, swallowing, and breathing in a control infant (101 days old) during nutritive sucking. Note expanded time-scale in **right panel.**

mechanisms of the pathogenesis of SIDS suggests that we can probably predict the risk of SIDS by defining the risk for disorders in respiratory control and/or automatic control. Subsequently, we must try to find measurable parameters for the confirmation of our hypothesis. The ultimate goal of this process is the prevention of SIDS.

In our investigations we introduced the probability for the occurrence of an apnea of a particular duration with respect to the age of the infant. Thus, the different diagnostic meanings of extremely prolonged apneas in contrast to physiologically occurring short apneas is taken into account when we try to describe the respiratory pattern by a numeric value, the GA-value. Because of the age-specific weighting function of the GA-value, infants of different ages may be compared with respect to respiratory pattern.

One of the reasons for the different apneic behavior of control infants and infants at

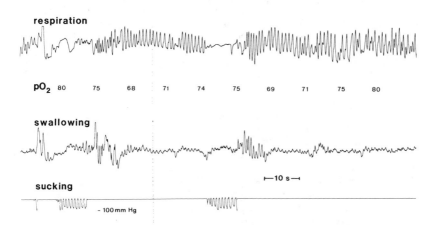

FIGURE 7. Recording showing the coordination of sucking, swallowing, breathing, and transcutaneous pO_2-values of a near-miss-for-SIDS infant (74 days old) during nutritive sucking.

risk could be differences in the maturing pattern of neurons in the medulla oblongata, as has been shown by Quattrochi et al.,[20] who found significantly higher dendritic spine densities in brainstems of SIDS victims than in controls. Takashima and Becker[21] discuss the possibility that the postnatal decrease of dendritic spines in medullary respiratory centers may be related to the functional development of central respiratory control from intrauterine to extrauterine life.

Postmortem examinations of victims of SIDS have revealed morphological findings that are consistent with chronic hypoxemia.[1,2] Therefore, to see whether at-risk infants do hypoventilate during sleep, we plotted the frequency distribution of breath-to-breath intervals for control and risk infants and also found a higher incidence of increased intervals in at-risk infants during non-apneic periods. In addition, the mean pO_2-values during sleep were significantly lower in at-risk infants compared to controls, and we also could demonstrate a long-term effect of the chronic hypoxemia on certain properties of the erythrocytes, such as increased 2,3-DPG-concentrations and decreased mean red-blood cell density.

In analogy to the treatment of apneas of prematurity, infants at risk were treated with aminophylline. Within the first week of treatment, the GA-values and transcutaneous pO_2-values improved significantly; they then remained in the normal range in most of the infants, even after termination of therapy. The effects of aminophylline on respiration have been attributed to a direct action on the respiratory center by an increase in the level of cyclic AMP, which plays a role in mediating the effect of neurotransmitters,[22] or to an increase of CO_2-sensitivity[23] and respiratory drive.[24] Recently, the participation of neuromodulators such as endorphins and adenosine has been discussed with respect to respiratory control.[25] By using naloxone as opiate antagonist, we could not support the assumption that endorphins play a major role in the pathogenesis of sleep apnea syndrome in infancy.[26] On the other hand, Lagercrantz et al.[27] could demonstrate that the respiratory depression caused by adenosine or adenosine agonists could be completely reversed by aminophylline. These findings suggest that the therapeutic effect of aminophylline could be exerted via blockade of adenosine receptors. This proposal is supported by the observation that the adenosine antagonist, 8-phenyl-theophylline, which is essentially devoid of phosphodiesterase-inhibitory effect, is as potent as aminophylline.[27]

In a couple of studies, siblings of SIDS victims have been regarded to be at increased risk for SIDS (for a review, see Ref. 28). The estimate of risk of SIDS for siblings varies considerably between several research groups, from very low risk estimates in Norway (4.8 SIDS events/1000 siblings) to very high ones in the United States (19.0/1000) and South Australia (20.0/1000). Peterson et al.[28] emphasize that although the risk of SIDS in siblings is almost 4 times that of the SIDS risk among births at large, one has to consider the combined effects of maternal age and birth rank. The authors believe that siblings of SIDS victims have no higher risk of SIDS than infants in families of comparable size and with mothers of similar age. To evaluate possible hereditary components in conjunction with respiratory disorders, we calculated the GA-values of siblings of SIDS victims, of SAS infants, and of near-miss infants. Most of our siblings of SIDS victims had no conspicuous respiratory symptoms, which is in a very good agreement with a study of Curzi-Dascalova et al.[29] concerning respiratory rates. The finding of elevated GA-values in near-miss siblings and SAS siblings raises the question of whether identification of respiratory disorders and supposed "risk-factors for SIDS" really helps to discriminate between low-risk and high-risk infants.

One of the mechanisms which it seems could ultimately lead to SIDS is the specific reaction to hypoxia in infants with SAS. A prolonged apnea could be the trigger mechanism for a "circulus vitiosus," by provoking hypoxemia with subsequent depression of the respiratory center. Bureau et al.[30] discuss the hypothesis that in the postnatal period chemoreceptors which have an immature response to hypoxia also inhibit the ability to adapt during steady-state hypoxia. This fact could explain the biphasic ventilatory response of neonates to hypoxia. Again, in at-risk infants the maturing process seems to be delayed in comparison to controls.

Since the sleep apnea syndrome seems to be a consequence of an immaturity of respiratory control mechanisms,[8,9] we also investigated the control of other autonomic functions of the medulla oblongata. The centers for the ability to coordinate sucking and swallowing during feeding are closely linked to respiratory control.[10,11] In contrast to control infants, for most of the at-risk infants, normal simultaneous sucking and breathing seems to be difficult. In addition, when we interviewed parents of SIDS victims, in a surprisingly large number of cases parents reported that their babies had revealed problems with feeding before death.

In conclusion, the current methods of testing allow us to find group differences when we compare control infants and infants assumed to be at risk for SIDS. The methods used are not specific or sensitive enough to prospectively identify infants in the "at risk group" who are most likely to die. Abnormal results of oxycardiorespirograms do not necessarily correlate with the severity of subsequent episodes of respiratory difficulties or with the outcome.

SUMMARY

We have examined in a group of normal infants and in an "at-risk" group with clinical sleep apnea syndrome the duration and frequency distribution of apneas during sleep. In order to improve the estimation of an apnea factor, we introduced a weighting function which is based on the expected frequency distribution of apnea durations of normal infants. We were able to observe a good agreement between clinical rating, based on anamnestic symptoms, and numerical scoring. All infants of the at-risk group were treated with aminophylline, and the respiratory state improved significantly in nearly all cases. Breathing hypoxic gas mixtures tended to depress respiration, especially in the at-risk group, with a pronounced drop of pO_2-values. Investigations on the coordination of respiration, sucking, and swallowing during nutritive sucking demonstrated a correspondence between disturbed coordination ability and the sleep apnea syndrome (SAS). This relationship is interpreted to be a result of an immaturity of the autonomic nervous system. In order to evaluate possible hereditary components in conjunction with respiratory disorders and, possibly, SIDS, we studied siblings of SIDS victims, of near-miss infants, and of infants with SAS. Only siblings of SAS and near-miss infants showed clinical signs of respiratory disorders with a rather high prevalence, whereas most of the siblings of SIDS victims were completely lacking conspicuous respiratory symptoms. Our results suggest that not all infants with sleep apnea syndrome are necessarily at increased risk for SIDS.

REFERENCES

1. NAEYE, R. L. 1976. Brain-stem and adrenal abnormalities in the sudden infant death syndrome. Am. J. Clin. Pathol. **66:** 526–569.
2. VALDES-DAPENA, M. A., M. M. GILLANE & R. CATHERMAN. 1976. Brown fat retention in sudden infant death syndrome. Arch. Pathol. Lab. Med. **100:** 547–549.
3. KELLY, D. H. & D. C. SHANNON. 1979. Periodic breathing in infants with near-miss sudden infant death syndrome. Pediatrics **63:** 355–360.

4. GUILLEMINAULT, C., R. PERAITA, M. SOUQUET & W. C. DEMENT. 1975. Apneas during sleep in infants: Possible relationship with sudden infant death syndrome. Science **190:** 677–679.
5. SHANNON, D. C., D. H. KELLY & K. O'CONNELL. 1977. Abnormal regulation of ventilation in infants at risk for sudden infant death syndrome. N. Engl. J. Med. **297:** 747–750.
6. HUNT, C. E. 1981. Abnormal hypercarbic and hypoxic sleep arousal responses in near-miss SIDS infants. Pediatr. Res. **15:** 1462–1464.
7. ARIAGNO, R., L. NAGEL & C. GUILLEMINAULT. 1980. Waking and ventilatory responses during sleep in infants near-miss for sudden infant death syndrome. Sleep **3:** 351–359.
8. BABA, N., J. QUATTROCHI, C. B. REINER, W. ADRION, P. T. MCBRIDE & A. J. YATES. 1983. Possible role of brain stem in sudden infant death syndrome. J. Am. Med. Assoc. **249:** 2789–2791.
9. GUNBY, P. 1978. Brain stem abnormalities may characterize S.I.D.S. victims. J. Am. Med. Assoc. **240:** 2138–2144.
10. PEIPER, A. 1938. Das Zusammenspiel des Saugzentrums mit dem Atemzentrum beim menschlichen Säugling. Pfluegers Arch. **240:** 312–324.
11. WILSON, S. L., B. T. THACH, R. T. BROUILLETTE & Y. K. ABU-OSBA. 1981. Coordination of breathing and swallowing in human infants. J. Appl. Physiol. **50:** 851–858.
12. KERSCHHAGGL, P., R. HAIDMAYER, R. KERBL, K. P. PFEIFFER, R. KURZ & T. KENNER. 1986. Computer-assisted evaluation of respiration in newborns and infants during sleep. *In* Neonatal Physiological Measurements. P. Rolfe, Ed.: 301–307. Butterworths & Co. London.
13. HAIDMAYER, R., K. P. PFEIFFER, T. KENNER & R. KURZ. 1982. Statistical evaluation of respiratory control in infants to assess possible risk for the sudden infant death syndrome (SIDS). Eur. J. Pediatr. **138:** 145–150.
14. HAIDMAYER, R., R. KURZ, T. KENNER, H. WURM & K. P. PFEIFFER. 1982. Physiological and clinical aspects of respiration control in infants with relation to the sudden infant death syndrome. Klin. Wochenschr. **60:** 9–18.
15. PFEIFFER, K. P., R. HAIDMAYER, P. KERSCHHAGGL, R. KURZ & T. KENNER. 1984. Statistical evaluation of the respiratory pattern as a risk factor for the sudden infant death syndrome. Method. Inf. Med. **23:** 41–46.
16. KENNER, T., H. LEOPOLD & H. HINGHOFER-SZALKAY. 1977. The continuous high-precision measurement of the density of flowing blood. Pfluegers Arch. **370:** 25–29.
17. KELLY, D. H., L. M. STELLWAGEN, E. KAITZ & D. C. SHANNON. 1985. Apnea and periodic breathing in normal full-term infants during the first twelve months. Pediatr. Pulmonol. **1:** 215–219.
18. STEINSCHNEIDER, A., S. L. WEINSTEIN & E. DIAMOND. 1982. The sudden infant death syndrome and obstructive apnea during neonatal sleep and feedings. Pediatrics **70:** 858–863.
19. GUILLEMINAULT, C., R. L. ARIAGNO, L. S. FORNO, L. NAGEL, R. BALDWIN & M. OWEN. 1979. Obstructive sleep apnea and near-miss SIDS: Report of an infant with sudden death. Pediatrics **63:** 837–843.
20. QUATTROCHI, J. J., P. T. MCBRIDE & A. J. YATES. 1985. Brainstem immaturity in sudden infant death syndrome: A quantitative rapid Golgi study of dendritic spines in 95 infants. Brain Res. **325:** 39–48.
21. TAKASHIMA, S. & L. E. BECKER. 1986. Prenatal and postnatal maturation of medullary "respiratory centers." Dev. Brain Res. **26:** 173–177.
22. GABRIEL, M., C. WITOLLA & M. ALBANI. 1978. Sleep and aminophylline treatment of apnea in preterm infants. Eur. J. Pediatr. **128:** 145–149.
23. DAVI, M. J., K. SANKARAN, K. J. SIMONS, F. E. R. SIMONS, M. M. SESHIA & H. RIGATTO. 1978. Physiologic changes induced by theophylline in the treatment of apnea in preterm infants. J. Pediatr. **92:** 91–95.
24. GERHARDT, T., J. MCCARTHY & E. BANCALARI. 1979. Effect of aminophylline on respiratory center activity and metabolic rate in premature infants with idiopathic apnea. Pediatrics **63:** 537–542.
25. MOSS, I. R., M. DENAVIT-SAUBIE, F. L. ELDRIDGE, R. A. GILLIS, M. HERKENHAM & S. LAHIRI. 1986. Neuromodulators and transmitters in respiratory control. Fed. Proc. Fed. Am. Soc. Exp. Biol. **45:** 2133–2147.
26. HAIDMAYER, R., R. KERBL, U. MEYER, P. KERSCHHAGGL, R. KURZ & T. KENNER. 1986.

Effects of naloxone on apnoea duration during sleep in infants at risk for SIDS. Eur. J. Pediatr. **145:** 357–360.

27. LAGERCRANTZ, H., Y. YAMAMOTO, B. B. FREDHOLM, N. R. PRABHAKAR & C. VON EULER. 1984. Adenosine analogues depress ventilation in rabbit neonates. Theophylline stimulation of respiration via adenosine receptors? Pediatr. Res. **18:** 387–389.

28. PETERSON, D. R., E. E. SABOTTA & J. R. DALING. 1986. Infants mortality among subsequent siblings of infants who died of sudden infant death. J. Pediatr. **108:** 911–914.

29. CURZI-DASCALOVA, L., R. FLORES-GUEVARA, S. GUIDASCI, G. KORN & N. MONOD. 1983. Respiratory frequency during sleep in siblings of sudden infant death syndrome victims. A comparison with control, normal infants. Early Hum. Dev. **8:** 235–241.

30. BUREAU, M. A., A. COTE, P. W. BLANCHARD, S. HOBBS, P. FOULON & D. DALLE. 1986. Exponential and diphasic ventilatory response to hypoxia in conscious lambs. J. Appl. Physiol. **61:** 836–842.

Analysis of Long-Term Cardiorespiratory Recordings from Infants Who Subsequently Suffered SIDS[a]

A. J. WILSON,[b] V. STEVENS,[b] C. I. FRANKS,[b] AND
D. P. SOUTHALL[c]

[b]Department of Medical Physics and Clinical Engineering
Royal Hallamshire Hospital
Sheffield S10 2JF
England
[c]Department of Paediatrics
Cardiothoracic Institute
University of London
Fulham Road
London SW3 6HP
England

INTRODUCTION

Evidence from all aspects of research into the sudden infant death syndrome (SIDS) has suggested that a defect in the cardiorespiratory control mechanisms may be an underlying problem in some SIDS cases.[1] Physiological studies designed to investigate this possibility have primarily been carried out on 2 groups of infants who are believed to be at increased risk for SIDS. The first group are those infants who are the siblings of SIDS cases and the second group are those infants who have had an episode of bradycardia, cyanosis or pallor (the "near-miss" infants). The results from cardiorespiratory and polygraphic studies using both of these groups have demonstrated respiratory and heart-rate differences between these "at-risk" cases and controls.[2-8] The major problems with these studies is that they have been carried out on infants who are believed to be at increased risk for SIDS, rather than on infants who subsequently died. In the case of the "near-miss" infants, the findings may represent the effects of the episode itself rather than some underlying problem.

Southall et al. (the Multicentre Study Group[9]) carried out a prospective study into SIDS in which 24-hr electrocardiogram (ECG) and respiratory waveform (abdominal wall movement) recordings were obtained on a group of full-term infants who subsequently suffered SIDS. In the current study, respiratory and heart-rate patterns were analyzed in these recordings to determine 3 factors: firstly, whether differences in these patterns existed between subsequent SIDS cases and a control group; secondly, if such differences did exist, whether they were of sufficient magnitude to allow prediction of which infants would subsequently die; and, thirdly, whether the pattern of any differences which existed provided an insight into the mechanism or mechanisms which may underlie SIDS.

[a]This work was supported by the Medical Research Council.

390

METHODS

The data from the prospective study into SIDS[9] consisted of 24-hr recordings of the ECG and respiratory waveform (abdominal wall movement) made on 6,914 full-term infants. The aim of the study for the majority of infants was to obtain 2 recordings: the first within the first week of life and the second within the sixth week of life. In a small number of infants, the aim was to obtain a single recording within the third week of life. The majority of these recordings were made within the home, except for those made during the first week of life, which were done in the maternity wards. From this population of infants, 13 subsequently died with a postmortem diagnosis of SIDS. Simultaneous research being carried out yielded recordings on a further 3 infants who also subsequently suffered SIDS. Twenty-two recordings were available on 16 full-term infants who subsequently suffered SIDS. A control group against which to compare these infants consisted of 324 recordings randomly selected from the remaining population. Infants who had died of other causes, who had congenital abnormalities, or who had major postnatal complications were not included in this control group. The control group consisted of 120 recordings taken at one week of age, 97 recordings taken at 3 weeks of age, and 107 recordings taken at 6 weeks of age. Age and birthweight details of the individual SIDS cases and the control groups are given in TABLE 1. Each of the SIDS cases has been allocated a code number for identification purposes; these numbers will be used throughout the paper.

Each of the recordings in the study was first processed by a microprocessor-based version of the Sheffield Respiration Analysis System.[10] This system determined the instantaneous heart rate and breath-to-breath interval distributions for non-overlapping time epochs of 100-sec duration throughout a recording. The R waves in the ECG were detected and the R–R interval determined by a clock and counter. The R–R interval was represented by a 10-bit binary word. This 10-bit binary word, together with the digitized respiratory waveform, was inputted to the computer, sampling at 1.2 kHz for data replayed at 60-times real time. The instantaneous heart rate (IHR) was then determined from the R–R interval values using a software procedure. Breaths were detected by the detection of "peaks" and "troughs" in the respiratory waveform. Amplitude differences between these had to exceed a "threshold" level determined from the preceding 60 sec of respiratory waveform before a breath could be detected. The time interval between breaths (TIBB) was taken as the time between the half-amplitude points on the inspiratory phase of two consecutive breaths. The peak-trough searching procedure essentially "identified" cycles in the respiratory waveform. Movement artifact was distinguished by identifying cycles which had a larger amplitude, a larger high-frequency content, and a different shape than breaths detected from the preceding 60 sec of respiratory waveform.

Once the IHR and TIBB values had been determined, the median and interquartile ranges of both these were computed for 100-sec, non-overlapping time epochs throughout a recording. These quantities, which described the average value of the "rate" and its variability for that epoch, were used in place of the mean and standard deviation, because they were less sensitive to the presence of extreme values in the data. An epoch length of 100 sec was selected to be sufficiently long to allow reliable estimates of the rate and variability to be obtained whilst being sufficiently short to allow short-term pattern changes to become apparent.

When the data have been processed in this manner, the results can then be plotted in form of a graph (FIG. 1). Data from 24-hr recordings processed in the manner described yielded approximately 850 data values for each of 4 measures: the average heart rate (HRA), the heart-rate variability (HRV), the average time interval between breaths (TIBBA) and the variability of the time interval between breaths (TIBBV). Each of these measures was considered as a sampled data series, where the sampling interval was 100

TABLE 1. Birthweight Data and Age at Time of Recordings for Control Groups and Infants Who Subsequently Suffered SIDS

Infants	1-Week Group[a]			3-Week Group[a]			6-Week Group[a]		
	Recordings (n)	Age[b] (days)	Birthweight (g)	Recordings (n)	Age[b] (days)	Birthweight (g)	Recordings (n)	Age[b] (days)	Birthweight (g)
Controls (n = 324)[c]	120			97			107		
Mean ± SD		5 ± 3	3,376 ± 482		23 ± 4	3,338 ± 569		49 ± 9	3,401 ± 551
SIDS cases (n = 16)[d]	10			5			7		
	Code#[e]			Code#[e]			Code#[e]		
	8	2	4,790	11	30	2,350	1	47	2,920
	3	2	3,740	9	19	2,980	8	41	4,790
	12	12	1,890	5	24	3,770	10	40	3,960
	6	5	3,030	13	16	2,780	5	63	3,770
	16[f]	5	2,000	15	16	2,320	9	61	2,980
	7	3	3,080				6	40	3,030
	2	6	3,490				4	52	2,810
	4	8	2,810						
	1	5	2,920						
	14	2	2,700						
Mean ± SD		5 ± 3	3,045 ± 839		21 ± 6	2,840 ± 591		49 ± 10	3,465 ± 735

[a] A pair of recordings were made for most infants, one each during the first and sixth weeks of life; for some infants a recording was made during the third week of life.
[b] Age at time of recording.
[c] Total number of randomly selected control recordings analyzed (see text).
[d] A total of 22 recordings were available from 16 infants who subsequently suffered SIDS (but see footnote f).
[e] Code numbers assigned to identify individual SIDS cases, for whom age and birthweight data are listed.
[f] Infant #16 had no respiration on the recording; therefore TIBBA and TIBBV are presented on 21 recordings.

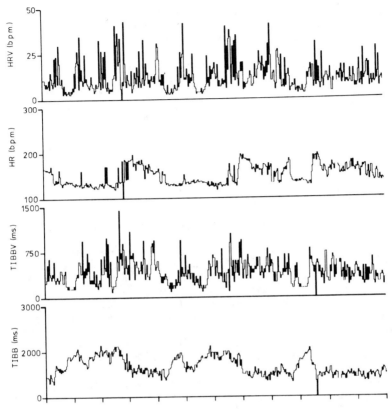

FIGURE 1. 12-hr graphs of data values for (**bottom** to **top**, respectively) average TIBB, TIBB variability (TIBBV), average heart rate (HR), and heart-rate variability (HRV) plotted against time (hr). TIBB and TIBBV in msec (ms.); HR and HRV in beats per minute (b.p.m.).

sec and the amplitude of each sample was the value of one of the 4 "rate" and variability measures. The problem then became one of processing each of these 4 data series to obtain numerical descriptors of the "rate" and variability measures that could be statistically compared between SIDS cases and controls.

The simplest numerical descriptor of a series of data values is the mean. For each of the 4 measures of "rate" and variability, the mean value measured over the 24-hr period was determined. Because of the rapid and non-linear changes in heart rate which occur during the early part of life,[11,12] it was impossible to make a simple statistical comparison between SIDS cases and controls. Therefore, a modified Wilcoxon rank sum test, suitably adjusted for age stratification, was used, allowing group comparison to be made between SIDS cases and controls. The postnatal ages of the infants were divided into a series of groups such that within each group there was no change in the measure being studied with age. For the TIBBA, TIBBV, and HRV, the age groupings used were 2, 3, 4–6, 7–9, 10–15, 16–18, 19–39, 40–47 and ≥ 48 days. For the HRA, a different set of age groupings were used to allow for the very rapid rise in heart rate during the first few weeks of life: 2, 3, 5, 6, 8, 10–15, 16–18, 19–39, 40–47 and ≥ 48 days. To avoid introducing a possible bias into the results because some of the SIDS cases did not have 2 recordings, only the first recording on each of the SIDS cases was used in this comparison.

The mean value of each of the 4 data series yields a single-valued descriptor of that series. However, this descriptor is only a good measure of the "average" value of a data series for a data series that is normally distributed. The results from associated research have shown that in the majority of cases such data are not normally distributed.[13] Therefore, in order to investigate the distribution of data values, the probability density function (PDF) was constructed for each of the 4 data series. This function, which defines the probability that the signal has a particular amplitude value, is calculated from the following formula:

$$P(y, y + \delta y) = \frac{1}{T} \sum_0^T t(y)$$

where $P(y, y + \delta y)$ is the probability that a signal has an amplitude value between y and $y + \delta y$; $t(y)$ is the total time that a signal is within the amplitude band between y and $y + \delta y$; and T is the total duration of the signal. Thirty amplitude intervals were used for each of the data series. For the TIBBA and TIBBV data series, the amplitude intervals used were 120 msec and 50 msec, respectively. For the HRA and HRV data series, the amplitude intervals used were 10 b. p. m. (beats per min) and 2 b. p. m., respectively. A typical example of the PDF for the average heart rate (HRA) data series is given in FIGURE 2. In order to compare the SIDS cases and the controls, the data were analyzed for the age groups given in TABLE 1. None of the groups contained more than a single recording on an infant who had suffered SIDS. The PDFs for each of the 4 data series in each of the 3 age groups were processed independently by a principal-components factor analysis in order to obtain a data reduction and to classify the data.[13,14] Principal-components analysis performs P orthogonal transformations on a set of M data records, where each data record contains P values. Each orthogonal transformation is performed on the residual records from the previous cycle to give the best approximation to the most prominant structures ("shape") in those records. The "shape" identified is the principal component, and the amount of that component present in a particular record is the coefficient for that record. On completion of each transformation cycle, the residual record for each of the M data records is calculated by subtracting the principal component, scaled by the coefficient for that record, from the current record. If $M > P$, then an efficient description of each data record can be obtained by using J principal components, where $J < P$. The first 3 principal components were used to describe the PDFs. The first 3 coefficients were plotted against each other in pairs and the plots inspected visually to identify any separation in the values of the coefficients between SIDS cases and control subjects. Where a separation of the SIDS cases and controls could be identified, a Fisher exact probability test was applied to determine the statistical significance.

The mean values and PDFs describe the statistical properties of the 4 data series, but they do not describe the time ordering of the values. In order to investigate this, we performed a Fourier transformation on each of the 4 data series after we did some necessary data preparation and preprocessing.[13] Part of the data analysis performed by the Sheffield Respiration Analysis system identified movement artifacts in both the IHR and TIBB data independently. This led to epochs in which there were too few breaths or heartbeats to obtain a reliable estimate of the median and interquartile range values of either the TIBB or the IHR. Thus, many of the data series effectively contained missing values. These missing values were inserted into the data series using a linear interpolation algorithm. Clearly, the presence of an excessive number of interpolated values would

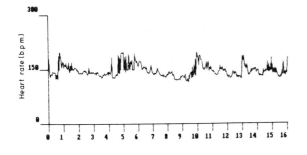

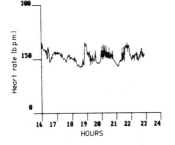

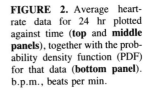

FIGURE 2. Average heart-rate data for 24 hr plotted against time (**top** and **middle panels**), together with the probability density function (PDF) for that data (**bottom panel**). b.p.m., beats per min.

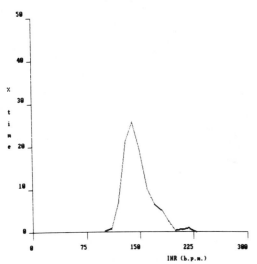

have led to an erroneous result.[13] In order to preserve the frequency content of a signal, each cycle must be sampled at least twice (Nyquist sampling theorem). A visual inspection of the data series suggested that the highest major frequency component present was at about 1 cycle/hr (36 data samples). Therefore, any data series which contained more than 18 consecutively interpolated points was eliminated from further analysis. In addition to this, each data series was "deglitched" to remove any transient spikes which would contain broadband spectral energy. Each data series was then filtered with a

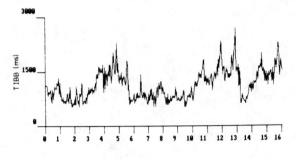

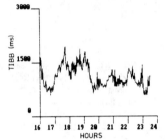

FIGURE 3. Average TIBB data for 24 hr plotted against time (**top** and **middle panels**), together with its power spectral density function (PSD; **bottom panel**). c/hr, cycles/hr.

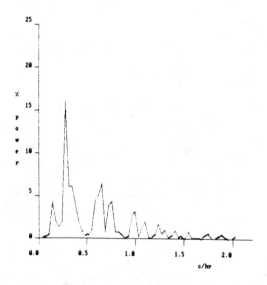

0.25–4.0 cycle/hr bandpass filter to remove any circadian rhythm and to smooth the data. Finally, a cosine taper window was applied to each data series for 10% of its length at either end to prevent spectral leakage. Having performed this preprocessing, we padded each of the data series with zeros to give 1,024 data values, which were then processed by an FFT algorithm and the result used to calculate the power spectral density (PSD) function. A typical example of the PSD for the TIBBA data series is given in FIGURE 3.

The process of eliminating recordings because of artifacts reduced the number of infants available for study. In addition, infants eliminated from the analysis for the respiratory measures (TIBBA and TIBBV) were not necessarily eliminated from the analysis of the heart-rate measures (HRA and HRV). Similarly, infants eliminated from the analysis of the heart-rate measures were not necessarily eliminated from analysis of the respiratory measures. The details of the individual SIDS cases and the control group used for the TIBBA and TIBBV analysis are given in TABLE 2, and those used for the HRA and HRV analysis are given in TABLE 3. Statistical comparisons between SIDS cases and controls were made in terms of the age groups given in TABLES 2 and 3.

In order to make comparisons between SIDS cases and controls, the integrated power in 4 spectral bands was obtained: 0.25–0.75 cycles/hr, 0.75–1.25 cycles/hr, 1.25–1.75 cycles/hr, and 1.75–2.25 cycles/hr. The power within each of these bands, expressed as a percentage of the total integrated power, was then compared between SIDS cases and controls in each of the 3 age groups, using a Wilcoxon rank sum test. Because there are effectively 4 correlated measures for each of the parameters studied, a probability level of $p \leq 0.01$ was required to obtain statistical significance. In addition to this, the total power in the signal (its variance) and the percentage of power described by the frequency range of 0.25–2.25 cycles/hr were compared between SIDS cases and controls, using a Wilcoxon rank sum test.

RESULTS

FIGURE 4 gives the mean value for the average TIBB data series (TIBBA) measured over 24 hr for the SIDS cases and the control subjects. The results of the Wilcoxon rank sum test showed no statistically significant difference between SIDS cases and controls ($p > 0.05$). None of the recordings from the SIDS cases have mean values of TIBBA that represent extreme values relative to the controls of a similar postnatal age. However, infants 7, 13 and 11 had values that are near the maximum values found in the control group at the appropriate postnatal ages.

FIGURE 5 gives the mean values for the TIBB variability data series (TIBBV) measured over 24 hr for the SIDS cases and the control subjects. The results of the Wilcoxon rank sum test showed no statistically significant difference between the cases and controls in terms of the mean TIBBV ($p > 0.05$). All the SIDS cases, with the exception of infant 7 and infant 5 (the first recording), had values that were appropriate for their postnatal ages. The second recording on infant 5 was well within the range of the control group.

FIGURE 6 gives the mean value for the average heart-rate data series (HRA) measured over 24 hr for the SIDS cases and the control subjects. The results of the Wilcoxon rank sum test showed that there was a statistically significant difference between the SIDS cases and controls in terms of the mean HRA ($p < 0.05$). FIGURE 6 shows that, as a group, the SIDS cases tended to have a higher overall heart rate than the controls and that this difference is most pronounced during the first 2 weeks of life. None of the SIDS cases had heart-rate values that were outside the range of the control subjects appropriate for their postnatal ages, with the exception of infant number 9, whose second recording had a mean HRA value outside the range of the control subjects appropriate for that postnatal age.

FIGURE 7 shows the mean values of the heart-rate variability data series (HRV) for the SIDS cases and the control subjects. The results of the Wilcoxon rank sum test showed no significant difference between the SIDS cases and the controls in terms of the mean HRV ($p > 0.05$). All the recordings from the SIDS cases had mean HRV values that were within the range of the control subjects of appropriate postnatal age, with the exception

TABLE 2. Recordings Used in Spectral Analysis of TIBBA and TIBBV Data Series: Birthweight Data and Age at Time of Recordings for Control Groups and Infants Who Subsequently Suffered SIDS

Infants	1-Week Group[a]			3-Week Group[a]			6-Week Group[a]		
	Recordings (n)	Age[b] (days)	Birthweight (g)	Recordings (n)	Age[b] (days)	Birthweight (g)	Recordings (n)	Age[b] (days)	Birthweight (g)
Controls									
Mean ± SD	94	5 ± 3	3,321 ± 512	73	22 ± 4	3,195 ± 559	81	49 ± 9	3,390 ± 466
SIDS cases	8			4			6		
	Code#[c]			Code#[c]			Code#[c]		
	8	2	4,790	11	30	2,350	1	47	2,920
	12	12	1,890	9	19	2,980	8	41	4,790
	6	5	3,030	13	16	2,780	10	40	3,960
	7	3	3,080	15	16	2,320	9	61	2,980
	2	6	3,490				6	40	3,030
	4	8	2,810				4	52	2,810
	1	5	2,920						
	14	2	2,700						
Mean ± SD	14	5 ± 3	3,311 ± 877		20 ± 7	2,607 ± 325		47 ± 8	3,415 ± 791

[a] A pair of recordings were made for most infants, one each during the first and sixth weeks of life; for some infants a recording was made during the third week of life.
[b] Age at time of recording.
[c] Code numbers assigned to identify individual SIDS cases, for whom age and birthweight data are listed.

TABLE 3. Recordings Used in Spectral Analysis of HRA and HRV Data Series: Birthweight Data and Age at Time of Recordings for Control Groups and Infants Who Subsequently Suffered SIDS

Infants	1-Week Group[a] Recordings (n)	Age[b] (days)	Birthweight (g)	3-Week Group[a] Recordings (n)	Age[b] (days)	Birthweight (g)	6-Week Group[a] Recordings (n)	Age[b] (days)	Birthweight (g)
Controls	86			67			88		
Mean ± SD		5 ± 3	3,341 ± 533		23 ± 4	3,319 ± 445		49 ± 10	3,439 ± 466
SIDS cases	9			5			7		
	Code#[c]			*Code#[c]*			*Code#[c]*		
	8	2	4,790	11	30	2,350	1	47	2,920
	3	2	3,740	9	19	2,980	8	41	4,790
	12	12	1,890	5	24	3,770	10	40	3,960
	6	5	3,030	13	16	2,780	5	63	3,770
	16	5	2,000	15	16	2,320	9	61	2,980
	7	3	3,080				6	40	3,030
	4	8	2,810				4	52	2,810
	1	5	2,920						
	14	2	2,700						
Mean ± SD		5 ± 3	2,995 ± 874		21 ± 6	2,840 ± 591		49 ± 10	3,465 ± 735

[a] A pair of recordings were made for most infants, one each during the first and sixth weeks of life; for some infants a recording was made during the third week of life.

[b] Age at time of recording.

[c] Code numbers assigned to identify individual SIDS cases, for whom age and birthweight data are listed.

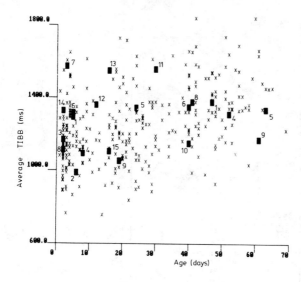

FIGURE 4. Scatter plot of the mean values of the average TIBB data series versus postnatal age for the SIDS cases (■) and the subjects in the control group (X).

of infant number 10 and infant number 8 (second recording), whose values were towards the higher extreme of the control group, and infant number 5 (second recording), whose value was less than the lowest value in the control group.

In order to make comparisons between the SIDS cases and the control groups for the PDFs of each of the data series, a principal-components factor analysis was used to provide data reduction and classification. The first 3 principal components described in excess of 80% of the information present in the PDFs for each data series. At no age was there any separation between the SIDS cases and controls in the values of the first 3 coefficients for either of the respiratory rate measures (TIBBA and TIBBV) or for the average heart rate (HRA). For the heart-rate variability (HRV) data series, there was no

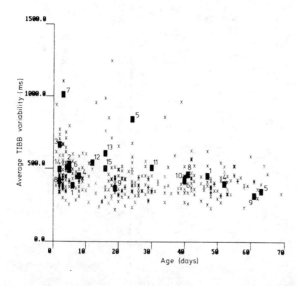

FIGURE 5. Scatter plot of the mean values of the TIBB variability data series versus postnatal age for the SIDS cases (■) and the subjects in the control group (X).

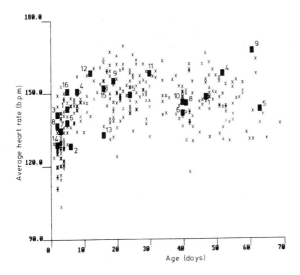

FIGURE 6. Scatter plot of the mean value of the average heart-rate data series versus postnatal age for the SIDS cases (■) and the subjects in the control group (X).

separation in the values of the first 3 coefficients between the SIDS cases and control subjects for infants within the 1- and 3-week age groups. However, at 6 weeks of age, the plot of the first coefficient against the second coefficient for the PDF of the HRV data series showed that a line of separation could be drawn (line AA' in FIG. 8). This line of separation identified 3 of the 6 SIDS cases, and this separation is statistically significant ($p < 0.01$). In order to investigate whether this result was due to postnatal age effects, a Kendall rank correlation was performed between postnatal age and each of the first 3 coefficients for the PDF of the HRV. This showed no significant correlations ($p > 0.05$), and, therefore, this result is not due to postnatal age effects. In order to investigate what property of the PDF gave rise to this separation, the PDFs of the 3 SIDS cases identified

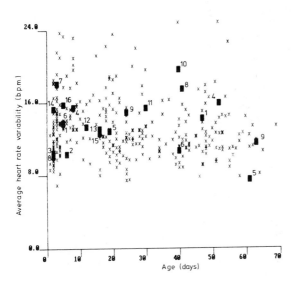

FIGURE 7. Scatter plot of the mean values of the heart-rate variability data series versus postnatal age for the SIDS cases (■) and the subjects in the control group (X).

(infants number 9, 4 and 10) and the mean PDF of the control group were plotted (FIG. 9). From FIGURE 9 it can be seen that 2 of the SIDS cases (numbers 4 and 10) had an increased variability in heart rate and the third (number 9) had a reduced variability in heart rate.

The results of the spectral analysis of the 4 data series showed that the frequency range 0.25–2.25 cycles/hr described in excess of 65% of the variance in each of the data series in each of the age groups studied. No significant difference was found ($p > 0.05$) between the SIDS cases and the control group in either the total power or in the percentage of the

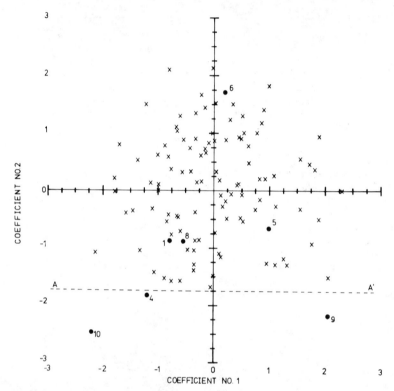

FIGURE 8. Plot of the first coefficient against the second coefficient for the principal-components analysis of the PDFs of the heart-rate variability data series from SIDS cases (●) and control infants (X) at 6 weeks of age, showing a separation of values at AA′ (**dashed line**). (Reprinted from V. Stevens *et al.*,[14] with permission from *Pediatric Research.*)

power described in the frequency range of 0.25–2.25 cycles/hr for any of the 4 data series in any of the 3 age groups studied.

The results for the spectral analysis of the average TIBB data series are given in TABLE 4. These showed no significant differences between SIDS cases and controls in any of the frequency bands studied for infants at 1 and 3 weeks of age. For infants at 6 weeks of age, the power in the 0.25–0.75 cycle/hr band was found to be significantly lower in the SIDS cases ($p < 0.01$), whilst the power in the 1.75–2.25 cycle/hr frequency band was found to be significantly higher ($p < 0.01$). FIGURES 10 and 11 give the percentage of power in

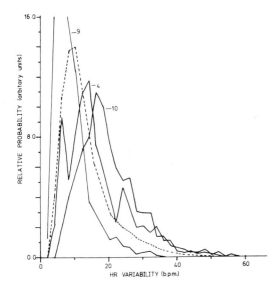

FIGURE 9. Plot of the mean probability density function curve for the heart-rate variability data series for the 6-week control group (**dashed line**) and for the 3 SIDS cases (numbers 4, 9, and 10: **solid lines**) lying below line AA′ in FIGURE 8 (Reprinted from V. Stevens *et al.*,[14] with permission from *Pediatric Research.*)

the average TIBB data series for the frequency ranges of 0.25–0.75 cycles/hr and 1.75–2.25 cycles/hr, respectively, for the individual SIDS cases and the control subjects. From FIGURE 10 it can be seen that all the SIDS cases, with the exception of infant number 10, have a low percentage power in the 0.25–0.75 cycles/hr band for the 6-week age range, whilst this infant, along with the other SIDS cases, has a higher power in the 1.75–2.25 cycle/hr band (FIG. 11) for the 6-week age group.

The results from the spectral analysis of the TIBB variability data series can be seen in TABLE 5. From these results it can be seen that there are no significant differences between SIDS cases and controls in the power in any frequency band at any of the postnatal ages studied.

From results of the spectral analysis of the average heart-rate data series, given in

TABLE 4. Spectral Analysis of the Average TIBB Data Series for SIDS Cases and Control Groups

	Mean % Power in Average TIBB for Frequency Range			
Postnatal Age	0.25–0.75 cycles/hr	0.75–1.25 cycles/hr	1.25–1.75 cycles/hr	1.75–2.25 cycles/hr
1-Week group				
Controls	41.4	25.3	11.0	4.7
SIDS cases	47.2[a]	22.3[a]	9.5[a]	4.1[a]
3-Week group				
Controls	46.1	22.0	8.8	4.1
SIDS cases	49.6[a]	15.9[b]	9.2[a]	4.8[a]
6-Week group				
Controls	48.7	23.5	8.5	3.6
SIDS cases	38.6[c]**	27.5[a]	9.4[a]	5.9[c]**

[a]$p > 0.1$, Wilcoxon rank sum test.
[b]$p < 0.1$, Wilcoxon rank sum test.
[c]**$p < 0.01$, Wilcoxon rank sum test.

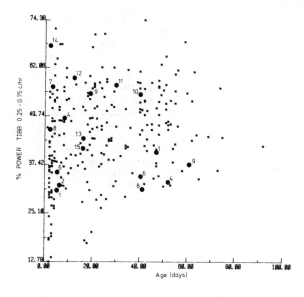

FIGURE 10. Scatter plot for the percentage of power in the 0.25–0.75 cycle/hr (c/hr.) frequency band for the average TIBB data series versus postnatal age of SIDS cases (●) and control subjects (■).

TABLE 6, it can be seen that there is no significant difference between the SIDS cases and the controls for infants at 1 and 6 weeks of age. For infants at 3 weeks of age, the power in the frequency band of 1.25–1.75 cycles/hr was significantly lower in the SIDS cases than in the control group ($p < 0.01$). The power was not significantly higher in the SIDS cases in any of the other 3 frequency bands within that age group. A scatter plot showing the percentage of power in the 1.75–2.25 cycle/hr band for the individual SIDS cases and the control subjects is given in FIGURE 12.

The results from the spectral analysis of the heart-rate variability (HRV) data series

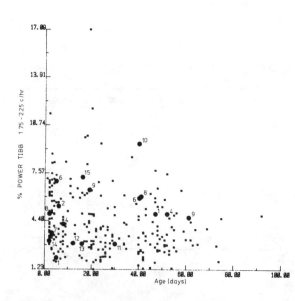

FIGURE 11. Scatter plot for the percentage of power in the 1.75–2.25 cycle/hr (c/hr.) frequency band for the average TIBB data series versus postnatal age of SIDS cases (●) and control subjects (■).

TABLE 5. Spectral Analysis of the TIBB Variability Data Series for SIDS Cases and Control Groups

	Mean % Power in TIBB Variability for Frequency Range			
Postnatal Age	0.25–0.75 cycles/hr	0.75–1.25 cycles/hr	1.25–1.75 cycles/hr	1.75–2.25 cycles/hr
1-Week group				
Controls	26.4	26.7	13.9	7.3
SIDS cases	29.9^a	26.4^b	12.8^b	7.7^b
3-Week group				
Controls	24.0	25.3	15.6	7.7
SIDS cases	22.5^b	31.0^a	12.8^a	8.5^b
6-Week group				
Controls	22.1	31.0	15.9	7.3
SIDS cases	24.9^b	26.2^b	12.4^c	8.3^b

$^a p < 0.1$, Wilcoxon rank sum test.
$^b p > 0.1$, Wilcoxon rank sum test.
$^c p < 0.05$, Wilcoxon rank sum test.

given in TABLE 7 indicate that there are no significant differences between the SIDS cases and controls for infants at 3 and 6 weeks of age. However, for infants at 1 week of age, the power in the 1.25–1.75 cycle/hr frequency band is significantly reduced in the SIDS cases when compared with the controls, but is not significantly increased in any of the other bands. FIGURE 13 shows a scatter plot of the percentage of power in the 1.25–1.75 cycle/hr band of the HRV data series for the individual SIDS cases and the control subjects.

CONCLUSIONS

In this paper we have reported the analysis of average heart rate (HRA), heart-rate variability (HRV), average time interval between breaths (TIBBA) and variability of the time interval between breaths (TIBBV) data series measured for 100-sec, non-overlapping time epochs over a 24-hr period in SIDS cases and control subjects. Three different types of analysis have been independently applied to these 4 data series. Firstly, the mean value

TABLE 6. Spectral Analysis of the Average Heart-Rate Data Series for SIDS Cases and Control Groups

	Mean % Power in Average Heart Rate for Frequency Range			
Postnatal Age	0.25–0.75 cycles/hr	0.75–1.25 cycles/hr	1.25–1.75 cycles/hr	1.75–2.25 cycles/hr
1-Week group				
Controls	50.0	18.3	7.9	4.1
SIDS cases	51.5^a	18.2^a	7.5^a	4.0^a
3-Week group				
Controls	51.7	17.0	8.2	4.3
SIDS cases	54.4^a	18.0^a	5.0^{b**}	3.8^a
6-Week group				
Controls	51.3	17.4	7.7	4.2
SIDS cases	48.9^a	19.2^a	8.4^a	4.2^a

$^a p > 0.1$, Wilcoxon rank sum test.
$^{b}**p < 0.01$, Wilcoxon rank sum test.

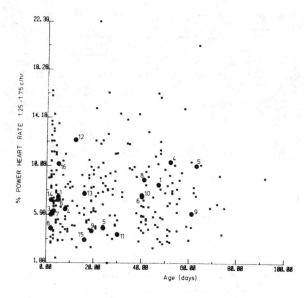

FIGURE 12. Scatter plot for the percentage of power in the 1.25–1.75 cycle/hr (c/hr.) frequency band for the average heart-rate data series versus postnatal age of SIDS cases (●) and control subjects (■).

of each of the data series was determined and the values obtained compared between SIDS cases and control subjects. This showed a significantly elevated mean HRA in the SIDS cases, but no significant difference was found in the mean value of any of the other data series. Secondly, the probability density function for each of the data series was constructed and a principal-components factor analysis showed that 3 SIDS cases studied at 6 weeks of age had significantly different heart-rate variability patterns compared to the age-matched control subjects. Finally, a spectral analysis of each of the 4 data series showed that the SIDS cases at 6 weeks of age had a significantly reduced power for the TIBBA data series in the 0.25–0.75 cycle/hr frequency band with a significantly

TABLE 7. Spectral Analysis of the Average Heart-Rate Variability Data Series for SIDS Cases and Control Groups

	Mean % Power in Heart-Rate Variability for Frequency Range			
Postnatal Age	0.25–0.75 cycles/hr	0.75–1.25 cycles/hr	1.25–1.75 cycles/hr	1.75–2.25 cycles/hr
1-Week group				
Controls	23.9	24.8	14.4	7.0
SIDS cases	26.0[a]	28.3[b]	10.1[c**]	6.9[a]
3-Week group				
Controls	22.4	27.0	15.0	6.9
SIDS cases	22.2[a]	28.4[a]	13.5[a]	7.9[a]
6-Week group				
Controls	21.9	29.0	14.3	6.8
SIDS cases	19.3[a]	30.5[a]	13.5[a]	8.3[d]

[a] $p > 0.1$, Wilcoxon rank sum test.
[b] $p < 0.1$, Wilcoxon rank sum test.
[c**] $p < 0.01$, Wilcoxon rank sum test.
[d] $p < 0.05$, Wilcoxon rank sum test.

increased power in the 1.75–2.25 cycle/hr frequency band. The SIDS cases also had significantly reduced power in the HRA data series for the 1.25–1.75 cycle/hr frequency band for infants at 3 weeks of age and significantly reduced power in the same frequency band of the HRV data series for infants at 1 week of age. Thus there are statistically significant differences in the heart-rate and respiratory-rate patterns in 24-hr recordings obtained from infants who subsequently suffered SIDS compared to control subjects. However, these differences are group differences and are not of sufficient magnitude to provide a discriminant for those infants who subsequently died. For the mean values of the 4 data series, we have previously shown that the number of SIDS cases where the mean values are at the extremes of the distribution for the control group are not sufficient to develop a discriminant based on these measures.[12] The probability density function analysis did provide a separation of 3 infants who subsequently suffered SIDS at 6 weeks of age. Of these 3 infants, only infant number 10 had a mean value for the HRV data

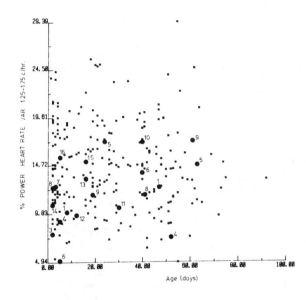

FIGURE 13. Scatter plot for the percentage of power in the 1.25–1.75 cycle/hr (c/hr.) frequency band for the heart-rate variability data series versus postnatal age of SIDS cases (●) and control subjects (■).

series which was near the extreme of the values found in the control group. Infants number 4 and 9, however, did have values which were near the extremes of the distribution for the mean values of the HRA data series.

For the spectral analysis of the TIBBA data series for infants at 6 weeks of age, all the SIDS cases, with the exception of SIDS case number 10, were near the lower extreme values in the control group for the power in the 0.25–0.75 cycle/hr frequency band. All the SIDS cases were near the upper extreme of the values in the control group for the power in the 1.75–2.25 cycle/hr band for infants at 6 weeks of age. However, these differences once again represent group differences and are not of sufficient magnitude to form the basis of a discriminant function for those infants who would subsequently die. The SIDS cases also had a significantly reduced power in the 1.25–1.75 cycle/hr band for the spectral analysis of the HRV data series for infants at 1 week of age. No significant differences were detected in any of the other 3 frequency bands in the analysis of the HRV data series. Since no significant difference was found between the SIDS cases and controls for the total power in the HRV data series for infants within the 1-week age group, the power in the remaining 3 frequency bands must have tended to be higher in the SIDS cases without attaining a statistically significant difference. This trend can be seen in TABLE 7. Once again, this is a group difference, and the magnitude of the difference is not sufficient to provide a discriminant for those infants who subsequently suffered SIDS. The final significant difference found between the SIDS cases and the control groups was that the power in the 1.25–1.75 cycle/hr band of the spectral analysis of the HRA data series was lower in the SIDS cases for infants at 3 weeks of age. No significant differences were detected in any of the other 3 frequency bands of the spectral analysis of the HRA data series for infants at 3 weeks of age. Since there was no significant difference in the total power in the HRA data series between SIDS cases and controls for infants at 3 weeks of age, the power in the remaining 3 frequency bands must have tended to be higher in the SIDS cases without attaining a statistically significant difference. This trend can be seen in TABLE 6. Once again, this difference is a group difference and does not provide a method of identifying those infants who subsequently suffered SIDS.

The second objective in analyzing the cardiorespiratory data from the prospective study into SIDS was to determine whether the magnitude and pattern of any group differences provided a method for predicting which infants were to subsequently suffer SIDS. Although some infants appear as "outliers" on the scatter plots, the total number of SIDS cases available for analysis was small and therefore care must be taken in making predictions. Since no systematic pattern emerged in considering the statistical differences, it is our conclusion that this analysis does not provide a method of predicting those infants who would subsequently suffer SIDS.

One of the major factors affecting heart-rate and breathing patterns in infants is sleep. One of the problems in interpreting the results that we have reported is that they have not taken into account the effects of sleep. The measurements were made on recordings containing only the ECG and respiratory waveform. In order to assign a sleep stage to the data formally, it is necessary to have recordings that contain the EEG, electro-oculogram, and electromyogram. Harper and his co-workers[15] have recently developed a technique for assigning sleep stage to recordings containing only the ECG and respiration pattern. Using this system on the same recordings of the same SIDS cases reported in this paper, they have shown that there is no difference in time spent in different sleep states between the SIDS cases and a control group.[15] Therefore the results we report cannot be due to the effects of sleep.

Perhaps the most interesting of all the differences we have reported is the significantly increased mean heart rate in the SIDS cases, which is particularly prominent during the first week of life, and the decreased power in the SIDS cases in the 1.25–1.75 cycle/hr band of the heart-rate variability during the first week of life. The 1.25–1.75 cycle/hr band, together with the 0.75–1.25 cycle/hr band, covers the frequency range associated with REM (rapid eye movement)/non-REM sleep cycles. These findings may be of many origins, and the current data are not adequate to investigate them fully. However, one possibility is that there is a difference in the lung mechanics between infants who suffer SIDS and control subjects. If this were the case, then differences in the mean respiratory rate (mean TIBBA) and respiratory-rate variability (mean TIBBV), together with differences in the PDFs of these data series, would have been expected, since these are sensitive to changes in lung mechanics.[16] Therefore, we feel that our results are unlikely to be due to differences in lung mechanics. A second possibility is that the differences are of a central origin. If there was a significant difference between SIDS cases and controls in all the data series in the frequency bands associated with REM/non-REM sleep-cycle changes, it would suggest that there was a major disturbance in the sleep rhythm of the infants who subsequently suffered SIDS. However, this was not found, and, therefore, the findings suggest that there may be some difference in central cardiorespiratory control during sleep. Yet another possibility is that the infants who suffer SIDS have more body movements which would give rise to the differences reported. At 3 weeks of age, the power in the 1.25–1.75 cycle/hr band is significantly reduced in the SIDS cases in the average heart-rate data series but not in the heart-rate variability data series. This finding, too, supports the concept that there may either be a difference in central cardiorespiratory control during sleep or that there are more body movements in the infants who subsequently suffered SIDS. At 6 weeks of age, there was a reduced power in the TIBBA data series at 0.25–0.75 cycles/hr with an increased power in the frequency range 1.75–2.25 cycles/hr. The power in the lower of these two frequency bands results from respiratory-rate changes associated with feeding, whilst the power in the second of these two frequency bands is at the first harmonic of the REM/non-REM sleep-cycle changes. From TABLE 4 it can be seen that in the control group the power in the band associated with feeding tends to increase during the first 6 weeks of life whilst the power in the 1.75–2.25 cycles/hr band tends to decrease. The SIDS cases show the reverse of this trend. This difference may arise because of a different rate of maturation in the SIDS cases than in the control subjects. Three of the 6 SIDS cases also had significantly different heart-rate variability patterns at 6 weeks of age. It may be that these are yet another manifestation of either deficient central cardiorespiratory control or the presence of more body movements in the subsequent victims of SIDS. The fact that the significant differences we have reported are found in different measures at different postnatal ages may reflect changes in cardiorespiratory control with age. As yet there is insufficient data to investigate this possibility further.

The third question raised in analyzing the data from the prospective study was: If there are statistically significant differences between the SIDS cases and control subjects, are there patterns in these differences which suggest a possible mechanism or mechanisms for SIDS? The findings described suggest that there may be differences in either central cardiorespiratory control or in the level of activity of infants who subsequently die of SIDS. Most important of all is that some of these findings occur in the very early part of life, which suggests that a physiological disturbance exists from birth, which is several weeks or months before the majority of SIDS cases occur. Therefore, we need to investigate the patterns of sleep in normal infants and in infants with a variety of known pathologies to determine what maturational changes occur in cardiorespiratory control during sleep and what their effects are on the respiratory and heart-rate patterns we have studied, in order to be able to interpret more adequately the findings described in this paper.

REFERENCES

1. VALDES-DAPENA, M. A. 1980. Sudden infant death syndrome: A review of the medical literature 1974–1979. Pediatrics **66:** 597–614.
2. FRANKS, C. I., J. B. G. WATSON, B. H. BROWN & E. F. FOSTER. 1980. Respiratory patterns and risk of sudden unexpected death in infancy. Arch. Dis. Child. **55:** 595–599.
3. KELLY, D. H., D. C. SHANNON & K. O'CONNELL. 1978. Care of infants with near miss sudden infant death syndrome. Pediatrics **61:** 511–514.
4. SOUTHALL, D. P., J. M. RICHARDS, P. G. B. JOHNSTON, M. DE SWIET & E. A. SHINEBOURNE. 1980. 24 hour tape recordings of ECG and respiration in the newborn infant with findings related to sudden death and unexplained brain damage in infancy. Arch. Dis. Child. **55:** 7–16.
5. STEINSCHNEIDER, A. 1972. Prolonged apnoea and the sudden infant death syndrome: Clinical and laboratory observations. Pediatrics **50:** 646–654.
6. LEISTNER, H. L., G. G. HADDAD, R. A. EPSTEIN, T. L. LAI, M. A. EPSTEIN & R. B. MELLINS. 1980. Heart rate and heart rate variability during sleep in aborted sudden infant death syndrome. J. Pediatr. **97:** 51–55.

7. HOPPENBROUWERS, T., J. E. HODGMAN, D. J. McGINTY, R. M. HARPER & M. B. STERMAN. 1980. Sudden infant death syndrome: Sleep apnoea and respiration in subsequent siblings. Pediatrics **66:** 205–214.

8. HARPER, R. M., B. LEAKE, T. HOPPENBROUWERS, M. B. STERMAN, D. J. McGINTY & J. HODGMAN. 1978. Polygraphic studies of normal infants and infants at risk for the sudden infant death syndrome: Heart rate and variability as a function of state. Pediatr. Res. **12:** 778–785.

9. MULTICENTRE STUDY GROUP. 1983. Identification of infants destined to die unexpectedly during infancy: Evaluation of predictive importance of prolonged apnoea and disorders of cardiac rhythm and conduction. Br. Med. J. **286:** 1092–1096.

10. WILSON, A. J. & C. I. FRANKS. 1982. The Sheffield respiration analysis system. IEE Proc. (London) Part A. **129:** 702–706.

11. HARPER, R. M., T. HOPPENBROUWERS, M. B. STERMAN, D. J. McGINTY & J. HODGEMAN. 1976. Polygraphic studies of normal infants during the first six months of life. I. Heart rate and variability as a function of state. Pediatr. Res. **10:** 945–951.

12. WILSON, A. J., V. STEVENS, C. I. FRANKS, J. ALEXANDER & D. P. SOUTHALL. 1985. Respiratory and heart rate patterns in infants destined to be victims of sudden infant death syndrome: Average rates and variabilities measured over 24 hours. Br. Med. J. **290:** 497–501.

13. STEVENS, V., A. J. WILSON, D. P. SOUTHALL & C. I. FRANKS. Techniques for the analysis of long term cardio-respiratory recordings from infants. Med. Biol. Eng. Comput. In press.

14. STEVENS, V., A. J. WILSON, D. P. SOUTHALL, D. C. BARBER & C. I. FRANKS. 1985. Analysis of heart rate and breathing patterns of infants destined to suffer SIDS: Probability density function analysis. Pediatr. Res. **19:** 1327–1332.

15. SCHECHTMAN, V. L., R. M. HARPER, K. A. KLUGE, A. J. WILSON, H. J. HOFFMANN & D. P. SOUTHALL. Cardiac and respiratory patterns in normal infants and victims of SIDS. Sleep. In press.

16. SELSTAM, U. 1975. The rate of ventilation as a basis for evaluating respiratory patterns in the neonatal period. Research report. Department of Pediatrics, University of Goteborg. Goteborg, Sweden.

Seizure-Induced Apnea

N. MONOD,[a] P. PEIRANO,[a,b,f] P. PLOUIN,[b,c]
B. STERNBERG,[d] AND C. BOUILLE[e]

[a]Hôpital Port Royal, [b]INSERM U-29, [c]Hôpital Saint Vincent de Paul,
and [d]Hôpital International de l'Université de Paris, Paris, France,
and [e]Hôpital Longjumeau, Longjumeau, France

INTRODUCTION

The frequency of apneic seizures (AS) is closely age-related. Newborns show a higher frequency of AS as compared to infants > 1 month old, and AS are rarely observed after the neonatal period.

Dreyfus-Brisac et al.,[1] in a polygraphic study of 121 cases of neonatal seizures, reported that the most common events during electrical discharges are motor (28%) and respiratory (25%) phenomena. They remarked that these events cannot be recognized as seizures in the absence of simultaneous EEG or polygraphic data.

In the present report, we present 5 cases of full-term infants with AS, without antecedents of acute fetal distress or cerebral anoxia, using EEG or polygraphic recordings (FIG. 1).

CASE REPORTS

Case 1 was a boy born at Port Royal Hospital at 38 weeks of gestation, after a materno-fetal infection, and weighing 3,200 g. The Apgar score was 9 at 1 min and 10 at 5 min. There was no family history of epileptic disorders. At 4 hr of life, he presented the first episodes of cyanosis. The clinical examination showed a full-term infant with a normal appearance, but repetitive cyanotic attacks requiring stimulation were observed. The cerebrospinal fluid (CSF) was red in the 3 samples examined. Apnea appeared every 5 min, with clonic eyeball movements. No other convulsive clinical manifestation was observed. The polygraphic recording during quiet sleep showed an electrical seizure in the right temporal area consisting of delta waves or slow spikes at around 2 Hz, associated with apnea and cyanosis (without bradycardia) lasting for 16 min and requiring assisted ventilation (FIGS. 2–6). Treatment with phenobarbital (2 cg/kg) was started. He did not experience any other apneic and/or convulsive episodes. The CT scan was normal.

Case 2 was a girl born after an uncomplicated pregnancy and delivery. She was a full-term newborn with a birthweight of 4,015 g. The Apgar score was 9 at 1 min and 10 at 5 min. There was no family history of epilepsy. At 2 months of age, after an acute rhinopharyngitis, the mother observed attacks of cyanosis on the lips and extremities of the infant after each bottle-feeding, followed by several seconds of hypotonia while the baby was awake. She was hospitalized at the age of 2.5 months. The clinical examination showed a normal and eutrophic infant, but at the end of the examination an episode of

[f]To whom correspondence should be addressed at: INSERM U-29, Hôpital Port Royal, 123, Bd. Port Royal, Paris 75014, France.

cyanosis and hypotonia lasting for 10 sec was observed. The EEG recording obtained immediately after this event was normal. The EEG recording performed on the next day showed an electrical seizure in the right temporal area, which occurred simultaneously with apnea and cyanosis (FIGS. 7–9). Treatment with phenobarbital was started and the seizure stopped. The CT scan showed a hypodensity of the right temporo-occipital area. The angiography did not reveal any element suggesting a vascular pathology.

After several attacks of apnea with cyanosis, hypotonia, and fixed gaze, the anticonvulsive treatment was changed to carbamazepine with good results. At 8 months of age, the infant showed a normal clinical and psychomotor development. The CT scan

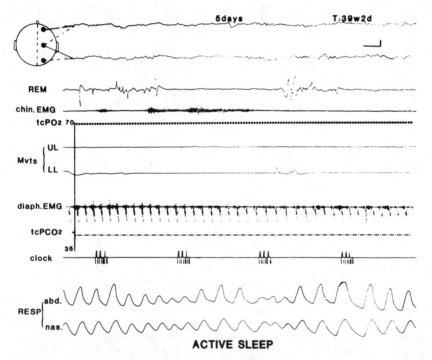

FIGURE 1. Example of a polygraphic tracing of active sleep in a normal full-term newborn aged 5 days. REM, rapid eye movements; chin. EMG, chin electromyogram; tcPO$_2$, transcutaneous oxygen tension (mm Hg); Mvts UL & LL, movements of the upper and lower limbs; diaph. EMG, diaphragmatic electromyogram; tcPCO$_2$, transcutaneous carbon dioxide tension (mm Hg); clock, binary clock; RESP abd. & nas., abdominal and nasal respiration.

revealed an opaque mass in the right temporoparietal area. Surgery revealed a malignant mixed sarcoma and a gliosic tumor. The infant died during the early postsurgical period.

Case 3 was a full-term boy born normally after an uneventful pregnancy. The neonatal period was uncomplicated. There was no family history of epilepsy. At the age of 3 weeks of life, he manifested several episodes of apnea with a bluish colour. The polygraphic recording during active sleep showed an electrical seizure in the left temporo-occipital area, consisting of slow spikes at around 3–4 Hz, associated with a 2-min apnea, preceded by periodic breathing. There was no cardiac activity change or other clinical manifestation of seizure. Phenobarbital treatment was initiated, and 2 months later no other seizure or apneic episode was observed. The cerebral echography and CT scan were normal.

Case 4 was a full-term boy born after a pregnancy with threatened premature delivery. The amniotic fluid was colored. The Apgar score at 1 min of life was 9 and at 5 min was 10. There was no family history of epilepsy. The neonate was normal until the fifth day of life, when he presented a clinical left hemiconvulsion, followed by atonia. The polygraphic recording showed several episodes of apnea lasting for 20 to 120 sec occurring during active sleep and electrical seizures that occurred during quiet sleep. The interictal EEG tracing showed predominantly rhythmic theta waves. These seizures, as well as apnea, were completely controlled with phenobarbital treatment. The day following the incident, the polygraphic recording did not show any EEG or respiratory abnormality. Follow-up at the ages of 2 and 4 yr showed a child with a completely normal development.

Case 5 was a boy born at 40 weeks of gestation, after an uncomplicated pregnancy and delivery, and weighing 4,000 g. The Apgar score was 10 at 1 and 5 min. There was no family history of epilepsy. The first day of life he presented an episode of cyanosis followed by hypotonia for some minutes, after which the clinical examination was completely normal. The fifth day of life, another episode of cyanosis associated with apnea, bradycardia and hypotonia was observed. The EEG recording obtained immediately was normal. The TOGD examination showed an antral dyskinesia without gastroesophageal reflux. Antireflux treatment was started. At the age of 2.5 months, he was hospitalized for prolonged attacks of generalized cyanosis, apnea, ocular revulsion, and hypotonia. The EEG recording, as well as the ECG, Holter recording, oculocardiac reflex, echocardiography, CT scan, and esophagoscopy were normal. The polygraphic recording performed on the next day showed during active sleep an electrical seizure in the left occipital area, consisting of alpha waves, associated with apnea and cyanosis (without bradycardia or other clinical manifestation), lasting for 1 min and requiring stimulation (FIG. 10). Treatment with depakine (30 mg/kg) was started and the seizure stopped. Three months after the beginning of the anticonvulsive treatment, no other seizure or apneic episode was detected.

COMMENT

This report confirms that apneic episodes during infancy which occur as a manifestation of partial seizures require prolonged and repeated EEG or polygraphic recordings for their diagnosis. It is well known that apnea is a common phenomenon in premature and full-term sick newborns with various underlying disorders and that polygraphic recordings are mandatory for its differential diagnosis.

During the neonatal period, antecedents of acute fetal distress or cerebral anoxia are often observed in cases of AS.[1-4] In our population, as well as in the cases reported by Watanabe *et al.*,[5] most pregnancies, deliveries, and neonatal periods were uncomplicated. There is agreement that respiratory phenomena are the most common critical events during electrical seizures in the neonatal period. However, their incidence varies according to different authors: 25% for Dreyfus-Brisac *et al.*[1] and Torricelli *et al.*,[4] 18% for Giroud *et al.*,[3] and 6% for Watanabe *et al.*[2] These disagreements may be due to the populations studied. Dreyfus-Brisac *et al.*[1] included a great number (40/121) of premature

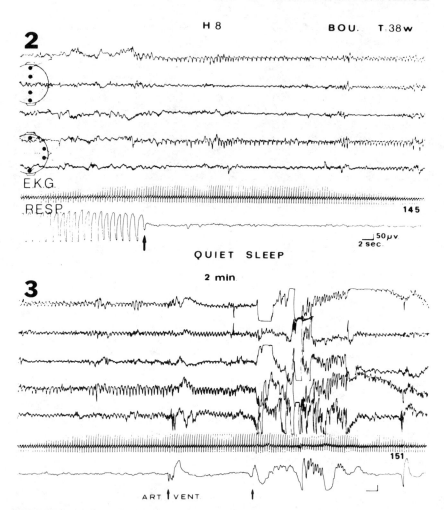

FIGURES 2–6. Polygraphic tracing of quiet sleep in the full-term infant of Case 1, aged 8 hr. See FIGURE 2 for identification of individual tracings. (**2,** *top panel*) Beginning of a seizure in the right temporal area. **Arrow** (*bottom tracing*) indicates the start of the apnea. E.K.G., electrocardiogram (heart rate: 145 beats/min); RESP., respiration. (**3,** *bottom panel*) The second minute of the apneic seizure. Slow artifacts in respiratory and EEG activity involve artifacts of mechanical ventilation (some of them are indicated by **arrows,** ART. VENT.). Heart rate: 151 beats/min. (**4,** *facing page, top panel*) The ninth minute of the apneic seizure. Heart rate: 152 beats/min. (**5,** *facing page, center panel*) The thirteenth minute of the apneic seizure. Heart rate: 166 beats/min. (**6,** *facing page, bottom panel*) The end of the apneic seizure at 16 min and the renewal of autonomous respiratory activity. Heart rate: 151 beats/min.

infants (even those receiving mechanical ventilation) and remarked that most cases were selected from a group with neonatal anoxia or asphyxia. Watanabe *et al.*[2] studied a population of 326 newborns and found 21 cases presenting AS (only 2 cases were premature infants). However, they reported that it was difficult to determine the overall

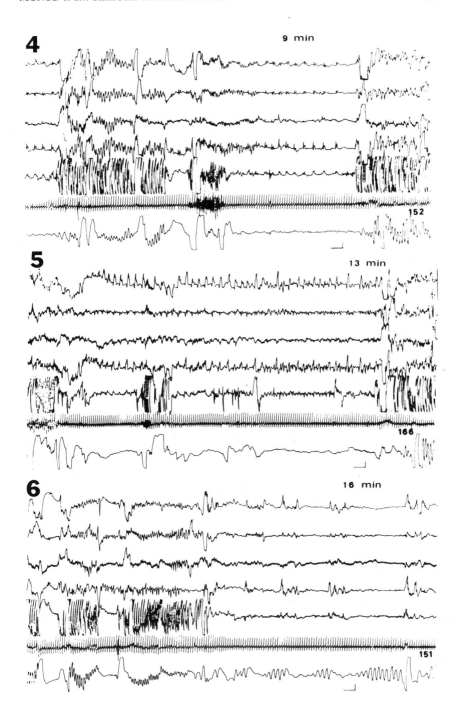

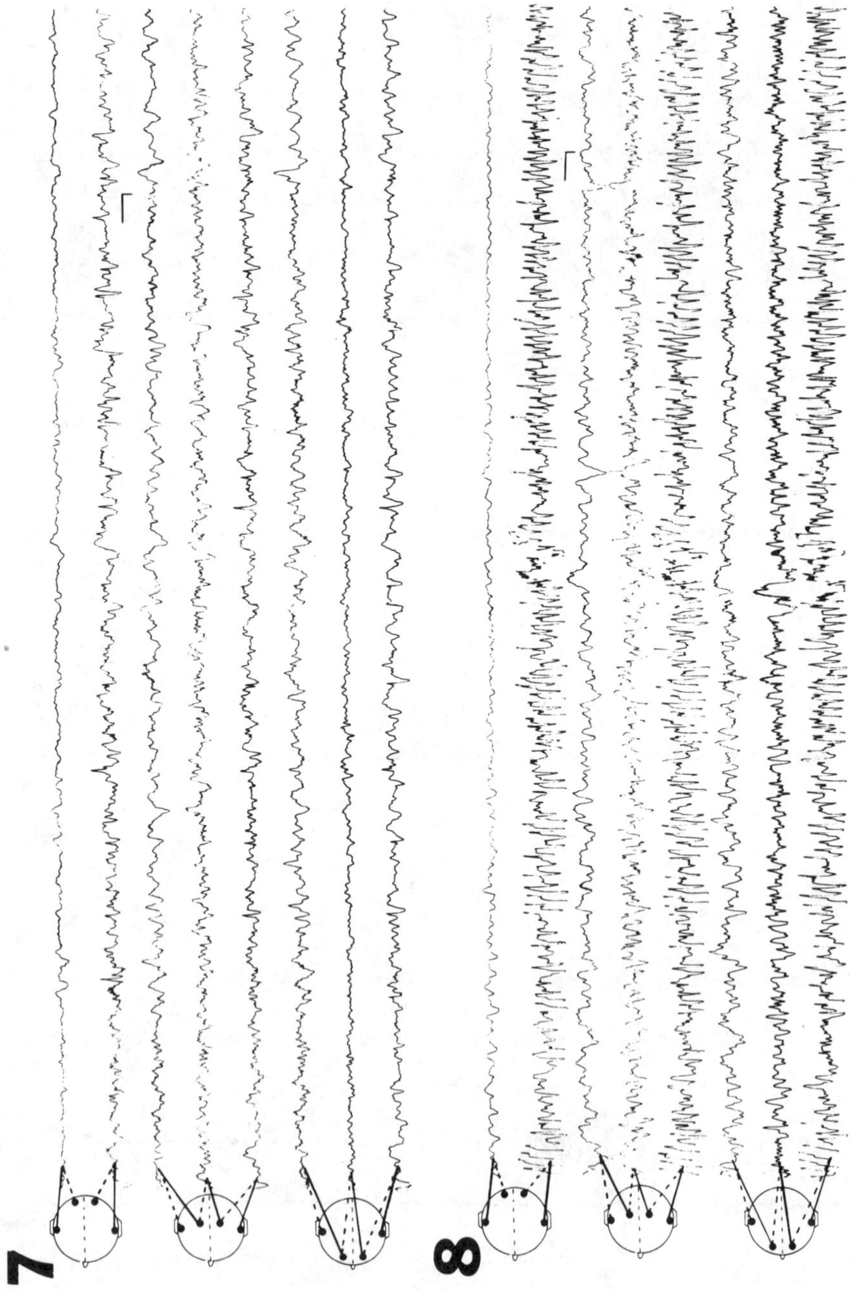
7
8

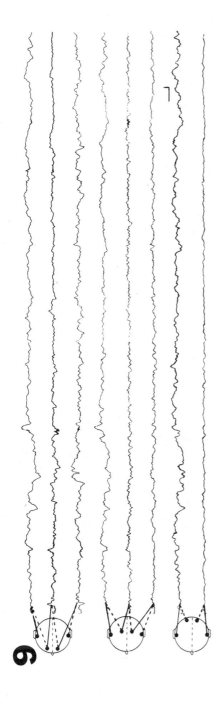

FIGURES 7–9. EEG recording in the full-term infant of Case 2, aged 2.5 months, (**7**, *top panel*) at 3 min before the beginning of a seizure; (**8**, *center panel*) during an electrical seizure in the right temporal area which occurred simultaneously with apnea and cyanosis; and (**9**, *bottom panel*) 3 min after the end of the seizure.

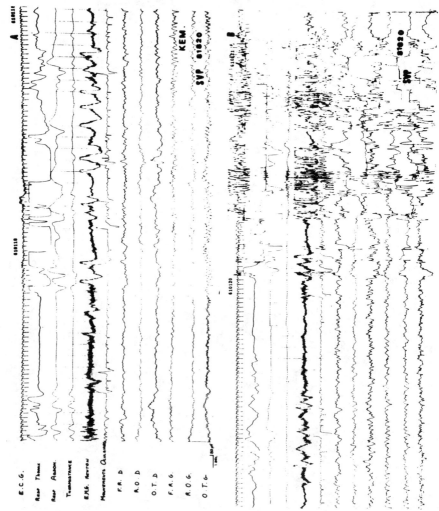

FIGURE 10. Polygraphic recording of active sleep in infant of Case 5 showing an electrical seizure in the left occipital area consisting of alpha waves associated with apnea and cyanosis. Lower panel is a continuation of the tracings in the upper panel. E.C.G. = electrocardiogram; RESP THORAX = thoracic respiration; RESP ABDOM. = abdominal respiration; THERMISTANCE = nasal respiration; E.M.G. MENTON = chin electromyogram; MOUVEMENTS OCULAIRES = rapid eye movements; F.R.D. = right fronto-central area; R.O.D. = right centro-occipital area; O.T.D. = right occipitotemporal area; F.R.G. = left frontocentral area; R.O.G. = left centro-occipital area; O.T.G. = left occipitotemporal area.

incidence of AS because not all newborns with apneic episodes were subjected to polygraphic examinations. Giroud *et al.*[3] found 6 newborns (4 full-term and 2 premature) presenting AS, in a population of 148 newborns with neonatal apnea during the first month of life. These cases represented 4% of the neonatal apnea population and 18% of the population exhibiting neonatal seizures. Torricelli *et al.*[4] studied 12 full-term newborns presenting early status epilepticus (within the first 5 days of life).

It has been reported that AS rarely last longer than 10 sec.[3] Watanabe *et al.*[2] reported that those lasting more than 20 sec were the exception rather than the rule during the neonatal period, and they usually lasted 1 to 2 min (characterized by respiratory embarrassment rather than complete arrest) during infancy.[5] However, we have recorded polygraphically an AS lasting for 16 min in which the only clinical manifestation was the apnea. Interestingly, this AS was not associated with variation in the heart rate. Watanabe *et al.*[5] described heart-rate variation in AS lasting longer than 1 min, and San Marti (personal communication) reported that ECG variations such as tachycardia, low amplitude and morphological variations of the QRS complex exist only during long AS. Fenichel *et al.*[6] stated that prolonged apneic spells without bradycardia suggest the possibility of a convulsion.

Watanabe *et al.*[2] reported that in most cases it was not possible to determine in which state of sleep AS occurred. However, they remarked that AS never occurs during quiet sleep. Nevertheless, some of our AS cases occurred during quiet sleep.

The ictal discharge often occurred initially in the temporal area, suggesting the origin of AS in the limbic system. This finding agrees with results previously reported in animal as well as in clinical studies (references in Kaada & Jasper,[7] Nelson *et al.*,[8] and Watanabe *et al.*[5]).

The relationship between seizures and alphalike EEG rhythm has been previously reported.[9–11] Willis & Gould[12] observed this phenomenon in a single case and Watanabe *et al.*[2] reported that rhythmic alpha waves were the most frequent ictal discharges in their newborns (15/21). Knauss & Carlson[13] studied 13 newborns showing rhythmic alpha-wave discharge on EEG and reported that this discharge was not usually associated with clinical manifestations. Moreover, they mentioned apnea as one of the clinical findings, but they could not correlate it with EEG discharge. In the present study, only one case (Case 5) presented rhythmic alpha-wave discharge associated with apnea.

Kelly *et al.*[14] have described an infant presenting episodes of apnea with cyanosis for whom an ictal EEG recording showed rhythmic 3 to 4 Hz sharp wave activity in the left temporal area. This infant was later found to have a brain tumor (astrocytoma) in the left temporal lobe. One of our infants (Case 2) presenting a similar history was also found to have a brain tumor.

Recently, Davis *et al.*[15] reported 2 infants with near-miss sudden infant death syndrome events exhibiting seizure disorders after caffeine treatment. They suggested that there is a subgroup of infants diagnosed as having near-miss sudden infant death syndrome who have apnea with seizures and that the threshold of these seizures could be lowered by central nervous system stimulants like caffeine. Navelet *et al.*[16] described 3 cases of infants with well-treated gastroesophageal reflux who presented important apneic events associated with cyanosis and bradycardia. These events were diagnosed initially as gastroesophageal reflux accidents; however, electrical or electroclinical seizures were demonstrated by polygraphic recordings. They concluded that initial epileptic disorders may be suspected in infants with well-treated gastroesophageal reflux presenting repetitive apneic events. Therefore, it is very important to detect the cause of apneic episodes so that we will be able to provide a suitable anticonvulsive therapy for those few infants with near-miss SIDS events.

ACKNOWLEDGMENTS

We gratefully acknowledge the valuable technical assistance of Françoise Morel-Kahn. Thanks are due to A. Strickland for reviewing the English.

REFERENCES

1. DREYFUS-BRISAC, C., N. PESCHANSKI, M. F. RADVANYI, F. CUKIER-HEMEURY & N. MONOD. 1981. Convulsions du nouveau-né. Aspects clinique, électrographique, étiopathogenique et pronostique. Rev. E.E.G. Neurophysiol. **11:** 367–378.
2. WATANABE, K., K. HARA, S. MIYAZAKI, S. HAKAMADA & M. KURONAYAGI. 1982. Apneic seizures in the newborn. Am. J. Dis. Child. **136:** 980–984.
3. GIROUD, M., J. B. GOUYON, D. SANDRE, J. L. NIVELON & M. ALISON. 1983. Les apnées épileptiques en période néonatale. Arch. Fr. Pédiatr. **40:** 719–722.
4. TORRICELLI, A., F. FERRARI, A. SFERRAZZA PAPA, R. MANZOTTI, R. CAVALLO, A. BENATTI, A. M. GIUSTARDI, L. CAPPELLA, L. ORI & L. DE CARIS. 1986. Le apnee nelle convulsioni del neonato a termine: Studio preliminare. *In* Le Apnee del Neonato e del Lattante. G. B. Cavazzuti, Ed.: 73–80. Humana Italia. Milan.
5. WATANABE, K., K. HARA, S. HAKAMADA, T. NEGORO, M. SUGIURA, A. MATSUMOTO & M. MAEHARA. 1982. Seizure with apnea in children. Pediatrics **79:** 87–90.
6. FENICHEL, G. M., B. J. OLSON & J. E. FITZPATRICK. 1980. Heart rate changes in convulsive and nonconvulsive apnea. Ann. Neurol. **7:** 577–582.
7. KAADA, B. R. & H. JASPER. 1952. Respiratory responses to stimulation of temporal pole, insula, and hyppocampal and limbic gyri in man. Arch. Neurol. Psychiatry **68:** 601–611.
8. NELSON, D. A., W. DEL & C. D. RAY. 1968. Respiratory arrest from seizure discharges in the limbic system. Arch. Neurol. (Chicago) **19:** 199–207.
9. DREYFUS-BRISAC, C. & N. MONOD. 1964. Electroclinical studies of status epilepticus and convulsions in the newborn. *In* Neurological and electroencephalographic correlative studies in infancy. P. Kellaway & I. Petersen, Eds.: 250–272. Grune & Stratton. New York.
10. SCHULTE, F. J. & U. JÜRGENS. 1969. Apnoen bei reifen und unreifen neugeborenen. Monatsschr. Kinderheilkd. **117:** 595–601.
11. MONOD, N., N. PAJOT & S. GUIDASCI. 1972. The neonatal EEG: Statistical studies and prognostic value in full-term and pre-term babies. Electroencephalog. Clin. Neurophysiol. **32:** 529–544.
12. WILLIS, J. & J. B. GOULD. 1980. Periodic alpha seizures with apnea in a newborn. Develop. Med. Child Neurol. **22:** 214–222.
13. KNAUSS, T. A. & C. B. CARLSON. 1978. Neonatal paroxysmal monorhythmic alpha activity. Arch. Neurol. (Chicago) **35:** 104–107.
14. KELLY, D. H., K. S. KRISHNAMOORTHY & D. C. SHANNON. 1980. Astrocytoma in an infant with prolonged apnea. Pediatrics **39:** 563–568.
15. DAVIS, J. M., K. METRAKOS & J. V. ARANDA. 1986. Apnoea and seizures. Arch. Dis. Child **61:** 791–793.
16. NAVELET, Y., M. TARDIEU, D. DEVICTOR, P. LANDRIEU & S. FALLEFRANQUE. 1986. Reflux gastro-oesophagien et malaises graves d'origine comitiale. *In* Abstracts of the Réunion du Groupe d'Etude Langue Française de la Mort Subite Inexpliquée du Nourrisson, Lausanne, 12–13 Sept. 1986: 20–21.

Cardiac and Respiratory Mechanisms That Might Be Responsible for Sudden Infant Death Syndrome

Ideas for Future Research

P. FROGGATT,[a] J. B. BECKWITH,[b] P. J. SCHWARTZ,[c]
M. VALDES-DAPENA,[d] AND D. P. SOUTHALL[e,f]

[a]The Queen's University of Belfast
Belfast, Northern Ireland

[b]Department of Pathology
The Children's Hospital
Denver, Colorado 80218

[c]Centro di Fisiologia Clinica e Ipertensione
Istituto Clinica Medica II
Centro SIDS
Università di Milano
Milan, Italy

[d]Department of Pathology
School of Medicine
University of Miami
Miami, Florida 33101

[e]Cardiothoracic Institute
Brompton Hospital
London SW3 6HP
United Kingdom

This international conference sought to piece together what is already known and what should be determined concerning the possible role of cardiac and respiratory mechanisms in the pathogenesis of sudden infant death syndrome (SIDS). Selection of the speakers was designed not only to include researchers who had previously or were now actively engaged in research into SIDS, but also eminent physiologists who, through their understanding of basic cardiac, respiratory, and neural mechanisms, could help guide us into directions likely to further our progress in determining underlying mechanisms.

The meeting covered a period of 4 days and was based upon relatively short presentations followed by long periods of discussion. On the fourth day, a series of workshops was held to allow the presenters from the first 3 days of the meeting and their

[f]Address correspondence to D. P. Southall.

associate researchers to discuss and formulate some form of consensus on 4 questions. The statement below represents our own attempt to summarize these discussions. The views expressed are therefore not necessarily those of all members of each workshop.

QUESTION 1
How can we best proceed in the identification of infants at risk for SIDS?

This workshop was moderated by Dr. P. Froggatt.

It was felt that with the resources available the "epidemiological" factors so far known to be associated with an increased risk for SIDS, even in combination, are not sufficiently specific or sensitive to identify infants for special treatment. Nevertheless, it was felt that research studies using clinical physiological or biochemical techniques should be performed on infants with certain epidemiological risk factors, especially when these were present in combination. The risk factors considered most important were previous treatment in the neonatal intensive care unit, drug-dependence of the mother during pregnancy, teenage or multiple pregnancy in the mother, and a history of a previous sibling dying suddenly and unexpectedly. In order for any kind of physiological or biochemical study to have an impact on identifying "at-risk" infants, it was felt that the ideal approach would be prospective, without intervention, and would involve large numbers of infants, some of whom would subsequently suffer SIDS, thus allowing their physiological or biochemical data to be compared with surviving control infants or "low" and "high risk." If evidence of their benefit is to be meaningfully demonstrated, it was also felt that intervention programs implemented on the basis of high and low risk status, as identified by epidemiological risk factors alone, *must* consist of controlled studies.

It was also considered that the physiological factors which have to date been reported in association with subsequent SIDS are—like the epidemiological factors—insufficiently specific or sensitive to be used to segregate infants for special treatment. Thus, conventional analyses of breathing patterns (namely, the frequency and duration of apneic pauses or of periodic breathing: the "pneumogram") have not been shown capable of distinguishing subsequent SIDS victims from controls. Increased levels of sinus tachycardia and higher heart rates have been found in subsequent SIDS victims, but before these criteria can be applied, they require validation by further prospective studies. It was felt that the recording of arterial oxygen saturation levels using the new technique of pulse oximetry, combined with analysis of breathing patterns and electrocardiograms, could provide, in a prospective study without intervention, the greatest hope of finding a sensitive and specific physiological predictor for SIDS.

Other recently observed clinical features which become apparent only after the perinatal period may also provide information relevant to prediction of risk. Thus, excessive sweating, certain patterns of infant behavior (possibly including sudden changes in weight), and the presence of respiratory tract infections are situations warranting physiological studies that might enhance identification of the "at-risk" infant.

QUESTION 2
With due regard to the recent consensus statement on home apnea monitoring, what are our views on this activity and on the use of methylxanthine drugs?

This workshop was moderated by Dr. B. Beckwith.

It was felt that in certain countries there is still substantial overuse of home monitoring and that the specific indications for monitoring need better definition. The group fully supported the recommendations of the consensus panel convened by the National Institute of Child Health and Human development.[1]

It was considered by the group that there are major technical limitations to existing monitors with regard to their detection of prolonged hypoxemia or acute reductions in cardiac output. Thus, without some form of oxygen or airflow monitoring they will not identify obstructive or prolonged expiratory apnea. It was considered to be somewhat unethical for monitors to be supplied which did not include a recording device to inform the parents and their physician of the cause of any alarms. An ability to document the pathophysiology leading to an alarm would also provide a better understanding of any underlying potentially harmful events.

A physician must not be pressured into providing a monitor if, in his opinion, it is not indicated. But when he does prescribe such a system, he has a responsibility to explain to the parents its limitations, provide support to the parents, and ensure that they know how to use the monitor and how to resuscitate their baby in the event of a severe apneic event. Since the efficacy of home monitoring has *not* been established, there is no ethical contradiction to a controlled trial of this form of treatment. The control for this study should ideally be the use of a monitor which does not detect apnea but which has randomly occurring alarms at the average frequency of those occurring in the monitor under test.

With regard to methylxanthine preparations, there is considerable evidence of their efficacy in treating apnea of prematurity. However, their value in treating infants with apparent life-threatening events has not been subject to controlled trials. Nor are the changes in breathing patterns which they produce, for example, reduction of periodic breathing on "pneumogram" recordings, of any proven relevance to a decreased subsequent risk of SIDS or of further apparent life-threatening events. Of most importance are the known side effects of methylxanthines, some of which may be harmful or even dangerous. For this latter reason, it was felt that these preparations should not be used in treating infants suffering apparent life-threatening events except as part of research studies subject to the usual scientific principles and accompanied by informed parental consent.

QUESTION 3
What is known concerning the role of various possible cardiac mechanisms in SIDS, and in what directions should we focus our future research in this area?

This workshop was moderated by Dr. P. J. Schwartz.

The group considered that both theoretical considerations and the factual knowledge about SIDS were not opposed to the possibility of primary cardiac death being responsible for a number of SIDS cases.[2] The group felt that the implications of a cardiac mechanism acting in a portion of SIDS cases would be important, if subgroups at high risk could be identified, because sudden cardiac death can often be prevented. The data presented and discussed during the conference indicated that during the first week of life a percentage, yet to be defined with accuracy, of future SIDS victims already had electrocardiographic abnormalities potentially useful for risk stratification. These abnormalities involved a prolongation of the Q–T interval and a reduction of heart rate variability, and both reflect abnormalities in the autonomic control of the heart. Prolongation of the Q–T interval may suggest an imbalance in cardiac sympathetic innervation resulting in inappropriate modulation of ventricular repolarization, while reduced heart rate variability indicates an impairment in cardiac vagal efferent activity. Of relevance to SIDS is the fact that both these abnormalities have been shown to be associated with a markedly increased risk for sudden cardiac death in adults. The group viewed the data gathered in infants who subsequently became SIDS victims as very promising but still numerically insufficient; thus, extension of these studies is encouraged to allow the drawing of firm conclusions.

The absence of adequate information on the cardiac rhythm present at the time of death represents a major limitation for understanding the mechanisms of SIDS in general and for assessing the cardiac hypothesis in particular. The group felt that documentation of the final cardiorespiratory events that cause SIDS is of such importance as to justify even major efforts. One possible approach would be the use of monitors that record and store both respiratory activity and the electrocardiogram with a memory system that allows the recording of the events *preceding* the alarm, which should be triggered not only by cessation of respiration and by profound bradycardia, but also by the onset of ventricular fibrillation. To the group's knowledge, the latter is a critical feature not yet available for commercial cardiorespiratory monitors.

Based on the relative rarity of a SIDS event, large data bases are needed and simple screening techniques should be applied. Centers could be identified for handling data sets, electrocardiograms, 24-hr ECG recordings, etc. of those rare cases of SIDS which had been, by chance, studied before the event. This would progressively make available useful and interpretable material which otherwise would remain entirely anecdotal. The identification of countries whose health-care systems could run a mass screening study would be useful for planning targeted cooperative research projects; this may provide the opportunity for large-scale studies with a reasonable cost-benefit ratio.

The group felt strongly that in order to make progress in ascertaining the role of a cardiac mechanism in SIDS, a series of basic research studies was needed. Two main areas were identified with specific issues enumerated for each:

A. *Autonomic Nervous System*

  1. normal growth and development: afferent and efferent limbs
  2. development of cardiac and cardiovascular reflexes
  3. neurohumoral synthesis, release and reuptake mechanisms
  4. relation to sleep and waking states
  5. central control of autonomic functions
  6. receptor mechanisms
  7. regulatory proteins
  8. effector responses, including sympathetic-parasympathetic interactions

B. *Primary Cardiac Mechanisms*

  1. normal growth and development
  2. cardiac conduction and impulse formation: developmental changes
  3. development of channels and ionic pump mechanisms
  4. metabolic changes
  5. relationship of cardiac and respiratory mechanisms

QUESTION 4

What is known concerning the role of various possible respiratory mechanisms in SIDS, and in what directions should we focus our future research in this area?

This workshop was moderated by Dr. D. P. Southall.

The first possibility considered was obstructive apnea. The presence and characteristic distribution of petechial hemorrhages supports acute airway obstruction at end expiration as a potentially important mechanism for SIDS. However, the petechial hemorrhages also could be adequately explained by prolonged expiratory apnea (see below). There is a need to obtain more data on petechial hemorrhages, perhaps using an animal model or, if technically possible, by studies in the human infant. The presence of deposits of hemosiderin in the lungs of SIDS victims, suggesting previous petechial hemorrhages, is also of importance and needs further study.

The studies of Thach (this volume) and recently reported "death scene" investigations by Bass and colleagues have suggested that accidental suffocation must still be considered a possible cause of SIDS and that the avoidance of this potentially preventable problem must be pursued. The designers of cots must remain aware of this rare cause of SIDS and parents must be warned that, if they have consumed alcohol or any form of sedation, it is dangerous to sleep within the same bed as their baby.

The specter of non-accidental injury, imposed asphyxia, has also to be born in mind, as shown by the studies of Rosen *et al.*[3] and Southall *et al.*;[4] but all the available evidence continues to suggest that this is likely to be only a rare cause of SIDS.

There is a need to learn more about the functional development of the airway musculature and the infant's response to upper airway occlusion, including nasal occlusion, with increasing age. Lung reflexes associated with laryngeal closure, as described at this meeting by Widdicombe (this volume), must also be studied in the human infant. In addition, the possibility that acute airway closure may not be limited to the upper airway, but may occur down to the level of the bronchioles, should be considered in further studies.

Seizure-induced apnea, as described by Monod and by Southall (this volume), was further discussed in the workshop. It was pointed out by Harper that, apart from the direct suppression of inspiratory efforts generated by a seizure in the limbic system, a primary disturbance of cerebral function in certain areas of the brain might also produce a sudden catastrophic disturbance of the respiratory or cardiovascular control system. There is a need to develop non-invasive techniques for studying the electrophysiology of deeper brain structures. There is a need to relate sleep-state organization to cardiorespiratory function and chart its development in infants subsequently suffering SIDS. New techniques involving metabolic scanning may be of value in determining underlying disturbances deep within the brain, and ongoing postmortem studies of central nervous system neurotransmitters within the brain and brain stem may be of value.

Many groups have studied aspects of cardiorespiratory control systems in infants but have usually confined their investigations to one particular aspect of this highly integrated and complex system. There is need to study how, for example, sleep state, thermoregulation, respiratory pattern and cardiovascular function develop as an integrated system during the first 6 months of life. Such a study must first involve recordings of as many variables as possible on healthy, randomly selected, "normal" infants. Only when normal limits have been established will it be advisable to investigate infants at risk of SIDS. Non-invasive techniques for studying certain aspects of the control system, for example, lung reflexes, have yet to be developed. The impact of the environment on these studies must also be considered, for example, ambient temperature, the degree of clothing, etc.

Prolonged expiratory apnea has many characteristics; of most importance are the rapidity of onset and severity of progression of the arterial hypoxemia, which suggest it could play a major role in SIDS. Its relationship to a primary defect in lung surfactant and its associated disturbances of lung reflexes need further research; which may be best pursued by the development of a suitable animal model. Further studies must examine the possible effects of respiratory tract infections on the lung surfactant system and determine how this latter system is modified by autonomic input. There is also a need to develop non-invasive techniques for analyzing the biochemistry and function of lung surfactant from living "normal" infants as well as from those with prolonged expiratory apnea.

As described for possible cardiac mechanisms in Question 3, above, there is a need to document the mode of death in SIDS. Animal models may help, as might appropriately designed monitoring systems which would record all near-fatal or even fatal events so that they could subsequently be analyzed.

Some additional aspects were considered:

Infection, both respiratory and at other sites, appears to be linked with SIDS. More investigators should try to determine whether it plays a direct role, affects arousal from sleep, affects metabolic rate, or acts as a trigger to sudden death.

Conceptual mathematical models might be applied in attempts to unravel the complex interreacting components of cardiorespiratory control. They may allow each step of a potentially catastrophic event to be analyzed (see Southall and Talbert[5] and Fleming *et al.*[6] for examples).

There is a need to find out more about the origin of the pulmonary edema which is found in SIDS. Could this result from a respiratory mechanism, for instance alveolar atelectasis, as in prolonged expiratory apnea or acute upper airway obstruction?

There is also a need to find out whether enzyme deficiencies of the type recently described in SIDS may be acting through some disturbance of respiration, in particular through the surfactant system.

Postmortem studies of the innervation of the lungs may also be of value.

Finally, there is a need to document the repeatability and reproducibility of the tests used to evaluate cardiorespiratory function and, if possible, to standardize what is measured between laboratories, thus allowing the results of different studies to be more appropriately compared.

REFERENCES

1. NATIONAL INSTITUTES OF HEALTH. 1986. Infantile apnea and home monitoring. National Institutes of Health Consensus Development Conference Statement. Vol. 6, No. 6.
2. SCHWARTZ, P. J. 1987. The quest for the mechanisms of the sudden infant death syndrome: doubts and progress. Circulation **75:** 677–683.
3. ROSEN, C. L., J. D. FROST, JR., T. BRICKER, J. D. TARNOW, P. C. GILLETTE & S. DUNLAVY. 1983. Two siblings with recurrent cardiorespiratory arrest: Munchausen syndrome by proxy or child abuse? Pediatrics **71:** 715–720.
4. SOUTHALL, D. P., V. A. STEBBENS, S. V. REES, M. H. LANG, J. O. WARNER & E. A. SHINEBOURNE. 1987. Apnoeic episodes induced by smothering: Two cases identified by covert video surveillance. Br. Med. J. **294:** 1637–1641.
5. SOUTHALL, D. P. & D. G. TALBERT. 1987. Sudden alveolar atelectasis braking syndrome (SAABS). *In* Current Topics in Pulmonary Pharmacology. M. A. Hollinger, Ed.: 210–281. Elsevier. New York.
6. FLEMING, P. J., M. R. LEVINE, A. M. LONG, *et al.* 1986. The maturation of the control of respiration in infancy. *In* Physiology of the Fetal and Neonatal Lung. D. V. WALTERS, L. B. STRANG & F. GEUBELLE, Eds. MJP Press Ltd. Lancaster, England.

SIDS Family International
Introduction

MARTA BROWN[a,b]

National Sudden Infant Death Syndrome Foundation
Landover, Maryland

An international workshop, "The Sudden Infant Death Syndrome: Practical Management of Infants at Higher Risk," was held in Brussels, Belgium, on October 15–18, 1985. This meeting was organized by WHO Europe and the Belgian Association for the Study of Sleep and was financed by Healthdyne. Twenty-six experts in the clinical management of SIDS met to discuss high-risk populations, screening techniques, and the management of high-risk infants.

At the same time and in the same location, another group also assembled—representatives of SIDS parents' organizations. These organizations had been started by SIDS parents determined to communicate with and help other SIDS families. Some groups had raised money to support research on SIDS or to purchase monitors to help parents who needed them. Many of the associations had little money and even less structure. Others, especially the groups in the United States and Great Britain, had been in existence for longer periods of time and seemed to be better organized. Many parents came to Brussels because they wanted to hear clinical experts speaking at the international workshop—there was particular interest in the debate concerning monitoring of high-risk infants. But most of all, parents came because they felt the need to communicate beyond national boundaries. Thus, the University of Brussels became the site of the First International Parents' Association Meeting, held on the last day of the international workshop, October 18, 1985.

Unlike the second meeting, which was organized far in advance and held at Lake Como nearly 2 years later, that first international meeting of parents' groups was an almost spontaneous event, with little formal agenda. Nevertheless, it served its purposes well. Representatives of associations dedicated to helping SIDS families came from Belgium, France, Luxemburg, Germany, Holland, Denmark, Great Britain, and the United States. They shared their experiences in managing SIDS in their various countries and expressed a primary aim to help SIDS families and support infant monitoring at home. Most importantly, they initiated links of *international* communication and cooperation which have continued to develop and grow in the years since.

[a]Mrs. Brown is president of the National Sudden Infant Death Syndrome Foundation (U.S.A.). She served as chairman of the Second Meeting of SIDS Family International, held at Lake Como, Italy, on May 27, 1987.

[b]Address for correspondence: National Sudden Infant Death Syndrome Foundation, 8200 Professional Place, Suite 104, Landover, MD 20785-2264 U.S.A.

After this initial meeting in Brussels, the representatives of the parents' associations determined to meet again in 2 years. This second meeting was organized and, as already mentioned, was held in Lake Como, Italy, on May 27, 1987, in conjunction with the Lake Como conference on SIDS, whose proceedings are reported in this volume.

The extensive agenda for this second parents' meeting (see Appendix 1) and the large number of countries represented (see Appendix 2 for a list of attendees) give some indication of the development of parents' groups over the time since the first international meeting. Much was accomplished at the second meeting. Round-table discussions among the representatives from the various countries reviewed the status of local and national parents' groups and summarized statistics concerning SIDS in those countries (see Appendix 3). Several topics on the agenda were discussed in detail, resulting in the adoption of recommendations concerning goals and procedures for the groups. It was recommended that an autopsy be performed in all cases of sudden unexpected infant death and that the information obtained in the procedure be thoroughly explained to the parents by the physician(s) involved. Cooperation between parents and researchers, a goal already achieved in many countries, was held to be desirable. Methods for providing information and support to SIDS parents and to other parents who might benefit were examined, and procedures for training and organizing parent "contact" and support groups were also discussed. Finally, strategies for communicating to the news media information about SIDS and about parents' groups were considered. The minutes of the meeting, which follow this introduction, provide a summary of the discussions which took place.

Representatives of all countries expressed interest in research, counseling, and education as aims for their associations. Some groups were still small and in their formative stages, whereas others were larger and more organized. The climate of acceptance and warmth at this meeting allowed representatives the freedom to share problems they were having in their own associations. Smaller groups had time to talk with one another, which they indicated was beneficial to them. Some larger organizations offered to send information to help the smaller groups solve their problems. The National SIDS Foundation sent manuals on "How to Start a Chapter" to eight different countries. Packets of background information were provided by groups from the various countries represented at the meeting. The overall feeling of the representatives at this meeting was an eagerness to establish some way to stay in touch with one another. Therefore, the highlight of the meeting was the formation of SIDS Family International. A steering committee was named to plan the next meeting in Great Britain in 1989. More information about this meeting can be obtained from the chairman of the committee, June Reed.[a] Plans are underway and a large attendance is expected.

Networking among parents' groups in the various countries has increased since the Lake Como meeting. Three members of SIDS Family International, from Canada, Scotland, and Germany, respectively, attended the 25th Anniversary Conference of the National SIDS Foundation (U.S.A.), in September. The friendships formed in Italy were renewed at that conference. Representatives have corresponded regularly with one another seeking advice and offering support. Newsletters are crossing this country and being read eagerly by other groups struggling to assist parents and inform the public. There is so much to share and so much to learn from one another. SIDS Family International wishes to communicate with its members; therefore, an international newsletter is being published. The editor of this publication is Carrie Sheehan, Western Regional Director,

---

[a]Information about the 1989 meeting may be obtained from June Reed, The Foundation for the Study of Infant Deaths, 15 Belgrave Square, London, SW1X 8PS, U.K.

National SIDS Foundation. More information about the newsletter can be obtained from Carrie, and articles for publication should be sent to her.[b]

It is obvious that a need exists for an international network, and, through SIDS Family International, a way is finally being provided to meet that need. After all, grief is universal and knows no boundaries. It speaks a common language by the bond it forms when these parents reach out, one to another.

[b]Address correspondence concerning the international newsletter to Carrie Sheehan, Western Regional Director, National SIDS Foundation, 915 16th Street East, Seattle, WA 98112 U.S.A.

SIDS Family International

Minutes of the Second SIDS International Parents' Meeting[a]
Lake Como, Italy
27 May 1987

ATTENDEES:	Australia, Austria, Britain, Canada, Denmark, France, Germany, Italy, New Zealand, Norway, Scotland, Sweden, United States (See APPENDIX 2 for names and affiliations of attendees.)
APOLOGIES:	Belgium, Ireland, Switzerland
CHAIRMAN:	Mrs. Marta Brown, United States
SECRETARY:	Mrs. Kaaren Fitzgerald, Australia

GENERAL DISCUSSION

The morning session was devoted to the outlining of programs and problems by representatives from each country. From this list, an agenda was drawn up (see APPENDIX 1). Groups from all countries had research, counseling and education as their aims. Tabulation of data from the 13 countries attending the meeting indicated that they represented a total population of 499.5 million people and an average total of 18,050 sudden unexpected infant deaths per annum (see APPENDIX 3).

AGENDA ITEMS

1. AUTOPSIES

A great deal of discussion centered around 3 problems:

    a. The fact that autopsies are not performed in some SIDS cases
    b. The variability of procedures used by pathologists in SIDS cases
    c. Notification of parents.

[a]Minutes of the meeting were recorded and prepared by Mrs. Kaaren Fitzgerald, Executive Director, Sudden Infant Death Research Foundation Inc., Melbourne, Australia.

Concerning the first and second problems, there was an extremely wide range of practices used in the various countries. For the third issue, it was found that notification ranged from a phone call immediately after the autopsy to no contact at all.

Recommendations

    A. Every baby dying suddenly and unexpectedly should have a thorough autopsy undertaken by an appropriately trained pathologist (pediatric, if possible).
    B. Preliminary results of the autopsy should be given to the parents either by telephone or letter within 24 hr of the autopsy.
    C. Either the pathologist, pediatrician or general practitioner should be available, free-of-charge, to explain the final medical results to the parents.

2. EMERGENCY RESPONDERS

Recommendation

That all emergency responders, and in particular the police, should receive appropriate training in crisis intervention and interviewing techniques.

3. SETTING UP NEW GROUPS

The group from the United States offered the use of their manual on setting up a group to any representatives requiring this information.

4. PARENTS WORKING WITH RESEARCHERS

In many countries there was full cooperation between parents and researchers. However, it was felt that some researchers may request parent assistance in the wrong way. Representatives from New Zealand suggested that occasionally parents feel comfortable with the ''mystery of SIDS'' and prefer not to be involved in research.

Recommendations

Most parents would be happy to consider participating in responsible SIDS research projects if offered the opportunity. Parents would like to aid research on SIDS.

5. NOTIFICATION OF PARENTS' GROUPS WHEN SIDS OCCURS

In the majority of cases parents' groups receive the names of new parents in an informal manner via either newspaper accounts, neighbors, the distribution of parent information sheets by health professionals, or radio programs. Many organizations have individually negotiated with their local coroners or medical examiners in order to receive official notification. It was agreed that representatives from each country would document their parent-contact procedure for distribution.

Recommendations

A. Within 24 hr of a SIDS death, health professionals should provide to all newly bereaved parents a copy of their local SIDS Foundation's information booklet and phone number.

B. Health professionals should ask newly bereaved parents if they would like to have their names, addresses and phone numbers given to the local SIDS Foundation.

6. NON-SIDS PARENTS

Parent's groups from Australia, Britain, Canada, the United States, and New Zealand have information available for the education of non-SIDS parents, i.e., those whose babies have died suddenly, but of recognized causes. The United States government also has available for distribution a pamphlet on SIDS designed especially for pregnant women.

Recommendations

A. Those families whose infants have died suddenly and unexpectedly of a disease identified at autopsy should receive the same care and support as SIDS parents.

B. Those families concerned about the possibility of a SIDS death occurring should receive appropriate information and support.

[After a lunch break and a short talk by Dr. Fred Mandell, Children's Hospital (Boston, Massachusetts, U.S.A.), the meeting continued its consideration of items on the agenda.]

7. PARENT CONTACT

The problems of parent contact and support were discussed at length. The difficulties of recruiting, training, supervising and matching parent supporters were recognized. It was recommended that business meetings should be kept separate from parent support meetings. It was highly recommended that one central phone number for SIDS information be used in each country or state.

Representatives from several countries commented on the problem of parents leaving support work for SIDS organizations but still having their phone numbers in circulation. In some countries, health professionals assist local support groups. Several groups have appointed regional coordinators (either volunteer or paid).

Recommendations

A. All parent supporters should have training or, at least, guidelines for their work. They should be accountable to their supervisors through a main office.

B. Closer liaison must be established between health professionals, parent supporters, and foundations.

C. The different needs of parents should be recognized. For instance, parent-to-parent and parent-to-group sessions should be provided.

8. Media

On the whole the media were considered to be responsible in regard to this subject. However, some suggestions were made, as follows: First, if there is an inaccurate report, correct information should be sent to the reporter and an attempt should be made to have a second article written. Second, the media should always be thanked. Finally, a phone number should be given in every article and a central location should be used for meetings to enable the press to attend.

[After a short slide presentation by the New Zealand group and afternoon tea, the assembly broke up into 2 working parties to discuss items 9 and 10 of the agenda.]

9. International Group

It was decided to form an international SIDS group whose aims would be to

a. Facilitate the sharing of information
b. Improve services to families
c. Increase public awareness of SIDS
d. Encourage liaison with all professionals
e. Encourage research to eliminate the sudden and unexpected deaths of infants.

Names suggested for the international group were

a. International SIDS Support Council
b. International SIDS Parent Council
c. SIDS International
d. SIDS Family International

The last 2 names were nominated and SIDS Family International was approved, with 1 dissenting vote, as the new name for the international group. Some discussion centered around the use of the word "family" in the title. All of the health professionals present (who were not SIDS parents themselves) expressed the feeling that they were part of the "family of SIDS."

International Conference of Parents' Groups

The First Conference of SIDS Family International will be held in either Cambridge or Glasgow, in September, 1989.

It was decided that each group should seek its own financial support to attend this conference (through fund-raising within their own countries). The Steering Committee will also approach various sponsors, as necessary, to finance speakers' airfares and accommodations.

The Steering Committee for this conference comprises Hazel Brook, Scotland; Marta Brown, United States; Kaaren Fitzgerald, Australia; June Reed, United Kingdom; and Marie Thenard, France.

International Newsletter

This newsletter is to be edited by Marta Brown and Geraldine Norris-Funke; it will be printed and mailed by the SIDS Clearinghouse, U.S.A. Each group should send relevant news items to Marta Brown by December 1, 1987, for the first international newsletter in January 1988. The assembly acknowledged the generous offer of assistance from Mrs. Norris-Funke and the SIDS Clearinghouse.

It was also suggested that each group could send its newsletter and annual general meeting reports to others affiliated with the SIDS Family International.

It was also recommended that each national group issue a press release announcing the formation of SIDS Family International.

10. RUNNING AN ORGANIZATION

Carrie Sheehan, United States, led a general discussion, in which much useful information was exchanged. It was agreed that many more hours would be needed to cover the wide range of subjects and problems inherent in the topic.

AGENDA ITEMS 11–20

It was not possible to discuss the remaining items on the agenda (11–20), because there was not enough time. It was decided to consider using them as agenda items for the next international conference.

GENERAL BUSINESS

A list of attendees was compiled (APPENDIX 2).

The meeting closed at 4:50 P.M.

APPENDIX 1.

Agenda of the Second SIDS International Parents' Meeting Lake Como, Italy 27 May 1987

1. AUTOPSIES
   Standards
   All babies to receive

2. EMERGENCY RESPONDERS
   Training

3. SETTING UP NEW GROUPS

4. PARENTS WORKING WITH RESEARCHERS

5. NOTIFICATION OF PARENTS' GROUPS WHEN SIDS OCCURS

6. NON-SIDS PARENTS AND THEIR PROBLEMS

7. PARENT CONTACT/SUPPORT/BEFRIENDERS

8. MEDIA

9. FORMATION OF INTERNATIONAL GROUP
   International conference
   International newsletter

10. RUNNING AN ORGANIZATION
    What happens when someone wants to resign
    Parents moving on
    Part-time involvement; coping with the work
    Financial responsibility

11. GOVERNMENT ORGANIZATIONS AND THEIR SUPPORT OF PARENTS, PARENTS' ORGA-
    NIZATIONS, AND RESEARCH

12. FUND-RAISING

13. STANDARDS FOR SCIENTIFIC RESEARCH GRANT-FUNDING BODIES

14. BOARDS OF MANAGEMENT

15. PARENT QUESTIONNAIRE

16. COUNSELING PROBLEMS
    Subsequent children
    Isolation

17. MONITORING POLICIES FOR PARENTS

18. ROLE OF PROFESSIONALS
    Information-giving vs. counseling

19. RESEARCH/THEORIES

20. EDUCATION

Attendees of the Second SIDS International Parents' Meeting Lake Como, Italy 27 May 1987

AUSTRALIA
KAAREN FITZGERALD
Executive Director
Sudden Infant Death Research Foundation Inc.
1227 Malvern Road
Malvern, 3144, Victoria,Australia
(Secretary, National SIDS Council of Australia)

AUSTRIA
ADELHEID KREMSER
Dillacher Str. 22
A-8,580 Koflach, Austria
Association: Physiologisches Institut
Harrachgasse 21
8010 Graz, Austria

DR. CHRISTA EINSPIELER
Institute of Physiology
University of Graz

BRITAIN
JUNE REED
The Foundation for the Study of Infant Deaths
15 Belgrave Square
London SWIX 8PS, U.K.

CANADA
BEVERLEY DE BRUYN
Executive Director
Canadian Foundation for the Study of Infant Deaths
P.O. Box 190 Station R
Toronto, Ontario M4G 3Z9, Canada

DENMARK
ULLA LIBERG
Bergreensgade 54
2100 Kobenhavn, Denmark

FRANCE
MARIE-ANNICK CORNU THENARD
Presidente de "Naitre & Vivre"
(Federation des Associations pour l'etude et la prevention de la MSIN)
1 Rue d'Edinbourg 75008, Paris, France

JACQUES HONORE
9 Allee du Bosquet
59650 Villeneuve d'Ascq, France
(information, newsletters)

GERMANY
WERNER BAESSLER
Gesellschaft zur Erfaschung des ploetzichen
Sauglingstods (GEPS) e V
Stiftsbogen 156 D-8000
Munchen 70, Germany

ITALY
ALESSANDRA CAMPISI GARBAGNATI
Associazione SIDS per lo Studio e la Prevenzione della Morte Improvvisa nell'Infanzia
Via Gherardini 6
20146 Milan, Italy

CARLA & FRANCO UCELLI CATTANEO
Via Cappuccio
20123 Milan, Italy

NEW ZEALAND
SHIRLEY DOWDING
Box 20
Te Karaka, New Zealand

DR. SHIRLEY TONKIN
27 Eastbourne Road
Remuera, Auckland 5, New Zealand

NORWAY
SVERRE SLOERDAHL, M.D.
Dept. of Pediatrics
University Hospital of Trondheim
700 Trondheim, Norway

SCOTLAND
HAZEL BROOKE
DR. ANGUS GIBSON
SHEILA BARTHOLOMEW
Scottish Cot Death Trust
Royal Hospital for Sick Children
Yorkhill, Glasgow G3 8SJ, Scotland

SWEDEN
INGELE BENDT
Swedish SIDS Parent Group
Box 19045 S-16119
Bkomma, Sweden

UNITED STATES
MARTA BROWN
5504 Spearmint Drive
Charlotte, North Carolina 28212, U.S.A.
(President, National SIDS Foundation)

JUDY JACOBSON
National Center for the Prevention of SIDS
330 N. Charles Street
Baltimore, Maryland 21201, U.S.A.

CARRIE SHEEHAN
Western Regional Director
National SIDS Foundation
915/16th East
Seattle, Washington 98112, U.S.A.

Current International Statistics on SIDS and on Parents' Groups (March 1988)[a]

Compiled for SIDS Family International
by Kaaren Fitzgerald[b]
Sudden Infant Death Syndrome Foundation Inc.
Melbourne, Australia

Country	Population (millions)	Date Group Formed (yr)		Sudden Unexpected Infant Deaths		
		First Group	National Group	Ave. No./yr	Autopsy Performed	Incidence[c] (per 1,000 live births)
Australia	16	1977	1986	560	Yes	1.9–3.7[1]
Austria	8	1986	1986	350	Sometimes	?[d]
Belguim	10	1981	1981	240	Sometimes	?[d]
Britain	55	1971	1971	1500	Yes	2.0–2.78[2]
Canada	25	1973	1973	600	Yes	3.0[2]
Czechoslovakia	15	?[d]	?[d]	?[d]	?[d]	0.8[2]
Denmark	5	1986	1986	100	Yes	0.92[2]
Finland	5	?[d]	?[d]	80	Yes	0.31–0.51[3]
France	54	1984	1986	2000	Sometimes	2.71[4]
Germany	60	1984	1984	2500	Sometimes	?[d]
Hong Kong	?[d]	none	none	3	No	0.36[5]
Ireland	3.5	?[d]	?[d]	30	Usually	2.67[6]
Israel	4.3	1988	1988	?[d]	?[d]	0.31[2]
Italy	60	1987	?[d]	1400	Sometimes	0.8[7]–2.6[2]
Netherlands	14.5	?[d]	?[d]	?[d]	?[d]	0.42[2]
New Zealand	3.5	1979	1979	200	Yes	1.9[2]
Norway	4.5	1982	1985	100	Usually	?[d]
Scotland	4	1985	1985	140	Yes	?[d]
Sweden	8	1986	1986	100	Yes	0.4–0.8[2]
United States	200	1962	1962	8500	Usually	1.7–3.06[2]

[a]This summary has been amended slightly from the version originally presented at the second international meeting to reflect some changes in population and to include information not available at that time and data from countries not represented at the meeting.

[b]Please address correspondence to Mrs. Kaaren Fitzgerald, Executive Director, Sudden Infant Death Research Foundation Inc., 1227 Malvern Rd., Malvern, 3144, Australia.

[c]See list of references for sources of information.

[d]Information is being sought but is not yet available.

REFERENCES

1. DWYER, T. SIDS in Tasmania—A prospective cohort study of possible courses. Unpublished paper.
2. SCHWARTZ, P.J. 1981. The sudden infant death syndrome. Rev. Perinat. Med. 4: 475–524.
3. RINTAHAKA, P.J. & J. HIRVONEN. 1986. The epidemiology of SIDS in Finland. Forensic Sci. Int. 30: 219–233.
4. WAGNER, M., D. SAMSON-DOLLFUS & J. MENARD. 1984. Sudden unexpected infant death in a French county. Arch. Dis. Child. 59: 1082–1097.
5. DAVIES, D.P. Cot death in Hong Kong: A rare problem? Child Health.

6. MATTHEWS, T. 1985. Perinatal epidemiological characteristics of SIDS in an Irish population.
    Ir. Med. J. **9:** 251–253.
7. RUSINENTI, P., F. GRANCINI, A. SEGANTINI, V. CARNELLI, D. PORTALEONE, P. CAREDDU &
    P.J. SCHWARTZ. 1988. The incidence of SIDS in Italy: A prospective study. Ann. N.Y. Acad.
    Sci. (This volume).

Changing Patterns of SIDS in Southeast Scotland

SHEILA BARTHOLOMEW[a] AND BARTON MacARTHUR[b]

[a]Department of Pathology
Royal Hospital for Sick Children
Edinburgh EH9 1LF
Scotland
[b]University of Auckland
New Zealand

A systematic inquiry concerning various epidemiological characteristics of SIDS victims and their families has been carried out over the past decade (1977–1986) by the same team of investigators. Cases of SIDS were defined according to Bergman *et al.*[1] and classified only after a thorough pediatric autopsy. A personal visit to the home of each bereaved family was made 2–3 weeks after the death. Epidemiological data were analyzed by comparing the quinquennia to determine any changing patterns. The infant mortality rate for the area, per 1,000 live births, fell from 14.6 to 12.4 (1977–1981) and from 11.5 to 9.7 (1982–1986).[2] The average rate for SIDS during these periods was 2.9 and 2.7, respectively. Overall, several of the variables associated with the SIDS cases matched the usual picture of SIDS[3]: 80% of deaths occurred in infants younger than 8 months of age, peaks of death occurred in winter (48% November through February), male infants predominated (64%), and the majority of the mothers of SIDS victims had previous children (71%). In comparing the 2 periods, however, some differences were demonstrated. The second half of the decade revealed significant increases ($p < 0.01$) for SIDS victims and their families in unemployment, in registration of the mother for prenatal health care at >12 weeks gestation, and in mothers with previous fetal loss and deaths of newborn children at 2 months of age. Increases ($p < 0.05$) were also observed in the numbers in social classes (SES)[4] IV and V, in single mothers, and in deaths of newborns in May through July. Decreases in 1982–1986 were observed in the numbers of infants dying at 4 months of age ($p < 0.05$) and in mothers aged 30–34 ($p < 0.05$).

The majority of factors for which a change had occurred appeared to have been related to socioeconomic status. There was a significant increase in 1982–1986 in the percentage of the population in SES IV and V ($p < 0.05$) and a decrease in SES I, II and III (74% to 61%; see FIG. 1). Since the variables showing significant differences in their association with SIDS between the first and second 5-yr period either were frequently used as measures of social class or had been associated with SES in the literature,[5] further analysis was undertaken to determine whether the changes in their association with SIDS were reflected in all SES groups or whether some SES groups were contributing preferentially to the modification of the pattern of significant factors for SIDS observed in the earlier phase.

Significant increases peculiar to SIDS cases in SES IV and V were the numbers of fathers who were unemployed ($p < 0.01$), mothers who registered for prenatal care at >12 weeks gestation ($p < 0.05$), infants who were bottle-fed ($p < 0.05$), and infants who had a birthweight of 2,501–3,500 g ($p < 0.05$). Significant decreases appearing only in SES IV and V were the number of firstborns ($p < 0.05$) and the number who died in September through October ($p < 0.05$). The only significant change not demonstrated in

SES IV and V but present in SES I and II was a decrease in the number of male infants ($p < 0.05$).

As there was not an increase overall in the numbers of SIDS cases, but rather an increased representation in groups IV and V, the question arises as to whether this is an indication of the effect of increased disadvantage in the last 5 yr. To achieve a reliable data base of socioeconomic factors for SIDS subjects, it is recommended that relatively long-term studies, ideally by the same group of investigators, be undertaken to enable any changing patterns to be observed and put in perspective.

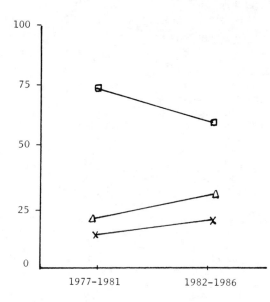

FIGURE 1. Changes in the distribution of population by socioeconomic status between the periods of 1977–1981 and 1982–1986 and the proportion of the total infant deaths attributable to SIDS (x). Percentage of population in SES I, II, or III (□); percentage in SES IV or V (△).

REFERENCES

1. BERGMAN, A. B., J. B. BECKWITH & G. C. RAY, Eds. 1970. Sudden Infant Death Syndrome. Proceedings of the Second International Conference on Causes of Sudden Death in Infants. University of Washington Press. Seattle, WA.
2. REGISTRAR GENERAL. 1985. Annual report of the Registrar General for Scotland. HMSO. London.
3. KELLY D. H. & D. C. SHANNON. 1982. Sudden infant death syndrome and near sudden infant death syndrome: A review of the literature 1964–1982. Pediatr. Clin. North Am. **29**: 1241–1261.
4. OFFICE OF POPULATION CENSUSES AND SURVEYS. Classification of Occupations. 1970. HMSO. London.
5. MOORE, A. 1986. Preventable childhood deaths in Wolverhampton. Br. Med. J. **293**: 656–658.

SIDS in Sweden

S. G. NORVENIUS AND G. WENNERGREN

Department of Pediatrics I
Gothenburg University
Sweden

SIDS has increased in Sweden in 1973–1986, from 0.41 to 0.94 cases per 1,000 live births, as shown in 2 independent studies.[1,2] The increased incidence is real and is based upon strictly uniform diagnosis of SIDS, according to Beckwith's criteria, but including "delayed" SIDS.

A change of the time of death from SIDS was recorded during the period. An increasing proportion of SIDS victims now die during the day. The incidence of SIDS in own bed/cot was relatively constant, but the incidence of SIDS occurring rose for outdoors, in the back seats of cars, and in bed with 1–2 adults. "Attacks of lifelessness" (AL) had epidemiological characteristics similar to SIDS with regard to age distribution, sex-ratio, and place of occurrence. Further apneic spells were rather common in the AL group during the following 2–3 days but uncommon still later, indicating a short, transient period of unstable autonomic control.

REFERENCES

1. Norvenius, S. 1987. Sudden infant death syndrome in Sweden in 1973–1977 and 1979. Acta Paediatr. Scand. Suppl. **333.**
2. Wennergren, G., J. Milerad, H. Lagercrantz, *et. al.* 1987. The epidemiology of sudden infant death syndrome and attacks of lifelessness in Sweden. Acta Paediatr. Scand. **76:** 898–906.

The Incidence of SIDS in Italy

A Prospective Study

P. RUSINENTI, F. GRANCINI, A. SEGANTINI,
V. CARNELLI, D. PORTALEONE, P. CAREDDU, AND
P. J. SCHWARTZ

Clinica Pediatrica I and Centro SIDS
Clinica Medica Generale e Terapia Medica
University of Milan
Italy

Although the incidence of SIDS has been described for many countries, no direct data have ever been reported for Italy. The only exception is a retrospective study for the years 1970–1976[1] conducted by our own group using, however, the surrogate method proposed by Peterson et al.[2] We have now studied prospectively the incidence of SIDS in an area of northern Italy, i.e., the city of Milan and 19 suburban towns. The population studied includes 46,793 live births in the period 1984–1986. We analyzed all the deaths which occurred between 7 days and 1 yr of age, as recorded at the bureau of vital statistics of each area included in the study. This procedure made possible the acquisition of an accurate diagnosis of the cause of death in each case and the identification of the real SIDS group (TABLE 1).

The global incidence of SIDS in the period observed is 0.55/1,000, with an infant mortality of 10.4/1,000. The SIDS group differs statistically ($p < 0.001$) from the group of deaths from other causes by (1) the age at death (mean 14.8, median 10.7 weeks for SIDS vs. mean 8.4, median 3.9 weeks for non-SIDS) (FIG. 1), and (2) the prevalence of death during the cold season (85% for SIDS vs. 51% for non-SIDS). SIDS is more frequent in males (62%) and is distributed homogeneously during the weekdays. There is not a substantially different incidence between the city of Milan (29,882 live births, 18 cases of SIDS: 0.6/1,000) and the suburban area (16,471 live births, 8 cases of SIDS: 0.49/1,000). The striking difference between this direct estimate of incidence and the previous indirect one could be explained by the fact that the surrogate method proposed by Peterson does not fit with our population characteristics and also by the fact that the total infant mortality in Italy has impressively decreased in the last years (1970: 29/1,000; 1977: 17.9/1,000; 1985: 10.5/1,000).[3–5]

SIDS seems to have a surprisingly low incidence in this part of Italy. An extrapolation from these data to the whole Italian population should be done with caution, considering the small sample studied (about 3% of total live births in the entire country) and the significant socioeconomic gaps existing between northern and southern Italy. Nonetheless, the methodology of this study can be utilized in the entire country and we should soon be able to determine the SIDS incidence in a larger and more representative population. All other epidemiologic features are in agreement with previous reports. SIDS is confirmed to be the most frequent single cause of death during the first year of life after the neonatal period.

TABLE 1. Distribution by Cause of Death of All Infant Deaths in the City of Milan and 19 Suburban Towns in 1984–1986

Cause of Death	n	% of Total
Prematurity and perinatal problems	309	66
Congenital anomalies	99	21
SIDS	29	6
Infections	13	3
Others	11	2
Metabolic Diseases	5	1
Neoplasias	3	1
Total[a]	469	100

[a]Total infant deaths in the population of 46,793 live births.

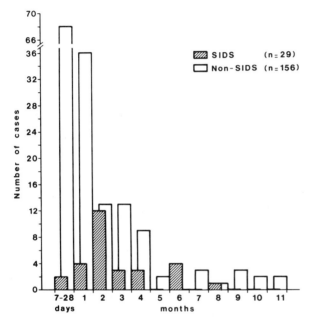

FIGURE 1. Age distribution of SIDS (**hatched bars**) and non-SIDS (**open bars**) deaths which occurred between 7 days and 1 yr of age in a population of 46,793 live births in the city of Milan and 19 suburban towns in the period 1984–1986.

REFERENCES

1. MONTEMERLO, M., N. NEGRINI, D. ROSTI & P. J. SCHWARTZ. 1977. Elettrocardiografia neonatale e sindrome della morte improvvisa nell'infanzia (SIDS). Boll. Soc. Ital. Cardiol. **22:** 1917–1934.
2. PETERSON, D. R., D. J. THOMPSON, N. M. CHINN. 1974. A method for assessing the geographic distribution and temporal trends of the sudden infant death syndrome in the United States from vital statistics data. Am. J. Epidemiol. **100:** 373–379.
3. ANNUARIO STATISTICO ITALIANO. 1974. Istituto Centrale di Statistica (ISTAT), Roma: 54.
4. ANNUARIO STATISTICO ITALIANO. 1980. Istituto Centrale di Statistica (ISTAT), Roma: 16.
5. BOLLETTINO MENSILE DI STATISTICA. 1986. Istituto Centrale di Statistica (ISTAT). **12:** 13.

Conspicuous Modifications of Behavioral Patterns in Infants at Risk for SIDS Because of Pathological Cardiorespiratory Mechanisms[a]

C. EINSPIELER, A. HOLZER, AND T. KENNER

Institute of Physiology
University of Graz
Austria

In a detailed retrospective study on SIDS victims who died between 1982 and 1986 in the Austrian province of Styria, semistructured open-ended interviews were used. The parents were asked questions concerning family socioeconomic condition, health history, pregnancy and perinatal problems, the infant's somatic development, feeding practice, and the infant's behavior.

In comparison to a control group matched for age and sex (n = 80) we found the following significant differences ($p \leq 0.01$): feeding difficulties (51%), vomiting (40%), paleness (35%) and cyanosis (15%), high-pitched crying (33%), and excessive night sweating (49%). 58% of the parents described their infants as apathetic, moving little, placid, anxious, shy and withdrawn, and easily tired. A contrasting picture of their babies was provided by 15% of the parents, who characterized their infants as being irritable and easily startled. Previously in the literature weak sucking, general hypotonia, and low activity[1-3] had been reported.

We have taken up a prospective study to investigate behavioral characteristics of at-risk infants for SIDS and compared these results with matched controls, aged 6–24 weeks. This study comprised 29 at-risk infants and 33 healthy infants (matched for conceptional age, sex, birthweight and social background). The at-risk group consisted of 13 siblings of SIDS victims, 6 near-miss infants, and 10 infants with a severe sleep apnea syndrome (SAS: prolonged apneas $\geq$ 15 sec, periodic breathing attacks of bradycardia, and decreased Po_2).

Detailed behavioral analyses have been carried out with the aid of video-recording, lasting 10–15 min, when the infants were lying in a supine position in their cots. Behavioral observation was based on the scoring system of Hopkins and Prechtl.[4] The motor activity (general and fine distal movements) as well as more specific behavior, such as smiling, vocalization, and visual exploration, were scored separately for each infant. Special attention was paid to the quality of motor activity, e. g., fluency, elegance, and variability.

Striking differences could be demonstrated in the behavioral characteristics in the at-risk infants when compared with the healthy controls. Seventy-two percent of the at-risk infants, i. e., 11 siblings of SIDS victims (85%), 5 near-miss infants (83%) and 7

[a] This study was supported by the Austrian Research Fund.

SAS infants (70%), showed conspicuously different behavior from the controls. The deviant behavior observed was that the infants moved very little (34%) or moved continuously throughout the whole observation period (38%). Even more striking than these quantitative differences was the qualitative difference of movements present in both groups. Of the infants suffering cardiorespiratory problems, 40% were found to be apathetic, inactive and possibly showing delayed maturation; 30% of the SAS infants were hyperactive, agitated, moving restlessly, and had a low threshold for responses to stimulation. The other 30% showed inconspicuous patterns of behavior.

Our results stress the importance of behavioral assessment by means of an analysis of the quantity and, especially, the quality of movement, in addition to the widely employed cardiorespiratory monitoring.

REFERENCES

1. ANDERSON-HUNTINGTON, R.B. & J.F. ROSENBLITH. 1976. Central nervous system damage as a possible component of unexpected deaths in infancy. Dev. Med. Child Neurol. **18:** 480–492.
2. VALDES-DAPENA, M. 1986. Sudden infant death syndrome. Morphology update for forensic pathologists—1985. Forensic Sci. Int. **30:** 177–186.
3. NAEYE, R.L., J. MESSMER, T. SPECHT & T.A. MERRITT. 1976. Sudden infant death syndrome temperament before death. J. Pediatr. **88:** 511–515.
4. HOPKINS, B. & H.F.R. PRECHTL. 1984. A qualitative approach to the development of movements during early infancy. *In* Continuity of Neural Functions from Prenatal to Postnatal Life. H.F.R. Prechtl, Ed.: 179–198. Blackwell Scientific Publications. Oxford.

QT Interval, Total Calcium Blood Levels, and SIDS

A Prospective Study

P. AUSTONI, R. MISSAGLIA, M. V. INNOCENTI,
G. B. DANZI, V. CONSOLE, M. MONTEMERLO,
A. SEGANTINI, T. VARISCO, AND P. J. SCHWARTZ

Ospedale Niguarda
Milan, Italy
and
Clinica Medica Generale e Terapia Medica
and Centro SIDS
University of Milan
Milan, Italy

In our ongoing electrocardiographic prospective study,[1-3] we have enrolled more than 13,000 newborns, with a standard ECG recorded on the fourth day of life. The follow-up at 1 yr, completed for 10,431 infants, has revealed 9 SIDS victims: 6 of them (66%) had a QTc exceeding the mean by more than 2 SD. A prolonged QT interval, usually associated with electrical instability of the heart, may be due to an imbalance in cardiac sympathetic innervation or to electrolyte disorders. In the neonatal period hypocalcemia is of particular interest. To test the relationship between QT interval and total calcium blood levels (Ca) in a large population of infants, we have initiated a new specific prospective study (at Niguarda Hospital, Milan). QTc and Ca are determined on the fourth day of life; so far, 818 healthy newborns have been enrolled. For technical reasons, it was not possible to determine the ionized calcium fraction in such a large population. The distribution of QTc and Ca is summarized in TABLE 1. In this population, there is a negative but weak correlation between QTc and Ca ($r = -0.21$). By examining the Ca of the newborns ($n = 92$) with QTc values between 427 and 449 msec ($\bar{X} + 1$ SD and $\bar{X} + 2$ SD), and the Ca of those ($n = 19$) with QTc values exceeding 449 msec ($\bar{X} + 2$ SD), one can observe statistically significant reductions ($p < 0.005$ and $p < 0.02$, respectively) of Ca in comparison to newborns with QTc < 427 msec ($n = 707$). In the group with prolonged QT interval (QTc > 449 msec), only 5 of 19 (26.3%) had a low Ca (< 8 mg/dl).

These data indicate that the classic correlation between QT interval and Ca is very weak and becomes significant only for high QTc values. Furthermore, in the majority of cases (almost 75%), prolongation of QT interval cannot be explained by a low Ca.

Thus, the rational basis and interest for the prognostic evaluation of a prolonged QT interval at birth in relationship with SIDS does not involve the question of calcium blood levels.

TABLE 1. Distribution of QTc Values in the Population of Newborn Infants and Its Relationship to Total Blood Calcium Levels (Ca)

| | Total Population | Infants with | | |
		QTc < 427	427 < QTc < 449	QTc > 449
n	818	707	92	19
QTc (msec)[a]	405 ± 22	400 ± 17	433 ± 5	467 ± 24
Ca (mg/dl)[a]	—	9.04 ± 0.67	8.78 ± 0.73[b]	8.65 ± 0.71[c]

[a] $\overline{X}$ ± SD.

[b] $p < 0.005$ in comparison to newborn infants with QTc < 427 msec.

[c] $p < 0.02$ in comparison to infants with QTc < 427 msec. In this group only 5 cases (26.3%) showed a Ca ≤ 8 mg/dl.

REFERENCES

1. SCHWARTZ, P. J., M. MONTEMERLO, M. FACCHINI, P. SALICE, D. ROSTI, G. L. POGGIO & R. GIORGETTI. 1982. The Q–T interval throughout the first 6 months of life: A prospective study. Circulation **66**: 496–501.
2. SEGANTINI, A., T. VARISCO, E. MONZA, V. SONGA, M. MONTEMERLO, P. SALICE, G. L. POGGIO, D. ROSTI & P. J. SCHWARTZ. 1986. QT interval and sudden infant death syndrome. A prospective study. J. Am. Coll. Cardiol. **7**:118A.
3. SCHWARTZ, P. J. 1987. The quest for the mechanisms of the sudden infant death syndrome: Doubts and progress. Circulation **75**:677–683.

Epidemiologic Comparisons of Sudden Infant Death Syndrome with Infantile Apnea

NORA DAVIS,[a,d] LEE BOSSUNG SWEENEY,[b] AND
DONALD R. PETERSON[c]

[a]Department of Pediatrics
University of Washington
Seattle, Washington

[b]Department of Ambulatory Services
Children's Hospital and Medical Center
Seattle, Washington

[c]Department of Epidemiology
University of Washington
Seattle, Washington

Previous investigators have assumed that infantile apnea and sudden infant death syndrome (SIDS) are related.[1-3] This relationship has never been defined epidemiologically. The Apnea Program at Children's Hospital and Medical Center (CHMC) evaluates, manages, and follows infants referred for apparent life-threatening events (ALTE). In 1980–1983, virtually all infants with clinically recognized ALTE events in King County (which includes Seattle) were referred; we were the only provider of this service in the region.

METHODS

Resident apnea cases from King County were identified from patient records and selected for epidemiologic comparison with resident SIDS cases in the county. A diagnosis of ALTE was based on the history of at least one unexplained episode of apnea which was observed by caretakers and was associated with cyanosis, pallor or limpness. Infants with "apnea of prematurity" (prematurity defined as $\leq$ 37 weeks gestation) whose apneic episodes did not resolve prior to discharge from the hospital were excluded from the study. Only infants whose episodes occurred after discharge were included. SIDS cases were identified from linked infant birth-death computer tapes. All live births were identified from tapes supplied by the King County Office of Vital Statistics.

Of 132 infants referred for ALTE, 63 had a treatable condition and, after appropriate intervention, no longer had episodes. Apnea monitors were not prescribed for these infants. All infants were followed for 1 yr. Sixty-nine infants with idiopathic apnea were

[d]To whom correspondence should be addressed at: Children's Hospital and Medical Center, P. O. Box C5371, Seattle, WA 98105.

450

managed as follows: monitor alone (40 infants), methylxanthines (8), methylxanthines and monitor (20), and refused intervention (1). The infants remained on these regimens until free of episodes for at least 2 months and were followed for at least 1 yr.

All sudden unexpected infant deaths in King County are autopsied at CHMC using a uniform death investigation and autopsy protocol. In 1980–1983, ascertainment, prosectors, and diagnostic criteria for SIDS were unchanged. Epidemiologic variables studied were age at death (SIDS) or onset (ALTE), sex, ethnicity, birthweight, birth rank and season of onset.

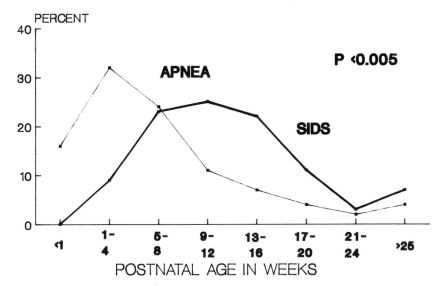

FIGURE 1. Age distribution of apnea and SIDS cases in King County, 1980–1983.

RESULTS

There were 174 deaths of infants born in King County and certified as SIDS after postmortem examination. During the same period, 132 infants born in King County were referred for ALTE. Live births were 81,776. SIDS incidence was 2.1 per 1,000 live births and ALTE incidence 1.6 per 1,000 live births. The distribution patterns of ALTE do not differ significantly for those of SIDS except for age (TABLE 1). The frequency distribution of apnea peaks during the first month of life, in contrast to the SIDS peak during the third month of life (FIG. 1).

All but 2 of the apnea patients survived: 98.5% survival. Both infants who died were diagnosed to have idiopathic apnea, and monitoring was prescribed for use at home. One infant, a sibling of SIDS, was not on a monitor at the time of death; the other had multiple severe obstructive episodes and died during one such episode, despite appropriate intervention.

TABLE 1. Comparison of Epidemiologic Features of SIDS and Infantile Apnea

Epidemiologic Factors	No. of Infants		No. per 1,000 Live Births		p^c
	SIDS[a]	Apnea[b]	SIDS	Apnea	
Infant's sex					> 0.1
Male	101	68	2.4	1.6	
Female	73	64	1.8	1.6	
Ethnicity					> 0.5
White	140	109	2.2	1.7	
Black	16	9	3.9	1.7	
Native American	6	5	5.1	4.3	
Other	12	9	1.6	1.2	
Birthweight (g)					> 0.1
<1,500	8	9	8.7	9.8	
1,500–2,000	7	6	6.8	5.8	
2,001–2,500	17	6	5.8	2.1	
2,501–3,000	34	31	3.2	3.1	
3,001–3,500	51	46	1.8	1.7	
3,501–4,000	42	18	1.6	0.7	
≥4,001	15	13	1.3	1.2	
Unlisted	0	3	0	0	
Birth rank					> 0.5
1st	68	53	1.8	1.4	
2nd	56	45	2.1	1.7	
3rd or more	49	33	2.9	2.0	
Unlisted	1	1	0	0	
Season of onset[d]			% of Cases		< 0.5
Dec.–Feb.	55	40	31.6	30.3	
Mar.–May	36	32	20.7	24.2	
Jun.–Aug.	34	32	19.5	24.2	
Sep.–Nov.	49	28	28.2	21.2	
Postnatal age (weeks)[d]					< 0.005
<1	0	21	0	15.9	
1–4	15	43	8.6	32.6	
5–8	40	31	23.0	23.5	
9–12	43	14	24.7	10.6	
13–16	39	9	22.4	6.8	
17–20	19	5	10.9	3.8	
21–24	6	3	3.4	2.3	
≥ 25	12	6	6.9	4.5	

[a]Total no. of infants with SIDS was 174.
[b]Total no. of infants with apnea was 132.
[c]Comparison of SIDS and apnea; differences not significant except for age.
[d]Season and postnatal age at time of death (SIDS) or onset (apnea).

DISCUSSION

This study took advantage of a period of time when CHMC was the sole provider of apnea services in King County, providing an opportunity to compare apnea and SIDS epidemiologically. Our estimate of apnea incidence in non-institutionalized infants of 1.6/1,000 live births is based on referrals. We surmise that most infants with an ALTE episode had been referred. The figure of 1.6/1,000 probably underestimates the actual incidence to some degree. Despite this, the incidence of infantile apnea is at approximately the same level as the incidence of SIDS. Except for age at onset, the distribution patterns of the variables used in this study for comparison of SIDS with ALTE were similar. The 2 infants who died represent 1.5% of infants with apnea and 1.2% of SIDS victims. The contribution of infantile apnea to the SIDS population is very small.

REFERENCES

1. KRAUS, J. F. & N. O. BORHANI. 1972. Post-neonatal sudden unexplained death in California: A cohort study. Am. J. Epidemiol. **95:** 497–510.
2. OREN, J., D. H. KELLY, & D. C. SHANNON. 1986. Identification of a high-risk group for sudden infant death syndrome among infants who were resuscitated for sleep apnea. Pediatrics **77:** 495–499.
3. STANDFAST, S. J., S. JEREB & D. T. JANERICH. 1980. The epidemiology of sudden infant death in upstate New York. II. Birth characteristics. Am. J. Public Health **70:** 1061–1067.

A Screening Program for Identification of Respiratory Risk Factors for SIDS

N. MONOD, P. PLOUIN, B. STERNBERG, P. PEIRANO,[a]

N. PAJOT, V. VARILLE, S. LINNETT, B. KASTLER,

C. SCAVONE, S. GUIDASCI, AND J. LACOMBE

Hôpital Port Royal
Paris, France

The relationship between sleep apnea and SIDS has long been suggested.[1,2] A prospective study was conducted on a group of 204 control infants (C) and compared with groups of infants at higher than normal epidemiological risk for SIDS: 650 siblings of SIDS victims (SS) and 146 infants who had had one or more life-threatening events, so-called near-miss for SIDS (NM) infants, but in whom no etiology was found for the dramatic episode after a complete pediatric team check-up. Infant groups did not differ in gestational, legal and conceptional age, total recording time, and duration of sleep states.

METHODS

Recordings for these 1,000 appropriate-for-gestational age full-term infants were done between 1973 and 1984 by day-polysomnography: DPSG (417 recordings) (FIG. 1), night-polysomnography: NPSG (257 recordings), and cardiopneumography (over 2 successive nights): CPG (2,600 recordings). Successive recordings were done in many infants, but only the data derived from the first recording were used for this study. Records were visually analyzed. In DPSG and NPSG, the total amount of central (≥ 2, 2–5, ≥ 5, ≥ 10, and ≥ 15 sec), mixed, and obstructive apnea, as well as the percentage of periodic breathing, were studied in each sleep state (active: AS, quiet: QS, indeterminate: IS, and total sleep: TS) and over total recording time (TRT). In CPG, only the total amount of central apnea (≥ 5, ≥ 10, and ≥ 15 sec) and the percentage of periodic breathing over TRT were studied. Since results of the first and second nights studied by CPG were not significantly different, only the data from the first night were used for this study. Infants were grouped according to postnatal age: < 5, ≥ 5 but < 13, and ≥ 13 but < 26 weeks. For each age-group, the results were compared as follows: C vs. SS, C vs. NM, and SS vs. NM for each parameter studied.

RESULTS AND CONCLUSIONS

Before 5 and after 13 weeks of age, differences were not observed between C and SS, C and NM, and SS and NM in DPSG and NPSG for all categories of central, mixed, and

[a]To whom correspondence should be addressed at: INSERM U-29, Hôpital Port Royal, 123, Bd. Port Royal, Paris 75014, France.

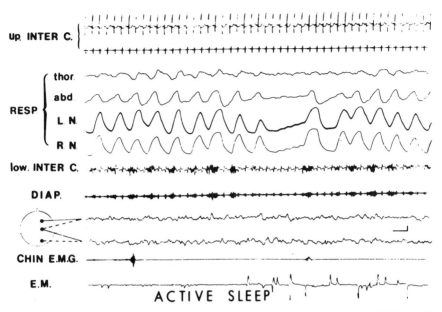

FIGURE 1. Example of polysomnographic tracing of active sleep in a full-term normal infant aged 6 weeks, showing a 3-sec central apnea. Up. INTER C.: upper intercostal electromyogram; RESP thor., abd., L.N., and R.N.: thoracic, abdominal, left and right nasal respiration; low. INTER C.: lower intercostal electromyogram; DIAP.: diaphragmatic electromyogram; CHIN E.M.G.: chin electromyogram; and E.M.: rapid eye movements.

obstructive apnea, as well as for the percentage of periodic breathing in different sleep states and over TRT. Similar results were obtained in CPG for all categories of central apnea and for the percentage of periodic breathing over TRT. Between 5 and 13 weeks of age, results were comparable with those given above, except that central apneas of

TABLE 1. Central Apnea and Periodic Breathing in Day-Polysomnographic Recordings during Active, Quiet and Total Sleep in Different Infant-Groups Aged between 5 and 13 Weeks

Sleep State[a]	Controls[b]	Siblings of SIDS Victims[b]	Near-Miss for SIDS[b]
Active sleep			
Central apnea (n)[c]	33 ± 34	66 ± 54	68 ± 48
Periodic breathing (%)[d]	0.8 ± 2.5	1.4 ± 4.5	2.1 ± 4.8
Quiet sleep			
Central apnea (n)[c]	11 ± 23	11 ± 21	14 ± 22
Periodic breathing (%)[d]	4.0 ± 17.1	0.2 ± 0.8	1.2 ± 6.4
Total sleep			
Central apnea (n)[c]	18 ± 21	32 ± 29	33 ± 27
Periodic breathing (%)[d]	1.6 ± 6.4	0.5 ± 2.4	1.3 ± 4.7

[a]Values are calculated per 100 min of recording.

[b]Values are presented as means ± SD. For level of statistical significance between different comparisons, see text.

[c]Central apnea of between 2 and 5 sec.

[d]Percentage of periodic breathing over total recording time.

between 2 and 5 sec in DPSG were more numerous in both SS and NM as compared to C in AS ($p < 0.01$ and < 0.001, respectively) and TS ($p < 0.001$ and < 0.01, respectively) (TABLE 1).

The group of NM infants were compared according to whether they subsequently had no NM event (117 infants) or 1 or more NM events (29). No difference which could allow the risk of a subsequent NM event to be predicted was found between the 2 groups (in DPSG, NPSG and CPG). The same study was done in the SS group (650 infants). Five of these infants subsequently had 1 or more NM events; their PSG or CPG recordings were no different from the recordings of the other 645 SS infants.

Thus, the role of sleep apnea in SIDS is probably less important than it was thought. SIDS may have many causes and probably multifactorial causes. In any case, the ability to predict an individual risk for SIDS remains very poor with these techniques.

REFERENCES

1. STEINSCHNEIDER, A. 1972. Prolonged apnea and the sudden infant death syndrome. Pediatrics **50:** 646–654.
2. GUILLEMINAULT, C., W. C. DEMENT & N. MONOD. 1973. Syndrome mort subite du nourrisson. Apnées au cours du sommeil. Nouv. Press. Med. **2:** 1355–1357.

Vulnerability and Stabilization of the Cardiorespiratory System in Infants at Risk for SIDS and in the Animal Model

M. E. SCHLAEFKE,[a] T. SCHAEFER,[a] A. BAEUMER,[a]
D. SCHAEFER[a] AND H. KRONBERG[b]

[a]Abteilung fuer Angewandte Physiologie
der Ruhr-Universitaet Bochum
D-4630 Bochum 1
Federal Republic of Germany

[b]Hellige GmbH
D-7800 Freiburg im Breisgau
Federal Republic of Germany

In cats the role of the ventral medullary surface as an important stabilizing system for cardiorespiratory function has been well established.[1] With respect to the involvement of the cardiorespiratory system in the sudden infant death syndrome (SIDS), the ventral medullary surface has been studied in SIDS victims and in controls. The area medial and rostromedial of the hypoglossal root showed a significant reduction of nerve cells compared to controls. Bilateral lesions of area S medial and rostromedial of the hypoglossal root in cats cause the symptoms known as the Ondine's Curse Syndrome.[2] Area S was coagulated unilaterally in cats in order to simulate a possible disposition for SIDS. These models were observed while they were asleep. Periodic breathing and bradycardia were found, together with a reduced function of chemoreflexes.

During their first year of life, more than 400 infants at risk for SIDS, including siblings of SIDS victims who had life-threatening episodes and infants who had near-miss for SIDS episodes, were studied polygraphically while they were asleep. Peripheral and central chemoreflexes were tested. Besides periodic breathing and bradycardia in most of these cases, chemoreflexes were transiently weak or missing. There was a striking instability of arterial Po_2 within the first 3 months of life and a reduced respiratory response to CO_2 within the third 3 months. In both phases we frequently observed hypoxemia while the infants were asleep.

As recently described, lack of chemosensitivity of the respiratory system can be overcome by conditioning.[3] We used a nonspecific stimulus (1 sec), driving respiration during sleep, followed by a jet of oxygen or of 2% CO_2 in oxygen (1.5 sec) after a pause of 0.5 sec. Stimulation was triggered by either transcutaneous Po_2, heart frequency, or end tidal Pco_2. The paired stimulation was repeated every 10 sec for as long as the trigger remained below threshold. In order to prove the value of the method, e.g., the duration of the conditioned reflexes, analogous studies were performed in the cat model described above. The data obtained so far show that training of chemoreflexes during sleep may be a useful preventive measure against SIDS by avoiding hypoxemia during sleep (FIG. 1) and by training the hydrogen ion homeostasis of the brain and thus the stabilizing function of the cardiorespiratory system. This may be valid for otherwise healthy infants.

457

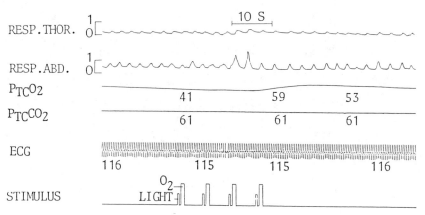

FIGURE 1. "Training" of chemoreflexes by paired stimulation during sleep in an infant with hypoventilation during sleep. In this example a nonspecific stimulus (light) is followed by a short jet of oxygen. Stimulation is triggered by the transcutaneous P_{O_2} ($P_{TC}O_2$).

REFERENCES

1. SCHLAEFKE, M. E. 1981. Central chemosensitivity: A respiratory drive. Rev. Physiol. Biochem. Pharmacol. **90:** 171–244.
2. SCHLAEFKE, M. E., J. F. KILLE & H. H. LOESCHCKE. 1979. Elimination of central chemosensitivity by coagulation of a bilateral area on the ventral medullary surface in awake cats. Pfluegers Arch. **378:** 231–241.
3. SCHLAEFKE, M. E., T. SCHAEFER, H. KRONBERG, G. J. ULLRICH & J. HOPMEIER. 1987. Transcutaneous monitoring as trigger for therapy of hypoxemia during sleep. Adv. Exp. Med. Biol. **220:** 95–100.

A New On-Line Ambulatory Monitoring System for Studying Cardiorespiratory Development in Infants at Home[a]

P. JOHNSON, P. SANDS, J. HEAD, F. D. STOTT, AND
S. HUMPHREYS

Department of Obstetrics
University of Oxford
Oxford OX3 9DU
United Kingdom

There is a peak incidence of death in full-term infants at 2–3 months of age, similar to that claimed for sudden infant death syndrome (SIDS). The possibility of important changes in cardiorespiratory control occurring at this age is supported by newer research in sleep state organization, temperature control, and chemical regulation of breathing. Risk factors for SIDS, if any, are ill-defined, whereas the influence of environmental factors at home has largely been uninvestigated. It is therefore planned to carry out a prospective study in the home of cardiorespiratory control in 100 randomly selected infants during the first 6 months of life.

A monitor based on pulse oximetry and inductance plethysmography, but also able to detect body movements and temperatures (body and ambient) and accept signals from measurements of transcutaneous or respired CO_2 or O_2, and pneumotachograph, ECG, and EMG measurements for more detailed studies, has been developed. This non-invasive monitor (which samples, part-analyzes, and stores data in a 20-min-updating digital memory) can be used to transmit data via modem telephone or cell phone link to an IBM-compatible PC (Amstrad PC1512), forming a two-way link controlled by preset criteria (e.g., SaO_2 at 80% for 5 min), an automatic data acquisition time clock, or a portable graphics terminal monitored by the on-call investigator.

The system stores data on oxygen saturation, heart rate, and respiratory frequency and amplitude each second. Additionally, respiratory waveforms (sampled at 25 Hz) and two auxiliary channels sampled at either 25 Hz or 1 Hz can also be stored. This information is recorded onto a disk. The stored data can be reviewed and analyzed on the computer or printed out on a dot matrix printer at a wide range of timescales. Analysis programs for detecting frequencies and breath patterns (e.g., inspiratory or expiratory obstruction) have been developed.

Observations made during use of the system in preliminary studies in normal infants at home, and more particularly in infants with (1) sleep-related obstructive apnea (micrognathia), (2) central alveolar hypoventilation (Ondine's curse), (3) "silent" seizure-induced apnea ("near-miss SIDS"), and (4) marked periodic breathing (apnea), demonstrate the need for using data on both SaO_2 and thoracoabdominal movements in order to determine the nature of any abnormality or adaptive change in cardiorespiratory

[a] This work was funded by The Foundation for the Study of Infant Deaths.

control during sleep or respiratory compromise. (Simply measuring the magnitude of antiphase thoracic abdominal breathing—as does the Vitalog—is not appropriate for detecting airway obstruction, since out-of-phase thoracoabdominal breathing occurs normally during REM sleep in infants.)

With these new monitors and analytical software, a unique low-cost system now exists so that critical failures in cardiorespiratory development can be determined. In addition, multicenter studies can be carried out by use of telephone modem links or cheap storage media.

Pulmonary Neuroendocrine Cells in SIDS

An Immunohistochemical and Quantitative Study[a]

ERNEST CUTZ,[b] WILSON CHAN,
AND DONALD G. PERRIN

Department of Pathology and Research Institute
The Hospital for Sick Children and
University of Toronto
Toronto, Ontario
Canada

The system of pulmonary neuroendocrine (PNE) cells consists of amine- (serotonin) and peptide- (bombesin, calcitonin, leu-enkephalin) containing cells distributed as single cells and as innervated clusters (neuroepithelial bodies, NEB).[1–3] While single PNE cells are scattered throughout the epithelium of the tracheobronchial tree, NEB are localized mainly within the epithelium of intrapulmonary airways.[1] The precise role and function of these cells and their amine and peptide mediators is presently unknown.

Experimental studies in neonatal rabbits have shown increased exocytosis of dense core granules (site of amine and peptide storage) from NEB cells in response to acute hypoxia.[3,4] Other recent studies suggest that this response is mediated by vagal innervation.[5] Furthermore, hyperplasia of PNE cells and NEB has been documented in animals exposed to chronic hypoxia.[6] It has been suggested that NEB may represent airway chemoreceptors (analogous to carotid bodies) involved in autonomic regulation of breathing. Since NEB are prominent in fetal/neonatal lungs and decline with postnatal age, this role may be particularly important during neonatal respiratory adaptation.[7]

In this study we have investigated the immunohistochemical profile, distribution, and frequency of PNE cells and NEB in lungs of infants who died of SIDS ($n = 7$, 1.5–5 months of age, mean 3.3 months) and compared them with age-matched controls (previously healthy infants who suffered sudden death; $n = 5$, 2.5–6 months of age, mean 4.5 months). The lung tissue was fixed in formalin, and deparaffinized sections (after trypsinization) were immunostained with monoclonal antibodies against bombesin, calcitonin (Hybritech, U.S.A.), serotonin, and leu-enkephalin (Sera Lab, U.K.).

For quantitative assessment of PNE cells and NEB in lungs of SIDS and control infants, random sections (3–5 per case), immunostained for bombesin, were analyzed. To determine the frequency of bombesin-immunoreactive (BI) cells in airways, areas of airway epithelium and immunoreactive epithelium were outlined on paper using a projecting microscope. The surface areas were measured by an IBAS image analyzer and expressed as percent immunoreactive epithelium (% IRA). An average of 40 airways per

[a]This work was supported by grants from NICHD (1 R01 HD22713-01) and the Medical Research Council of Canada (MT-7641).

[b]To whom correspondence should be addressed at: Department of Pathology, The Hospital for Sick Children, 555 University Avenue, Toronto, Ontario, Canada M5G 1X8.

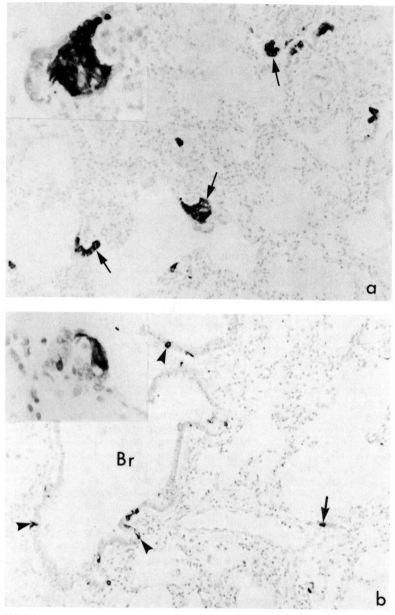

FIGURE 1. **(a)** Several large bombesin-immunoreactive NEB (*arrows*) located at bronchiole-alveolar junctions in a lung from a 4-month-old SIDS victim (×250). *Inset*: Close-up view of an NEB (shown in **a**) made up of tightly packed bombesin-immunoreactive cells (×450).**(b)** Lung section from a control (4-month-old infant) shows a few single bombesin-immunoreactive PNE cells (*arrowheads*) scattered within the epithelium of the small bronchioles (Br). Only a single, small NEB (*arrow*) is evident in the alveolar duct region (×250). *Inset*: Close-up view of a NEB (in control lung) composed of a few elongated bombesin-immunoreactive cells in close proximity to the alveolar duct surface (×450). All magnifications were reduced 10% at reproduction of figure.

case were measured; final values were expressed as mean % IRA ($\pm$ SEM). The number of NEB in peripheral airways (bronchiole-alveolar junctions, B-A) were counted and expressed per total surface area of lung section (NEB/cm^2). The size of NEB (NEB μm^2) was measured directly on sections using IBAS. An average of 20 NEB per case were assessed. Statistical analysis and comparison of data between SIDS and controls was performed using Student's *t* test.

The sections of lungs from all SIDS and control infants contained scattered single and groups of bombesin-immunoreactive PNE cells and NEB within the epithelium of most airways. However, in lungs of SIDS infants, compared to control lungs, BI cells appeared more numerous and NEB were larger, particularly those at B-A junctions (FIGS. 1a and 1b). Immunostaining for other PNE cell markers (serotonin, calcitonin, leu-enkephalin) was variable, with no distinct differences between SIDS samples and controls.

The quantitative assessment of BI cells revealed an almost 2-fold increase in the frequency of these cells in lungs of SIDS victims (mean % IRA: 7.6 $\pm$ 0.5 in SIDS vs. 4.3 $\pm$ 0.4 in controls; $p < 0.01$); the number of NEB at B-A junctions was also significantly increased (mean: 58.9 $\pm$ 7.2/cm^2 in SIDS vs. 31.0 $\pm$ 6.1/cm^2 in controls; $p < 0.05$), as was NEB size (mean: 859.3 $\pm$ 88.9 μm^2 in SIDS vs. 427.4 $\pm$ 53.6 μm^2 in controls; $p < 0.01$).

Our findings indicate that bombesin-immunoreactive PNE cells and NEB are increased in lungs of SIDS victims compared to age-matched controls. This suggests "activation" and/or hyperplasia of the PNE cell system in the lungs of SIDS victims. The possible factors involved include chronic hypoxia or relative immaturity of this chemoreceptor system in the lungs of SIDS infants. We have previously found that, during normal lung development, the number of BI cells and the amount of bombesin-like peptide (measured by radioimmunoassay) peaks at the time of birth and declines postnatally.[7] The increased number of BI cells observed in lungs of SIDS infants may also be reflected by an increased amount of bombesin-like peptide in lung tissue, making this peptide a potentially useful biochemical marker for SIDS. Since NEB are presumed to be intrapulmonary hypoxia-sensitive chemoreceptors, their dysfunction, compounded by other abnormalities in the autonomic regulation of breathing, may play a role in the pathogenesis of SIDS.

REFERENCES

1. CUTZ, E. 1982. Exp. Lung Res. **3:** 185–208.
2. CUTZ, E., W. CHAN & N. S. TRACK. 1981. Experientia **37:** 765–767.
3. LAUWERYNS, J. M. & M. COKELAERE. 1973. Z. Zellforsch. **145:** 521–540.
4. LANWERYNS, J. M., M. COKELAERE, M. DELEERSNIJDER, & M. LIEBENS. 1977. Cell Tissue Res. **182:** 425–440.
5. LANWERYNS, J. M. & A. VAN LOMMEL. 1986. Exp. Lung Res. **11:** 319–339.
6. KEITH, I. M. & J. A. WILL. 1981. Thorax **36:** 767–773.
7. CUTZ, E., J. E. GILLAN & N. S. TRACK. 1984. *In* Endocrine Lung in Health and Disease. K. L. Becker & A. F. Gazdar, Eds.: 210–231. W. B. Saunders Co. Philadelphia.

Distinctive Pattern of Pulmonary Neuroendocrine Cells in Sudden Infant Death Syndrome

J. E. GILLAN AND S. F. CAHALANE

Departments of Pathology
Rotunda Hospital and
The Children's Hospital
Temple Street
Dublin, Ireland

The hypothesis of ventilatory dysfunction is currently favored as the pivotal pathophysiological mechanism in SIDS. This view derives from clinical studies in near-miss cases and pathological studies demonstrating, respectively, carotid body insensitivity to elevated levels of carbon dioxide and gliosis of the dorsal nucleus of the vagus. The latter offers a possible pathological correlate for the central apnea noted clinically.

The pulmonary neuroendocrine (PNE) system consists of specialized innervated cells in the lining epithelium of the bronchial tree. A recent study[1] has demonstrated an association between birth asphyxial brainstem dysfunction and the pulmonary neuroendocrine system. This study has suggested that the brainstem controls release of bombesin-like immunoreactive peptide from the PNE cells via vagal innervation. This has prompted the present study which examines the possibility that brainstem dysfunction in SIDS might cause changes in the PNE system.

The study comprised 18 cases of SIDS, ranging from 48 hr to 6 months of age, and 20 controls, ranging from 3 weeks to 12 months of age, who had died from some acute fatal insult which did not involve respiratory and intracerebral disease. A minimum of 100 airways were examined on routine postmortem lung sections stained by the Grimelius technique, and the neuroendocrine- (NE) positive airways expressed as a percent of the total airways. The SIDS cases had $64.22 \pm 28.88\%$ (mean and SD) NE-positive airways with a range of 2–97%. Controls had $20.39 \pm 15.03\%$ with a range of 0–44%. The SIDS results were significantly different from controls ($p > 0.001$). In addition, the quantity of NE-stainable cell cytoplasm, while not formally quantified in this study, was clearly increased, as shown in FIGURES 1 and 2. A number of cases also showed NE-positive cells within the respiratory units, i.e. respiratory bronchioles and alveoli, a feature not present in controls.

This pattern of increased numbers of airways containing PNE cells is similar to that noted in birth asphyxial brainstem dysfunction, i.e., increased numbers of NE-positive airways and increased cytoplasmic staining, suggesting a defect in PNE innervation.[1] Chronic hypoxia, which causes hyperplasia of the PNE system, could also account for these changes.[2,3] While the presence of neodevelopment of PNE cells within the respiratory units would favor the latter hypothesis, the 2 explanations offered are not mutually exclusive, i.e., both mechanisms may be operative. Regardless of the precise mechanism, this distinction between SIDS and controls may provide a new marker which may prove useful to the practicing pathologist.

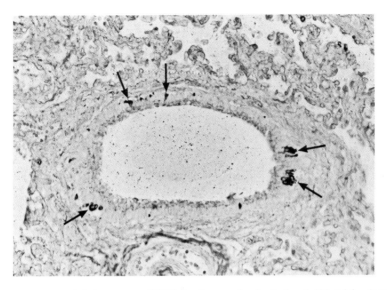

FIGURE 1. Bronchiole from a case of SIDS showing prominent cytoplasmic NE-staining (**arrows**) in the epithelial lining.

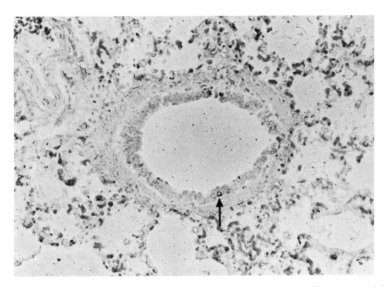

FIGURE 2. Bronchiole from a control autopsy showing significantly less NE-positive staining of cells (**arrow**) compared to the SIDS case in FIGURE 1.

REFERENCES

1. GILLAN, J. E., K. E. PAPE & E. CUTZ. 1986. Association of changes in bombesin immunoreactive neuroendocrine cells in lungs of newborn infants with persistent fetal circulation and brainstem damage due to birth asphyxia. Pediatr. Res. **20:** 828–833.
2. MOOSAVI, H., P. SMITH & D. HEATH. 1973. The Feyrter cell in hypoxia. Thorax **28:** 729–741.
3. PACK, R. J., S. BARKER & A. HOWE. 1986. The effect of hypoxia on the number of amine containing cells in the lung of the adult rat. Eur. J. Respir. Dis. **68:** 121–130.

Size of the Tongue in Sudden Infant Death Syndrome

JOSEPH R. SIEBERT[a] AND JOEL E. HAAS

Departments of Pathology and Pediatrics
Children's Hospital and Medical Center and
University of Washington
Seattle, Washington 98105

In 1975, Tonkin suggested that an enlarged tongue could be important in the pathogenesis of airway obstruction in sudden infant death syndrome (SIDS). An enlarged tongue might occlude the airway, within the context of other phenomena, including tone of suprahyoid and pterygoid muscles, sleep mechanisms, suckling, and the infant's normally hypermobile mandible and elevated larynx.

This hypothesis, as it pertains to enlargement of the tongue in victims of SIDS, has not been tested previously. We therefore conducted a morphometric study of the tongue, using a method developed previously.[1] The excised tongue was studied in 100 victims of SIDS and 40 control infants matched for age and body size; illnesses in the latter group were brief and not thought to affect body or tongue size. Length, width, and thickness of the tongue were measured to 1.0 mm with helios calipers; weight was obtained to 0.1 g. Other variables examined were body weight and length, head circumference, age, sex, and postmortem interval. Linear regression provided a measure of size and cross-sectional growth; analysis of covariance permitted the examination of lingual dimensions without the effects of body size. Representative samples were examined histologically; others were desiccated and the fluid content was determined.

Nearly all tongue weights in SIDS were greater than expected. For the 2 groups of infants, regression lines of tongue weight upon body weight were separated by more than one standard error of the y-estimate (FIG. 1). Mean tongue length, width, and thickness were also significantly increased in victims of SIDS (TABLE 1). Histological examination and determination of dry weights revealed no evidence of increased fluid in the SIDS tongue; no correlation between tongue weight and postmortem interval was identified.

Our findings document significant enlargement of the tongue in SIDS. Desiccation, statistical studies, histological examination, and care taken in the selection of control

TABLE 1. Size of the Tongue in SIDS and Control Infants

Dependent Variable	SIDS[a]	Control[a]	p
Tongue weight (g)	14.1 (0.20)	11.0 (0.30)	<0.001
Tongue length (cm)	4.8 (0.04)	4.5 (0.06)	<0.001
Tongue width (cm)	3.2 (0.02)	3.0 (0.04)	<0.001
Tongue thickness (cm)	1.4 (0.01)	1.2 (0.02)	<0.001

[a]Adjusted group means (±SE), derived by analysis of covariance, are free of the effects of the independent variable (body weight).

[a]To whom correspondence should be addressed at: Department of Laboratories, Children's Hospital and Medical Center, P. O. Box C-5371, Seattle, WA 98105.

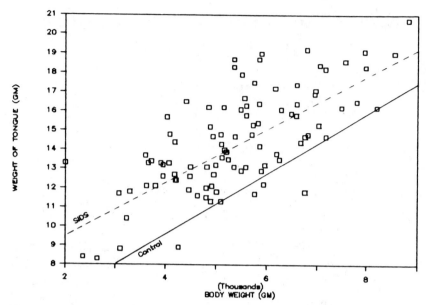

FIGURE 1. Regression analysis of tongue weight upon body weight in SIDS (**dashed line**) and in control (**solid line**) infants. The regression lines are separated by more than one SE of the y-estimate.

infants allow us to reject such explanations as agonal change in fluid content, effect of postmortem interval, and smallness of control tongues. Effects of a large tongue upon the airway of SIDS victims are unclear. The importance of the normal tongue in maintaining a patent airway is, however, recognized in normal and abnormal infants, during feeding, other wakeful periods, and sleep. Mechanisms responsible for enlargement of the tongue in SIDS also remain unclear, but might include alterations in morphogenesis or hypertrophy. Further studies—of the tongue *in situ* and of developmental and pathogenetic mechanisms—are necessary to determine the significance of lingual enlargement in SIDS.

REFERENCES

1.   SIEBERT, J. R. 1985. A morphometric study of normal and abnormal fetal to childhood tongue size. Arch. Oral Biol. **30:** 433–440.

Evaluation of Near-Miss Sudden Infant Death

The Importance of Investigations to Determine Etiology

A. BOCHNER, G. VEEREMAN, AND
M. VAN CAILLIE-BERTRAND

Algemeen Kinderziekenhuis Antwerpen
Albert Grisarstraat 19-2018 Antwerpen
Belgium

INTRODUCTION

Sudden infant death syndrome (SIDS) remains the most common cause of death in the first year of life following the neonatal period. The purpose of this study was to emphasize the importance of complementary investigations in the identification of a high-risk group for SIDS.[1,2]

PATIENTS AND METHODS

Between January 1984 and August 1986, 407 infants were admitted to our center for an all-night sleep study. On admission the infants were about 8 weeks old. There were 130 infants who had experienced an unexplained episode of sleep apnea accompanied by a change in tone and color (group I), 74 siblings born to women who had lost an infant to SIDS (group II), and 203 asymptomatic infants, either prematurely born or with overanxious parents, but with no personal or family history of SIDS (group III). The data were recorded on an 8-channel Alvar model polygraph. Only in group I the following investigations were done: complete blood cell count; measurement of serum calcium, magnesium, glucose, electrolytes, and BUN; and metabolic, neurological, cardiological, gastrointestinal and toxicological screening. Further investigations, such as thyroid tests, lumbar puncture, CT-scan or pH-probe, were also performed when required.[3] In groups II and III no further investigations were done for ethical reasons. A polysomnographic recording was considered abnormal (A.R.) at the age of 8 weeks if it showed central apneas of more than 10 sec, periodic breathing for more than 5% of the total sleep time, and obstructive apnea longer than 3 sec. These A.R. were considered to be the "risk factors."[4-6]

RESULTS

The number of infants with A.R. in each group is indicated in TABLE I. In group I, the number of infants with abnormal observations in the complementary investigations, and the number in each of these categories who also had A.R., is as follows: 56 had an

TABLE 1. The Number of Infants In Each Group with an Abnormal Polysomnographic Recording (A.R.)

Category	Group		
	I	II	III
No. of infants studied	130	74	203
No. of infants with A.R.	27	12	42

abnormal esophagogram and/or esophageal pH-measurements (AR : 10/56), 22 had neurological disturbances (AR : 6/22), 11 had respiratory problems (AR : 5/11), 6 had intoxications (AR : 0/6), 1 had metabolic abnormality (AR : 0/1), 1 had a Pierre Robin syndrome (AR : 1/1), and 2 had nose- throat- ear-infection (AR : 1/2). Of 31 who had no abnormalities (AR : 4/31), 4 required vigorous stimulation and resuscitation and 6 had clinical symptoms of gastroesophageal reflux, but complementary investigations of these 6 infants could not be done.

FOLLOW-UP AND CONCLUSIONS

Two deaths were observed in group I; both had normal polygraphic recording and were treated for gastroesophageal reflux. At the time of death, both children had been discontinued from treatment for a week or longer by the decision of their parents. In groups II and III there were no deaths. Only 34 children (8%) were selected for home monitoring. Not one infant died while being monitored. Forty-eight infants (12%) were treated with methylxanthines. If the polygraphic recording is combined with a systematic protocol of complementary investigations, an etiology can be found in 99 of 130 (76%) infants admitted for an event suggestive of near-miss SIDS. In group I, gastroesophageal reflux was the most common abnormality observed (43%).[7]

REFERENCES

1. KAHN, A., D. BLUM, P. HENNART, C. SELLENS, D. SAMSON-DOLFUS, J. TAYOT, R. GILLY, J. DUTRUGE, R. FLORES & B. STERNBERG. 1984. A critical comparison of the history of sudden death infants and infants hospitalised for near-miss for SIDS. Eur. J. Pediatr. **143:** 103–107.
2. OREN, J., D. KELLY & D.C. SHANNON. 1986. Identification of a high risk group for sudden infant death syndrome among infants who were resuscitated for sleep apnea. Pediatrics **77:** 495–499.
3. BOIX-OCHOA, J., J.M. LAFLUENTE & J.M. GIL-VERMET. 1980. Twenty-four hours esophageal pH-monitoring in gastroesophageal reflux. J. Pediatr. Surg. **15:** 74–78.
4. KAHN, A., D. BLUM & L. MONTAUK. 1986. Polysomnographic studies and home monitoring of siblings of SIDS victims and of infants with no family history of sudden infant death. Eur. J. Pediatr. **145:** 351–356.
5. KAHN, A. & D. BLUM. 1982. Home monitoring of infants considered at risk for the sudden infant death syndrome. Four years experience (1977–1981).Eur. J. Pediatr. **139:** 94–100.
6. KELLY, D.H. & D.C. SHANNON. 1979. Periodic breathing in infants with near-miss sudden infant death syndrome. Pediatrics **63:** 355–360.
7. HERBST, J.J., L.S. BOOK & P.F. BRAY. 1978. Gastroesophageal reflux in the near-miss sudden infant death syndrome. J. Pediatr. **92:** 73–75.

Is Anemia a Cause of Apnea?

J. J. SHAH, L. T. BUSH, S. KNOBLAUCH,
M. DENSBERGER, AND J. KROGMAN

Saint Francis Medical Center and
University of Illinois College of Medicine
530 N.E. Glen Oak Avenue
Peoria, Illinois 61637

Anemia is frequently mentioned as a cause of apnea in preterm infants.[1-3] However, a thorough search of the literature revealed no evidence of any studies to substantiate this premise. Thirteen preterm infants with a mean gestational age of 29.8 weeks (range, 28–35 weeks) and a mean weight of 1,169 g (range, 794–2240 g) were studied. No infant was considered to be critically ill. A pneumocardiogram (PCG) was done for a minimum of 6 hr before each infant received a blood transfusion. The PCG was then repeated 6–24 hr after the transfusion. Mean pre- and posttransfusion hematocrits (6 hr posttransfusion) were 29.4 and 41.6, respectively ($p < 0.001$). The following apnea-related variables were determined pre- and posttransfusion: (1) A6/D% (total time for apneas of duration ≥ 6 sec as a percentage of total sleep time), (2) # apneas/100 min sleep (number of apneas of duration ≥ 6 sec/100 min of sleep time), (3) % PB (total periodic breathing time as a percentage of total sleep time, (4) # PB/100 min sleep (number of periodic breathing episodes/100 min of sleep time), and (5) duration of the longest apnea. The results are presented in TABLE 1.

Even though the hematocrit increased significantly after a transfusion, no statistically significant changes occurred in any of the apnea variables in these preterm infants. Based on these results, we conclude that anemia may not have a direct causal relationship to apnea in the preterm infant.

TABLE 1. Effect of Blood Transfusion on Apnea-Related Variables Determined by Pneumocardiogram

	Mean Values[b]	
Apnea Variables[a]	Pretransfusion[c]	Posttransfusion[c]
A6/D% (%)	1.45	1.16
# apneas/100 min sleep	11.42	8.75
%PB (%)	3.36	2.32
# PB/100 min sleep	3.78	3.22
longest apnea (sec)	12.70	12.39

[a]For definitions of variables, see text.
[b]Mean for 13 preterm infants who each received a transfusion after the pretransfusion pneumocardiogram was recorded.
[c]Mean pre- and posttransfusion hematocrits were 29.4 and 41.6, respectively ($p < 0.001$).

REFERENCES

1. LEE, J. & S.E. DOWNING. 1979. Effects of anemia and growth retardation on respiratory activity in the piglet. Biol. Neonate **36:** 255–263.

2. KATTWINKEL, M.D. 1976. Neonatal apnea: Pathogenesis and therapy. J. Pediatr. **90**(3): 342–347.
3. DELIVARIA-PAPADOPOULOS, M., L.D. MILLER, R.E. FORSTER & F.A. OSKI. 1975. The role of exchange transfusion in the management of low-birth weight infants with and without severe respiratory distress syndrome. J. Pediatr. **89**(2): 273–278.

Index of Contributors